CEN

REVIEW MANUAL

PLUS 2 ONLINE EXAMS

FIFTH EDITION

ENA™
EMERGENCY NURSES ASSOCIATION

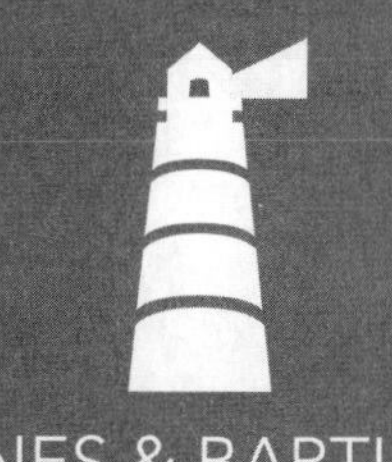

JONES & BARTLETT
LEARNING

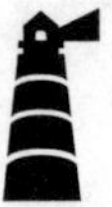

World Headquarters
Jones & Bartlett Learning
5 Wall Street
Burlington, MA 01803
978-443-5000
info@jblearning.com
www.jblearning.com

EMERGENCY NURSES ASSOCIATION
Emergency Nurses Association
930 E. Woodfield Road
Schaumburg, IL 60173
847-460-4000
education@ena.org
www.ena.org

16983-6

Production Credits
VP, Product Management: David D. Cella
Director of Product Management: Amanda Martin
Product Manager: Teresa Reilly
Product Assistant: Christina Freitas
Production Editor: Vanessa Richards
Associate Production Editor, Navigate: Rachel DiMaggio
Marketing Communications Manager: Katie Hennessy
Product Fulfillment Manager: Wendy Kilborn
Composition: S4Carlisle Publishing Services
Cover Design: Denise Wawrzyniak, Kristin E. Parker
Text Design: Kristin E. Parker
Rights & Media Specialist: John Rusk
Cover Image (Title Page, Chapter Opener): © Antishock/iStock/Getty Images Plus
Printing and Binding: McNaughton & Gunn
Cover Printing: McNaughton & Gunn

Library of Congress Cataloging-in-Publication Data
Names: Emergency Nurses Association, issuing body.
Title: CEN review manual : plus 2 online exams / Emergency Nurses Association.
Other titles: Certification Examination for Emergency Nurses review manual & 2 online exams | CEN review manual and 2 online exams
Description: Fifth edition. | Burlington, Massachusetts : Jones & Bartlett Learning, [2020] | Preceded by CEN review manual / Emergency Nurses Association. 3rd ed. c2001. | Includes bibliographical references.
Identifiers: LCCN 2018031449 | ISBN 9781284169713 (pbk.)
Subjects: | MESH: Emergency Nursing | Emergencies--nursing | Examination Questions
Classification: LCC RC86.9 | NLM WY 18.2 | DDC 616.02/5076--dc23
LC record available at https://lccn.loc.gov/2018031449

6048

Printed in the United States of America
23 22 21 20 10 9 8 7 6 5 4 3

Contents

Preface

The goal of the *CEN Review Manual: Plus 2 Online Exams, Fifth Edition* is to provide the emergency nurse with a comprehensive resource containing current practice information in a format that will enhance their preparation for the Certification in Emergency Nursing examination and becoming a certified emergency nurse (CEN). Many individuals have made this edition a reality, including section editors, numerous item writers, ENA staff, and the staff of Jones & Bartlett Learning.

The *CEN Review Manual: Plus 2 Online Exams, Fifth Edition* would not have been possible without the expertise of each item writer and section editor. Their willingness to write items, review them, rewrite them, and meet deadlines was the cornerstone of the success of this publication. Each of your contributions to this publication will be remembered for many years to come as a gift to emergency nurses, both present and future. I would also like to include a special recognition of Kathie Carlson, the project's board liaison. Thank you for your unending support.

Most importantly I want to recognize the time that this project has taken away from friends, family, and especially my very patient husband, Rob. I am grateful to each of them for letting me complete this project that will benefit so many others.

—Louise Hummel,
MSN, RN, CNS, CEN, TCRN, FAEN

Acknowledgments

Lead Editor

Louise Hummel, MSN, RN, CNS, CEN, TCRN, FAEN
Lecturer/Clinical Faculty
School of Nursing
California State University, San Marcos
San Marcos, California
Clinical Educator
St. Joseph Hospital
Orange, California

Board of Directors Liaison

Kathleen E. Carlson, MSN, RN, CEN, FAEN
Staff Nurse
Sentara Virginia Beach General Hospital
Virginia Beach, Virginia

Section Editors

Benjamin E. Marett, EdD, MSN, RN-C, CEN, CCRN, NE-BC, FAEN, FAHA
Clinical Nurse Executive
Emergency Care Consultants of the Carolinas
Rock Hill, South Carolina

Dawn M. Specht, PhD, MSN, RN, APN, CEN, CPEN, FAEN
Assistant Professor
American Sentinel University
Aurora, Colorado

Jacqueline Stewart, DNP, RN, CEN, CCRN, FAEN
Associate Professor
Passan School of Nursing
Wilkes University
Wilkes Barre, Pennsylvania

Jennifer Van Cura, DNP, MBA, MPH, RN, CEN, CPEN, TCRN
Emergency Department Clinical Nurse Educator
Centura Penrose St. Francis Hospital Systems
Colorado Springs, Colorado
Emergency Department Staff Nurse
UCHealth Memorial Central Hospital
Colorado Springs, Colorado

Melissa L. Weir, MS, BSN, RN, CEN, CPEN, CNE
Faculty
College of Nursing
Howard University
Washington, DC
RN II
Children's National Medical Center
Washington, DC

ENA Staff

Nicole Williams, MSN, RN-BC
Director, Institute of Emergency Nursing Education
Emergency Nurses Association
Des Plaines, Illinois

LaToria Woods, MSN, APRN, CCNS
Senior Associate
Emergency Nurses Association
Des Plaines, Illinois

Chris Zahn, PhD
Developmental Editor
Emergency Nurses Association
Des Plaines, Illinois

Contributing Authors

Anthony M. Angelow, PhD, CRNP, ACNP, ACNPC, AGACNP-BC, CEN
Assistant Clinical Professor
College of Nursing and Health Professions
Drexel University
Philadelphia, Pennsylvania

Kathy Bowen, BSN, RN, CEN, TCRN
Staff Nurse
Emergency Department
Advocate Christ Medical Center
Oak Lawn, Illinois

Andrew J. Bowman, MSN, RN, ACNP-BC, ACNP-C, TNS, CEN, CPEN, CTRN, CFRN, TCRN, CCRN-CMC, CVRN-I-BC, NREMTP, FAEN
Boone County Emergency Physicians
Acute Care Nurse Practitioner—Emergency Department
Lebanon, Indiana
Emergency Medicine Specialists
Acute Care Nurse Practitioner—Emergency Department
Danville, Iowa

Brenda Braun, MSN, RN, CEN, CPEN, FAEN
Shore Medical Center

Kathleen Carlson, MSN, RN, CEN, FAEN
Staff Nurse
Sentara Virginia Beach General Hospital
Virginia Beach, Virginia

Pat Clutter, MEd, RN, CEN, FAEN
ED Staff Nurse/Independent Educator/Journalism
Mercy Lebanon
Lebanon, Missouri

Caitlin Costello, BSN, RN, CEN
RN Clinical Leader
Geisinger Community Medical Center
Scranton, Pennsylvania

Lisa Dukes, MSN, RN, CEN, CPEN, TCRN, NREMT-P
Trauma Educator/Outreach Coordinator
Doctors Hospital
Augusta, Georgia

Lauren Dreiling, BSN, RN, CEN
Emergency Department RN, Charge Nurse
Penrose Hospital
Colorado Springs, Colorado

Don Everly, MSN, MBA, RN-BC, CEN, CPEN, CCRN-CMC, CCNS, ONC, OCNS-C
Nursing Education Specialist/Director of Life Support Training Center
Cooper University Hospital
Camden, New Jersey

Lynette R. Fair, RN, NE-BC, CEN

Col. Kathleen M. Flarity, PhD, DNP, RN, CEN, CFRN, FAEN
Emergency CNS/Nurse Scientist
Memorial Health System
Colorado Springs, Colorado

Cathy C. Fox, RN, CEN, CPEN, TCRN, FAEN
Quality and Safety Nurse Consultant
Emergency Services and Cardiovascular Services, Catheter Lab, Vascular and CT Surgery
Naval Medical Center
Portsmouth, Virginia

Katelynn Garner-Cooke, MS, MBA, RN, CEN
Registered Nurse
Wake Forest Baptist Medical Center
Winston-Salem, North Carolina

Robin Gilbert, MSN, RN, CEN, CPEN
Regional Education Manager
Central Maine Medical Center
Lewiston, Maine

Michael D. Gooch, DNP, RN, ACNP-BC, FNP-BC, ENP-BC, CEN, CFRN, CTRN, TCRN, NREMT-P
Assistant Professor of Nursing
School of Nursing
Vanderbilt University
Nashville, Tennessee
Flight Nurse
Vanderbilt University Medical Center—LifeFlight
Nashville, Tennessee
Emergency Nurse Practitioner
TeamHealth
Columbia, Tennessee
Faculty
Middle Tennessee School of Anesthesia
Madison, Tennessee

Mary Gronberg, BSN, RN, CEN
Nurse Educator/Supervisor
Penrose Hospital
Colorado Springs, Colorado

Diane Gurney, MS, RN, CEN, FAEN
Emergency Nursing Education Professional and Consultant
Athol, Massachusetts

Carol Hightower, MSN, RN, CEN
Nurse Educator
Emergency Department
Hunter Holmes McGuire Veterans Administration Medical Center
Richmond, Virginia

Renee Semonin Holleran, PhD, FNP-BC, CEN, CCRN, CTRN, FAEN
Nurse Practitioner
Holistic Medicine
SLC Veterans Health Administration
Volunteer Nurse Practitioner
Hope Free Clinic
Midvale, Utah

Louise Hummel, MSN, RN, CNS, CEN, TCRN, FAEN
Lecturer/Clinical Faculty
School of Nursing
California State University, San Marcos
San Marcos, California
Clinical Educator
St. Joseph Hospital
Orange, California

Michelle Inglis, ASN, RN, CEN
Clinical Nurse III
Emergency Department
Orlando Regional Medical Center
Orlando, Florida

Linell Jones, BSN, RN, CEN, CPEN
Lakewood, WA
Contract Educator
Cascade Training Center
Lakewood, Washington

Mary Kamienski, PhD, APN, FAEN, FAAN
Professor
Rutgers School of Nursing
Specialty Director
FNP in Emergency Care
Newark, New Jersey

Marylou Killian, DNP, RN, FNP-BC, ENP, CEN, FAEN
Lead APC
Ascension Lourdes Hospital
Binghamton, New York

Kathleen Klunk, MSN, BSN, RN, FNP-C
Emergency Department Nurse Practitioner
West Suburban Hospital
Oak Park, Illinois

Jill LeBeau, MSN, RN, CEN
Manager
Emergency Services
UCHealth Grandview Hospital
Colorado Springs, Colorado

Mary Jo Lombardo, DNP, RN, CEN
Clinical Education Program Manager
Howard County General
Columbia, Maryland

Benjamin E. Marett, EdD, MSN, RN-C, CEN, CCRN, NE-BC, FAEN, FAHA
Clinical Nurse Executive
Emergency Care Consultants of the Carolinas
Rock Hill, South Carolina

Rhonda Miller, MS, RN, CEN, CCRN
Emergency Department
Education/QI Coordinator
CGH Medical Center
Sterling, Illinois

Daniel Misa, MSN, RN, CEN, CPEN
Clinical Shift Supervisor
The Valley Hospital
Lincoln Park, New Jersey

Elizabeth Mizerek, MSN, RN, FN-CSA, CEN, CPEN, CNE
Director of Nursing Education
Mercer County Community College
West Windsor, New Jersey

Lisa A. Moment, APRN, FNP-BC, AFN-BC, CEN, SANE-A
Advanced Practice Provider
Carle Foundation Hospital
Urbana, Illinois

Jason Moretz, MHA, BSN, RN, CEN, CTRN
Senior Managing Consultant
Berkeley Research Group
North Carolina Area
Emeryville, California

Tim Murphy, MSN, RN, CEN, TCRN, FAEN
Trauma Performance Improvement Coordinator
Robert Wood Johnson University Hospital
New Brunswick, New Jersey

Kellyn Pak, MSN, RN, CEN, TCRN, MICN
Senior Nursing Instructor
Disaster Program Manager
Los Angeles County USC Medical Center
Los Angeles, California

Andrea L. Pawlak, MSN, RN, FNP-BC, CEN
Emergency Department
Loyola University Medical Center
Maywood, Illinois

Janis Farnholtz Provinse, MS, RN, CNS, CEN, TCRN, FAEN
Emergency Department Clinical Nurse Specialist
Alameda Health System
Highland Hospital
Oakland, California

Elizabeth Saska, MSN, RN, CEN
Emergency Department
St. Vincent's Medical Center
Bridgeport, Connecticut

Chris Sharpe, DNP, MSN, FNP-BC, NP-C, CEN, CPEN, CTRN, NRP, NCEE, TP-C
Training Manager
Advanced Practice Nurse Virtua EMS
Mt. Laurel, New Jersey

Mary Anne Silcox, BSN, RN, CEN
Registered Nurse
Penrose Hospital
Colorado Springs, Colorado

Melinda Smith, MSN, BBS, RN, CEN
Comanche, Oklahoma

Amy Smith-Peard, MSN, RN, CNS, CEN, ENP
Clinical Nurse Specialist
Sentra Leigh Emergency Department
Norfolk, Virginia

Dawn M. Specht, PhD, MSN, RN, CNS, CEN, CCNS, CCRN, FAEN
Assistant Professor
American Sentinel University
Aurora, Colorado

Jacqueline Stewart, DNP, MSN, RN, CEN, CCRN, FAEN
Associate Professor
Passan School of Nursing
Wilkes University
Wilkes Barre, Pennsylvania

Vicki Sweet, MSN, RN, CEN, MICN, FAEN
ALS/CQI Coordinator
Orange County Emergency Medical Services
Santa Ana, California
Associate Faculty
Health Sciences/Human Services
Saddleback College
Mission Viejo, California

Michele Swida, MS, RN, CEN
Nursing Supervisor/Coordinator Clinical Affiliates
Geisinger Wyoming Valley Medical Center
Wilkes Barre, Pennsylvania
Adjunct Clinical Instructor
Wilkes University
Wilkes Barre, Pennsylvania
Adjunct Clinical Instructor
Misericordia University
Dallas, Pennsylvania

Anna Maria Valdez, PhD, RN, CEN, CFRN, CNE, FAEN
Associate Dean of Nursing
Santa Rosa Junior College
Santa Rosa, California
Senior Contributing Faculty
Walden University
Santa Rosa, California

Jennifer Anne Van Cura, DNP, MBA, MPH, RN, CEN, CPEN, TCRN
Emergency Department Clinical Nurse Educator
Centura Penrose St. Francis Hospital Systems
Colorado Springs, Colorado
Emergency Department Staff Nurse
UCHealth Memorial Central Hospital
Colorado Springs, Colorado

Kathy Van Dusen, MSN, RN, CEN, CPEN, NHDP-BC
Nurse Specialist II
Emergency Services
St. Joseph Health, Mission Hospital
San Clemente, California

Mary Alice Vanhoy, MSN, RN, CEN, CPEN, NRP, FAEN
Emergency Center Nurse Manager
University of Maryland
College Park, Maryland
Shore Emergency Center at Queenstown
Queenstown, Maryland

Suzanne M. Wall, MSN, RN, CEN, FNP-BC, ANP-BC
Nurse Practitioner
Yorktown, Virginia

Melissa L. Weir, MS, BSN, RN, CPEN, CNE
Faculty
College of Nursing
Howard University
Washington, DC
RN II
Children's National Medical Center
Washington, DC

Mary E. Wilson, MS, RN, FNP-C, CEN, COHN-S, FAEN
Regional Health Services Manager
Avery Dennison
Brunswick, Ohio

Lisa A. Winchester, MSN, RN, CEN
Clinical Nurse Educator
Lourdes Health System
Camden, New Jersey

Jalean Zettlemoyer, BSN, RN, CEN
Registered Nurse
Vascular Center of Colorado
Colorado Springs, Colorado

Polly Gerber Zimmerman, MS, MBA, RN, CEN, FAEN
Assistant Professor
Ivy Tech Community College—Lawrence Campus
Chicago, Illinois

CHAPTER 1

Introduction

What Is the CEN?

The Certification Examination for Emergency Nurses is developed and administered by the Board of Certification for Emergency Nursing (BCEN). On successful completion of the certification examination, the nurse earns the mark of distinction of the Certified Emergency Nurse (CEN) credential. The Emergency Nurses Association acknowledges the American Board of Nursing Specialties definition of certification: "Certification is the formal recognition of the specialized knowledge, skills, and experience demonstrated by the achievement of standards identified by a nursing specialty to promote optimal health outcomes."[1,2]

Why Should I Be Certified as a CEN?

The BCEN emergency nursing certification promotes professionalism and informs the public that the Certified Emergency Nurse possesses essential knowledge to deliver care competently. The CEN certification:

- signifies your expertise and adherence to nursing specialty standards,
- validates your qualifications and competencies to current and potential employers, and
- communicates your commitment to delivering high-quality, current patient care.[3]

What Is the Purpose of the *CEN Review Manual*?

As in previous editions of the *Certified Emergency Nurse (CEN) Review Manual*, this fifth edition is intended to serve as a preparatory aid for nurses who wish to take the CEN examination. The manual is intended for use by both first-time certifying nurses and nurses who are preparing for recertification as a CEN.

The main focus of the manual is to provide a means of self-assessment in the topic areas found within the CEN examination itself. Another purpose is to provide a review and overview of emergency nursing knowledge by presenting an explanation (rationale) for each of the four multiple-choice answers to every question—the single correct answer, as well as the three incorrect responses. Although the *CEN Review Manual, Fifth Edition* offers the opportunity to take practice examinations in both a paper-and-pencil and computer-based format, the BCEN offers the actual CEN examination in a computer-based format only.

How Is the *CEN Review Manual* Constructed?

The *CEN Review Manual, Fifth Edition* has more than 1,500 new questions that are unique to this edition, and each question was written by emergency nursing experts who hold the CEN credential. Although there are practice variations among emergency departments, the content of the questions represents and reinforces current standards and practices in the emergency department setting in the United States and worldwide.

The format of the fifth edition of the *CEN Review Manual* is as follows. Chapters 6–10 each consist of a simulated 150-question test. Each test has been organized according to the BCEN blueprint content categories to facilitate focusing on specific areas of interest. Every sample test has been carefully constructed to have the same proportion of items as that found in each content category of the actual CEN examination (see Chapter 2). Your score, which you may record in the charts provided in Chapter 5, should clearly indicate any subject areas that require further study. The answer key also reveals the content category of each question.

How Can Using the CEN *Review Manual* Help Me?

Using the *CEN Review Manual* will:

- help you identify your strong and weak subject areas so that you can most efficiently study for the certification examination,
- enhance your knowledge of how to manage many specific situations that you may encounter in your clinical practice, and
- give you experience taking multiple examinations that are similar to the CEN examination in content and length.

What Are Some Other Advantages of Using the *CEN Review Manual*?

You can derive many benefits from reading the four chapters between this introduction and the practice examinations themselves, which begin with Chapter 6.

- **Test blueprint.** Chapter 2 explains the BCEN test blueprint on which the CEN examination is based.
- **Nursing process.** Chapter 3 provides an overview of the nursing process. This section delineates ways in which the nursing process is integrated into the CEN testing questions.
- **Test preparation.** Use Chapter 4 as a general review of strategies in preparing for the certification exam. It includes suggestions to help you improve your test-taking skills.
- **Using the *CEN Review Manual*.** Chapter 5 offers advice on how you can gain the most benefit from taking the practice examinations. Chapter 5 also provides a grid that you can use to evaluate your areas of identified strength as well as areas in which you would benefit from additional study.

The *CEN Review Manual, Fifth Edition* includes five traditional paper-and-pencil sample tests as well as computerized Web-based versions of simulated tests. Each of the two computerized Web-based simulation examinations consists of 150 questions. Taking these sample tests on a computer will simulate the experience of taking the CEN examination online.

Times built into the computerized tests establish the same time constraints as the actual examination: 3 hours. You can earn 3.0 continuing nursing education contact hours for each completed examination with a passing score of 70%. Additional information regarding how to obtain your continuing nursing education contact hours will be provided when you access the online examinations.

The *CEN Review Manual, Fifth Edition* can be used in several ways. Choose the method that best suits your needs as you prepare for the CEN examination. This book provides an overview of the CEN blueprint, practice examinations representative of content areas on the CEN examination, methods for self-assessment of your areas of CEN content knowledge, and an opportunity to take computer-based simulation tests. Make this manual work for you as an excellent resource in preparing for the CEN examination.

REFERENCES

1. American Board of Nursing Specialties. (n.d.). About us. Retrieved from http://nursingcertification.org/about
2. Emergency Nurses Association. (2014). Position statement: Emergency Nursing Certification. Retrieved from https://www.ena.org/docs/default-source/resource-library/practice-resources/position-statements/encertification.pdf?sfvrsn=b3563eb6_12
3. Board of Certification for Emergency Nursing. (2017). *Candidate handbook*. Oak Brook, IL: Author.

CHAPTER 2

Test Blueprint

Emergency nursing certification provides a method to measure attainment of a defined body of knowledge that an emergency nurse must have to function at the *competent* level.[1] Measurement of this knowledge through a certification examination encourages the application of knowledge to clinical practice.

The basis for any certifying examination is a test blueprint that reflects specific content areas covered in the examination. The Certified Emergency Nurse (CEN) test blueprint was developed based on a practice analysis of emergency nurses throughout the United States. The use of a test blueprint ensures the consistent application of emergency nursing knowledge and minimizes variability in the measurement of that knowledge.

The Board of Certification for Emergency Nursing (BCEN) determines the component of the test blueprint for the CEN examination based on feedback from practicing emergency department nurses throughout the country. The test blueprint is revised periodically to ensure that the test remains an accurate reflection of current emergency nursing knowledge. The test blueprint used as the basis for the CEN examination is protected by copyright held by the BCEN.

Clinical and professional practices are the cornerstones of the CEN test blueprint. Clinical knowledge is the dominant content area covered within the CEN examination. The test blueprint does not address age-specific knowledge. Knowledge required for various age groups is tested within each content area or dimension of the examination. Therefore, age-specific content is distributed throughout the examination. Similarly, nursing process is integrated into all aspects of the test blueprint and tested within each content area or dimension of the test.

Certified Emergency Nurse Detailed Content Outline Effective July 6, 2016*

1. **Cardiovascular Emergencies (20 Questions)**
   - A. Acute coronary syndrome
   - B. Aneurysm/dissection
   - C. Cardiopulmonary arrest
   - D. Dysrhythmias
   - E. Endocarditis
   - F. Heart failure
   - G. Hypertension
   - H. Pericardial tamponade
   - I. Pericarditis
   - J. Peripheral vascular disease (e.g., arterial, venous)
   - K. Thromboembolic disease (e.g., deep vein thrombosis [DVT])
   - L. Trauma
   - M. Shock (cardiogenic and obstructive)
2. **Respiratory Emergencies (16 Questions)**
   - A. Aspiration
   - B. Asthma
   - C. Chronic obstructive pulmonary disease (COPD)
   - D. Infections
   - E. Inhalation injuries
   - F. Obstruction

*__Note:__ The Board of Certification for Emergency Nursing (BCEN®) does not endorse any resources or have a proprietary relationship with any publishing company. BCEN is the sole owner of the 2016 CEN Content Outline and did not contribute to the development of the content or exam questions in this product.

G. Pleural effusion
H. Pneumothorax
I. Pulmonary edema, noncardiac
J. Pulmonary embolus
K. Respiratory distress syndrome
L. Trauma

3. **Neurological Emergencies (16 Questions)**
   A. Alzheimer's disease/dementia
   B. Chronic neurological disorders (e.g., multiple sclerosis, myasthenia gravis)
   C. Guillain-Barré syndrome
   D. Headache (e.g., temporal arteritis, migraine)
   E. Increased intracranial pressure (ICP)
   F. Meningitis
   G. Seizure disorders
   H. Shunt dysfunctions
   I. Spinal cord injuries, including neurogenic shock
   J. Stroke (ischemic or hemorrhagic)
   K. Transient ischemic attack (TIA)
   L. Trauma
4. **Gastrointestinal, Genitourinary, Gynecology, and Obstetrical Emergencies (21 Questions)**
   A. Gastrointestinal
      1. Acute abdomen (e.g., peritonitis, appendicitis)
      2. Bleeding
      3. Cholecystitis
      4. Cirrhosis
      5. Diverticulitis
      6. Esophageal varices
      7. Esophagitis
      8. Foreign bodies
      9. Gastritis
      10. Gastroenteritis
      11. Hepatitis
      12. Hernia
      13. Inflammatory bowel disease
      14. Intussusception
      15. Obstructions
      16. Pancreatitis
      17. Trauma
      18. Ulcers
   B. Genitourinary
      1. Foreign bodies
      2. Infection (e.g., urinary tract infection, pyelonephritis, epididymitis, orchitis, STD)
      3. Priapism
      4. Renal calculi
      5. Testicular torsion
      6. Trauma
      7. Urinary retention
   C. Gynecology
      1. Bleeding/dysfunction (vaginal)
      2. Foreign bodies
      3. Hemorrhage
      4. Infection (e.g., discharge, pelvic inflammatory disease, STD)
      5. Ovarian cyst
      6. Sexual assault/battery
      7. Trauma
   D. Obstetrical
      1. Abruptio placenta
      2. Ectopic pregnancy
      3. Emergent delivery
      4. Hemorrhage (e.g., postpartum bleeding)
      5. Hyperemesis gravidarum
      6. Neonatal resuscitation
      7. Placenta previa
      8. Postpartum infection
      9. Preeclampsia, eclampsia, HELLP syndrome
      10. Preterm labor
      11. Threatened/spontaneous abortion
      12. Trauma
5. **Psychosocial and Medical Emergencies (25 Questions)**
   A. Psychosocial
      1. Abuse and neglect
      2. Aggressive/violent behavior
      3. Anxiety/panic
      4. Bipolar disorder
      5. Depression
      6. Homicidal ideation
      7. Psychosis
      8. Situational crisis (e.g., job loss, relationship issues, unexpected death)
      9. Suicidal ideation
   B. Medical
      1. Allergic reactions and anaphylaxis
      2. Blood dyscrasias
         a. Hemophilia
         b. Other coagulopathies (e.g., anticoagulant medications, thrombocytopenia)
         c. Leukemia
         d. Sickle cell crisis
      3. Disseminated intravascular coagulation (DIC)

4. Electrolyte/fluid imbalance
5. Endocrine conditions
    a. Adrenal
    b. Glucose-related conditions
    c. Thyroid
6. Fever
7. Immunocompromise (e.g., HIV/AIDS, patients receiving chemotherapy)
8. Renal failure
9. Sepsis and septic shock

6. **Maxillofacial, Ocular, Orthopedic, and Wound Emergencies (21 Questions)**
    A. Maxillofacial
        1. Abscess (i.e., peritonsillar)
        2. Dental conditions
        3. Epistaxis
        4. Facial nerve disorders (e.g., Bell's palsy, trigeminal neuralgia)
        5. Foreign bodies
        6. Infections (e.g., Ludwig's angina, otitis, sinusitis, mastoiditis)
        7. Acute vestibular dysfunction (e.g., labyrinthitis, Ménière's disease)
        8. Ruptured tympanic membrane
        9. Temporomandibular joint (TMJ) dislocation
        10. Trauma
    B. Ocular
        1. Abrasions
        2. Burns
        3. Foreign bodies
        4. Glaucoma
        5. Infections (e.g., conjunctivitis, iritis)
        6. Retinal artery occlusion
        7. Retinal detachment
        8. Trauma (e.g., hyphema, laceration, globe rupture)
        9. Ulcerations/keratitis
    C. Orthopedic
        1. Amputation
        2. Compartment syndrome
        3. Contusions
        4. Costochondritis
        5. Foreign bodies
        6. Fractures/dislocations
        7. Inflammatory conditions
        8. Joint effusion
        9. Low back pain
        10. Osteomyelitis
        11. Strains/sprains
        12. Trauma (e.g., Achilles tendon rupture, blast injuries)
    D. Wound
        1. Abrasions
        2. Avulsions
        3. Foreign bodies
        4. Infections
        5. Injection injuries (e.g., grease gun, paint gun)
        6. Lacerations
        7. Missile injuries (e.g., guns, nail guns)
        8. Pressure ulcers
        9. Puncture wounds
        10. Trauma (i.e., including degloving injuries)

7. **Environment and Toxicology Emergencies, and Communicable Diseases (15 Questions)**
    A. Environment
        1. Burns
        2. Chemical exposure (e.g., organophosphates, cleaning agents)
        3. Electrical injuries
        4. Envenomation emergencies (e.g., spiders, snakes, aquatic organisms)
        5. Food poisoning
        6. Parasite and fungal infestations (e.g., giardia, ringworm, scabies)
        7. Radiation exposure
        8. Submersion injury
        9. Temperature-related emergencies (e.g., heat, cold, and systemic)
        10. Vector-borne illnesses
            a. Rabies
            b. Tick-borne illness (e.g., Lyme disease, Rocky Mountain spotted fever)
    B. Toxicology
        1. Acids and alkalis
        2. Carbon monoxide
        3. Cyanide
        4. Drug interactions (including alternative therapies)
        5. Overdose and ingestions
        6. Substance abuse
        7. Withdrawal syndrome
    C. Communicable Diseases
        1. *C. difficile*
        2. Childhood diseases (e.g., measles, mumps, pertussis, chickenpox, diphtheria)
        3. Herpes zoster

4. Mononucleosis
5. Multi-drug-resistant organisms (e.g., MRSA, VRE)
6. Tuberculosis

8. **Professional Issues (16 Questions)**
   A. Nurse
      1. Critical incident stress management
      2. Ethical dilemmas
      3. Evidence-based practice
      4. Lifelong learning
      5. Research
   B. Patient
      1. Discharge planning
      2. End-of-life issues
         a. Organ and tissue donation
         b. Advance directives
         c. Family presence
         d. Withholding, withdrawing, and palliative care
      3. Forensic evidence collection
      4. Pain management and procedural sedation
      5. Patient safety
      6. Patient satisfaction
      7. Transfer and stabilization
      8. Transitions of care
         a. External handoffs
         b. Internal handoffs
         c. Patient boarding
         d. Shift reporting
      9. Cultural considerations (e.g., interpretive services, privacy, decision making)
   C. System
      1. Delegation of tasks to assistive personnel
      2. Disaster management (i.e., preparedness, mitigation, response, and recovery)
      3. Federal regulations (e.g., HIPAA, EMTALA)
      4. Patient consent for treatment
      5. Performance improvement
      6. Risk management
      7. Symptom surveillance
         a. Recognizing symptom clusters
         b. Mandatory reporting of diseases
   D. Triage

REFERENCE

1. Board of Certification for Emergency Nursing. (2016). *Certified Emergency Nurse Detailed Content Outline.* Retrieved from http://www.bcencertifications.org/BCENMain/media/CEN/2016-CEN-Content-Outline.pdf

SUGGESTED READINGS

Emergency Nurses Association. (2012). *Emergency Nursing Pediatric Course: Provider manual* (4th ed.). Des Plaines, IL: Author.

Emergency Nurses Association. (2014). *Trauma Nursing Core Course: Provider manual* (7th ed.). Des Plaines, IL: Author.

Hammond, B. B., & Zimmermann, P. G. (Eds.). (2013). *Sheehy's manual of emergency care* (7th ed.). St. Louis, MO: Elsevier Mosby.

Howard, P. K., & Steinmann, R. A. (Eds.). (2010). *Sheehy's emergency nursing: Principles and practice* (6th ed.). St. Louis, MO: Mosby Elsevier.

Hoyt, K. S., & Selfridge-Thomas, J. (Eds.). (2007). *Emergency nursing core curriculum* (6th ed.). St. Louis, MO: Saunders Elsevier.

CHAPTER

3

Nursing Process

The *CEN Review Manual, Fifth Edition* provides you with questions and answers, rationales for the correct and incorrect answers, and references to help you prepare for the Certified Emergency Nurse (CEN) examination. As you study, remember that the entire nursing process is an integral part of emergency nursing and therefore a part of the CEN examination.

Nursing Process

The steps of the nursing process[1] provide the framework for the essential components of emergency nursing practice. These steps are called slightly different thing in various models but invariably involve assessment and data gathering; analysis; planning; intervention; and evaluation. It has also been suggested that reassessment is another critical step in the nursing process.

Assessment

Assessment is defined as the collection of data performed using a systematic approach regarding patients' actual or potential health problems and their potential needs. The nurse gathers two types of information when performing the patient assessment: subjective data and objective data.

Subjective data represent information offered by the patient or others. This information may include descriptions of the current health concern or concerns, the patient's report of past medical history, and events and perceptions surrounding the precipitating event that brought the patient to seek treatment. Caregivers, friends, bystanders, and past medical records may provide subjective data, especially when patients cannot provide such information themselves.

Objective data include vital signs, other physical findings, and nursing observations. Emergency nursing assessment differs from other types of nursing assessment in that it begins with a primary assessment. Included in the primary assessment is the determination of the patient's airway, breathing, and circulatory status (ABCs). If the primary assessment identifies any area of concern, attention is given to correcting life-threatening conditions before the assessment is continued.

Once the primary assessment has been completed and emergent problems, if any, have been identified and addressed, a secondary assessment is performed. Secondary assessment is a systematic head-to-toe examination of the patient centering on a search for signs of illness or injury. Particular attention is paid to areas of concern that the patient has identified.

Both subjective and objective assessment are ongoing processes in emergency nursing. Assessment is an ongoing process throughout the patient's stay in the emergency setting. Examination questions reflecting assessment may focus on the candidate's ability to ask the right questions, gather the right information, or perform the appropriate examination.

Analysis

When initial data collection has been completed, the next phase of the nursing process calls for the nurse to analyze all assessment data in order to identify and prioritize the patient's actual or potential health problems. Using critical thinking skills and assessment data, laboratory values, and alterations in pathophysiology, the nurse formulates a judgment or conclusion about the patient's condition.

In essence, the nurse identifies a patient's problem or problems for which he or she is held responsible. Although the satisfactory resolution of many health problems requires a collaborative effort—and indeed, nurses are actively involved in the treatment of the patient's medical diagnosis—medical and nursing diagnoses differ. A nursing diagnosis is based on the priorities of care delivered by the nurse. Multiple nursing diagnoses may be applicable to the patient, but the nurse and patient must prioritize the diagnoses to plan care that will be most effective. Possible analysis examination items may list assessment findings in the stem, followed by statements such as: "the nurse should suspect...," "the nurse concludes...," "... are due to," and so on.

Intervention

Analysis leads to the development of a plan of care. In busy emergency settings, it is not unusual for this plan, or components of it, to be unwritten. It is clear, however, that the nurse must formulate a plan to proceed with the appropriate interventions for a particular patient. The plan includes the priorities of the patient as well as the nurse.

Implementation of the plan follows the priorities already established. The interventions should be patient oriented, goal directed, and based on established psychological and/or physiological principles. The nurse selects interventions based on the likelihood of success in achieving desired outcomes.

Interventions can be independent or collaborative. Independent interventions are those activities that the nurse is licensed to implement and responsible for implementing based on his or her education and experience. Collaborative interventions are those activities performed by the nurse in conjunction with members of other healthcare disciplines. For example, if the patient is experiencing pain, independent nursing interventions might include positioning and anxiety reduction, while collaborative interventions might include administration of pain medications. Administration of pain medication is a collaborative intervention because the nurse may not administer the medication until a physician has written an order for it.

The stem of intervention questions may end with "the nurse prepares," "the nurse assists with," "the nurse anticipates the administration of," "the nurse should not," or "the nurse should first," followed by a variety of intervention options.

Evaluation

As the plan is being developed and implemented, the nurse must be aware of the outcome that is desired as a result of the intervention(s) to be made. The evaluation component of the nursing process involves the time when the nurse assesses the attainment of the desired outcome as a result of the interventions(s). The criteria by which the efficacy of the intervention will be measured should be predetermined as part of the plan of care. Criteria should be outcome focused and based on patient response.

If the interventions suggested for pain relief are implemented, certain outcomes are expected to result; for example, "Patient will experience pain relief within 30 minutes." Evaluation in this case would consist of the nurse's reassessment of the patient's pain status 30–40 minutes after the interventions had been made and comparing that with the level of pain experienced before the interventions took place. If satisfactory pain relief has not been accomplished, the steps of the nursing process should be repeated. In this way, additional assessment data, analysis, or interventions as a result of ongoing assessment may lead to a more satisfactory outcome. Both in practice and on the examination, outcomes are not always positive and may identify the need for additional interventions or modifications in the plan of care.

Reassessment

Emergency patients should be assessed regularly while they are in the emergency setting. The analysis should be reviewed and additional independent and collaborative interventions implemented if planned outcomes were achieved or if changes were noted in reassessment. Following these steps, the patient's response to the interventions would be evaluated once again. The steps of the nursing process should be repeated as frequently as needed to meet the goals established by the patient and nurse.

Documentation

All nursing assessments, interventions, and evaluations must be documented. This process allows the nurse to share his or her findings with other caregivers. It is important to consider all steps of the nursing process in preparing documentation, both for legal reasons and to ensure clear communication with other caregivers.[2]

REFERENCES

1. American Nursing Association (2018). The nursing process. Retrieved from https://www.nursingworld.org/practice-policy/workforce/what-is-nursing/the-nursing-process/
2. Emergency Nurses Association. (2017). *Emergency nursing scope and standards of practice* (2nd ed.) Des Plaines, IL: Author.

CHAPTER

4

Test-Taking Strategies

When you decide to take the Certified Emergency Nurse (CEN) certification examination, it is important that you begin to prepare both your mind and your emotions for success. Maintaining strong study habits and positive attitudes will help to strengthen your efforts.

Preparing for the CEN Examination

Since 2000, the CEN examination has been offered in a computer-based testing (CBT) format. The CBT version of the CEN is administered in a designated testing center, where the candidate sits in a private cubicle to take the examination. If you require special accommodations to take the CEN examination, contact the BCEN (bcen@bcencertifications.org).

No prior computer experience is required for taking a CBT examination. Before the CEN examination begins, each candidate reviews a tutorial program that explains how to take the test online. Once the candidate feels comfortable with the computer, he or she can begin to take the examination.

The CBT version of the CEN examination must be completed within 3 hours. (This period does not include the time needed to complete the tutorial program before the test begins.) The CEN examination comprises 175 multiple-choice questions; 150 of these items are scored, and 25 are pretest questions of varying content that are analyzed to determine whether certain questions should be used in future examinations. Because pretest questions reflect area of need in the overall bank, the content of the examination may not appear to reflect the exact blueprint provided by BCEN. On completing the examination, the examinee receives a report that identifies the total score as passing or failing. In addition, candidates who do not pass the examination will receive a subscore in each major subject area; this subscore alerts them to areas of knowledge proficiency and knowledge deficit, thereby providing information for further study.

Test Blueprint

Preparation for a test like the CEN examination begins with determining what material you will be required to know. The BCEN provides a blueprint (outline) for the test items on the CEN examination. Review the outline in Chapter 2 of this manual to become aware of the broad content areas of the CEN. Further information is available on the BCEN website (www.bcencertifications.org).[1]

Organizing and Using Resources

Once you know the broad content areas to be covered on the CEN examination, gather emergency nursing resources that will be useful as you prepare. Examples include textbooks on emergency nursing, *Emergency Nursing Core Curriculum*, and journal articles on content related to the topics in the CEN test blueprint. Additional resources that may help in preparing for the examination include:

- Emergency Nurses Association. (2012). *Emergency Nursing Pediatric Course: Provider manual* (4th ed.). Des Plaines, IL: Author.

- Emergency Nurses Association. (2014). *Trauma Nursing Core Course: Provider manual* (7th ed.). Des Plaines, IL: Author.
- Hammond, B. B., & Zimmermann, P. G. (Eds.). (2013). *Sheehy's manual of emergency care* (7th ed.). St. Louis, MO: Elsevier Mosby.
- Hoyt, K. S., & Selfridge Thomas, J. (Eds.). (2007). *Emergency nursing core curriculum* (6th ed.). St. Louis, MO: Saunders Elsevier.

Next, prepare some notes on central ideas of the examination. The act of writing may help you organize your thoughts and aid you in remembering the material. Describe key concepts and explain how the information ties together. Write down important names, relationships, formulas, and examples that will jog your memory as you review them (flash cards can be helpful memory joggers). Then rewrite your notes and organize them into major categories that make sense to you. Organizing your notes based on the CEN test blueprint may also be helpful.

Pacing Yourself

Cramming as the examination date nears may cause anxiety. Developing a study plan in advance and using it over time is far more effective and less stressful. Determine how much material you need to cover before your CEN examination is scheduled. Plot a timeline on a calendar. By doing this, you will gain a realistic perspective for reviewing your materials and resources. Be sure to allow extra time in your plan for the more difficult content areas and for areas that you are less familiar with.

Overstudy! When you believe you have retained 100% of the material, it may be helpful to study more. Scrupulously following your study and review schedule will prevent procrastination and let you relax on occasion without guilt.

Part of your strategy for review may include joining a CEN study group or taking a formal CEN review course. All members of the study group should have an equal grasp of the material. Coming into the study group with baseline knowledge will guard against inadvertently learning incorrect information. Study groups can provide a forum in which to think out loud, clear up misunderstandings, and put together relationships between facts. Group discussion will reinforce your long-term memory, too.

Strategies for Taking Multiple-Choice Examinations

Carefully read the stem of each question. Then, think about what the question is asking. Next, answer each item on the examination, searching for the closest answer among the choices given. Some general test-taking tips:

- Eliminate the answers that are obviously wrong.
- Do not eliminate an answer unless you know what every word means.
- Implausible answers may be partly right.
- Some responses may be correct in themselves but are not related to the stem of the question.
- Don't read between the lines. Well-written certification questions are intended to be straightforward and to the point, and contain no ambiguity.
- Read each question carefully.
- Try to reason out the answers to tough questions.
- Analyze the wording in a question's stem. The correct answer may be one that uses words similar to those in the question.
- Choose the closest answer—the one that is definitely better than the rest.
- It is usually best to follow your first impulse in determining your response to a question. Changing answers often leads to incorrect responses.
- Make an educated guess. Doing this increases your odds of answering correctly from 0% to 25% when you aren't sure of the answer.
- Don't look for any pattern to correct items on the examination. Letters (A, B, C, or D) that precede the correct answers on the certification examination are chosen at random.

The Night Before the Examination

The night before you take your examination, get a good night's rest. On the day of your scheduled CEN examination, take essential materials with you (e.g., photo identification, admission ticket) and be sure you have had some nourishment. Tell yourself that you are going to be successful in taking this examination. Imagine yourself doing well on the CEN examination. You will have spent plenty of time preparing for the event. Believe in yourself and that you will remain calm and perform well.

Using Practice Examinations for Testing Assessment

Another major strategy for success on the CEN certification examination is to take practice examinations that simulate the experience. Besides helping you to identify areas of emergency nursing content that you will want to review before taking the examination, taking practice examinations can motivate you and enhance your confidence. Additionally, the rationale offered after each response may provide new knowledge that will prove useful when you take the actual examination.

In certification examinations like the CEN, all test items are multiple choice. They contain a stem followed by several options. The stem presents a problem or asks a question. Options are potential answers to the questions. Options include both the correct answer and the distracters (incorrect answers). Although all the options often seem plausible, the correct answer represents the best response to the question.

By taking practice examinations, you will identify strengths and weaknesses in your emergency nursing knowledge while gaining insight into your own test response patterns. After you have completed a practice CEN examination, reread the items that you answered incorrectly and ask yourself the questions on the following grid. Consider using some of the strategies identified to enhance future performance when taking an examination or test.

Contributing Factors: Why do you think you answered an item incorrectly?	**Possible Strategies**
Did I really know the right answer but marked it incorrectly on the scoring sheet?	Take time to review your answers after you have marked your scoring sheet to ensure that you have marked the item you intended.
Did I not have the knowledge to answer the question?	Review the rationale for the correct response, which usually contains succinct information to help you fill gaps in your ED knowledge base. Read the reference list at the end of the manual. You can use these references to update or refresh your knowledge of particular content areas.
Did I misunderstand the question?	After reading the rationale, reread the stem of the question and all the distracters. Does the correct answer now make sense to you, or do you have a knowledge gap?
Did I miss a key word or concept in the stem (body of the question)?	After reading the rationale, reread the stem of the question and all the distracters. Does the correct answer now make sense to you, or do you have a knowledge gap?
Did I change my answer?	If you find that you often change your answer on a test or exam, determine whether the changed answer tends to be correct. If you tend to change incorrect answers to correct ones, it may be to your advantage to continue the practice. If you tend to change correct answers to incorrect ones, reevaluate the usefulness of this practice.

BCEN Examination Scoring

Scores will be reported to you in a written format in person at the testing center on completion of the examination. The reported score will indicate your test results as pass/fail. A raw score indicating the number of questions you answered correctly will be provided. A breakdown of questions in each category will be provided to you that indicates how you scored within each content area.

The BCEN uses the Angoff technique for determining pass/fail decisions on the CEN examination. The Angoff philosophy makes a distinction between the standard set and its relationship to item difficulty. This process establishes an objective decision that is criterion referenced and consistent with the intent of the examination. Therefore, your individual ability to successfully pass the examination is based on the knowledge and skill you displayed, not on the performance of other candidates who have taken the examination. For this reason, passing scores may vary slightly for each form of the examination.

REFERENCE

1. Board of Certification for Emergency Nursing. (2017). *Candidate handbook*. Oak Brook, IL: Author.

CHAPTER

5

Using the *CEN Review Manual*

Organization

This manual is organized into two parts. The first part consists of five chapters that provide information on how you can prepare to take the Certified Emergency Nurse (CEN) examination. You are encouraged to read the first five chapters to better prepare you to take the practice tests that begin in Chapter 6.

- Chapter 1 addresses questions that nurses ask about the CEN examination and how to prepare for it.
- Chapter 2 describes the test blueprint concept and the content areas contained in the CEN examination, which are based on the BCEN test blueprint.
- Chapter 3 describes the nursing process with an emphasis on how the concepts of the nursing process are integrated into the CEN examination.
- Chapter 4 has information and strategies to maximize test-taking skills for the CEN examination.
- Chapter 5 helps you benefit optimally from using this book's practice examinations as a method to prepare for the CEN test.

Using the Rationale Section of the *CEN Review Manual*

A very useful aspect of this manual is the rationale section that follows each practice examination. To enhance your preparation for the CEN examination, read the rationales for each correct answer and each incorrect answer (distracter). By reviewing these materials, you are using a highly effective study technique to reinforce your emergency nursing knowledge.

Another strategy for using the rationale section to identify possibly insufficient content knowledge is to evaluate the items you have answered incorrectly. Determine whether the content is really unfamiliar to you or if there was some other reason that you answered the item incorrectly. Studying the rationales carefully may provide you with enough review of content. If not, you may decide to use other resources to review the areas in which your emergency nursing knowledge is least strong.

Getting the Most Out of the Practice CEN Examinations

This manual consists of five practice CEN examinations, each with 150 questions. General subjects (content categories) in these practice examinations are proportional to those found within the CEN test blueprint.

Blank answer sheets for the practice examinations are provided at the back of the manual. Follow the steps in the next section to develop strategies to assist you in assessing your emergency nursing knowledge. What you learn in these self-assessments will serve as the basis for implementing additional test-taking strategies and identifying areas for additional study.

Determine Content Areas for Further Study

Follow these steps to determine the content areas where you need to do more studying:

1. Begin by completing the first examination. Some prefer to look at the rationale section as they answer each question, while others prefer

to complete the whole examination and then go through the rationale section.

2. The content category for each question is found following each rationale. They are:
   - Cardiovascular emergencies (items 1–20)
   - Respiratory emergencies (items 21–36)
   - Neurological emergencies (items 37–52)
   - Gastrointestinal, genitourinary, gynecology, and obstetrical emergencies (items 53–73)
   - Psychosocial and medical emergencies (items 74–98)
   - Maxillofacial, ocular, orthopedic, and wound emergencies (items 99–119)
   - Environment and toxicology emergencies and communicable diseases (items 120–134)
   - Professional issues (items 135–150)
3. Use the self-assessment worksheet as you look at the rationale section. You can also go through the answer sheet and transfer the number of each incorrect answer into the column for the corresponding content area on the self-assessment worksheet.
4. Count the number of incorrect questions in each content category and total them in the appropriate column.
5. Refer to the last column of the self-assessment worksheet for the number of incorrect answers that constitute 30% of the total number of questions in that content area. If your incorrect answers are equal to or greater than that number (or the total number of all questions in the blueprint is greater than 30%), you should identify this as an indicator that you should focus your study efforts more intensely on this content area. (You can also divide the number incorrect by the content outline content category total to give you the % incorrect.)

Sample Self-Assessment Worksheet

In the example that follows, the reader answered cardiovascular content category questions 4, 7, 9, 18, and 21 incorrectly. The total number of incorrect answers is 5. The content outline total number in that category is 21. In the example, the reader answered medical content category questions 47, 51, 53, 57, 58, 60, and 61. The total number of incorrect answers is 7. The blueprint total number in that category is 15. In both examples, the learner can determine areas where he or she can benefit from further content study.

Content Category	Questions Answered Incorrectly	Total Number of Questions Answered Incorrectly in Each Category	Total Number of Questions in Each CEN Blueprint Category
Cardiovascular Emergencies	4, 7, 9, 18, 21	5	21
Medical Emergencies	47, 51, 53, 57, 58, 60, 61	7	15

Sample Self-Diagnostic Content Area Worksheet

How to Use the Self-Assessment Worksheet

1. Indicate on your answer sheet whether your answers are correct or incorrect.
2. Note the items you answered incorrectly.
3. Count the total number of items you answered incorrectly in each category.
4. Compare the total number of items you answered incorrectly in each category with the total number of items per category. This information will give you an idea of where you need to focus your continued study.

Summary

This manual can serve as an invaluable study aid as you prepare to take the CEN examination. You may discover additional strategies for using the manual constructively besides those described in this and previous chapters.

Review the manual and reflect on your own learning preferences, and then use the manual to prepare for the CEN examination. Good luck!

Content Category	Questions Answered Incorrectly	Total Number of Questions Answered Incorrectly in Each Category	Total Number of Questions in Each CEN Content Outline Category
Cardiovascular Emergencies			20
Respiratory Emergencies			16
Neurological Emergencies			16
Gastrointestinal, Genitourinary, Gynecology, and Obstetrical Emergencies			21
Psychological and Medical Emergencies			25
Maxillofacial, Ocular, Orthopedic, and Wound Emergencies			21
Environment and Toxicology Emergencies, and Communicable Diseases			15
Professional Issues			16

CHAPTER 6

Practice Examination 1

PART 1

1. A patient presents to the emergency department with chest pain and diaphoresis, and denies dyspnea. Vital signs are BP 148/70 mm Hg, HR 72 beats/minute, RR 18 breaths/minute, SpO_2 98% on room air. Breath sounds are clear and equal. The electrocardiogram shows an inferior wall ST segment elevation. You anticipate the following oxygen order.
   A. No supplemental oxygen at this time
   B. Nasal cannula at 6 L per minute
   C. Partial rebreather mask at 10 L per minute
   D. Nonrebreather mask at 15 L per minute

2. A patient complains of chest pain, dyspnea, and diaphoresis. Which of the following assessment factors would indicate a possible diagnosis of acute coronary syndrome?
   A. Pleuritic chest pain
   B. Positional chest pain
   C. Chest pain that radiates to the shoulders, with pain in the right shoulder worse than pain in the left shoulder
   D. Pain reproducible with chest wall palpation

3. Which of the following human compensatory mechanisms to the presence of shock triggers glycogenolysis?
   A. Chemoreceptor activation
   B. Clotting cascade activation
   C. Cerebral autoregulation stimulation
   D. Adrenal gland stimulation

4. A patient presents to the emergency department with abdominal pain and "ripping" back pain. Which condition places the patient at risk for abdominal aortic dissection?
   A. Down syndrome
   B. Romano–Ward syndrome
   C. Jervell and Lange-Nielsen syndrome
   D. Ehler–Danlos syndrome

5. A patient presents via emergency medical services in cardiopulmonary arrest, following 15 minutes of cardiopulmonary resuscitation (CPR). On completion of the initial nursing assessment, which of the following findings would indicate that termination of resuscitation efforts should be considered?
   A. Decreased compliance while performing bag-mask device ventilation
   B. An end-tidal carbon dioxide level reading less than 10% after 20 minutes of high-quality CPR
   C. An initial rhythm of pulseless electrical activity
   D. An initial presentation of a shockable rhythm

6. A 7-year-old suddenly develops ventricular fibrillation. The child weighs 66 lbs (30 kg). Cardiopulmonary resuscitation is started immediately. What is the correct defibrillation dose for the initial shock to be used by the emergency nurse?
   A. 60 joules
   B. 30 joules
   C. 120 joules
   D. 90 joules

7. The emergency nurse is participating in the care of an obtunded patient presumed to have taken an overdose of a tricyclic antidepressant. The patient has a palpable pulse, and an electrocardiogram (ECG) is obtained. The nurse would anticipate the presence of which ECG finding?
   A. Sinus bradycardia with normal QRS and QT intervals
   B. Ventricular fibrillation
   C. Narrow complex supraventricular tachycardia
   D. Sinus tachycardia with both a widened QRS interval and prolonged QT interval

8. During triage, the patient states the pacemaker only fires when the patient's heart rate slows below a certain number of beats/minute. The nurse anticipates that the patient has a(n):
   A. asynchronous pacemaker.
   B. demand pacemaker.
   C. dual-chamber pacemaker.
   D. fixed-rate pacemaker.

9. A patient being evaluated in the emergency department is noted to have Janeway lesions, Roth's spots, and Osler's nodes along with an elevated body temperature and elevated white blood cell count. Patient assessment reveals the presence of several recent body piercings. The emergency nurse suspects the patient has:
   A. endocarditis.
   B. pericarditis.
   C. myocarditis.
   D. leukemia.

10. A conscious pulseless patient with a continuous-flow left ventricular assist device and a history of end-stage heart failure presents to the emergency department because of a "low-flow" alarm. The nurse anticipates performing which intervention first?
    A. Obtain a blood pressure using a Doppler and sphygmomanometer
    B. Auscultate over the pump to ascertain if the device is working
    C. Administer intravenous fluids
    D. Begin chest compressions

11. A heart failure patient with profound dyspnea, lung crackles, and pink frothy sputum presents to the emergency department. The physician orders for the patient to be placed on bilevel positive airway pressure at an end-expiratory pressure of 10 cm H_2O and an inspiratory pressure of 5 cm H_2O. Which of the following findings demonstrates that the patient's symptoms and work of breathing have been reduced?

    A. Increasing the blood returned to the right side of the heart
    B. Decreasing cardiac output
    C. Decreasing the preload
    D. Increasing the afterload

12. Intravenous nitroprusside (Nipride) has been ordered for blood pressure reduction in a patient with a hypertensive emergency. The patient's blood pressure is 280/124 mm Hg with a mean arterial pressure (MAP) of 176 mm Hg. When titrating the nitroprusside for this patient, which order has the safest parameter to follow?

    A. Titrate nitroprusside to a MAP of 124 mm Hg over the next hour
    B. Titrate nitroprusside to a MAP of 106 mm Hg over the next hour
    C. Titrate nitroprusside to a MAP of 158 mm Hg over the next hour
    D. Titrate nitroprusside to a MAP of 132 mm Hg over the next hour

13. The assessment of a patient involved in a motor vehicle collision reveals muffled heart sounds and distended neck veins. The nurse understands that the treatment for this life-threatening situation is to:

    A. minimize the administration of intravenous fluids.
    B. prepare for a 3- to 4-cm incision to the left of the xiphoid process.
    C. prepare for insertion of a 14-gauge needle into the midclavicular line second intercostal space.
    D. prepare for chest tube insertion at the 5th intercostal space.

14. What is the best position to place a patient, in order to assess for the presence of a cardiac friction rub?

    A. Ask the patient to stand up and then squat, then place the stethoscope at the left sternal border and listen at midsystole.
    B. Ask the patient to lie or sit quietly, then place the stethoscope at the right sternal border and listen for radiation to the neck.
    C. Ask the patient to lean forward, then place the stethoscope at the left sternal border and listen at end-expiration.
    D. Ask the patient to lie or sit quietly, then place the stethoscope at the apex of the heart and listen for radiation to the axilla.

15. Raynaud's disease is characterized by which assessment findings?

    A. Severe leg cramps and redness
    B. Carpopedal spasms and intense heat
    C. Intense vasospasms and pallor of the digits
    D. Numbness and tingling of the wrist and elbow

16. Which of the following statements made by a patient recently diagnosed with peripheral vascular disease indicates that the patient has an accurate understanding of the disease?

    A. "When my leg starts to cramp, I should stop walking and rest."
    B. "When pain develops in my leg, I should apply an ice pack."
    C. "When my leg starts to cramp, I should elevate it on two pillows."
    D. "I will limit my cigarette smoking to a half-pack a day."

17. Which of the following patients would demonstrate the presence of delayed venous return resulting from increased intra-abdominal pressure, creating a high risk for deep venous thrombosis and pulmonary embolus?
   A. 57-year-old hypertensive male
   B. 48-year-old diabetic female
   C. 26-year-old bariatric female
   D. 32-year-old male with peripheral vascular disease

18. A patient has sustained a stab wound to the left parasternal anterior chest. Emergency medical services treatment has included intubation and intravenous therapy with crystalloid solution. The patient exhibited vital signs during transport; however, as the patient is being wheeled into the trauma room, pulses are no longer detected. Cardiopulmonary resuscitation is initiated. Breath sounds are present bilaterally. The nurse anticipates the following procedure to be immediately performed.
   A. Point-of-care cardiac ultrasound
   B. Chest radiograph
   C. Open thoracotomy
   D. Needle pericardiocentesis

19. Emergency medical services arrives with an unrestrained driver who was involved in a multivehicle collision. The patient is diagnosed with a pelvic fracture and left tibial fracture. Which classification of hypovolemic shock would most likely occur as the result of these injuries?
   A. Class IV
   B. Class III
   C. Class II
   D. Class I

20. Following the insertion of an intraosseous (IO) device, which of the following findings by the emergency nurse would indicate that the IO has been properly placed?
   A. The needle has slight movement after insertion.
   B. Bright red blood is noted in the cannula after insertion.
   C. The fluid will only infuse with the use of positive pressure.
   D. A reddish frothy aspirate is noted after insertion.

21. When caring for a child who has been treated for an asthma exacerbation, the emergency nurse identifies that the patient is ready for discharge when:
   A. the patient is awake and alert.
   B. the patient can demonstrate proper use of a rescue inhaler without assistance.
   C. the patient's peak expiratory flow is greater than 70% and response is sustained for 60 minutes following the last bronchodilator treatment.
   D. the patient demonstrates SpO_2 of 93% on room air (21% oxygen).

22. An adult patient with a history of asthma presents to triage stating they are experiencing an acute asthma exacerbation. The emergency care provider orders an electrocardiogram (ECG). The patient asks the nurse why this procedure is necessary. The nurse explains to the patient:
   A. "In adults, underlying cardiac conditions can often present as, or exist with, respiratory complaints."
   B. "It is a part of our order set for patients with respiratory complaints."
   C. "ECGs can show us how well you are breathing."
   D. "I don't know. I just do what the provider orders."

23. A patient is being discharged after being treated for the presence of a cough for 3 months and increasing shortness of breath with excretion. The patient has been diagnosed with chronic obstructive pulmonary disease (COPD). The emergency nurse knows that the only proven medical therapy shown to reduce the progression and mortality of COPD is:

A. smoking cessation.
B. short-acting inhaled bronchodilator.
C. inhaled corticosteroids.
D. pulmonary rehabilitation.

24. The emergency nurse would anticipate arterial blood gas values from a patient in a severe chronic obstructive pulmonary disease exacerbation to illustrate:

A. metabolic acidosis.
B. respiratory alkalosis.
C. respiratory acidosis.
D. metabolic alkalosis.

25. The nurse ensures that the mechanically ventilated patient is placed in a semirecumbent position to:

A. prevent the development of a decubitus pressure ulcer.
B. make the patient more comfortable.
C. allow for oral care to be more easily performed.
D. prevent aspiration.

26. A patient arrives via emergency medical services following a house fire. The patient has a Glasgow Coma Scale score of 15. The emergency nurse understands that the patient's airway is patent because:

A. the pulse oximetry reads at 100%.
B. the patient is able to state their name clearly.
C. the patient's respiratory rate is 20.
D. the patient is not able to cough.

27. A patient with severe respiratory distress has been intubated, and mechanical ventilation has been initiated. The ventilator is alarming, indicating high airway pressures. As the emergency nurse, you are aware that this alarm indicates the importance to assess for the:

A. signs of a pneumothorax.
B. need for additional sedation.
C. change in the patient's oxygen saturation level.
D. presence of secretions.

28. A patient presents to triage with a complaint of difficulty breathing, presence of a nonproductive cough, and "stabbing" chest pain. The patient reports a history of congestive heart failure. On assessment, the emergency nurse auscultates diminished breath sounds, bilaterally. What additional information would be the most pertinent to obtain from the patient?

A. Recent sick contacts
B. Medications prescribed and compliance
C. Vaccination history
D. Recent travel history

29. Which assessment finding would best indicate that chest tube insertion has been successful in relieving a tension pneumothorax?

A. Presence of bloody drainage in the chest tube
B. Decrease in discomfort
C. Improvement in hemodynamics
D. Improved ability to deep breathe

30. A tube thoracostomy has been placed for a patient with a hemothorax. Initially after placement, what output amount would alert the nurse to anticipate that the patient would be taken to the operating room for an emergency thoracotomy?

A. 1000 mL
B. 750 mL
C. 500 mL
D. 200 mL

31. A patient presents to the emergency department pale and diaphoretic with VS: BP 130/85 mm Hg; HR 135 beats/minute; RR 40 breaths/minute; SpO_2 48% room air; T 37.2°C (99.0°F). Lungs sounds are diminished bilaterally throughout, with crackles at the bases. The patient is visiting from Florida and has been in town for 4 days; the current elevation is 9500 feet. What condition should the emergency nurse be most concerned about?

A. Pulmonary embolism
B. Pneumonia
C. Pneumothorax
D. High-altitude pulmonary edema

32. A patient arrives complaining of a sudden onset of chest pain. The patient is anxious and tachypnic. The initial priority intervention for the emergency nurse to perform for this patient would be to:

A. obtain an echocardiogram.
B. obtain intravenous access.
C. obtain arterial blood gas.
D. administer supplemental oxygen.

33. Which is the term used to describe a form of shock that occurs following a large pulmonary embolism that has resulted in unstable patient hemodynamics with decreased tissue perfusion?

A. Cardiogenic shock
B. Distributive shock
C. Hypovolemic shock
D. Obstructive shock

34. An appropriate intervention in the treatment of acute respiratory distress syndrome is:

A. mechanical ventilation.
B. treating the underlying cause.
C. decreasing fluid intake to avoid pulmonary edema.
D. using high tidal volumes to open collapsed alveoli.

35. Which diagnostic finding is consistent with the presence of an esophageal injury?
   A. Widening of the mediastinum on chest radiograph
   B. Esophageal tissue in the nasogastric tube
   C. Elevated central venous pressure
   D. Abnormal echocardiogram

36. A patient presents to triage with complaints of runny nose, headache, and a nonproductive cough for 3 days. The patient is able to speak without difficulty and reports a history of moderate to severe chronic obstructive pulmonary disease. Vitals signs are BP 158/88 mm Hg, HR 106 beats/minute, RR 22 breaths/minute, SPO_2 88% room air, T 37.1°C (98.8°F). The priority intervention for the emergency nurse to implement for this patient is which of the following?
   A. Apply low flow supplemental oxygen
   B. Call a code because the patient is hypoxic
   C. Obtain a chest radiograph
   D. Obtain an arterial blood gas analysis

37. When caring for an elderly patient with dementia, the emergency nurse is aware that a patient with dementia will directly exhibit which of the following first?
   A. Inaccurate medical history
   B. Disruptive behavior
   C. Impaired communication
   D. Sensory overload

38. In caring for a patient with multiple sclerosis, the emergency nurse is aware that a common healthcare issue that affects the quality of life in this patient population is:
   A. hypertension.
   B. diabetes.
   C. depression.
   D. elevated cholesterol.

39. A patient arrives to the emergency department with a 2-week history of repeatedly falling, accompanied by ascending weakness and tingling in the feet and fingers. There is loss of the knee-jerk reflex, and the patient is complaining of being unable to take a deep breath and of overall difficulty in breathing. Vital signs are BP 120/70 mm Hg, HR 72 beats/minute, RR 22 breaths/minute, SpO_2 96% on room air. The emergency nurse suspects the patient may have which of the following?
   A. Myasthenia gravis
   B. Guillain–Barré syndrome
   C. Bell's palsy
   D. Botulism

40. A patient with a history of chronic headaches presents to the emergency department (ED) with a severe headache that has grown in intensity over the last 2 weeks. A computed tomography angiography of the brain reveals no acute pathology. The patient typically uses nonsteroidal anti-inflammatories (NSAIDs) for pain relief and notes that over the last 2 weeks, they have had to increase the frequency of NSAID use to 4–5 days per week. The ED provider decides to place the patient on propranolol (Inderal) for prophylactic pharmacologic therapy. Which of the following statements by the patient would indicate a need for further education?
   A. "I will take my propranolol (Inderal) as needed with the onset of a headache."
   B. "I will not discontinue this medication without first notifying my healthcare provider."
   C. "The reason for this medication is to reduce my headache frequency and severity."
   D. "This medication may improve the effectiveness of my other headache medications."

41. The emergency nurse is reviewing the medication orders for a patient newly diagnosed with a subarachnoid hemorrhage. Which of the following orders would cause the emergency nurse to question the provider?
   A. Nimodipine 60 mg every 4 hours
   B. Infuse 0.9% NaCl at 150 mL/hour
   C. Dexamethasone 16 mg daily
   D. Atorvastatin 40 mg daily

42. A patient with a 2-year history of uncontrolled hypertension presents to the emergency department with a complaint of a severe headache. A computed tomography scan of the head reveals the presence of a large subarachnoid hemorrhage. Which of the following is a late sign of increased intracranial pressure?
   A. Tachypnea
   B. Narrowing pulse pressure
   C. Bradycardia
   D. Behavioral changes

43. A 3-week-old infant presents to the emergency department with a T 38.3°C (100.9°F). The infant has a normal physical exam, normal chest radiograph, and a white blood cell count of 15,000 and appears sleepy. The emergency provider decides to perform a lumbar puncture. What disease process can be confirmed by this procedure?
   A. Hyponatremia
   B. Meningitis
   C. Otitis media
   D. Subarachnoid hemorrhage

44. The emergency nurse is caring for a patient with the following symptoms: severe headache, neck stiffness, fever, and inability to tolerate bright light. The patient has been administered intravenous antibiotics and an antipyretic for fever. The nurse identifies that additional patient education is required for their diagnosis of bacterial meningitis when the patient states:
   A. "My girlfriend will need to be evaluated for this disease."
   B. "I will have to cancel my dinner plans with friends for this evening."
   C. "I need to take medication to reduce my fever."
   D. "I will take my antibiotics until my symptoms go away."

45. An elderly patient presents to the emergency department after demonstrating aggressive behavior in the patient's group home residence. The emergency nurse observes the patient to be pale and diaphoretic and displaying tonic–clonic movement. Which laboratory test has the greatest priority for this patient?
   A. Dilantin (phenytoin) level
   B. Blood glucose level
   C. Blood alcohol level
   D. Vitamin B_6 (thiamine) level

46. A patient presents to the emergency department complaining of two tonic–clonic seizure episodes within the previous 3 days despite being compliant with daily doses of levetiracetam (Keppra). Which of the following statements made by the patient indicates that additional education is required this medication?
   A. "I use the rowing machine at the gym every day."
   B. "I use meditation to help with sleep."
   C. "I keep hydrated to protect my kidneys."
   D. "I limit alcohol to two drinks each night."

47. A patient presents to the emergency department following a bar fight. The patient reports being punched in the face and having their neck forced backward. A few hours later, the patient began noticing upper extremity weakness with associated sensory loss. They also report being unable to urinate, and the bladder scan reveals 300 mL of urine in their bladder. The most likely cause of this patient's symptoms is:

A. Brown–Sequard syndrome.
B. anterior cord syndrome.
C. central cord syndrome.
D. posterior cord syndrome.

48. A patient presents to the emergency department via emergency medical services (EMS). The patient has cervical spine precautions in place because of suspected spinal cord injury. Per the EMS report, the patient initially was able to move their wrists bilaterally. On initial assessment, the emergency nurse determines that the patient is only able to shrug their shoulders. The priority intervention for this patient would be to:

A. notify the trauma team.
B. document these new findings.
C. determine the patient's pain level.
D. reassess patient function in 15 minutes.

49. A patient who weighs 100 kg is ordered to receive tissue plasminogen activator for an acute ischemic stroke. The emergency provider orders a dose of 100 mg, with 10% of the dose to be administered via intravenous push, with the remaining dose to be administered over an hour infusion. The emergency nurse verifies the weight dosing and identifies that 0.9 mg/kg is the recommended dosing for this medication in the presence of an acute ischemic stroke. The next action by the emergency nurse is to:

A. administer 10 mg over 1 minute, followed by the administration of 90 mg over 59 minutes via infusion pump.
B. verify with the emergency provider the medication order for the patient.
C. administer 9 mg over 1 minute, followed by the administration of 91 mg over 59 minutes via infusion pump.
D. administer 10 mg over 1 minute, followed by the administration of 90 mg over 60 minutes via the infusion pump.

50. The provider is considering the administration of alteplase (Activase/tPA) to an 82-year-old patient diagnosed with an acute ischemic stroke. In addition to the patient's age, which other factor would exclude the patient from the administration of alteplase within the recommended extended 3- to 4.5-hour time window?

A. A National Institutes of Health Stroke Scale greater than 20
B. A National Institutes of Health Stroke Scale of 3
C. Previous history of a ST-elevation myocardial infarction
D. History of diabetes

51. Which of the following patients would benefit from the administration of nimodipine (Nimotop) to decrease the risk of associated cerebral infarction?

A. A subarachnoid hemorrhage resulting from traumatic brain injury
B. A subdural hematoma in an elderly patient
C. A subarachnoid hemorrhage resulting from a cerebral aneurysm
D. A subdural hematoma in a patient who abuses alcohol

52. Which type of skull fracture would place the patient at the highest risk for developing an intracranial infection?
    A. Basilar skull fracture
    B. Linear skull fracture
    C. Depressed skull fracture
    D. Temporal bone fracture

53. A 32-year-old female who is 28 weeks pregnant presents with right upper quadrant pain that is radiating to the right scapula area. The patient states that the pain began a short time after having dinner. Based on the patient's presentation, the most likely diagnosis is:
    A. diverticulitis.
    B. cholecystitis.
    C. pancreatitis.
    D. gastroenteritis.

54. A patient with a history of esophageal varices presents to the emergency department complaining of weakness and diaphoresis. The patient suddenly has an emesis of bright red blood. The priority intervention for the emergency nurse to perform is:
    A. to insert a large-diameter gastric tube.
    B. to obtain a complete set of vital signs.
    C. to administer high-flow oxygen via nonrebreather mask.
    D. to establish intravenous (IV) access with two large-caliber IV catheters.

55. A child presents to the emergency department after choking on a chicken bone. The patient's airway is not obstructed, but swallowing is difficult, and the child is consistently drooling. The nurse anticipates which diagnostic test to be performed initially?
    A. Chest radiograph
    B. Bedside ultrasound
    C. End-tidal carbon dioxide measurement
    D. Direct laryngoscopy

56. A normal full-term newborn has been delivered in the emergency department. The newborn has been warmed, their temperature is being maintained, their airway is being positioned, secretions have been cleared, and they have been stimulated. To evaluate the effectiveness of these interventions, the nurse anticipates the infant's preductal oxygen saturation target after 1 minute to be approximately:
    A. 63%.
    B. 67%.
    C. 73%.
    D. 90%.

57. A 3-year-old child who weighs 20 kg is being treated for a 2-day history of vomiting and diarrhea. The child has been orally rehydrated and is now being discharged home with the parents. Which of the following would be most important to include in the initial home care discharge instructions?
    A. Administer 1–2 teaspoons of an oral rehydration solution (Pedialyte) every 5 minutes
    B. Resume normal meals in small amounts
    C. Start a BRAT (bananas, rice, applesauce, toast) diet
    D. Do not permit the child to have anything orally for the next 24 hours. If no vomiting occurs, the child may advance to having small amounts of clear liquids.

58. A patient presents to the emergency department with complaints of upper abdominal fullness, fatigue, and nausea for the past 2 weeks. When obtaining the patient's history, the triage nurse would be most concerned that the patient may have developed hepatitis A if the patient reports:

A. having engaged in unprotected sexual contact with an individual who may have hepatitis B.
B. having a history of intravenous (IV) drug use and having recently shared needles with other IV drug users.
C. having been camping recently and sustaining a tick bite.
D. having recently traveled overseas to assist in the clean-up activities in a town flooded by heavy rains.

59. A male presents to the emergency department with complaints of pain and swelling in his right groin area. The patient states the pain intensity has increased, and the swelling has become larger over the past several days. The emergency nurse should anticipate which diagnostic test to best identify the source of the patient's complaint?

A. Abdominal radiographs
B. Computed tomography scan
C. Magnetic resonance imaging of the abdomen
D. Abdominal ultrasound

60. Parents of a 7-month-old state that the infant has not been as active as usual and has been crying and drawing up their legs at intervals. The child's abdomen is distended, and a mass is palpable in the right upper quadrant. The parents state that earlier today, the child had a small bowel movement that looked dark red with mucous in it. The child's symptoms are most consistent with which of the following conditions?

A. Intussusception
B. Pyloric stenosis
C. Appendicitis
D. Incarcerated hernia

61. Correct placement of a nasogastric tube (NG) is best confirmed by which method?

A. pH determination of NG tube aspirate
B. Obtaining a chest radiograph
C. Placing the end of the NG tube in a container of water
D. Auscultating for air over the epigastric region

62. A patient has an elevated serum lipase level and left upper quadrant abdominal pain that radiates to their back. The emergency nurse recognizes these signs and symptoms as most likely being associated with which disease process?

A. Hepatitis C
B. Cholecystitis
C. Pyelonephritis
D. Pancreatitis

63. Following a motor vehicle collision, a patient arrives in the emergency department with a suspected blunt abdominal injury. Vital signs are BP 100/72 mm Hg, HR 106 beats/minute, RR 18 breaths/minute, T 36.2°C (97.2°F). The emergency nurse should anticipate which of the following to be performed as part of the patient's initial assessment?

A. Computed tomography scan
B. Hemoglobin and hematocrit
C. Focused assessment with sonography for trauma exam
D. Diagnostic peritoneal lavage

64. A patient presents to the emergency department with frequency and urgency of urination, associated with the presence of right flank pain. On physical assessment, the patient exhibits a temperature of 38.8°C (102°F) and tenderness over the right costovertebral angle. Which of the following conditions is most consistent with the patient's signs and symptoms?

A. Bladder infection
B. Nephrolithiasis
C. Pyelonephritis
D. Urethral stricture

65. The presence of a suspected testicular torsion is best evaluated using which diagnostic study?

A. Computed tomography scan
B. Doppler sonography
C. Urine culture and sensitivity
D. Testicular transillumination

66. Following a motor vehicle collision, an unresponsive and intubated patient is received in the emergency department. On assessment, a rigid and bruised abdomen is noted, and a bedside ultrasound examination identifies a ruptured bladder. Based on this information, what is the emergency nurse's priority action?

A. Establish two large-caliber IVs and begin fluid resuscitation
B. Insert a urinary drainage catheter
C. Prepare the patient for computed tomography scan
D. Administer intravenous antibiotics

67. A patient presents to the emergency department complaining of lower abdominal pain and the inability to void in the past 24 hours. What is the priority intervention the emergency nurse should perform?

A. Obtaining a full set of vital signs
B. Preparing the patient for an abdominal radiograph to assess for bladder calculi
C. Insertion of urinary catheter
D. Administering an intravenous fluid bolus of 500 mL of 0.9% sodium chloride

68. A patient who is 32 weeks pregnant is involved in a motor vehicle collision. On arrival to the emergency department, the patient is complaining of severe abdominal pain. Blood is noted on the sheets around the patient's lower extremities, and on assessment, the nurse determines the patient is bleeding vaginally. High-flow oxygen is administered via face mask. The emergency nurse's next action is to perform which of the following?

A. Insert two large-caliber IVs and administer intravenous crystalloid fluids
B. Perform a type and cross-match for a blood transfusion
C. Initiate continuous fetal monitoring
D. Prepare the patient for a cesarean section

69. A patient who is diagnosed with a *Chlamydia trachomatis* vaginal infection should also be screened for what other associated sexually transmitted disease?

A. Human papillomavirus
B. Bacterial vaginosis
C. Candidiasis
D. Gonorrhea

70. The emergency nurse is caring for a victim of sexual assault. Which of the following statements made by the victim indicates the need for further education regarding the sexual assault examination process?

A. "Once the exam is finished, I'd like to take a shower."
B. "I am so anxious, I don't know how I will get through all of this."
C. "I really don't want the police in the room with me during the exam."
D. "I will need to be seen again in about 1 week to have more cultures taken."

71. A patient who is 6 days postpartum and breastfeeding presents to the emergency department complaining of fever, with right-sided breast redness and tenderness. The patient is diagnosed with mastitis. In addition to antibiotic therapy, which of the following should be included in the discharge instructions for this patient?

A. Avoid hand-expressing or using a mechanical breast pump
B. Have the baby nurse from the unaffected breast only
C. Stop breastfeeding and supplement feedings with formula until the infection clears
D. Apply a warm compress to the breast before breastfeeding

72. A patient presents to the emergency department with symptoms of left lower quadrant abdominal cramping with frequent episodes of blood and mucus-containing diarrhea. The symptoms have been present for the past 3 weeks and the patient has noticed a recent weight loss. The emergency nurse anticipates the patient will most likely need further evaluation for which disorder?

A. Ulcerative colitis
B. Colon cancer
C. Salmonella infection
D. Crohn's disease

73. A woman who is 10 weeks pregnant presents to the emergency department complaining of vaginal spotting with mild abdominal cramping and is discharged to home after a diagnosis of threatened abortion is made. Which of the following statements, made by the patient, indicates a correct understanding of their discharge instruction?

A. "I will keep a count of the number of tampons I use to determine how much I'm bleeding."
B. "I will need to stay on bed rest for at least a day or two."
C. "I can expect the bleeding to get heavier in a day or two."
D. "While I'm on bed rest, my partner and I can have sexual intercourse as long as it isn't too rough."

74. When suspecting the presence of child maltreatment or neglect in a patient, the emergency nurse is required to:

A. document the names of the suspected abusers in the medical record.
B. inform the parent of the police notification.
C. report the suspected abuse or neglect to the police and child protective services.
D. review the pediatrician or family physician records.

75. A patient is brought to the emergency department after exhibiting aggressive behavior toward family members. To assess the patient's current mental state, which question would be most important for the emergency nurse to ask the patient?

A. "What are the voices telling you to do?"
B. "What medications are you currently taking?"
C. "What past medical history do you have?"
D. "What brought this behavior on today?"

76. A 65-year-old female reports a history of generalized anxiety disorder that is controlled with 0.5 mg of alprazolam (Xanax) three times daily as needed. Which of the following patient statements requires additional follow-up and patient education by the emergency nurse?

A. "I do not take the Xanax every day."
B. "I only take the Xanax before participating in stressful events, such as being in large crowds, in order to prevent anxiety."
C. "I drink several glasses of wine in one setting on a regular basis."
D. "I eat a lot of dairy products frequently and sometimes take the Xanax with milk."

77. Parents arrive to triage with their child, stating that the child has demonstrated recent behavior changes that include extreme anger with family members, no desire to complete required tasks (attend school or do chores), racing thoughts with rapid speech, and impulsive actions. The emergency nurse will be most concerned about which type of psychiatric disorder being demonstrated by the patient?

A. Psychosis
B. Attention-deficit hyperactivity disorder
C. Bipolar disorder
D. Panic disorder

78. Which diagnostic test should the emergency nurse anticipate to be performed in a patient with bipolar disorder who has been receiving antipsychotic medications for treatment of acute mania?

A. Complete blood count
B. Liver function testing
C. Bladder scan
D. 12-lead electrocardiogram

79. On review of a patient's current medications, the emergency nurse identifies that the patient has been prescribed an alternative drug for depression. Which of the following is an alternative medication used in the treatment of depression?

A. Bupropion (Wellbutrin)
B. Citalopram (Celexa)
C. Fluoxetine (Prozac)
D. Sertraline (Zoloft)

80. Which of the following interventions would be appropriate for an emergency nurse to perform following the transfer of a patient? The patient has experienced an acute psychotic episode and states, "I'm coming back here when I get released from the hospital, and I am going to kill Jane Smith."

A. Ignore the threat because this is normal behavior in patients who are psychotic
B. Alert proper law enforcement authorities
C. Tell the patient that it is inappropriate to make this statement
D. Request that the hospital chaplain come and talk to the patient

81. A homeless patient arrives in the emergency department by emergency medical services after being found wandering on the street and talking to himself. The patient is in possession of proper identification but will not answer to their name. Speech is clear, and the patient displays no signs of aggressive behavior, but will not make eye contact with the emergency nurse or follow simple commands. Which of the following signs and symptoms would alert the emergency nurse to an organic cause for their psychosis?

A. Signs of trauma
B. Normal vital signs
C. Auditory hallucinations
D. Clear speech patterns

82. A patient presents to triage with a complaint of a headache and appears anxious and restless. The patient tells the emergency nurse that the "man at the desk" has followed the patient from Russia, where the patient worked for the Central Intelligence Agency, and that the headache began after the tracking chip implanted in their brain was activated. The nurse observes no one at the desk, and the patient has identification that indicates a local address and that they are a student at a nearby college. There is no indication of recent travel or corroboration of the information. The emergency nurse suspects the cause of the patient's symptoms is related to:

A. an anxiety attack.
B. migraine headache.
C. dementia.
D. psychosis.

83. Ziprasidone (Geodon) is most appropriate for which of the following psychiatric scenarios? The adult patient:

A. who is exhibiting acute depressive disorder and is tearful and sobbing.
B. who is exhibiting acute manic behavior, is in handcuffs, and is being accompanied by police.
C. who is having auditory hallucinations and is being told not to move.
D. who is experiencing extrapyramidal effects related to their psychiatric medications.

84. A patient presents to the emergency department (ED) voicing thoughts of suicidal ideation. Why is it important to identify and address medical issues before treating the mental health issue?

A. Medical problems can mimic mental health problems.
B. Mental health problems do not lead to serious illness.
C. Medical problems can be resolved more quickly than behavioral problems.
D. Once in the ED, the patient is safe from suicide.

85. A patient presents to the emergency department with sudden onset of lip swelling, facial edema, and throat tightness. Vital signs are BP 90/60 mm Hg, HR 127 beats/minute, RR 22 breaths/minute, T 38.6°C (97.8°F). The emergency nurse anticipates which of the following to be administered to this patient for their signs and symptoms?

A. Epinephrine
B. High-flow oxygen
C. Corticosteroids
D. Aerosol albuterol

86. A patient presents to the emergency department stating they were hunting the previous day in a heavily wooded area. This morning the patient noticed a red, itchy rash with many blisters covering their face, neck, back, and arms. The emergency provider diagnoses the patient with poison ivy. What medication should the emergency nurse anticipate will be prescribed for this patient?

A. A narcotic analgesic
B. An oral antibiotic
C. A topical antifungal agent
D. An oral corticosteroid

87. Which statement is correct regarding hemophilia disorders?

A. There is an increased incidence of hemophilia in females.
B. Platelet administration is a common treatment in hemophilia.
C. Hemophilia is an inherited sex-linked genetic disorder.
D. Two common triggers of hemophilia are hypoxia and dehydration.

88. An elderly patient arrives to the emergency department following a fall at home. The patient's daily medication includes clopidogrel (Plavix) 300 mg daily. The patient is diagnosed with an intracranial bleed. The emergency nurse anticipates which of the following actions to be taken?

A. Administer vitamin K intravenous (IV) immediately
B. Administer protamine sulfate IV immediately
C. Discontinue the clopidogrel (Plavix) immediately
D. Decrease in the next dose of clopidogrel (Plavix)

89. A patient with a history of leukemia and who is currently undergoing chemotherapy treatment is being discharged from the emergency department (ED) following a facial laceration repair. Which statement best indicates to the emergency nurse the patient's understanding of the discharge instructions?

A. "I should return to the ED immediately for a temperature of 37.3°C (99.1°F)."
B. "I might not see the common signs of infection."
C. "Because I have a high white blood cell count, I am protected from getting an infection."
D. "Pus will be expected during the healing because of my high white blood cell count."

90. An African American patient presents to emergency department triage with a complaint of chest pain, shortness of breath, fever, cough, and wheezing. The patient's medications include lisinopril, metformin, and hydroxyurea. The patient is a poor historian and is refusing to answer questions. The emergency nurse should be most concerned about which potential diagnosis for this patient?

A. Acute chest syndrome
B. Acute myocardial infarction
C. Chronic obstructive bronchitis
D. Superior vena cava syndrome

91. Which of the following laboratory test values would alert an emergency nurse that a patient with disseminated intravascular coagulation is beginning to improve?

A. Elevated D-dimer
B. Increased platelet count
C. Prolonged partial thromboplastin time
D. Increased prothrombin

92. The emergency nurse anticipates heparin to be administered for the treatment of disseminated intravascular coagulation in which of the following situations?

A. Postpartum bleeding
B. Multiple traumatic injuries
C. Excessive fibrin that has caused digital ischemia
D. Envenomation from a snake bite

93. A patient complains of transient palpitations and occasional numbness and tingling of their fingers and nose. While vital signs are being obtained, the emergency nurse observes a sudden onset of carpal spasms on the arm on which the blood pressure cuff is being inflated. The nurse recognizes that this finding is consistent with the presence of:

A. hypocalcemia.
B. hypercalcemia.
C. hypokalemia.
D. hyperkalemia.

94. Which of the following conditions caused by an insufficient amount of available antidiuretic hormone results in the patient urinating large amounts of diluted urine?

A. Diabetes insipidus
B. Adrenal crisis
C. Syndrome of inappropriate antidiuretic hormone
D. Cushing's syndrome

95. Which assessment finding in a patient with adrenal crisis would alert the emergency nurse to prepare for an expected complication?

A. Hypokalemia
B. Hypotension
C. Hyperglycemia
D. Bradycardia

96. A patient arrives at the emergency department via emergency medical services with sudden onset of altered level of consciousness. The patient was found wandering at the local bus station, is able to answer questions only after much thought, and is unable to recognize that they are currently in a hospital. The patient appears very anxious, is diaphoretic, and has uncontrolled tremors to bilateral arms. Which of the following diagnostic testing would be the first priority for the emergency nurse to obtain in order to assist in proper diagnosis of this problem?

A. Serum creatinine
B. Urinalysis
C. White blood cell count
D. Serum glucose

97. When providing discharge instructions to the parents of a child, the nurse is aware that the parents have understood the importance of avoiding products that contain aspirin when they state which of the following?
   A. There is an association between the use of aspirin-containing products in febrile children and the development of Reye's syndrome.
   B. Aspirin is less effective in controlling fevers in the pediatric population because of their immature and developing neurologic system.
   C. Aspirin has been shown to increase the risk of febrile seizures given its slower onset of action.
   D. There is an association between the use of aspirin in febrile children and the development of asthma.

98. Which of the following may be a subtle sign of sepsis that should be considered by the triage nurse during the initial assessment of a patient presenting to the emergency department?
   A. Systolic blood pressure greater than 90 mm Hg
   B. Respiratory rate greater than 22 breaths/minute
   C. Temperature of 37°C (98.6°F)
   D. Capillary refill less than 2 seconds

99. A patient presents to the emergency department with possible signs and symptoms of compartment syndrome 2 days following surgery for a fractured left tibia/fibula. Which of the following would alert the emergency nurse that this patient may be experiencing possible organ failure?
   A. Rales
   B. Jaundice
   C. Dark, scanty urine
   D. Generalized edema

100. A patient presents to triage with a complaint of continuous chest pain for the past 3 days. Vital signs are BP 108/70 mm Hg, HR 68 beats/minute, RR 18 breaths/minute, SpO_2 99% on room air, T 37°C (98.6°F). The patient describes the pain as sharp, located on the right side of the chest, and made worse by breathing and arm movement. The patient denies shortness of breath and any trauma or recent surgeries but does report having an upper respiratory infection the previous week. The emergency nurse anticipates the cause of the patient's symptoms is which of the following?
   A. Pericarditis
   B. Pulmonary contusion
   C. Anxiety
   D. Costochondritis

101. A young mother presents to triage with her toddler, stating the child fell while walking and now will not move their left arm. However, the child fell on their right side. What should the emergency triage nurse do next?
   A. Order a radiograph of the right arm per standing orders
   B. Suspect child maltreatment because the story does not match the injury
   C. Ask the mother if she attempted to prevent the child from falling by holding onto the opposite arm
   D. Assess the injured left arm by using passive range of motion

102. A patient presents to triage complaining of pain in the right distal forearm after falling onto their outstretched arm. There is an obvious deformity above the patient's right wrist. Right radial pulse is present and color and sensation are intact distally, however, the patient is unable to sustain a wrist grip. The emergency nurse is aware that it is best to immobilize the right forearm using a(n):

A. traction splint.
B. padded rigid long arm splint.
C. soft splint.
D. ice application.

103. The emergency nurse is preparing to discharge a female geriatric patient who presented to the emergency department for severe "heartburn." Medication reconciliation reveals the patient is on alendronate (Fosamax). What information should the emergency nurse provide to the patient with the discharge instructions?

A. Always take alendronate with food
B. Sit or stand upright for 30 minutes after taking alendronate
C. Have calcium blood levels monitored monthly
D. Take alendronate at bedtime

104. A patient is observed walking into the emergency department with a severely increased thoracic curve, or "humpback." The emergency nurse knows that this condition is referred to as:

A. scoliosis.
B. lordosis.
C. genu varum.
D. kyphosis.

105. A motorcyclist arrives to the emergency department via emergency medical services following a collision with a motor vehicle. The motorcyclist, who was thrown across the hood of the car, was helmeted and wearing leather clothing. The patient's primary survey is within normal limits. The secondary survey reveals pain and paresthesia to the right arm and hand, with pronounced weakness but no swelling, pallor, or coolness in the extremity. The emergency nurse anticipates the patient has the signs and symptoms of which of the following?

A. Brachial plexus injury
B. Compartment syndrome
C. Fracture of the humerus
D. Brachial artery dissection

106. A construction worker is brought to the emergency department by their coworkers. The patient reports that while descending from a ladder, they unintentionally fired a nail gun into their right thigh. Immediately following, the patient was unable to straighten their leg, and their coworkers had to cut the patient's jeans off from around the nail head. A radiograph reveals the presence of a foreign body embedded in the patient's right femur. The nurse anticipates that this injury will be managed as a(n):

A. foreign body.
B. open fracture.
C. comminuted fracture.
D. high-pressure grease injury.

107. The emergency nurse is preparing to discharge a patient who has received treatment to close a facial laceration. The nurse recognizes the patient's understanding of the discharge instructions when stating the following:

A. "I will be sure to call my doctor in the morning for a prescription for an antibiotic."
B. "I need to place a thin layer of antibiotic ointment over the sutures daily."
C. "I will be sure to have my staples removed after 3 weeks."
D. "I will return to the emergency department in 14 days for suture removal."

108. The emergency nurse is caring for a patient who was found lying on the floor for 2 days, unable to get up following a fall. The patient's skin assessment reveals an area of purple discoloration along the patient's greater trochanter, which is boggy and warm to the touch. The emergency nurse recognizes this wound as a(n):

A. stage 1 pressure ulcer.
B. area of bruising.
C. potential deep tissue injury.
D. stage 4 pressure ulcer.

109. Which wound is the highest risk for development of osteomyelitis?

A. Laceration to the palmar surface of the hand resulting from a carving knife
B. Stage 1 pressure injury to the heel
C. Laceration to the elbow from breaking glass
D. Deep puncture wound in the foot from stepping on a nail

110. What is the priority assessment for a patient who has sustained a traumatic laceration to the upper arm?

A. Range of motion in the fingers
B. The presence of a distal or radial pulse
C. Capillary refill
D. Skin color and temperature

111. An elderly patient arrives to the emergency department via emergency medical services with profuse epistaxis that has persisted for over an hour. After initiating universal precautions, the next priority intervention for the emergency nurse to perform is which of the following?

A. Obtain blood pressure
B. Initiate intravenous access
C. Maintain airway patency
D. Initiate direct pressure by instructing the patient to pinch their nostrils

112. A patient presents to emergency triage and tells the emergency nurse that they are experiencing a severe throbbing-type headache pain located over the frontal left region. The patient has a history of polymyalgia rheumatica. The emergency nurse suspects the patient's current discomfort is related to the presence of which of the following?

A. Temporomandibular joint dislocation
B. Temporal arteritis
C. Cluster headache
D. Sinusitis

113. A patient with a history of diabetes presents to the emergency department complaining of increasing swelling and severe pain in the left eye with movement of the eye. On assessment, the patient demonstrates decreased visual acuity, decreased pupillary reflexes, and the presence of erythema and edema of the upper and lower eyelids and of the left cheek area. The emergency nurse anticipates the patient has signs and symptoms of:

A. conjunctivitis.
B. anterior uveitis.
C. iritis.
D. orbital cellulitis.

114. An unresponsive patient involved in a high-speed motor vehicle collision with multiple facial injuries arrives in the emergency department via emergency medical services. Because of the presence of numerous facial injuries, it is determined that the patient is at risk for an upper airway obstruction. Which of the following maneuvers is best to initiate to prevent an upper airway obstruction?

A. Maintain the patient in semi-Fowler's position at a 45-degree angle to maintain airway patency
B. Place airway adjunct into the patient
C. Place patient in a left lateral "recovery" position to maintain an open airway
D. Assist the emergency provider to control facial bleeding using vessel ligation to prevent the occlusion of the upper airway as the result of significant bleeding.

115. A patient presents to the emergency department after being splashed in the both eyes with a cleaning solution. During assessment, the emergency nurse notes the presence of bilateral corneal clouding and prepares to irrigate the eyes. The emergency nurse knows the irrigation may be discontinued when:

A. the ocular pH reaches 7.0 in each eye.
B. 1 hour has passed.
C. the pain in each eye has been relieved.
D. 1000 mL of irrigation solution has been used.

116. An elderly patient presents to the emergency department complaining of a severe boring type pain of the right eye. The patient reports nausea, seeing halos around objects, and the presence of a headache behind the right eye. The patient has been diagnosed with acute angle-closure glaucoma and has received both 500 mg of acetazolamide (Diamox) intravenously and a 500 mg dose orally. Timolol (Timoptic) was instilled topically into the right eye. The emergency nurse identifies that this therapy has been effective when which of the following occurs?

A. The patient's intraocular pressure (IOP) is 35 mm Hg.
B. The patient's IOP is 20 mm Hg.
C. The patient's nausea has been alleviated.
D. The patient no longer complains of pain in their right eye.

117. You are discharging a 3-year-old patient who has been diagnosed and treated for conjunctivitis. You ask the parent to repeat the instructions for care and determine the child will receive the appropriate care for when the parent states:

A. "My child may return to daycare when there is no crusting around the eyes upon awakening in the morning."
B. "Everyone must practice good handwashing techniques, and my child may not attend daycare until the eye infection has resolved."
C. "My child may continue to sleep in the same bed with his brother."
D. "My child may return to school tomorrow because it is only viral conjunctivitis."

118. An elderly patient presents to the emergency department complaining of blindness in the left eye. The patient reports a history of two prior episodes that resolved after a few seconds and denies pain or recent trauma. The emergency nurse anticipates the patient has experienced which of the following?

A. Retinal detachment
B. Acute angle-closure glaucoma
C. Anterior uveitis
D. Central retinal artery occlusion

119. A patient presents to triage stating that they were hit in the eye with a ball while playing softball. A Snellen visual acuity is performed and determines the patient has no loss of vision. While awaiting to be seen by the emergency provider, the patient begins to complain of "an aching" eye pain that is associated with sudden onset of blurred vision. Which statement made by the patient would cause the emergency nurse the greatest concern?

A. The patient complains of increased lacrimation.
B. A decreased ability for the patient to look upward.
C. The patient reports that everything is looking red.
D. The cornea appears cloudy.

120. An adult patient presents to the emergency department with a thermal burn to the right forearm. The burn is very painful and sensitive to air. The patient's forearm area is red, involving the first few layers of the dermis, with a large fluid-filled blister. The nurse would appropriately classify the burn as a:

A. superficial partial-thickness burn.
B. fourth-degree burn.
C. deep partial-thickness burn.
D. full thickness burn.

121. Which of the following patients should receive rabies prophylaxis?

A. The patient with a bite from a pet cat
B. The patient with a bite from a pet dog
C. The patient who may or may not have been bitten by a bat in the house
D. The patient who may or may not have been bitten by a guinea pig

122. Which of the following is considered an appropriate treatment for a patient with a venomous snake bite?

A. Immobilize the involved area at or below the level of the heart
B. Administer hepatitis B vaccine as soon as possible and continue recommended dosing
C. Immediately apply ice packs and elevate the extremity
D. Contact poison control to have a specific antivenin prepared from the individual snake

123. A patient is being discharged following treatment for excessive vomiting and diarrhea from a possible foodborne illness. You know the patient understands the discharge instructions when the patient states:

A. "I will drink clear liquids, such as sports drinks, for the next 24 hours."
B. "I am OK to eat my regular diet when I leave here."
C. "Drinking milk will settle my stomach."
D. "I will drink clear liquids, such as orange juice and milk, for the next 24 hours."

124. The nurse is providing discharge education for an adult patient diagnosed with an infestation of *Sarcoptes scabiei* (scabies). Which of the following patient statements indicates that the patient understands the discharge instructions?

A. "I should not go to work or school for 7 days following treatment."
B. "I must discard all of my clothing and linens prior to treatment."
C. "It is normal to continue to experience itching for up to 7 days following treatment."
D. "It is not necessary to treat my family members."

125. There are four classifications of radiation particles that can affect life: alpha particles, beta particles, gamma radiation, and neutrons. Of these four, which one is able to penetrate the most objects (paper, wood, concrete) and is therefore more dangerous to life?

A. Gamma radiation
B. Beta particles
C. Neutrons
D. Alpha particles

126. A child is brought to the emergency department after falling through the ice while skating on a lake. On arrival, the patient's core temperature is 26.8°C (80.2°F). The nurse would anticipate this patient to exhibit which signs or symptoms?

A. Slow or slurred speech
B. An increased respiratory rate and effort
C. An increased urinary output
D. A decreased medication effect

127. A patient presents with fever and a small, flat, pink, nonpruritic macular rash on the palms of their hands and soles of their feet. The patient describes removing a tick from their forearm several days ago. Which tickborne disease would you suspect this patient has?

A. Tularemia
B. Rocky Mountain spotted fever
C. Lyme disease
D. Colorado tick fever

128. A patient is being discharged from the emergency department (ED) for treatment of carbon monoxide poisoning. The emergency nurse knows that the patient understands their discharge instructions when the patient states:

A. "I will use the space heater in the bedroom sometimes."
B. "I will not use a space heater."
C. "I can continue to use the space heater with the door closed."
D. "I will return to the ED the next time I get a headache and feel tired."

129. The emergency nurse is aware that a potential sign associated with the presence of cyanide poisoning is:

A. cherry-red skin.
B. symmetrical descending muscular weakness.
C. excessive secretions.
D. the odor of bitter almonds.

130. An adolescent is brought in to the emergency department by ambulance. The patient was at a "rave" party and experienced a seizure. The patient is confused and agitated. Vital signs are BP 180/98 mm Hg, HR 136 beats/minute, RR 26 breaths/minute, SpO_2 97%, T 39.6°C (103.2°F). Which of the following would be the first nursing intervention for this patient?

A. Initiate an intravenous line with a large-caliber catheter
B. Obtain a urine sample for analysis
C. Place the patient in seizure precautions
D. Administer a short-acting benzodiazepine medication

131. An adolescent patient was brought in by ambulance from a party at a friend's house. Paramedics report that the patient was drinking an unknown amount of alcohol at the party. The patient is lethargic and only responds to painful stimuli by moaning. Vital signs are BP 110/60 mm Hg, HR 122 beats/minute, RR 14 breaths/minute, SpO_2 94%, T 36.2°C (97.1°F). Which of the following diagnostic studies has the highest priority for this patient?

A. Serum glucose level
B. Computed tomography of the head
C. Blood alcohol level
D. Urine analysis for drugs of abuse

132. The emergency nurse is caring for an adult patient who was brought in by ambulance after having a tonic–clonic seizure. The patient is confused, appears anxious, and has obvious hand tremors. The patient's vital signs are BP 140/90 mm Hg, HR 128 beats/minute, RR 26 breaths/minute, SpO_2 98%, T 37.4°C (99.3°F). The patient reports that they consume alcohol on a daily basis but stopped drinking alcohol about 2 days ago. What is the priority concern for this patient?

A. The patient is at risk for dehydration.
B. The patient is at risk for decreased cardiac output.
C. The patient is at risk for experiencing hallucinations.
D. The patient is at great risk for injury.

133. A patient presents with a 24-hour history of abdominal pain, fever, nausea, and watery diarrhea. On further questioning, the patient states that they have been prescribed sulfamethoxazole/trimethoprim (Bactrim) for a urinary tract infection. What would your primary intervention be for this patient?

A. Request a stool sample from the patient
B. Place the patient in a private room on contact isolation
C. Prepare to infuse a isotonic crystalloid solution bolus
D. Prepare to administer antibiotics

134. You answer a call from a primary care provider who is sending a 14-year-old patient to be evaluated. The provider tells you the patient is experiencing extreme fatigue, fever, sore throat, body aches, and rash, and there is a "knot" in the left axilla. You suspect the patient may have:

A. abscess to left axilla.
B. infectious mononucleosis.
C. strep throat.
D. meningitis.

135. The key to safe and effective care of the trauma patient is associated with which of the following?

A. Identified roles and responsibilities of the team members
B. Group diversity
C. Individual mental processes and individual leadership
D. Engage in individual member review of performance activities

136. The child of a hospital employee has died in the emergency department. The emergency staff and hospital employees are visibly upset and are having difficulty coping with the child's death. Hospital administration decides to conduct a critical incident stress management (CISM) debriefing for the staff. Ideally the CISM debriefing should take place within what time frame?

A. As soon as possible
B. Within 24–72 hours
C. Within 3–5 days
D. Within 1 week

137. The emergency nurse is aware that the practice of lifelong learning is an essential element leading to the achievement of which of the following?

A. Professional expertise
B. Promotion to a management position
C. Academic success
D. Personal fulfillment

138. In preparing the body of an organ donor for eye tissue donation, the emergency nurse should perform which of the following?

A. Close the eyes and cover the eyelids with dry, sterile gauze
B. Apply warm compresses to the eyelids to promote circulation
C. Elevate the head of the bed 20 degrees
D. Prepare the patient for transfer to the operating room

139. Accurate documentation of the "chain of custody" in the handling of forensic evidence is necessary to ensure which of the following?

A. Validating the competency of the individual who collected the evidence
B. Safeguarding the integrity of the evidence
C. Providing law enforcement with evidence needed to convict the suspected criminal
D. Limiting the number of individuals who handle the evidence

140. The nurse is aware that the most reliable method of assessing a patient's pain is which of the following?

A. Utilizing a nurse-initiated pain management protocol
B. Observing specific pain-associated behaviors such as grimacing or crying
C. Asking the patient to describe what pain-relieving medications have been effective for them in the past
D. Acknowledging the patient's self-report of pain

141. A 5-year-old patient presents to a general emergency department. The patient requires a dose of oral medication for the illness. The nurse understands that this patient is at increased risk for medication errors because of which of the following?

A. Inability to swallow medications
B. Parent being a poor historian
C. Patient having no known allergies
D. Weight-based dosing

142. A patient with an acute myocardial infarction is being prepared for transport by ground ambulance to the nearby medical center. The patient is stable but is receiving multiple intravenous vasoactive medications. The emergency nurse should be most concerned regarding which of the following?

A. The patient's spouse is insisting that they ride along in the ambulance.
B. The patient is being transferred via ground ambulance rather than helicopter.
C. The transport team comprises individuals with extensive training in basic life support.
D. The patient experiences motion sickness when flying or riding in a vehicle.

143. A non–English-speaking patient presents to the triage nurse. The best method for the emergency triage nurse to effectively communicate with the patient is to use which of the following?

A. A member of the healthcare staff who speaks the patient's native language
B. A member of the patient's family or friend
C. An illustrated chart for the patient to point at descriptors of the symptoms
D. A certified translator fluent in the patient's native language

144. The emergency nurse caring for an elderly patient delegates hourly vital signs to unlicensed assistive personnel. The unlicensed assistive staff member does not report a hypotensive blood pressure to the registered nurse and only documents it on the patient's chart. The patient suffers a poor outcome. Who is at fault for not reporting the hypotensive blood pressure to the emergency department provider?

A. The registered nurse who delegated the task of vital signs
B. The assistive staff member who took the patient's vital signs
C. The charge nurse
D. The physician assistant

145. Using the mass casualty START triage system for adults, which of the following patients would be classified as a yellow (delayed) patient?

A. A patient who is able to stand and walk to a designated area as instructed
B. A patient who is unable to ambulate, with a respiratory rate of 32 breaths/minute
C. A patient who is unable to ambulate, has no spontaneous respirations even with repositioning airway, has absent central pulse, and does not follow commands
D. A patient who is unable to ambulate and who can follow commands, with a respiratory rate under 30 breaths/minute

146. The National Incident Management System requires that hospitals have plans and procedures in place to be prepared for emergency management situations, such as mass casualty incidents and disasters. One system that helps hospitals to be prepared and creates a command structure is the:

A. Federal Emergency Management Agency
B. National Response Framework
C. Hospital Incident Command System
D. Disaster Medical Assistance Team

147. To be compliant with the United States Emergency Medical Treatment and Active Labor Act, all patients presenting to the emergency department must have had which of the following performed?

A. Triage assessment by a registered nurse
B. Emergency Severity Index acuity level assigned
C. Medical screening exam
D. At least one set of vital signs

148. An unresponsive trauma patient is brought to the emergency department (ED) by ambulance. There are no family members present, and no contact information is available for the patient's family. It is appropriate for ED personnel to treat this patient based on which type of consent?

A. Implied consent
B. Expressed consent
C. Involuntary consent
D. Informed consent

149. According to The Joint Commission, the overwhelming majority of serious medical errors that occur during patient handoff can be attributed to which type of mechanism?

A. Equipment failure
B. Inappropriate staffing mix at the receiving facility
C. Communication breakdown
D. Use of unapproved abbreviations

150. A patient who recently returned from a trip to East Africa presents to triage complaining of fever, abdominal pain, bloody diarrhea, and weakness. The triage nurse recognizes that this patient is most at risk for which of the following?

A. Ebola virus
B. Chickenpox
C. Gastroenteritis
D. Influenza

PART 2

1. A patient presents to the emergency department with chest pain and diaphoresis, and denies dyspnea. Vital signs are BP 148/70 mm Hg, HR 72 beats/minute, RR 18 breaths/minute, SpO_2 98% on room air. Breath sounds are clear and equal. The electrocardiogram shows an inferior wall ST segment elevation. You anticipate the following oxygen order.

   A. No supplemental oxygen at this time
   B. Nasal cannula at 6 L per minute
   C. Partial rebreather mask at 10 L per minute
   D. Nonrebreather mask at 15 L per minute

Rationale

A. The use of supplemental oxygen in normoxic patients has not been established. In patients with potential coronary artery syndrome, withholding of additional supplemental oxygen should be considered for those in the prehospital or in-patient hospital setting and the emergency department.

B. Supplemental oxygen has been shown to potentially extend the size of myocardial infarction in the setting of normoxia.

C. Supplemental oxygen in the setting of normoxia has not been shown to improve outcomes from myocardial infarction. The higher concentration oxygen would not be indicated with an oxygen saturation of 98% on room air.

D. The use of supplemental oxygen in patients who are not hypoxic and are not exhibiting signs or symptoms of respiratory distress has not been shown to improve outcomes and may actually increase the size of the myocardial infarction.

Category: Cardiovascular Emergencies/Acute coronary syndrome
Nursing Process: Intervention

Reference

O'Connor, R. E., Al Ali, A. S., Brady, W. J., Ghaemmaghami, C. A., Menon, V., Welsford, M., & Shuster, M. (2015). Part 9: acute coronary syndromes: 2015 American Heart Association Guidelines Update for Cardiopulmonary Resuscitation and Emergency Cardiovascular Care. *Circulation, 132*(Suppl. 2), S483–S500. https://doi.org/10.1161/CIR.0000000000000263

---

2. A patient complains of chest pain, dyspnea, and diaphoresis. Which of the following assessment factors would indicate a possible diagnosis of acute coronary syndrome?

   A. Pleuritic chest pain
   B. Positional chest pain
   C. Chest pain that radiates to the shoulders, with pain in the right shoulder worse than pain in the left shoulder
   D. Pain reproducible with chest wall palpation

Rationale

A. Pleuritic chest pain has a likelihood ratio of 0.2—low likelihood of predicting acute coronary syndrome.

B. Positional chest pain has a likelihood ratio of 0.3, which is a low likelihood of predicting acute coronary syndrome.

C. Chest pain that radiates to both shoulders has a likelihood ratio of 7.1, and pain that radiates to the right shoulder has a stronger likelihood ratio of 2.9 of predicting acute coronary syndrome, compared with pain that radiates only to the left shoulder.

D. Reproducible pain with palpation has a low likelihood ratio, 0.3, of predicting acute coronary syndrome.

Category: Cardiovascular Emergencies/Acute coronary syndrome

Nursing Process: Analysis

Reference

Panju, A. A., Hemmelgarn, B. R., Guyatt, G. H., & Simel, D. L. (1998). The rational clinical examination. Is this patient having a myocardial infarction? *Journal of the American Medical Association, 280*(14), 1256–1263. 10.1001/jama.280.14.1256

---

3. Which of the following human compensatory mechanisms to the presence of shock triggers glycogenolysis?
   A. Chemoreceptor activation
   B. Clotting cascade activation
   C. Cerebral autoregulation stimulation
   D. Adrenal gland stimulation

Rationale

A. Chemoreceptors are activated by changes in blood oxygen, carbon dioxide, and pH.

B. Activation of the clotting cascade is associated with the trauma triad of death: hypothermia, acidosis, and coagulopathy. It is not directly related to glycogenolysis.

C. Cerebral autoregulation maintains a constant cerebral blood flow and is not directly related to glycogenolysis.

D. Adrenal gland stimulation causes the adrenals to release two catecholamines: epinephrine and norepinephrine. Epinephrine increases heart rate and peripheral vasoconstriction and triggers glycogenolysis.

Category: Cardiovascular Emergencies/Shock

Nursing Process: Analysis

Reference

Pentecost, D. A. (2014). Shock. In D. Gurney (Ed.), *Trauma Nursing Core Course: Provider manual* (pp. 73–90). Des Plaines, IL: Emergency Nurses Association.

4. A patient presents to the emergency department with abdominal pain and "ripping" back pain. Which condition places the patient at risk for abdominal aortic dissection?

A. Down syndrome
B. Romano–Ward syndrome
C. Jervell and Lange-Nielsen syndrome
D. Ehler–Danlos syndrome

Rationale

A. Down syndrome is chromosomal condition that causes learning difficulties. Patients with Down syndrome are at increased risk for heart defects, digestive problems, hearing loss, and sometimes hypothyroidism.

B. Romano–Ward syndrome is an inherited cardiac disorder that causes long QT syndrome. Patients with Romano–Ward syndrome may have sudden death resulting from a dysrhythmia.

C. Jervell and Lange-Nielsen syndrome is a condition that causes profound hearing loss from birth and also long QT syndrome. Patients with Jervell and Lange-Nielsen syndrome may have sudden death resulting from a dysrhythmia.

D. Patients with Ehler–Danlos syndrome may be identified by hypermobile joints and skin that is hyper-extensible, has a soft velvety-like appearance, is fragile, and tears or bruises easily. Ehler–Danlos syndrome is a connective tissue disorder that places patients at risk for the presence of aortic aneurysm and dissection.

Category: Cardiovascular Emergencies/Aneurysm/dissection
Nursing Process: Analysis

References

Bradley, T. J., Bowdin, S. C., Morel, C. F., & Pyeritz, R. E. (2016). Review: The expanding clinical spectrum of extra-cardiovascular and cardiovascular manifestations of heritable thoracic aortic aneurysm and dissection. *Canadian Journal of Cardiology, 32,* 86–99. https://doi.org/10.1016/j.cjca.2015.11.007

Hammond, B. B. (2013). Cardiovascular emergencies. In B. B. Hammond & P. G. Zimmermann (Eds.), *Sheehy's manual of emergency care* (7th ed., pp. 201–211). St. Louis, MO: Elsevier Mosby.

---

5. A patient presents via emergency medical services in cardiopulmonary arrest, following 15 minutes of cardiopulmonary resuscitation (CPR). On completion of the initial nursing assessment, which of the following findings would indicate that termination of resuscitation efforts should be considered?

A. Decreased compliance while performing bag-mask device ventilation
B. An end-tidal carbon dioxide level reading less than 10% after 20 minutes of high-quality CPR
C. An initial rhythm of pulseless electrical activity
D. An initial presentation of a shockable rhythm

Rationale

A. Changes in bag-mask device compliance may indicate development of a pneumothorax, which requires immediate intervention to prevent development of a tension pneumothorax.

B. A low end-tidal carbon dioxide level indicates a lack of both end cellular perfusion and adenosine triphosphate production, resulting in cellular death.

C. With an initial rhythm of pulseless electrical activity, there should be a review of potential underlying causes with initiation of the appropriate interventions before discontinuing resuscitative efforts.

D. Early defibrillation of a shockable rhythm, such as ventricular tachycardia or ventricular fibrillation, is associated with a higher rate of survival.

Category: Cardiovascular Emergencies/Cardiopulmonary arrest

Nursing Process: Evaluation

Reference

American Heart Association. (2016). *Advanced cardiovascular life support: Provider manual* (pp. 39, 146, 148–149). Dallas, TX: Author.

---

6. A 7-year-old suddenly develops ventricular fibrillation. The child weighs 66 lbs (30 kg). Cardiopulmonary resuscitation is started immediately. What is the correct defibrillation dose for the initial shock to be used by the emergency nurse?

A. 60 joules
B. 30 joules
C. 120 joules
D. 90 joules

Rationale

A. The child weighs 30 kg. The correct initial joule dose is 2 joules per kg. The correct dose would be 60 joules for the initial shock and increasing to 4 joules per kg. This dose can be increased up to a maximum of 10 joules per kg.

B. This dose would be too low for the initial defibrillation of this child. The correct initial joule dose is 2 joules per kg.

C. This calculation would be using 4 joules per kg. This dose would be used for a second defibrillation attempt.

D. This calculation is not in accordance with current the pediatric advanced life support algorithm. The correct initial joule dose is 2 joules per kg.

Category (Pediatric): Cardiovascular Emergencies/Cardiopulmonary arrest

Nursing Process: Intervention

Reference

American Heart Association. (2015). *2015 handbook of emergency cardiovascular care for healthcare providers.* Dallas, TX: Author.

---

7. The emergency nurse is participating in the care of an obtunded patient presumed to have taken an overdose of a tricyclic antidepressant. The patient has a palpable pulse, and an electrocardiogram (ECG) is obtained. The nurse would anticipate the presence of which ECG finding?

A. Sinus bradycardia with normal QRS and QT intervals
B. Ventricular fibrillation
C. Narrow complex supraventricular tachycardia
D. Sinus tachycardia with both a widened QRS interval and prolonged QT interval

Rationale

A. Cyclic antidepressants typically cause a tachycardia with prolonged QRS and QT intervals.

B. Although delayed or inappropriate intervention in the setting of cyclic antidepressant overdose may result in cardiopulmonary arrest and ventricular fibrillation, this patient currently has a pulse, and this dysrhythmia would not be anticipated at this time.

C. Dysrhythmias from cyclic antidepressant toxicity typically are wide complex tachycardias.

D. Sinus tachycardia occurs frequently from the anticholinergic effects of tricyclic antidepressant toxicity. QRS complex widening occurs as a result of sodium channel blockade, and this delayed conduction may be seen more commonly involving the right side of the heart, manifesting as a right bundle branch block. In addition, QT interval prolongation can occur with these agents.

Category: Cardiovascular Emergencies/Dysrhythmias
Nursing Process: Assessment

Reference

Holstege, C., Eldridge, D. L., & Rowden, A. K. ECG manifestations: The poisoned patient. *Emergency Medicine Clinics of North America, 24*(1), 159–177. https://doi.org/10.1016/j.emc.2005.08.012

---

8. During triage, the patient states the pacemaker only fires when the patient's heart rate slows below a certain number of beats/minute. The nurse anticipates that the patient has a(n):

A. asynchronous pacemaker.
B. demand pacemaker.
C. dual-chamber pacemaker.
D. fixed-rate pacemaker.

Rationale

A. Asynchronous is another name for fixed-rate pacemaker. A fixed-rate pacemaker will continue to deliver an impulse to "fire" regardless of the patient's intrinsic heart rate.

B. A demand pacemaker has the capability to sense the patient's intrinsic heart rhythm and only delivers an impulse to "fire" when the patient's intrinsic heart rate falls below a given rate.

C. Dual-chamber pacemakers provide electrical stimulation to both atrial and ventricular chambers, based on the patient's intrinsic heart rate.

D. Fixed-rate pacemakers deliver an electrical impulse at a given rate regardless of the patient's intrinsic heart rate or rhythm.

Category: Cardiovascular Emergencies/Dysrhythmias
Nursing Process: Assessment

Reference

Garcia, T. B., & Miller, G. T. (2004). Artificially placed rhythms. In *Arrhythmia recognition: The art of interpretation* (pp. 507–520). Sudbury, MA: Jones and Bartlett Publishers.

---

9. A patient being evaluated in the emergency department is noted to have Janeway lesions, Roth's spots, and Osler's nodes along with an elevated body temperature and elevated white blood cell count. Patient assessment reveals the presence of several recent body piercings. The emergency nurse suspects the patient has:

A. endocarditis.
B. pericarditis.
C. myocarditis.
D. leukemia.

Rationale

A. The patient's symptoms are classic for endocarditis. Janeway lesions are petechial lesions found on the palms of the hands or soles of the feet. Osler's nodes are defined as painful fingertip lesions, and Roth's spots are retinal hemorrhages with the presence of whitish spots in the center. The patient may experience fevers along with an elevated white blood cell (WBC) count, and recent body piercings may be a source of infections leading to endocarditis. The endocarditic infection may also spread to valve structures in the heart, resulting in permanent valvular dysfunction.

B. Pericarditis, or inflammation of the pericardial sac, is characterized by an elevation in WBC count, a pericardial friction rub, and ST changes throughout the electrocardiogram. Pericarditis is not associated with the presence of Janeway lesions.

C. Myocarditis, or inflammation of the cardiac muscle, is characterized by chest pain, cardiac rhythm abnormalities, poor nutrition, and fatigue. Myocarditis is typically a viral infection that presents with fevers and elevated WBC count.

D. Leukemia, or cancer of the blood system, is diagnosed by abnormalities in WBC counts. A rash may also be present with certain types of leukemia.

Category: Cardiovascular Emergencies/Endocarditis
Nursing Process: Analysis

Reference

Criddle, L. M. (2007). Cardiovascular emergencies. In K. S. Hoyt & J. Selfridge-Thomas (Eds.), *Emergency nursing core curriculum* (6th ed., pp. 187–248). St. Louis, MO: Saunders Elsevier.

---

10. A conscious pulseless patient with a continuous-flow left ventricular assist device and a history of end-stage heart failure presents to the emergency department because of a "low-flow" alarm. The nurse anticipates performing which intervention first?

A. Obtain a blood pressure using a Doppler and sphygmomanometer
B. Auscultate over the pump to ascertain if the device is working
C. Administer intravenous fluids
D. Begin chest compressions

Rationale

A. The "low-flow" alarm may be because of decrease preload from hypotension, dehydration, obstruction of the inflow or outflow (which would cause an increase in afterload) cannula, or disconnection of percutaneous leads. A mean arterial blood pressure (MAP) should be obtained by placing a Doppler over the brachial or radial artery and then inflating the cuff until flow is no longer heard. Once the arterial flow is heard again, this is the MAP. Left ventricular assist device (LVAD) patients should have MAPs between 70 and 80 mm Hg. In a conscious patient, determining the patient's blood pressure will help guide therapy and troubleshooting. The patient's LVAD coordinator should also be contacted as soon as possible.

B. Auscultation of the pump is prudent to determine if the pump is functioning properly. Device failure has been reported as the second most common cause of death in LVAD patients. Signs of pump failure include absence of a power light on the controller, undetectable blood pressure while using the Doppler, and inability to auscultate the motor.

C. If the MAP is low, intravenous fluids would be indicated.

D. Chest compressions are not indicated in a conscious patient. Patients with continuous-flow LVADs often do not have a palpable pulse because the device is pumping constantly through the cardiac cycle; this causes aortic flow to be present during diastole, causing a reduced pulse pressure.

Category: Cardiovascular Emergencies/Heart failure

Nursing Process: Intervention

References

Rihal, C. S., Naidu, S. S., Givertz, M. M., Szeto, W. Y., Burke, J. A., Kapur, N. K., . . . Tu, T. (2015). 2015 SCAI/ACC /HFSA/STS clinical expert consensus statement on the use of percutaneous mechanical circulatory support devices in cardiovascular care. *Journal of the American College of Cardiology, 65*(9), e7–e26. https://doi.org/10.1016/j.jacc.2015.03.036

Robertson, J., Long, B., & Koyfman, A. (2016). The emergency management of ventricular assist devices. *American Journal of Emergency Medicine, 34,* 1294–1301.

---

11. A heart failure patient with profound dyspnea, lung crackles, and pink frothy sputum presents to the emergency department. The physician orders for the patient to be placed on bilevel positive airway pressure at an end-expiratory pressure of 10 cm H_2O and an inspiratory pressure of 5 cm H_2O. Which of the following findings demonstrates that the patient's symptoms and work of breathing have been reduced?

A. Increasing the blood returned to the right side of the heart
B. Decreasing cardiac output
C. Decreasing the preload
D. Increasing the afterload

Rationale

A. Noninvasive positive airway pressure ventilation (NIPPV) decreases preload and blood flow into the right side of the heart.

B. NIPPV improves cardiac output by the reduction in preload and afterload.

C. NIPPV includes both continuous positive airway pressure and bilevel positive airway pressure (BiPAP) devices. By increasing the pressure within the thoracic cavity through NIPPV, blood flow into the right heart is reduced; this results in a decreased preload, which helps to improve pulmonary congestion in the acute heart failure patient.

D. BiPAP decreases afterload indirectly; it enables forward flow of blood to occur more easily because of the increased intrathoracic pressure on the left ventricle.

Category: Cardiovascular Emergencies/Heart failure

Nursing Process: Evaluation

References

Hammond, B. B. (2013). Cardiovascular emergencies. In B. B. Hammond & P. G. Zimmermann (Eds.), *Sheehy's manual of emergency care* (7th ed., pp. 201–211). St. Louis, MO: Elsevier Mosby.

Rihal, C. S., Naidu, S. S., Givertz, M. M., Szeto, W. Y., Burke, J. A., Kapur, N. K., . . . Tu, T. (2015). 2015 SCAI/ACC /HFSA/STS clinical expert consensus statement on the use of percutaneous mechanical circulatory support devices in cardiovascular care. *Journal of the American College of Cardiology, 65*(19), e7–e26.

Yancy, C. W., Jessup, M., Bozkurt, B., Butler, J., Casey, D. E., Colvin, M. M., . . . Westlake, C. (2016). 2016 ACC/AHA /HFSA focused update on new pharmacological therapy for heart failure: An update of the 2013 ACCF/AHA guideline for the management of heart failure. *Circulation, 134.* https://doi.org/10.1161/CIR.0000000000000435

---

12. Intravenous nitroprusside (Nipride) has been ordered for blood pressure reduction in a patient with a hypertensive emergency. The patient's blood pressure is 280/124 mm Hg with a mean arterial pressure (MAP) of 176 mm Hg. When titrating the nitroprusside for this patient, which order has the safest parameter to follow?

A. Titrate nitroprusside to a MAP of 124 mm Hg over the next hour
B. Titrate nitroprusside to a MAP of 106 mm Hg over the next hour
C. Titrate nitroprusside to a MAP of 158 mm Hg over the next hour
D. Titrate nitroprusside to a MAP of 132 mm Hg over the next hour

Rationale

A. This is greater than the recommended 20–25% reduction of the MAP within the first hour of treatment and could result in organ hypoperfusion.

B. This is greater than the recommended 20–25% reduction of the MAP within the first hour of treatment and could result in organ hypoperfusion.

C. This is less than the recommended reduction of lowering the MAP by about 20–25% within the first hour for hypertensive emergency.

D. Hypertensive emergency is defined as severe hypertension with signs or symptoms of end organ dysfunction. It is recommended that the patient's MAP be reduced by about 20–25% within the first hour of treatment, and rapid reduction of blood pressure should be avoided to prevent organ hypoperfusion.

Category: Cardiovascular Emergencies/Hypertension

Nursing Process: Intervention

References

Adebayo, O., & Rogers, R. L. (2015). Hypertensive emergencies in the emergency department. *Emergency Medicine Clinics of North America, 33*, 539–551.

Hammond, B. B. (2013). Cardiovascular emergencies. In B. B. Hammond & P. G. Zimmermann (Eds.), *Sheehy's manual of emergency care* (7th ed., pp. 201–211). St. Louis, MO: Elsevier Mosby.

13. The assessment of a patient involved in a motor vehicle collision reveals muffled heart sounds and distended neck veins. The nurse understands that the treatment for this life-threatening situation is to:

A. minimize the administration of intravenous fluids.
B. prepare for a 3- to 4-cm incision to the left of the xiphoid process.
C. prepare for insertion of a 14-gauge needle into the midclavicular line second intercostal space.
D. prepare for chest tube insertion at the 5th intercostal space.

Rationale

A. Minimizing the administration of intravenous fluids in addition to possible intubation and ventilation support is the treatment for cardiac contusion but is not the immediate treatment for pericardial tamponade.

B. Muffled heart sounds and distended neck veins are classic signs of pericardial (cardiac) tamponade. A 3- to 4-cm incision to the left of the xiphoid process allows for pericardial decompression or release of pericardial tamponade, which is the treatment for this life-threatening situation.

C. Insertion of a 14-gauge needle into the second intercostal space midclavicular line on the affected side is the recommended treatment for immediate decompression of a tension pneumothorax.

D. Chest tube insertion at the 5th intercostal space at the anterior or midaxillary line is the treatment for a hemothorax.

Category: Cardiovascular Emergencies/Pericardial tamponade

Nursing Process: Intervention

Reference

Day, M. W. (2014). Thoracic and neck trauma. In D. Gurney (Ed.), *Trauma Nursing Core Course: Provider manual* (7th ed., pp. 137–150). Des Plaines, IL: Author.

14. What is the best position to place a patient, in order to assess for the presence of a cardiac friction rub?

A. Ask the patient to stand up and then squat, then place the stethoscope at the left sternal border and listen at midsystole.
B. Ask the patient to lie or sit quietly, then place the stethoscope at the right sternal border and listen for radiation to the neck.
C. Ask the patient to lean forward, then place the stethoscope at the left sternal border and listen at end-expiration.
D. Ask the patient to lie or sit quietly, then place the stethoscope at the apex of the heart and listen for radiation to the axilla.

Rationale

A. The murmur in a patient with hypertrophic cardiomyopathy will decrease with a change from standing to squatting and peaks at midsystole, and an S4 gallop may also be present.

B. The harsh crescendo-decrescendo murmur in a patient with aortic stenosis is best heard at the right sternal border with radiation to the neck.

C. It has been reported that up to 85% of patients with pericarditis will have a friction rub. Although the presence of a friction rub during the initial evaluation of a patient with pericarditis is unreliable, when present, it is best heard while the patient is leaning forward, with the stethoscope placed at the left sternal boarder at end-expiration. The sound that is made when inflamed layers of the pericardium rub against each other is thought to be the cause of the friction rub.

D. The pansystolic blowing murmur in a patient with mitral regurgitation is best heard at the apex and radiates to the axilla.

Category: Cardiovascular Emergencies/Pericarditis

Nursing Process: Assessment

References

Crowley-Koschnitzki, C. (2017). Valvular heart disease and cardiac murmurs. In T. M. Buttaro, J. Trybulski, P. Polgar-Bailey, & J. Sandberg-Cook (Eds.), *Primary care: A collaborative practice* (5th ed., pp. 611–622). St. Louis, MO: Elsevier.

Mattu, A., & Martinez, J. P. (2013). Pericarditis, pericardial tamponade, and myocarditis. In J. G. Adams, E. D. Barton, J. L. Collins, P. M. C. DeBlieux, M. A. Gisondi, & E. S. Nadel (Eds.), *Emergency medicine clinical essentials* (2nd ed., pp. 514–523). Philadelphia, PA: Elsevier Saunders.

---

15. Raynaud's disease is characterized by which assessment findings?

A. Severe leg cramps and redness
B. Carpopedal spasms and intense heat
C. Intense vasospasms and pallor of the digits
D. Numbness and tingling of the wrist and elbow

Rationale

A. Although leg cramps and redness may be associated with peripheral vascular disease, Raynaud's disease typically effects the fingertips.

B. Carpopedal spasms may be caused by low blood calcium levels and has been associated with electrolyte disturbances connected to the presence of tetanus infections.

C. Raynaud's disease affects blood vessels supplying the skin. Intense vasospasms are noted to the digits, tip of the nose, or ears. Because circulation is impaired, pallor is also noted, especially in cold environments. The disease effects women more than men and may also affect motor function.

D. Numbness and tingling are generally associated with the presence of a nerve injury.

Category: Cardiovascular Emergencies/Peripheral vascular disease

Nursing Process: Assessment

Reference

Criddle, L. M. (2007). Cardiovascular emergencies. In K. S. Hoyt & J. Selfridge-Thomas (Eds.), *Emergency nursing core curriculum* (6th ed., pp. 187–248). St. Louis, MO: Saunders Elsevier.

---

16. Which of the following statements made by a patient recently diagnosed with peripheral vascular disease indicates that the patient has an accurate understanding of the disease?

A. "When my leg starts to cramp, I should stop walking and rest."
B. "When pain develops in my leg, I should apply an ice pack."
C. "When my leg starts to cramp, I should elevate it on two pillows."
D. "I will limit my cigarette smoking to a half-pack a day."

Rationale

A. Pain from peripheral vascular disease (PVD) can develop while exercising, experiencing stress, and being in a cold environment. It can be relieved by removing or discontinuing the cause.

B. Pain is exacerbated by a cold environment; a warm environment will help relieve the pain. Application of a direct heat source to the ischemic area could result in further harm to tissue.

C. The affected limb should not be elevated above the level of the heart because this will result in increased pain and cramping because peripheral blood flow to that area has been decreased.

D. Cigarette smoking has been identified as a major risk factor for the development of PVD. Other risk factors include hypertension, hyperlipidemia, diabetes, obesity, and a sedentary lifestyle.

Category: Cardiovascular Emergencies/Peripheral vascular disease

Nursing Process: Evaluation

Reference

Criddle, L. M. (2007). Cardiovascular emergencies. In K. S. Hoyt & J. Selfridge-Thomas (Eds.), *Emergency nursing core curriculum* (6th ed., pp. 187–248). St. Louis, MO: Saunders Elsevier.

---

17. Which of the following patients would demonstrate the presence of delayed venous return resulting from increased intra-abdominal pressure, creating a high risk for deep venous thrombosis and pulmonary embolus?

A. 57-year-old hypertensive male
B. 48-year-old diabetic female
C. 26-year-old bariatric female
D. 32-year-old male with peripheral vascular disease

Rationale

A. This patient does not have delayed venous return that would put him at risk for increased intra-abdominal pressure, leading to a high risk for deep venous thrombosis (DVT) and pulmonary embolus (PE).

B. This patient does not have delayed venous return that would put her at risk for increased intra-abdominal pressure, leading to a high risk for DVT and PE.

C. The bariatric patient has delayed venous return resulting from increased intra-abdominal pressure, creating a high risk for DVT and PE.

D. This patient does not have delayed venous return that would put him at risk for increased intra-abdominal pressure, creating a high risk for DVT and PE. Any obstruction to blood flow is caused by fatty deposits, narrowing, or spasm, which are unrelated to increased intra-abdominal pressure.

Category: Cardiovascular Emergencies/Thromboembolic disease

Nursing Process: Analysis

Reference

Moore, J. M. (2014). Special populations: The bariatric trauma patient. In D. Gurney (Ed.), *Trauma Nursing Core Course: Provider manual* (pp. 269–282). Des Plaines, IL: Emergency Nurses Association.

---

18. A patient has sustained a stab wound to the left parasternal anterior chest. Emergency medical services treatment has included intubation and intravenous therapy with crystalloid solution. The patient exhibited vital signs during transport; however, as the patient is being wheeled into the trauma room, pulses are no longer detected. Cardiopulmonary resuscitation is initiated. Breath sounds are present bilaterally. The nurse anticipates the following procedure to be immediately performed.

A. Point-of-care cardiac ultrasound
B. Chest radiograph
C. Open thoracotomy
D. Needle pericardiocentesis

Rationale

A. Ultrasound at the bedside may be helpful with the diagnosis of life-threatening injuries such as pericardial tamponade but will only delay the initiation of a potentially life-saving open emergency department thoracotomy (EDT).

B. A chest radiograph may help define the presence of pneumothorax, hemothorax, or retained foreign objects but delays the initiation of an open EDT.

C. Patients with low velocity penetrating chest trauma with loss of signs of life on or just before arrival to the emergency department have the best chance of survival with an open EDT.

D. Needle pericardiocentesis is often ineffective in relieving traumatic pericardial tamponade and delays the initiation of an open EDT.

Category: Cardiovascular Emergencies/Trauma

Nursing Process: Intervention

Reference

Carden, L., Gibbs, M. A., & MacVane, C. Z. (2012). Penetrating and blunt cardiac trauma. *Trauma Reports, 13*(2). Retrieved from https://www.ahcmedia.com/articles/76732-penetrating-and-blunt-cardiac-trauma

---

19. Emergency medical services arrives with an unrestrained driver who was involved in a multivehicle collision. The patient is diagnosed with a pelvic fracture and left tibial fracture. Which classification of hypovolemic shock would most likely occur as the result of these injuries?

A. Class IV
B. Class III
C. Class II
D. Class I

Rationale

A. Class IV hypovolemic shock occurs with blood loss greater than 2000 mL. Estimated blood loss from a pelvic fracture is 3000 mL and from a tibial fracture is approximately 650 mL. Severe signs and symptoms of hypovolemia would be present.

B. Class III hypovolemic shock is defined as blood loss of 1500 to 2000 mL. With a possible blood loss of 3000 mL from the fractured pelvis and 650 mL from the tibia, the blood loss would be well beyond the Class III category.

C. Class II hypovolemic shock is defined as blood loss of 750 to 1500 mL. The anticipated blood loss from a combined pelvic and tibia fracture would exceed this classification.

D. Class I hypovolemic shock is defined as blood loss of less than 750 mL. An isolated tibia fracture might meet this criterion, but with the addition of a pelvic fracture, greater blood loss would be anticipated.

Category: Cardiovascular Emergencies/Trauma
Nursing Process: Assessment

References

Calder, S. (2013). Shock. In B. B. Hammond & P. G. Zimmermann (Eds.), *Sheehy's manual of emergency care* (7th ed., pp. 213–222). St. Louis, MO: Elsevier Mosby.
Pentecost, D. A., & Smith, S. G. (2014). Shock. In D. Gurney (Ed.), *Trauma Nursing Core Course: Provider manual* (7th ed., pp. 73–90). Des Plaines, IL: Emergency Nurses Association.

---

20. Following the insertion of an intraosseous (IO) device, which of the following findings by the emergency nurse would indicate that the IO has been properly placed?

A. The needle has slight movement after insertion.
B. Bright red blood is noted in the cannula after insertion.
C. The fluid will only infuse with the use of positive pressure.
D. A reddish frothy aspirate is noted after insertion.

Rationale

A. As the IO device is placed in the bone, no movement should occur. Movement of the IO device could indicate improper placement, or the insertion hole in the bone has been drilled too large for the device to be secure.

B. Bone marrow is reddish and frothy, not bright red blood. Blood present in the cannula could indicate unintentional placement of the IO needle into a blood vessel.

C. Following an initial isotonic crystalloid solution bolus to clear the cannula and open any connective tissue, fluid or medications administered through the IO needle should flow freely without the use of positive pressure. The fluid will only flow as accommodated by the diameter of the marrow cavity. The marrow cavity does not expand with the use of pressure to infuse medications or fluids.

D. As the IO device is inserted, marrow may be aspirated. Bone marrow is a reddish frothy substance. During emergent situations, the aspirated marrow may be used for some laboratory testing.

Category: Cardiovascular Emergencies/Trauma

Nursing Process: Evaluation

Reference

Infusion Nurses Society. (2010). *Recommendations for the use of intraosseous vascular access for emergent and nonemergent situations in various healthcare settings: A consensus paper* (pp. 1–8). Norwood, MA: Author.

---

21. When caring for a child who has been treated for an asthma exacerbation, the emergency nurse identifies that the patient is ready for discharge when:
   A. the patient is awake and alert.
   B. the patient can demonstrate proper use of a rescue inhaler without assistance.
   C. the patient's peak expiratory flow is greater than 70% and response is sustained for 60 minutes following the last bronchodilator treatment.
   D. the patient demonstrates SpO_2 of 93% on room air (21% oxygen).

Rationale

A. Physical and mental status is important, however, neither activity nor mental status is the best indicator for success at home.

B. Assessment findings and improved peak expiratory flow are better indicators of success at home than return demonstration of medication administration.

C. Results of interventions should be measurable and sustained. A peak expiratory flow or forced expiratory volume measurement is objective and reliable in assessing for airflow obstruction.

D. Oxygenation is not the only indicator of respiratory improvement, and heart rate may remain elevated for several hours after bronchodilator therapy. An improved peak expiratory flow of greater than 70% associated with no respiratory distress is a better indicator of the patient's success at home.

Category (Pediatric): Respiratory Emergencies/Asthma

Nursing Process: Evaluation

Reference

Howard, P. K. (2012). Respiratory emergencies. In *Emergency Nursing Pediatric Course: Provider manual* (4th ed., pp. 131–146). Des Plaines, IL: Emergency Nurses Association.

---

22. An adult patient with a history of asthma presents to triage stating they are experiencing an acute asthma exacerbation. The emergency care provider orders an electrocardiogram (ECG). The patient asks the nurse why this procedure is necessary. The nurse explains to the patient:

A. "In adults, underlying cardiac conditions can often present as, or exist with, respiratory complaints."
B. "It is a part of our order set for patients with respiratory complaints."
C. "ECGs can show us how well you are breathing."
D. "I don't know. I just do what the provider orders."

Rationale

A. Cardiac conditions, such as ST elevation myocardial infarctions (STEMI) and dysrhythmias, can cause respiratory distress. Respiratory inefficacies can lead to myocardial irritation. All adult patients should have an ECG to rule out any coexisting cardiac conditions.

B. This is explaining to the patient that an ECG is a standard of care; this can be reassuring to patients but does not explain the reasoning as to why the procedure is necessary.

C. ECGs show the electrical activity of the heart and cannot indicate a patient's respiratory effort.

D. This is never an acceptable answer for the professional nurse to provide to their patient. If the nurse does not understand why something has been ordered, they need to clarify with the provider. Patient education is a responsibility of the nurse throughout the patient's care in the emergency department, not just at the time of discharge.

Category: Respiratory Emergencies/Asthma
Nursing Process: Intervention

Reference

Hoyt, K. S., & Selfridge-Thomas, J. (2007). Respiratory emergencies. In K. S. Hoyt & J. Selfridge-Thomas (Eds.), *Emergency nursing core curriculum* (6th ed., pp. 685–720). St. Louis, MO: Saunders Elsevier.

---

23. A patient is being discharged after being treated for the presence of a cough for 3 months and increasing shortness of breath with excretion. The patient has been diagnosed with chronic obstructive pulmonary disease (COPD). The emergency nurse knows that the only proven medical therapy shown to reduce the progression and mortality of COPD is:

A. smoking cessation.
B. short-acting inhaled bronchodilator.
C. inhaled corticosteroids.
D. pulmonary rehabilitation.

Rationale

A. Studies have shown that the reduction of risk factors slows the progression of COPD. Eliminating cigarette smoking is the single most valuable therapy in the reduction of COPD.

B. Bronchodilators are used to control symptoms but have no effect on airway inflammation, which is a main cause of worsening disease.

C. Airway inflammation is a characteristic of COPD. Anti-inflammatory medications may decrease the frequency of exacerbations but have not been shown to improve lung function or decrease mortality.

D. Pulmonary rehabilitation can improve a patient's quality of life by increasing exercise tolerance, but it does not improve lung function.

Category: Respiratory Emergencies/Chronic obstructive pulmonary disease (COPD)

Nursing Process: Assessment

Reference

Rastogi, S., Jain, A., Basu, S. K., & Rastogi, D. (2015). Current overview of COPD with special reference to emphysema. In M. Glass (Ed.), *Chronic obstructive pulmonary disease* (pp. 105–140). New York, NY: Hayle Medical.

---

24. The emergency nurse would anticipate arterial blood gas values from a patient in a severe chronic obstructive pulmonary disease exacerbation to illustrate:

A. metabolic acidosis.
B. respiratory alkalosis.
C. respiratory acidosis.
D. metabolic alkalosis.

Rationale

A. This is seen in metabolic disturbances, such as diabetic ketoacidosis or tissue hypoxia, causing a lower pH level. Metabolic acidosis occurs because of a decrease in the kidneys' ability to buffer the blood, resulting in a decrease of bicarbonate (HCO_3) availability.

B. Respiratory alkalosis results from the presence of an increased blood pH and a decreased $PaCO_2$ from a respiratory-related cause, such as hyperventilation.

C. Damaged alveoli do not efficiently exchange oxygen and carbon dioxide (CO_2). Retained CO_2 lowers the overall pH of the blood, resulting in respiratory acidosis.

D. Metabolic alkalosis occurs from an increased pH because of metabolic causes, such as a loss of gastric secretions from excessive vomiting.

Category: Respiratory Emergencies/Chronic obstructive pulmonary disease (COPD)

Nursing Process: Analysis

Reference

Hanania, N. A., & Sharafkhaneh, A. (2016). Chronic obstructive pulmonary disease. In E. T. Bope & R. D. Kellerman (Eds.), *Conn's current therapy 2016* (pp. 385–389). Philadelphia, PA: Elsevier.

---

25. The nurse ensures that the mechanically ventilated patient is placed in a semirecumbent position to:

A. prevent the development of a decubitus pressure ulcer.
B. make the patient more comfortable.
C. allow for oral care to be more easily performed.
D. prevent aspiration.

Rationale

A. This position can increase the chance of a decubitus pressure ulcer. When clinically indicated, a patient should be turned at least every 2 hours to prevent decubitus pressure ulcers from occurring.

B. A patient may be more comfortable sitting up in bed; however, the reason to keep the patient in a semirecumbent position is to prevent gastroesophageal reflux, which can cause ventilator-associated pneumonia, resulting in morbidity and mortality.

C. Oral care is important to prevent ventilator-associated pneumonia and can be completed with the patient supine if necessary.

D. An intubated patient who is supine is more likely to experience gastroesophageal reflux of stomach contents that can result in aspiration pneumonia. A semirecumbent position has been shown to prevent ventilator-associated pneumonia when the head and torso are at an angle of 30 to 45 degrees.

Category: Respiratory Emergencies/Infections

Nursing Process: Intervention

Reference

Stacy, K. M. Pulmonary therapeutic management. In L. D. Urden, K. M. Stacy, & M. E. Lough (Eds.), *Critical care nursing* (7th ed., pp. 549–586). Philadelphia, PA: Wolters Kluwer Health.

---

26. A patient arrives via emergency medical services following a house fire. The patient has a Glasgow Coma Scale score of 15. The emergency nurse understands that the patient's airway is patent because:

A. the pulse oximetry reads at 100%.
B. the patient is able to state their name clearly.
C. the patient's respiratory rate is 20.
D. the patient is not able to cough.

Rationale

A. Pulse oximetry only detects saturated hemoglobin and does not differentiate between oxygen and carbon monoxide hemoglobin saturation, so the pulse oximetry reading will usually appear to be within normal limits. A carboxyhemoglobin level will be necessary to determine the presence of carbon monoxide in the patient's blood.

B. Clear, audible speech indicates that there is no immediate threat to the patient's airway. The presence of clear and audible speech is the easiest way to determine a patent airway when rapid assessments are needed. Signs of inhalation injury include hoarse voice, stridor, wheezing, cough, and presence of carbonaceous sputum.

C. This is a normal assessment of breathing and ventilation and does not specifically indicate the presence of a patent airway.

D. Coughing is a reaction to clear an element from the trachea or lungs. An absence of the patient's ability to cough is usually indicative of airway obstruction.

Category: Respiratory Emergencies/Inhalation injuries

Nursing Process: Analysis

Reference

Ribbens, K. A., & DeVries, R. (2013). Burns. In B. B. Hammond & P. G. Zimmermann, *Sheehy's manual of emergency care* (7th ed., pp. 453–462). St. Louis, MO: Elsevier Mosby.

---

27. A patient with severe respiratory distress has been intubated, and mechanical ventilation has been initiated. The ventilator is alarming, indicating high airway pressures. As the emergency nurse, you are aware that this alarm indicates the importance to assess for the:

A. signs of a pneumothorax.
B. need for additional sedation.
C. change in the patient's oxygen saturation level.
D. presence of secretions.

Rationale

A. If, after suctioning the endotracheal tube, the ventilator continues to give high-pressure alarms, you should look for signs of pneumothorax (subcutaneous emphysema, absent/decreased breath sounds over the affected side, asymmetrical chest movement, tracheal deviation), but only after the airway has been assessed and cleared.

B. The patient may need additional sedation to tolerate endotracheal intubation; however, the priority is to assess for airway clearance.

C. Although assessing the oxygen saturation level is important to avoid the presence of hypoxemia, the first priority is to assess for airway clearance.

D. The endotracheal tube can become occluded with secretions, resulting in an increase in pressure to deliver oxygen to the patient. The priority intervention is to assess for the need to suction the endotracheal tube and the patient's airway. High pressure alarms can be caused by coughing, gagging, secretions, ventilator asynchrony, kinked tubing, and tubing condensation.

Category: Respiratory Emergencies/Obstruction

Nursing Process: Assessment

References

O'Neal, J. V. (2013). Airway management. In B. B. Hammond & R. G. Zimmermann (Eds.), *Sheehy's manual of emergency care* (7th ed., pp. 77–88). St. Louis, MO: Elsevier Mosby.
Walsh, R. (2013). Respiratory emergencies. In B. B. Hammond & R. G. Zimmermann (Eds.), *Sheehy's manual of emergency care* (7th ed., pp. 185–200). St. Louis, MO: Elsevier Mosby.

---

28. A patient presents to triage with a complaint of difficulty breathing, presence of a nonproductive cough, and "stabbing" chest pain. The patient reports a history of congestive heart failure. On assessment, the emergency nurse auscultates diminished breath sounds, bilaterally. What additional information would be the most pertinent to obtain from the patient?

A. Recent sick contacts
B. Medications prescribed and compliance

C. Vaccination history
D. Recent travel history

Rationale

A. Sick contacts are assessed when patients report respiratory symptoms because many respiratory illnesses are viral or bacterial in nature. However, noting decreased breath sounds and the patient's medical history, it is more relevant to collect additional information regarding the patient's history of congestive heart failure.

B. Dyspnea, cough, and chest pain are symptoms caused by numerous respiratory conditions. However, lung sounds that are decreased may indicate fluid or air around the lungs. Congestive heart failure causes increased hydrostatic pressure in the pulmonary vasculature, which leads to excess fluid collecting in the pleural space, known as a pleural effusion. In this scenario, it is most pertinent to assess a patient's compliance related to managing their congestive heart failure because unmanaged heart failure is the leading cause of pleural effusions.

C. The nurse may assess if a patient has been vaccinated against diseases that cause respiratory symptoms, such as influenza and pneumonia. However, because congestive heart failure seems to be the cause of the respiratory complaints in this scenario, it is most pertinent to assess the management of the heart failure.

D. Recent travel is assessed because pulmonary embolisms caused by prolonged venous stasis may cause respiratory symptoms that mimic other respiratory conditions. However, because congestive heart failure seems to be the cause of the respiratory complaints in this scenario, it is most pertinent to assess the management of heart failure.

Category: Respiratory Emergencies/Pleural effusion

Nursing Process: Assessment

Reference

Walsh, R. (2013). Respiratory emergencies. In B. B. Hammond & R. G. Zimmermann (Eds.), *Sheehy's manual of emergency care* (7th ed., pp. 185–200). St. Louis, MO: Elsevier Mosby.

---

29. Which assessment finding would best indicate that chest tube insertion has been successful in relieving a tension pneumothorax?

A. Presence of bloody drainage in the chest tube
B. Decrease in discomfort
C. Improvement in hemodynamics
D. Improved ability to deep breathe

Rationale

A. A tension pneumothorax is a life-threatening emergency that occurs when air enters the pleural space during inspiration and is unable to escape during exhalation. Blood would not necessarily be present in the pleural space with a tension pneumothorax.

B. A decrease in discomfort and restlessness may occur as cardiac output is restored. The patient may still have discomfort related to chest tube placement and underlying injuries. The improvement of hemodynamics is the best way to assess the success of relieving a tension pneumothorax.

C. A tension pneumothorax is a life-threatening emergency that occurs when air enters the pleural space during inspiration and is unable to escape during exhalation. The increasing intrathoracic pressure compresses the lungs, heart, and great vessels, resulting in markedly decreased cardiac output. Noted signs and symptoms include severe respiratory distress, tachycardia, hypotension, and poor tissue perfusion. Successful relief of a tension pneumothorax will be best assessed through the improvement of cardiac output via hemodynamics.

D. Increased intrathoracic pressure causes bilateral lung collapse if left untreated, resulting in quickly progressing dyspnea and tachypnea. However, successful relief of a tension pneumothorax will be best assessed through the improvement of hemodynamics.

Category: Respiratory Emergencies/Pneumothorax

Nursing Process: Evaluation

Reference

Everson, F. P. (2013). Chest trauma. In B. B. Hammond & R. G. Zimmermann (Eds.), *Sheehy's manual of emergency care* (7th ed., pp. 407–418). St. Louis, MO: Elsevier Mosby.

---

30. A tube thoracostomy has been placed for a patient with a hemothorax. Initially after placement, what output amount would alert the nurse to anticipate that the patient would be taken to the operating room for an emergency thoracotomy?

A. 1000 mL
B. 750 mL
C. 500 mL
D. 200 mL

Rationale

A. If there is at least 1000 mL of blood in the chest initially or blood drainage greater than 200 mL per hour for 3–4 hours, then an emergency thoracotomy may be considered to identify and repair the bleeding source.

B. If there is at least 1000 mL of blood in the chest initially or blood drainage greater than 200 mL per hour for 3–4 hours, then an emergency thoracotomy may be considered to identify and repair the bleeding source.

C. If there is at least 1000 mL of blood in the chest initially or blood drainage greater than 200 mL per hour for 3–4 hours, then an emergency thoracotomy may be considered to identify and repair the bleeding source.

D. If there is at least 1000 mL of blood in the chest initially or blood drainage greater than 200 mL per hour for 3–4 hours, then an emergency thoracotomy may be considered to identify and repair the bleeding source.

Category: Respiratory Emergencies/Trauma

Nursing Process: Analysis

Reference

Fazio, J. (2007). Thoracic trauma. In K. S. Hoyt & J. Selfridge-Thomas (Eds.), *Emergency nursing core curriculum* (6th ed., pp. 929–954). St. Louis, MO: Saunders Elsevier.

31. A patient presents to the emergency department pale and diaphoretic with VS: BP 130/85 mm Hg; HR 135 beats/minute; RR 40 breaths/minute; SpO_2 48% room air; T 37.2°C (99.0°F). Lungs sounds are diminished bilaterally throughout, with crackles at the bases. The patient is visiting from Florida and has been in town for 4 days; the current elevation is 9500 feet. What condition should the emergency nurse be most concerned about?

A. Pulmonary embolism
B. Pneumonia
C. Pneumothorax
D. High-altitude pulmonary edema

Rationale

A. The patient's lung sounds are diminished bilaterally. This assessment finding is inconsistent with the presence of a pulmonary embolism. Findings consistent with pulmonary embolism include tachypnea, tachycardia, hypotension, and dyspnea.

B. Pneumonia is not associated with exposure to high altitude, and there is no recent history of a respiratory illness or fever.

C. The patient has bilateral lung sounds throughout the lung fields. A pneumothorax would result in the patient having absent or diminished breath sounds over the area of the pneumothorax.

D. The patient is visiting from another state with a near sea level elevation. Current lung sounds reveal diminished lung sounds throughout, with crackles present at the bases. This assessment finding is concerning because of shifting of fluid into the lungs due to maladaptation to high-altitude exposure (9500 feet elevation).

Category: Respiratory Emergencies/Pulmonary edema
Nursing Process: Analysis

Reference

Sedlak, S. K. (2013). Environmental emergencies. In B. B. Hammond & P. G. Zimmermann (Eds.), *Sheehy's manual of emergency care* (7th ed., pp. 333–344). St. Louis, MO: Elsevier Mosby.

---

32. A patient arrives complaining of a sudden onset of chest pain. The patient is anxious and tachypnic. The initial priority intervention for the emergency nurse to perform for this patient would be to:

A. obtain an echocardiogram.
B. obtain intravenous access.
C. obtain arterial blood gas.
D. administer supplemental oxygen.

Rationale

A. Although an appropriate intervention, it is not the priority. Ensuring adequate oxygen exchange through administration of supplemental oxygen is the priority intervention for this patient. An echocardiogram is an ultrasound diagnostic tool to determine the function and structure of the heart.

B. Although obtaining intravenous access is an appropriate intervention, it is not the priority. Ensuring adequate oxygen exchange through administration of supplemental oxygen is the priority intervention for this patient.

C. Although an appropriate intervention, it is not the priority. Ensuring adequate oxygen exchange through administration of supplemental oxygen is the priority intervention for this patient.

D. Ensuring adequate oxygen exchange through administration of supplemental oxygen is the priority intervention for this patient.

Category: Respiratory Emergencies/Pulmonary embolus

Nursing Process: Intervention

Reference

Walsh, R. (2013). Respiratory emergencies. In B. B. Hammond & P. G. Zimmermann (Eds.), *Sheehy's manual of emergency care* (7th ed., pp. 185–200). St. Louis, MO: Elsevier Mosby.

---

33. Which is the term used to describe a form of shock that occurs following a large pulmonary embolism that has resulted in unstable patient hemodynamics with decreased tissue perfusion?
    A. Cardiogenic shock
    B. Distributive shock
    C. Hypovolemic shock
    D. Obstructive shock

Rationale

A. Cardiogenic shock is the result of myocardial pump failure and would not be caused by a pulmonary embolism.

B. Distributive shock is caused by an abnormal distribution of intravascular volume and would not be caused by a pulmonary embolism.

C. Hypovolemic shock is caused by an insufficient amount of circulating blood and would not be caused by a pulmonary embolism.

D. In obstructive shock, cardiac output and tissue perfusion are inadequate because of an obstruction limiting venous return to the heart during diastole. A large pulmonary embolism would create such an obstruction.

Category: Respiratory Emergencies/Pulmonary embolus

Nursing Process: Assessment

Reference

Calder, S. A. (2013). Shock. In B. B. Hammond & P. G. Zimmermann (Eds.), *Sheehy's manual of emergency care* (7th ed., pp. 213–222). St. Louis, MO: Elsevier Mosby.

---

34. An appropriate intervention in the treatment of acute respiratory distress syndrome is:
    A. mechanical ventilation.
    B. treating the underlying cause.
    C. decreasing fluid intake to avoid pulmonary edema.
    D. using high tidal volumes to open collapsed alveoli.

Rationale

A. Acute respiratory distress syndrome (ARDS), a severe pulmonary disorder that can be sudden or progressive, results in infiltrates, dyspnea, and hypoxemia. Decreased compliance of the lungs along with alveolar collapse can lead to severe hypoxemia; therefore, the initiation of mechanical ventilation will aid in the patient receiving adequate oxygenation.

B. It is crucial to treat the underlying cause of ARDS; however, airway and breathing are always the first priority.

C. The treatment of sepsis may require aggressive fluid resuscitation to maintain blood pressure and adequate tissue perfusion.

D. Lower tidal volumes during mechanical ventilation will help protect the lungs from further injury.

Category: Respiratory Emergencies/Respiratory distress syndrome

Nursing Process: Intervention

Reference

Walsh, R. (2013). Respiratory emergencies. In B. B. Hammond & P. G. Zimmermann (Eds.), *Sheehy's manual of emergency care* (7th ed., pp. 185–200). St. Louis, MO: Elsevier Mosby.

---

35. Which diagnostic finding is consistent with the presence of an esophageal injury?

A. Widening of the mediastinum on chest radiograph
B. Esophageal tissue in the nasogastric tube
C. Elevated central venous pressure
D. Abnormal echocardiogram

Rationale

A. Air from an esophageal injury leaks into the thoracic area, allowing air into the mediastinum; this results in widening of the mediastinum. Widened mediastinum may also be seen with aortic disruption and a pneumothorax.

B. Esophageal tissue or matter may be visible in the chest tube. Patients with a possible ruptured esophagus should not have a nasogastric tube inserted because this can lead to further damage to the esophagus.

C. The central venous pressure (CVP) would not be elevated in the presence of an esophageal injury. The CVP will be elevated in conjunction with a tension pneumothorax or cardiac tamponade.

D. An echocardiogram is used to assess cardiac functions such as wall motion, valvular function, estimated cardiac output, and presence of pericardial fluid. It is not a diagnostic tool to assess for the presence of an esophageal injury.

Category: Respiratory Emergencies/Trauma

Nursing Process: Analysis

Reference

Day, M. W. (2014). Thoracic and neck trauma. In D. Gurney (Ed.), *Trauma Nursing Core Course: Provider manual* (7th ed., pp. 137–150). Des Plaines, IL: Emergency Nurses Association.

36. A patient presents to triage with complaints of runny nose, headache, and a nonproductive cough for 3 days. The patient is able to speak without difficulty and reports a history of moderate to severe chronic obstructive pulmonary disease. Vitals signs are BP 158/88 mm Hg, HR 106 beats/minute, RR 22 breaths/minute, SPO_2 88% room air, T 37.1°C (98.8°F). The priority intervention for the emergency nurse to implement for this patient is which of the following?

A. Apply low flow supplemental oxygen
B. Call a code because the patient is hypoxic
C. Obtain a chest radiograph
D. Obtain an arterial blood gas analysis

Rationale

A. This patient's pulse oximetry may be at or close to their normal baseline. However, the application of supplemental oxygen may increase their oxygenation to an acceptable level, and a full physical assessment can then proceed. Airway, breathing, and circulation should always be assessed first, along with providing supplemental oxygen.

B. The patient's baseline oxygen level may be chronically low due to their advanced lung disease. Initial assessment reveals the patient is talking comfortably and does not appear to be in acute respiratory distress. Calling a code blue would not be indicated at this time.

C. A chest radiograph is important for ruling out other causes of hypoxia, but it is not the first intervention that should be performed. The first priority is to place the patient on low-flow supplemental oxygen.

D. Based on the patient's history and clinical presentation, obtaining an arterial blood gas (ABG) may be part of the full assessment. However, application of supplemental oxygen should not be delayed to obtain an ABG as assessment of airway, breathing, and circulation are the initial actions that need to be performed.

Category: Respiratory Emergencies/Chronic obstructive pulmonary disease (COPD)
Nursing Process: Intervention

Reference

Walsh, R. (2013). Respiratory emergencies. In B. B. Hammond & P. G. Zimmermann (Eds.), *Sheehy's manual of emergency care* (7th ed., pp. 185–200). St. Louis, MO: Elsevier Mosby.

---

37. When caring for an elderly patient with dementia, the emergency nurse is aware that a patient with dementia will directly exhibit which of the following first?

A. Inaccurate medical history
B. Disruptive behavior
C. Impaired communication
D. Sensory overload

Rationale

A. The dementia patient will first require additional time to promote communication. Patients with dementia frequently cannot recall their past medical history, medications, and recent visits to providers. Thus, the medical history may be incomplete, and this increases the risk for medical error in this population.

B. The dementia patient will first require additional time to promote communication. The fast-paced and overwhelming emergency department (ED) environment increases confusion and distraction, impairs communication, and increases the risk of disruptive behaviors. This is the rationale that supports separate, quieter environments for the geriatric population.

C. Older adults require additional time in the ED to promote communication. In the busy, rapidly changing, noisy atmosphere of the ED, patients with dementia are easily distracted, and communication becomes difficult. This is the rationale that supports separate, quieter environments for the geriatric population.

D. The dementia patient will first require additional time to promote communication. In the busy, rapidly changing, noisy atmosphere of the ED, patients with dementia are easily distracted, and communication becomes difficult. This is the rationale that supports separate, quieter environments for the geriatric population.

Category: Neurological Emergencies/Alzheimer's disease/dementia

Nursing Process: Analysis

Reference

Clevenger, C. K., Chu, T. A., Yang, Z., & Hepburn, K. W. (2012). Clinical care of persons with dementia in the emergency department: A review of the literature and agenda for research. *Journal of the American Geriatrics Society, 60*(9), 1742–1748. https://doi.org/10.1111/j.1532-5415.2012.04108.x

---

38. In caring for a patient with multiple sclerosis, the emergency nurse is aware that a common healthcare issue that affects the quality of life in this patient population is:

A. hypertension.
B. diabetes.
C. depression.
D. elevated cholesterol.

Rationale

A. Hypertension may develop earlier in patients with multiple sclerosis, but the percentage of patients is no greater than in the general population.

B. As individuals with multiple sclerosis age, they have the same risk for comorbid conditions as the general population.

C. Depression is common among patients with multiple sclerosis and often goes undiagnosed.

D. As individuals with multiple sclerosis age, they have the same risk for comorbid conditions as the general population.

Category: Neurological Emergencies/Chronic neurological disorders

Nursing Process: Assessment

Reference

Buhse, M. (2015). The elderly person with multiple sclerosis: Clinical implications for increasing life-span. *Journal of Neuroscience Nursing, 47*(6), 333–339. https://doi.org/10.1097/jnn.0000000000000172

39. A patient arrives to the emergency department with a 2-week history of repeatedly falling, accompanied by ascending weakness and tingling in the feet and fingers. There is loss of the knee-jerk reflex, and the patient is complaining of being unable to take a deep breath and of overall difficulty in breathing. Vital signs are BP 120/70 mm Hg, HR 72 beats/minute, RR 22 breaths/minute, SpO_2 96% on room air. The emergency nurse suspects the patient may have which of the following?

A. Myasthenia gravis
B. Guillain–Barré syndrome
C. Bell's palsy
D. Botulism

Rationale

A. Myasthenia gravis is a defect in neuromuscular junction transmission of acetylcholine. Symptoms include, most notably, ocular, facial, and neck weakness, as well as weakness of the upper extremities. The patient may demonstrate an abnormal smile, dysphagia, and the inability to manage their oral secretions, as well as difficulty speaking.

B. Guillain–Barré syndrome (GBS), also called acute inflammatory demyelinating polyneuropathy (AIDP), is characterized by the rapid onset of numbness, weakness, and often paralysis of the legs, arms, breathing muscles, and face. Paralysis is ascending, meaning that it travels upward from the toes, upward along the lower extremities, and from fingers along the upper extremities toward the torso. Absence or loss of tendon reflexes is also evident as GBS progresses.

C. Bell's palsy is a unilateral facial paralysis involving cranial nerve VII (facial nerve) that may result from the presence of herpes simplex virus within the facial nerve.

D. Botulism is caused by the *Clostridium botulinum* toxin. Botulism can be spread from home-canned or preserved food that has been improperly prepared. Symptoms include diplopia, blurred vision, drooping eyelids, muscle weakness, and dry mouth. Foodborne botulism usually begins 18–36 hours after consuming the contaminated food item.

Category: Neurological Emergencies/Guillain–Barré syndrome (GBS)

Nursing Process: Analysis

References

Botulism. (n.d.). Centers for Disease Control and Prevention. Retrieved from https://www.cdc.gov/botulism/general.html

GBS/CIDP Foundation International. (n.d.). Retrieved from https://www.gbs-cidp.org/gbs/

Walsh, R. (2013). Neurologic emergencies. In B. B. Hammond & P. G. Zimmermann (Eds.), *Sheehy's manual of emergency care* (7th ed., pp. 265–274). St. Louis, MO: Elsevier Mosby.

---

40. A patient with a history of chronic headaches presents to the emergency department (ED) with a severe headache that has grown in intensity over the last 2 weeks. A computed tomography angiography of the brain reveals no acute pathology. The patient typically uses nonsteroidal anti-inflammatories (NSAIDs) for pain relief and notes that over the last 2 weeks, they have had to increase the frequency of NSAID use to 4–5 days per week. The ED provider decides to place the patient on propranolol (Inderal) for

prophylactic pharmacologic therapy. Which of the following statements by the patient would indicate a need for further education?

A. **"I will take my propranolol (Inderal) as needed with the onset of a headache."**
B. "I will not discontinue this medication without first notifying my healthcare provider."
C. "The reason for this medication is to reduce my headache frequency and severity."
D. "This medication may improve the effectiveness of my other headache medications."

Rationale

A. The use of a beta-blocker is started if the patient is using a headache relief product such as acetaminophen, aspirin, and nonsteroidal anti-inflammatories (NSAIDs) more than 3 days per week or having two or more disabling migraine headache symptoms per month. The patient in the question is using NSAIDs 4–5 days per week. Prophylactic medications must be taken daily, with or without the presence of headache, to be effective.

B. Any beta-blocker requires a 10- to 14-day taper upon discontinuing the medication. Without this taper period, the patient may experience life-threatening rebound hypertension and tachycardia.

C. The purpose of prophylactic headache medications is to control symptoms on a long-term basis by reducing the frequency and severity of headaches.

D. Because prophylactic headache medications such as beta-blockers decrease the severity and frequency of headaches, abortive medications become more effective in controlling intermittent headache symptoms.

Category: Neurological Emergencies/Headache

Nursing Process: Evaluation

References

McMurray, J. (2013). Beta-blockers in cardiovascular medicine: Still alive and kicking. *Prescriber, 24*(6), 6–7. https://doi.org/10.1002/psb.1026

Silberstein, S. D., Holland, S., & Freitag, F. (2012). Evidence-based guideline updated: Pharmacologic treatment for episodic migraine prevention in adults: Report of the quality standards subcommittee of the American Academy of Neurology and the American Headache Society. *Neurology, 78*(1), 1337–1345.

---

41. The emergency nurse is reviewing the medication orders for a patient newly diagnosed with a subarachnoid hemorrhage. Which of the following orders would cause the emergency nurse to question the provider?

A. Nimodipine 60 mg every 4 hours
B. Infuse 0.9% NaCl at 150 mL/hour
C. **Dexamethasone 16 mg daily**
D. Atorvastatin 40 mg daily

Rationale

A. Nimodipine is used to treat vasospasm that occurs in patients with an acute subarachnoid hemorrhage (SAH). This would be an appropriate order for this patient.

B. Isotonic intravenous fluids are used to hemodilute and increase blood volume, thereby resulting in an increase in cerebral blood flow in patients with an acute SAH.

C. High-dose corticosteroids are not recommended for patients with an acute SAH.

D. Some studies have shown that the administration of a statin will help to increase cerebral blood flow and reduce vasospasm in patients with an acute SAH.

Category: Neurological Emergencies/Stroke

Nursing Process: Intervention

Reference

Glisic, E., Gardiner, L., Josti, L., Dermanelian, E., Ridel, S., Dziodzio, J., . . . Seder, D. B. (2016). Inadequacy of headache management after subarachnoid hemorrhage. *American Journal of Critical Care, 25*(2), 136–143.

---

42. A patient with a 2-year history of uncontrolled hypertension presents to the emergency department with a complaint of a severe headache. A computed tomography scan of the head reveals the presence of a large subarachnoid hemorrhage. Which of the following is a late sign of increased intracranial pressure?

A. Tachypnea
B. Narrowing pulse pressure
C. Bradycardia
D. Behavioral changes

Rationale

A. Apnea, not tachypnea, would be a late sign of increased intracranial pressure. Late signs of intracranial pressure include the presence of Cushing's triad: (1) bradycardia, (2) widening pulse pressure, and (3) apnea. In addition, late signs of intracranial pressure may also include unresponsiveness, dilated nonreactive pupils, and posturing. Early signs of intracranial pressure include headaches, nausea/vomiting, changes in mental status, and behavioral changes.

B. A widened pulse pressure, not a narrowing pulse pressure, would be a late sign of increased intracranial pressure. Late signs of intracranial pressure include the presence of Cushing's triad: (1) bradycardia, (2) widening pulse pressure, and (3) apnea. In addition, late signs of intracranial pressure may also include unresponsiveness, dilated nonreactive pupils, and posturing. Early signs of intracranial pressure include headaches, nausea/vomiting, changes in mental status, and behavioral changes.

C. Late signs of intracranial pressure include the presence of Cushing's triad: (1) bradycardia, (2) widening pulse pressure, and (3) apnea. In addition, late signs of intracranial pressure may also include unresponsiveness, dilated nonreactive pupils, and posturing. Early signs of intracranial pressure include headaches, nausea/vomiting, changes in mental status, and behavioral changes.

D. Behavioral changes would be considered an early sign of increased intracranial pressure. Late signs of intracranial pressure include the presence of Cushing's triad: (1) bradycardia, (2) widening pulse pressure, and (3) apnea. In addition, late signs of intracranial pressure may also include unresponsiveness, dilated nonreactive pupils, and posturing. Early signs of intracranial pressure include headaches, nausea/vomiting, changes in mental status, and behavioral changes.

Category: Neurological Emergencies/Stroke

Nursing Process: Assessment

Reference

Marino, P. (2013). *The ICU book.* Philadelphia, PA: Lippincott Williams & Wilkins.

43. A 3-week-old infant presents to the emergency department with a T 38.3°C (100.9°F). The infant has a normal physical exam, normal chest radiograph, and a white blood cell count of 15,000 and appears sleepy. The emergency provider decides to perform a lumbar puncture. What disease process can be confirmed by this procedure?

A. Hyponatremia
B. Meningitis
C. Otitis media
D. Subarachnoid hemorrhage

Rationale

A. Hyponatremia is a cause of seizures in the neonate and is related to supplementation of breast milk with either water or formula that has been diluted with too much water.

B. Group B streptococcus pneumoniae is the most common cause of meningitis in newborns. Meningitis is the result of an inflammation of the meninges. The mortality can be as high as 56%.

C. Otitis media is a common cause of fever but is diagnosed with an ear exam and visualization of the tympanic membrane, not a lumbar puncture.

D. Subarachnoid hemorrhage can be diagnosed with a lumbar puncture; however, it is commonly diagnosed with a computed tomography scan. The use of a lumbar puncture in suspected subarachnoid hemorrhage can lead to herniation of the brain stem in the presence of increased intracranial pressure, and patient death.

Category (Pediatric): Neurological Emergencies/Meningitis

Nursing Process: Assessment

Reference

Richard, G. C., & Lepe, M. (2013). Meningitis in children: Diagnosis and treatment for the emergency clinician. *Clinical Pediatric Emergency Medicine*, *14*(2),146–156. https://doi.org/10.1016/j.cpem.2013.04.008

---

44. The emergency nurse is caring for a patient with the following symptoms: severe headache, neck stiffness, fever, and inability to tolerate bright light. The patient has been administered intravenous antibiotics and an antipyretic for fever. The nurse identifies that additional patient education is required for their diagnosis of bacterial meningitis when the patient states:

A. "My girlfriend will need to be evaluated for this disease."
B. "I will have to cancel my dinner plans with friends for this evening."
C. "I need to take medication to reduce my fever."
D. "I will take my antibiotics until my symptoms go away."

Rationale

A. Patients with meningeal disease are contagious, and chemoprophylaxis is required for anyone who is exposed directly to oral secretions of the infected individual.

B. Patients with meningeal disease are contagious and should limit their interactions with others until their symptoms are no longer evident.

C. Patients should take their fever-reducing medications until their fever is under control to minimize their discomfort and prevent further complications.

D. The patient's symptoms are indicative of viral meningitis. Patients with meningitis are contagious, requiring antibiotics and observation for potential complications.

Category: Neurological Emergencies/Meningitis

Nursing Process: Evaluation

Reference

Baxter, C. S. (2013). Neurological emergencies. In Emergency Nurses Association (Eds.), *Emergency nursing core curriculum* (7th ed., pp. 349–365). St. Louis, MO: Saunders Elsevier.

---

45. An elderly patient presents to the emergency department after demonstrating aggressive behavior in the patient's group home residence. The emergency nurse observes the patient to be pale and diaphoretic and displaying tonic–clonic movement. Which laboratory test has the greatest priority for this patient?

A. Dilantin (phenytoin) level
B. Blood glucose level
C. Blood alcohol level
D. Vitamin B_6 (thiamine) level

Rationale

A. The patient does not have a history of a seizure disorder, and therefore would not be prescribed this medication. The fastest test to obtain is blood glucose level, which has the greatest priority for this patient.

B. Obtaining a blood glucose level has the greatest priority for this patient and is the fastest laboratory test to obtain. The presence of hypoglycemia is a frequent cause of seizures and acute mental status changes.

C. A blood alcohol level is not a priority for this patient. Alcohol is a sedative, and seizures most often only occur in the presence of alcohol withdrawal. This patient does not have a history of alcoholism and did not experience seizure activity.

D. Thiamine level may be low in patients with a history of alcoholism. However, this patient does not have a history of alcoholism, so this laboratory test does not have the greatest priority for this patient.

Category: Neurological Emergencies/Seizure disorders

Nursing Process: Intervention

Reference

Yamamoto, L., Olaes, E., & Lopez, A. (2004). Challenges in seizure management: Neurologic versus cardiac emergencies. *Topics in Emergency Medicine, 26*(3), 212–224.

---

46. A patient presents to the emergency department complaining of two tonic–clonic seizure episodes within the previous 3 days despite being compliant with daily doses of levetiracetam (Keppra). Which of the following statements made by the patient indicates that additional education is required this medication?

A. "I use the rowing machine at the gym every day."
B. "I use meditation to help with sleep."
C. "I keep hydrated to protect my kidneys."
D. "I limit alcohol to two drinks each night."

Rationale

A. Regular exercise contributes to overall health status and may assist with stress and coping with chronic illness. Activities chosen should consider the potential for injury should a seizure occur.

B. Regular sleep promotes general health, reduces stress on the system, and aids with coping.

C. Levetiracetam is excreted by the kidneys. Dehydration may cause concentration of medication, resulting in enhanced medication effects.

D. Drinking alcohol may trigger seizures, even in small amounts. The central nervous system depressant effects of levetiracetam in combination with alcohol may enhance these effects, resulting in physical or mental impairment.

Category: Neurological Emergencies/Seizure disorders

Nursing Process: Evaluation

References

Baxter, C. S. (2007). Neurologic emergencies. In K. S. Hoyt & J. Selfridge-Thomas (Eds.), *Emergency nursing core curriculum* (6th ed., pp. 510–535). St. Louis, MO: Saunders Elsevier.

Criddle, L. M. (2007). Cardiovascular emergencies. In K. S. Hoyt & J. Selfridge-Thomas (Eds.), *Emergency nursing core curriculum* (6th ed., pp. 187–248). St. Louis, MO: Saunders Elsevier.

England, K. M., & Plueger, M. D. (2014). Seizures and epilepsy. In J. V. Hickey (Ed.), *The clinical practice of neurological and neurosurgical nursing* (7th ed.) [Kindle version]. Philadelphia, PA: Lippincott Williams & Wilkins.

---

47. A patient presents to the emergency department following a bar fight. The patient reports being punched in the face and having their neck forced backward. A few hours later, the patient began noticing upper extremity weakness with associated sensory loss. They also report being unable to urinate, and the bladder scan reveals 300 mL of urine in their bladder. The most likely cause of this patient's symptoms is:

A. Brown–Sequard syndrome.
B. anterior cord syndrome.
C. central cord syndrome.
D. posterior cord syndrome.

Rationale

A. Brown–Sequard syndrome is consistent with hemiparaplegia on the same side as the cord injury and hemianesthesia on the opposite side of the cord injury, but below the level of injury.

B. Anterior cord syndrome is consistent with motor paralysis and a loss of pain and temperature sensation below the level of the injury, with a preservation of proprioception, touch, and vibratory sense.

C. Central cord syndrome results from a hyperextension injury of the cervical spinal cord. Common symptoms include upper and lower extremity weakness, with deficits more pronounced in the upper extremities. In addition, the patient may experience varying degrees of sensory loss, impaired pain, temperature, light touch, and position sense below the level of the injury. These symptoms may also lead to a neurogenic bladder. Symptoms are usually self-limiting.

D. Posterior cord syndrome is consistent with preserved motor function below the level of the injury, with a loss of sensory function.

Category: Neurological Emergencies/Spinal cord injuries

Nursing Process: Analysis

References

Aarabi, B., Alexander, M., Mirvis, S. E., Shanmuganathan, K., Chesler, D., Maulucci, C., . . . Blacklock, T. (2011). Predictors of outcome in acute traumatic central cord syndrome due to spinal stenosis: Clinical article. *Journal of Neurosurgery: Spine, 14*(1), 122–130. https://doi.org/10.3171/2010.9.spine09922

Diabira, S., Henaux, P. L., Riffaud, L., Hamlat, A., Brassier, G., & Morandi, X. (2011). Brown-Sequard syndrome revealing intradural thoracic disc herniation. *European Spine Journal, 20*(1), 65–70. https://doi.org/10.1007/s00586-010-1498-3

Kirshblum, S. C., Burns, S. P., Biering-Sorensen, F., Donovan, W., Graves, D. E., Jha, A., . . . Schmidt-Read, M. (2011). International standards for neurological classification of spinal cord injury. *Journal of Spinal Cord Medicine, 34*(6), 535–546. https://doi.org/10.1007/978-0-387-79948-3_5034

Markandaya, M., Stein, D. M., & Menaker, J. (2012). Acute treatment options for spinal cord injury. *Current Treatment Options in Neurology, 14*(2), 175–187. https://doi.org/10.1007/s11940-011-0162-5

---

48. A patient presents to the emergency department via emergency medical services (EMS). The patient has cervical spine precautions in place because of suspected spinal cord injury. Per the EMS report, the patient initially was able to move their wrists bilaterally. On initial assessment, the emergency nurse determines that the patient is only able to shrug their shoulders. The priority intervention for this patient would be to:

A. notify the trauma team.
B. document these new findings.
C. determine the patient's pain level.
D. reassess patient function in 15 minutes.

Rationale

A. Movement of the wrists is a function of C7 innervation. Movement at only the shoulders would reveal a worsening condition because this motion would be the result of innervation at the level of C6 and the loss of C7 function. This patient will require immediate diagnostic studies and treatment as deemed necessary by the trauma team.

B. Documentation is important; however, the priority would be to notify the trauma team for the appropriate treatment(s).

C. Determining the patient's pain level is important, however, the priority would be to notify the trauma team.

D. This patient is not improving and has lost C7 function. Immediate notification of the trauma team is indicated.

Category: Neurological Emergencies/Spinal cord injuries

Nursing Process: Intervention

References

Crowley, M. (2014). Spinal cord and vertebral column trauma. In D. Gurney (Ed.), *Trauma Nursing Core Course: Provider manual* (pp. 173–192). Des Plaines, IL: Emergency Nurses Association.

Hickey, J. (2013). *The clinical practice of neurological and neurosurgical nursing* (p. 424). Philadelphia, PA: Lippincott Williams & Wilkins

Howard, P., & Steinmann, R. (2010). In P. K. Howard & R. A. Steinmann (Eds.), *Sheehy's emergency nursing: Principles and practice* (6th ed., pp. 274–280). St. Louis, MO: Mosby Elsevier.

49. A patient who weighs 100 kg is ordered to receive tissue plasminogen activator for an acute ischemic stroke. The emergency provider orders a dose of 100 mg, with 10% of the dose to be administered via intravenous push, with the remaining dose to be administered over an hour infusion. The emergency nurse verifies the weight dosing and identifies that 0.9 mg/kg is the recommended dosing for this medication in the presence of an acute ischemic stroke. The next action by the emergency nurse is to:

A. administer 10 mg over 1 minute, followed by the administration of 90 mg over 59 minutes via infusion pump.
B. verify with the emergency provider the medication order for the patient.
C. administer 9 mg over 1 minute, followed by the administration of 91 mg over 59 minutes via infusion pump.
D. administer 10 mg over 1 minute, followed by the administration of 90 mg over 60 minutes via the infusion pump.

Rationale

A. The maximum intravenous (IV) dose of tissue plasminogen activator (tPA) for ischemic stroke is 90 mg. The bolus is 10% of the recommended dose administered over 1 minute, and the remainder of the dose is given over 60 minutes via infusion pump.

B. The maximum IV dose of tPA for ischemic stroke is 90 mg. The bolus is 10% of the recommended dose administered over 1 minute, and remainder of the dose is given over 60 minutes via infusion pump.

C. The maximum IV dose of tPA for ischemic stroke is 90 mg. The bolus is 10% of the recommended dose administered over 1 minute, and the remainder of the dose is given over 60 minutes via infusion pump.

D. The maximum IV dose of tPA for ischemic stroke is 90 mg. The bolus is 10% of the recommended dose administered over 1 minute, and the remainder of the dose is given over 60 minutes via infusion pump.

Category: Neurological Emergencies/Stroke

Nursing Process: Intervention

Reference

Brown, A., & King, D. (2010). Neurological emergencies. In P. K. Howard & R. A. Steinmann (Eds.), *Sheehy's emergency nursing: Principles and practice* (6th ed., pp. 457–466). St. Louis, MO: Mosby Elsevier.

---

50. The provider is considering the administration of alteplase (Activase/tPA) to an 82-year-old patient diagnosed with an acute ischemic stroke. In addition to the patient's age, which other factor would exclude the patient from the administration of alteplase within the recommended extended 3- to 4.5-hour time window?

A. A National Institutes of Health Stroke Scale greater than 20
B. A National Institutes of Health Stroke Scale of 3
C. Previous history of a ST-elevation myocardial infarction
D. History of diabetes

Rationale

A. There is no upper limit within the National Institutes of Health (NIH) Stroke Scale for the administration of alteplase in the 3- to 4.5-hour time window.

B. There is no lower limit of the NIH Stroke Scale for the administration of alteplase.

C. A history of a ST-elevation myocardial infarction does not exclude the patient from receiving alteplase in the extended time window of 3 to 4.5 hours.

D. The exclusion criteria for the extended time window of 3 to 4.5 hours include both age greater than 80 years and a history of diabetes and/or a prior stroke.

Category: Neurological Emergencies/Stroke

Nursing Process: Assessment

Reference

American Heart Association. (2016). *Advanced cardiovascular life support: Provider manual* (16th ed.). Dallas, TX: Author.

---

51. Which of the following patients would benefit from the administration of nimodipine (Nimotop) to decrease the risk of associated cerebral infarction?
    A. A subarachnoid hemorrhage resulting from traumatic brain injury
    B. A subdural hematoma in an elderly patient
    C. A subarachnoid hemorrhage resulting from a cerebral aneurysm
    D. A subdural hematoma in a patient who abuses alcohol

Rationale

A. Nimodipine is a calcium channel blocker proved to improve outcomes in patients with nontraumatic subarachnoid hemorrhage by decreasing cerebral vasospasm and decreasing the incidence of cerebral infarction. This drug is not indicated, and shows no benefit, in traumatic subarachnoid hemorrhage or subdural hematoma, regardless of the cause.

B. Nimodipine is a calcium channel blocker proved to improve outcomes in patients with nontraumatic subarachnoid hemorrhage by decreasing cerebral vasospasm and decreasing the incidence of cerebral infarction. This drug is not indicated, and shows no benefit, in traumatic subarachnoid hemorrhage or subdural hematoma, regardless of the cause.

C. Nimodipine is a calcium channel blocker proved to improve outcomes in patients with nontraumatic subarachnoid hemorrhage by decreasing cerebral vasospasm and decreasing the incidence of cerebral infarction. This drug is not indicated, and shows no benefit, in traumatic subarachnoid hemorrhage or subdural hematoma, regardless of the cause.

D. Nimodipine is a calcium channel blocker proved to improve outcomes in patients with nontraumatic subarachnoid hemorrhage by decreasing cerebral vasospasm and decreasing the incidence of cerebral infarction. This drug is not indicated, and shows no benefit, in traumatic subarachnoid hemorrhage or subdural hematoma, regardless of the cause.

Category: Neurological Emergencies/Stroke
Nursing Process: Analysis

Reference

Bhat, P., Dretler, A., Gdowski, M., Ramgopal, R., & Williams, D. (2016). *The Washington manual of medical therapeutics* (35th ed.). Philadelphia, PA: Wolters Kluwer.

---

52. Which type of skull fracture would place the patient at the highest risk for developing an intracranial infection?

A. **Basilar skull fracture**
B. Linear skull fracture
C. Depressed skull fracture
D. Temporal bone fracture

Rationale

A. Basilar skull fractures include a fracture of any of the five bones at the base of the skull. These fractures can cause a laceration of the dura mater, resulting in an open passage of cerebrospinal fluid, which places the patient at risk for intracranial infections such as meningitis, encephalitis, and/or brain abscess. A linear skull fracture is a nondisplaced fracture of the cranium and does not increase the risk of intracranial infections. A depressed skull is a fracture extending below the surface of the skull and lacerating the dura mater, which may cause intracranial infections; however, the incidence of infection is statistically higher in basilar skull fractures. Temporal bone fractures increase the risk of epidural hematoma.

B. A linear skull fracture is a nondisplaced fracture of the cranium and does not increase the risk of intracranial infections.

C. A depressed skull is a fracture extending below the surface of the skull and lacerating the dura mater, which may cause intracranial infections. However, the incidence of infection is statistically higher in basilar skull fractures.

D. Temporal bone fractures increase the risk of epidural hematoma.

Category: Neurological Emergencies/Trauma
Nursing Process: Assessment

Reference

McLaughlin, J. C. (2014). Brain, cranial, and maxillofacial trauma. In D. Gurney (Ed.), *Trauma Nursing Core Course: Provider manual* (7th ed., pp. 105–122). Des Plaines, IL: Emergency Nurses Association.

---

53. A 32-year-old female who is 28 weeks pregnant presents with right upper quadrant pain that is radiating to the right scapula area. The patient states that the pain began a short time after having dinner. Based on the patient's presentation, the most likely diagnosis is:

A. diverticulitis.
B. cholecystitis.
C. pancreatitis.
D. gastroenteritis.

Rationale

A. Diverticulitis is caused when the diverticula become inflamed. Pain is persistent and localized to the left lower quadrant. It is commonly described as a "left-sided appendicitis."

B. Symptoms of cholecystitis include a sudden onset of abdominal pain that is usually associated with ingestion of fatty or fried foods. Pain is located in the epigastrium and/or upper right quadrant. Pain may be referred to the right shoulder or supraclavicular area.

C. Pain with pancreatitis is generally located in left upper abdomen or epigastrium and may radiate through to the back.

D. Gastroenteritis is a common gastrointestinal illness that may have a viral or bacterial origin and may occur following ingestion of contaminated food. Symptoms would include nausea, vomiting, diarrhea, and abdominal cramps.

Category: Gastrointestinal, Genitourinary, Gynecology, and Obstetrical Emergencies/Gastrointestinal/Cholecystitis

Nursing Process: Analysis

References

Herrington, A. (2010). Gastrointestinal emergencies. In P. K. Howard & R. A. Steinmann (Eds.), *Sheehy's emergency nursing: Principles and practice* (6th ed., pp. 467–477). St. Louis, MO: Mosby Elsevier.

Wolf, L., & Zimmermann, P. G. (2013). Abdominal pain and emergencies. In B. B. Hammond & P. G. Zimmermann (Eds.), *Sheehy's manual of emergency care* (7th ed., pp. 291–301). St. Louis, MO: Mosby Elsevier.

---

54. A patient with a history of esophageal varices presents to the emergency department complaining of weakness and diaphoresis. The patient suddenly has an emesis of bright red blood. The priority intervention for the emergency nurse to perform is:

A. to insert a large-diameter gastric tube.
B. to obtain a complete set of vital signs.
C. to administer high-flow oxygen via nonrebreather mask.
D. to establish intravenous (IV) access with two large-caliber IV catheters.

Rationale

A. Gastric tube insertion should be done carefully to avoid inadvertent esophageal rupture. Insertion may be indicated, but treatment of hypovolemia is the priority.

B. The evaluation of hemodynamic status through vital sign measurement is important in ongoing evaluation but is not a priority in light of the patient's active bleeding.

C. Administering oxygen to this patient is an important intervention, however, the use of a nonrebreather mask would not be effective for a patient who is actively vomiting blood.

D. Therapeutic interventions should focus on the management of bleeding and hypovolemic shock.

Category: Gastrointestinal, Genitourinary, Gynecology, and Obstetrical Emergencies/Gastrointestinal/Esophageal varices

Nursing Process: Intervention

References

Rossoll, L. W. (2007). Abdominal emergencies. In K. S. Hoyt & J. Selfridge-Thomas (Eds.), *Emergency nursing core curriculum* (pp. 159–186). St. Louis, MO: Saunders Elsevier.

Wolf, L., & Zimmermann, P. G. (2013). Abdominal pain and emergencies. In B. B. Hammond & P. G. Zimmermann (Eds.), *Sheehy's manual of emergency care* (7th ed., pp. 291–301). St. Louis, MO: Mosby Elsevier.

---

55. A child presents to the emergency department after choking on a chicken bone. The patient's airway is not obstructed, but swallowing is difficult, and the child is consistently drooling. The nurse anticipates which diagnostic test to be performed initially?

A. Chest radiograph
B. Bedside ultrasound
C. End-tidal carbon dioxide measurement
D. Direct laryngoscopy

Rationale

A. Unless the object can be observed in the upper airway, a chest radiograph is best to determine the object's location in the upper gastrointestinal system.

B. Ultrasound is a quick and accurate means to evaluate organ structure and identify vascular injuries. It is not a useful tool to evaluate the presence of a foreign body in the upper airway or gastrointestinal system.

C. The child's respiratory status does not require endotracheal intubation, so an end-tidal carbon dioxide measurement would not provide any useful information.

D. Once the foreign body is located, direct laryngoscopy can be used to visualize and remove the foreign body, but a radiograph will initially define the existence and location of the object.

Category (Pediatric): Gastrointestinal, Genitourinary, Gynecology, and Obstetrical Emergencies/Gastrointestinal/Foreign bodies

Nursing Process: Analysis

References

Smith, D. A. (2007). Dental, ear, nose and throat emergencies. In K. S. Hoyt & J. Selfridge-Thomas (Eds.), *Emergency nursing core curriculum* (6th ed., pp. 249–289). St. Louis, MO: Saunders Elsevier.

Wolf, L., & Zimmermann, P. G. (2013). Abdominal pain and emergencies. In B. B. Hammond & P. G. Zimmermann (Eds.), *Sheehy's manual of emergency care* (7th ed., pp. 291–301). St. Louis, MO: Mosby Elsevier.

56. A normal full-term newborn has been delivered in the emergency department. The newborn has been warmed, their temperature is being maintained, their airway is being positioned, secretions have been cleared, and they have been stimulated. To evaluate the effectiveness of these interventions, the nurse anticipates the infant's preductal oxygen saturation target after 1 minute to be approximately:

A. 63%.
B. 67%.
C. 73%.
D. 90%.

Rationale

A. According to neonatal resuscitation, the preductal oxygen saturation target 1 minute after birth should be in the range of 60–65%. After the baby's initial cries and deep breaths, fluid moves out of the airways, causing the ductus arteriosus to constrict, and blood now flows from the right side of the heart into the lungs. It typically takes approximately 10 minutes for a normal full-term newborn to achieve oxygen saturation greater than 90%.

B. According to neonatal resuscitation, the preductal oxygen saturation target 2 minutes after birth should be in the range of 65–70%.

C. According to neonatal resuscitation, the preductal oxygen saturation target 3 minutes after birth should be in the range of 70–75%.

D. According to neonatal resuscitation, the preductal oxygen saturation target 10 minutes after birth should be in the range of 85–95%.

Category: Gastrointestinal, Genitourinary, Gynecology, and Obstetrical Emergencies/Obstetrical/Neonatal resuscitation

Nursing Process: Evaluation

Reference

American Academy of Pediatrics & American Heart Association. (2016). Foundations for neonatal resuscitation. In *Textbook of neonatal resuscitation* (7th ed., pp. 1–16). Elk Grove Village, IL: American Academy of Pediatrics.

---

57. A 3-year-old child who weighs 20 kg is being treated for a 2-day history of vomiting and diarrhea. The child has been orally rehydrated and is now being discharged home with the parents. Which of the following would be most important to include in the initial home care discharge instructions?

A. Administer 1–2 teaspoons of an oral rehydration solution (Pedialyte) every 5 minutes
B. Resume normal meals in small amounts
C. Start a BRAT (bananas, rice, applesauce, toast) diet
D. Do not permit the child to have anything orally for the next 24 hours. If no vomiting occurs, the child may advance to having small amounts of clear liquids.

Rationale

A. Oral rehydration therapy can be continued at home. The parents should be instructed to administer the solution in sips of 1–2 teaspoons every 5 minutes to promote absorption and prevent vomiting.

B. After 2 days of vomiting and diarrhea, the priority for this patient is oral rehydration. The reintroduction of solid food too quickly is likely to induce additional vomiting.

C. Rehydration is the priority for this child, so initial home care instructions should include the administration of an oral rehydration solution.

D. Rehydration is the priority for this child, so initial home care instructions should include the administration of an oral rehydration solution.

Category (Pediatric): Gastrointestinal, Genitourinary, Gynecology, and Obstetrical Emergencies/ Gastrointestinal/Gastroenteritis

Nursing Process: Intervention

References

Golder, D. (2012). Childhood illness. In *Emergency Nursing Pediatric Course: Provider manual* (4th ed., pp. 147–170). Des Plaines, IL: Emergency Nurses Association.

Mecham, N. L. (2010). Pediatric emergencies. In P. K. Howard & R. A. Steinmann (Eds.), *Emergency nursing: Principles and practice* (6th ed., pp. 630–651). St. Louis, MO: Mosby.

---

58. A patient presents to the emergency department with complaints of upper abdominal fullness, fatigue, and nausea for the past 2 weeks. When obtaining the patient's history, the triage nurse would be most concerned that the patient may have developed hepatitis A if the patient reports:

A. having engaged in unprotected sexual contact with an individual who may have hepatitis B.
B. having a history of intravenous (IV) drug use and having recently shared needles with other IV drug users.
C. having been camping recently and sustaining a tick bite.
D. having recently traveled overseas to assist in the clean-up activities in a town flooded by heavy rains.

Rationale

A. In this case, it would be more likely that the patient would have contracted hepatitis A, but may have been exposed to hepatitis B, which is transmitted through contact with blood and body fluids.

B. Because hepatitis A is transmitted by the fecal–oral route, sharing used IV needles will not transmit the hepatitis A virus. The patient is at greater risk of contracting hepatitis B or human immunodeficiency virus from sharing used IV needles.

C. The bite of a tick may put the patient at risk for developing Lyme disease, but not hepatitis A.

D. Hepatitis A virus is transmitted by the oral–fecal route and is prevalent in areas of poor sanitation.

Category: Gastrointestinal, Genitourinary, Gynecology, and Obstetrical Emergencies/Gastrointestinal/ Hepatitis

Nursing Process: Assessment

Reference

Almeida, S. L. (2010). Communicable diseases. In P. K. Howard & R. A. Steinmann (Eds.), *Sheehy's emergency nursing: Principles and practice* (6th ed., pp. 513–524). St. Louis, MO: Mosby Elsevier.

---

59. A male presents to the emergency department with complaints of pain and swelling in his right groin area. The patient states the pain intensity has increased, and the swelling has become larger over the past several days. The emergency nurse should anticipate which diagnostic test to best identify the source of the patient's complaint?

A. Abdominal radiographs
B. Computed tomography scan
C. Magnetic resonance imaging of the abdomen
D. Abdominal ultrasound

Rationale

A. An abdominal radiograph would be helpful in diagnosing a bowel obstruction but would not provide enough information to validate a diagnosis of inguinal hernia.

B. A computed tomography (CT) scan of the abdomen would be helpful to identify the source of the patient's discomfort in the absence of any physical signs. This patient has an obvious bulge in the inguinal area, so a CT scan would yield little additional information.

C. A magnetic resonance imaging might show the hernia, but the preferred method to diagnose a hernia is an ultrasound.

D. The patient's symptoms are most likely a result of an inguinal hernia. The patient's physical examination usually is diagnostic, but an ultrasound can be performed to determine if strangulation or an intestinal obstruction is present.

Category: Gastrointestinal, Genitourinary, Gynecology, and Obstetrical Emergencies/Gastrointestinal/Hernia
Nursing Process: Analysis

References

Parswa, A. (n.d.). Hernias of the abdominal wall. *Merck Manual Online*. Retrieved from http://www.merckmanuals.com/professional/gastrointestinal-disorders/acute-abdomen-and-surgical-gastroenterology/hernias-of-the-abdominal-wall

Wedro, B. (2016). Abdominal hernia. *MedicineNet.com*. Retrieved from http://www.medicinenet.com/hernia_overview/page3.htm

Wolf, L., & Zimmermann, P. G. (2013). Abdominal pain and emergencies. In B. B. Hammond & P. G. Zimmermann (Eds.), *Sheehy's manual of emergency care* (7th ed., pp. 291–301). St. Louis, MO: Elsevier Mosby.

---

60. Parents of a 7-month-old state that the infant has not been as active as usual and has been crying and drawing up their legs at intervals. The child's abdomen is distended, and a mass is palpable in the right upper quadrant. The parents state that earlier today, the child had a small bowel movement that looked dark red with mucous in it. The child's symptoms are most consistent with which of the following conditions?

A. Intussusception
B. Pyloric stenosis
C. Appendicitis
D. Incarcerated hernia

Rationale

A. Intussusception is the telescoping or prolapse of a segment of bowel into an adjacent segment, causing the classic symptoms of abdominal pain, a palpable abdominal mass, and "currant-jelly stools" with bloody mucus. It is more commonly seen in children between the ages of 3 months and 5 years. Sudden, acute, cramping pain and the child drawing up their legs are the most commonly reported signs. The child may be pain free between episodes.

B. Pyloric stenosis causes muscular thickening of the pylorus, leading to a functional gastric outlet syndrome. This disorder is the most common cause of intestinal obstruction in infancy. The infant typically presents with a previously normal feeding history and suddenly develops projectile emesis after eating. Occasionally an olive-shaped mass can be palpated in the right upper quadrant.

C. Acute appendicitis is one of the most common causes of abdominal pain. Classic symptoms include constant abdominal pain, fever, and vomiting. The pain may start as periumbilical and migrate to the right lower quadrant. Appendicitis occurs in all age groups but is rare in infants.

D. An incarcerated hernia typically presents as an asymptomatic bulge of a bowel loop that becomes more prominent with crying, laughing, or coughing. If circulation to the bowel loop is compromised, symptoms would include pain and swelling at the site of herniation, nausea and vomiting, and signs of a bowel obstruction. In children, these hernias are most commonly found in the inguinal area, where firm, tender masses can be palpated in the inguinal canal or scrotal area.

Category (Pediatric): Gastrointestinal, Genitourinary, Gynecology, and Obstetrical Emergencies/ Gastrointestinal/Intussusception

Nursing Process: Analysis

References

Golder, D. (2012). Childhood illness. In *Emergency Nursing Pediatric Course: Provider manual* (4th ed., pp. 147–170). Des Plaines, IL: Author.

Wolf, L., & Zimmermann, P. G. (2013). Abdominal pain and emergencies. In B. B. Hammond & P. G. Zimmermann (Eds.), *Sheehy's manual of emergency care* (7th ed., pp. 291–301). St. Louis, MO: Mosby Elsevier.

---

61. Correct placement of a nasogastric tube (NG) is best confirmed by which method?

A. pH determination of NG tube aspirate
B. Obtaining a chest radiograph
C. Placing the end of the NG tube in a container of water
D. Auscultating for air over the epigastric region

Rationale

A. Measuring the pH value of stomach aspirate has limited value in the clinical setting because many patients are on acid-inhibiting medications. These medications will alter the pH level of the stomach contents.

B. Radiographic confirmation of proper NG tube position is the most reliable method to ensure correct placement.

C. Placing the end of the NG tube in a container of water and observing for "bubbling" is an inaccurate and potentially dangerous practice to confirm NG tube placement. If the NG tube is in the airway, the patient may aspirate on inhalation.

D. Instilling air into the NG tube while listening with a stethoscope over the epigastrium for the associated "whoosh" sound has been found to be an unreliable method of verifying NG tube placement.

Category: Gastrointestinal, Genitourinary, Gynecology, and Obstetrical Emergencies/Gastrointestinal/Obstructions

Nursing Process: Assessment

References

Emergency Nurses Association. (2015). *Clinical practice guideline: Gastric tube placement verification.* Retrieved from https://www.ena.org/docs/default-source/resource-library/practice-resources/cpg/gastrictubecpg7b5530b71c1e49e8b155b6cca1870adc.pdf?sfvrsn=a8e9dd7a_8

Lippincott Williams & Wilkins. (2003). *Critical care challenges: Disorders, treatments, and procedures.* Philadelphia, PA: Author.

---

62. A patient has an elevated serum lipase level and left upper quadrant abdominal pain that radiates to their back. The emergency nurse recognizes these signs and symptoms as most likely being associated with which disease process?

A. Hepatitis C
B. Cholecystitis
C. Pyelonephritis
D. Pancreatitis

Rationale

A. The pain associated with hepatitis is typically felt in the right upper quadrant of the abdomen. Serum lipase is not elevated.

B. The pain associated with cholecystitis is typically felt in the right upper quadrant of the abdomen and may radiate to the back. Serum bilirubin and liver enzyme (ALT and AST) levels may be elevated, but not serum lipase levels.

C. The pain associated with pyelonephritis originates in the flank or back at the costovertebral angle and may radiate to the groin. Serum lipase levels are not elevated.

D. The pain associated with pancreatitis is typically felt in the left upper quadrant of the abdomen and may radiate through the abdomen to the back. An elevated serum lipase level is specific to pancreatic disease or injury.

Category: Gastrointestinal, Genitourinary, Gynecology, and Obstetrical Emergencies/Gastrointestinal/Pancreatitis

Nursing Process: Assessment

References

Quallich, S. (2013). Genitourinary emergencies. In B. B. Hammond & P. G. Zimmermann (Eds.), *Sheehy's manual of emergency care* (7th ed., pp. 353–360). St. Louis, MO: Elsevier Mosby.

Wolf, L., & Zimmermann, P. G. (2013). Abdominal pain and emergencies. In B. B. Hammond & P. G. Zimmermann (Eds.), *Sheehy's manual of emergency care* (7th ed., pp. 291–301). St. Louis, MO: Mosby Elsevier.

63. Following a motor vehicle collision, a patient arrives in the emergency department with a suspected blunt abdominal injury. Vital signs are BP 100/72 mm Hg, HR 106 beats/minute, RR 18 breaths/minute, T 36.2°C (97.2°F). The emergency nurse should anticipate which of the following to be performed as part of the patient's initial assessment?

A. Computed tomography scan
B. Hemoglobin and hematocrit
C. Focused assessment with sonography for trauma exam
D. Diagnostic peritoneal lavage

Rationale

A. A computed tomography (CT) scan should only be indicated for the hemodynamically stable patient. Although it is useful in determining the management of nonoperative solid organ injuries, a CT scan is not useful in identifying injuries to the diaphragm or gastrointestinal tract.

B. Hemoglobin and hematocrit will not reflect recent hemorrhage and should only be used as a baseline to compare future levels, especially if the patient needs surgery.

C. A Focused assessment with sonography for trauma (FAST) exam is a quick, accurate, and noninvasive bedside assessment tool that provides a rapid evaluation of the peritoneum and is recommended by the American College of Surgeons for the initial assessment of the patient with blunt abdominal trauma.

D. Diagnostic peritoneal lavage is an invasive procedure reserved for the hemodynamically unstable patient. Vital signs for this patient do not suggest hemodynamic instability, so a FAST exam is appropriate.

Category: Gastrointestinal, Genitourinary, Gynecology, and Obstetrical Emergencies/Gastrointestinal/Trauma

Nursing Process: Analysis

References

Bacidore, V. (2010). Abdominal and genitourinary trauma. In P. K. Howard & R. A. Steinmann (Eds.), *Sheehy's emergency nursing: Principles and practice* (6th ed., pp. 301–312). St. Louis, MO: Mosby Elsevier.

Campbell, M. R. (2007). Abdominal and urologic trauma. In K. S. Hoyt & J. Selfridge-Thomas (Eds.), *Emergency nursing core curriculum* (6th ed., pp. 781–802). St. Louis, MO: Saunders Elsevier.

---

64. A patient presents to the emergency department with frequency and urgency of urination, associated with the presence of right flank pain. On physical assessment, the patient exhibits a temperature of 38.8°C (102°F) and tenderness over the right costovertebral angle. Which of the following conditions is most consistent with the patient's signs and symptoms?

A. Bladder infection
B. Nephrolithiasis
C. Pyelonephritis
D. Urethral stricture

Rationale

A. Bladder infection does have the symptoms of frequency, urgency, and burning on urination, but a bladder infection is not usually associated with fever and tenderness over the costovertebral angle.

B. Although symptoms of nephrolithiasis can include urinary frequency and urgency, the cardinal sign is usually pain in the flank, abdomen, or groin area, depending on where the stone is located. This condition is not usually accompanied by fever.

C. Symptoms of pyelonephritis usually include pain on urination, frequency and urgency of urination, and flank or back pain on the affected side. Fever is one of the cardinal signs of pyelonephritis and can include the presence of chills. The costovertebral angle is located at the angle made by the vertebral column and the costal margin. When the affected side is percussed over the costovertebral angle, the patient with pyelonephritis will report pain.

D. Characteristic symptoms of urethral stricture are painful urination and urinary frequency and urgency. Additionally, the patient may experience the feelings of bladder fullness accompanied by the inability to urinate.

Category: Gastrointestinal, Genitourinary, Gynecology, and Obstetrical Emergencies/Genitourinary/ Infection

Nursing Process: Analysis

References

Imam, T. H. (2018). Bacterial urinary tract infections. *Merck Manual Online*. Retrieved from http://www.merckmanuals.com/professional/genitourinary-disorders/urinary-tract-infections-utis/bacterial-urinary-tract-infections-utis

Preminger, G. M. (2018). Urinary calculi. *Merck Manual Online*. Retrieved from http://www.merckmanuals.com/professional/genitourinary-disorders/urinary-calculi/urinary-calculi

Shenot, P. J. (2018). Urethral stricture. *Merck Manual Online*. Retrieved from https://www.merckmanuals.com/professional/genitourinary-disorders/penile-and-scrotal-disorders/urethral-stricture

---

65. The presence of a suspected testicular torsion is best evaluated using which diagnostic study?

A. Computed tomography scan
B. Doppler sonography
C. Urine culture and sensitivity
D. Testicular transillumination

Rationale

A. The twisting of the testicle results in the strangulation of the blood supply to the testis. A computed tomography scan cannot determine adequacy of blood flow.

B. The diagnosis of testicular torsion is made by clinical findings and Doppler sonography, which will demonstrate a lack of blood flow to the affected testicle.

C. Testicular torsion most commonly results from a congenital abnormality of the testicle. Urinary tract infection is not the underlying cause.

D. Testicular transillumination is a useful diagnostic tool when a testicular mass is suspected.

Category: Gastrointestinal, Genitourinary, Gynecology, and Obstetrical Emergencies/Genitourinary/Testicular torsion

Nursing Process: Assessment

References

Jordan, K. S. (2007). Genitourinary emergencies. In K. S. Hoyt & J. Selfridge-Thomas (Eds.), *Emergency nursing core curriculum* (6th ed., pp. 387–408). St. Louis, MO: Saunders Elsevier.

Quallich, S. (2013). Genitourinary emergencies. In B. B. Hammond & P. G. Zimmermann (Eds.), *Sheehy's manual of emergency care* (pp. 355–356). St. Louis, MO: Elsevier Mosby.

---

66. Following a motor vehicle collision, an unresponsive and intubated patient is received in the emergency department. On assessment, a rigid and bruised abdomen is noted, and a bedside ultrasound examination identifies a ruptured bladder. Based on this information, what is the emergency nurse's priority action?

A. Establish two large-caliber IVs and begin fluid resuscitation
B. Insert a urinary drainage catheter
C. Prepare the patient for computed tomography scan
D. Administer intravenous antibiotics

Rationale

A. The bladder has an extensive blood supply that is derived from the iliac artery, and injuries resulting from a motor vehicle collision are often associated with a pelvic fracture. For this reason, patients with a ruptured bladder are at risk for ineffective tissue perfusion and deficient fluid volume, so intravenous fluid resuscitation is the priority intervention to avoid the patient becoming hypovolemic.

B. Accurate measuring of urinary output is crucial, however, initiating fluid resuscitation to avoid hypovolemia is the priority intervention.

C. A bedside ultrasound exam will detect fluid, including blood, in the abdomen. A computed tomography scan will most likely be required for further evaluation, but the results of the ultrasound provide sufficient information for the nurse to recognize that the patient is at risk for hypovolemia.

D. A patient with a ruptured bladder is at an increased risk for developing peritonitis, and antibiotics are indicated; however, the prevention of hypovolemia as a result of the injury is the priority intervention.

Category: Gastrointestinal, Genitourinary, Gynecology, and Obstetrical Emergencies/Genitourinary/Trauma

Nursing Process: Intervention

References

Campbell, M. R. (2007). Abdominal and urologic trauma. In K. S. Hoyt & J. Selfridge-Thomas (Eds.), *Emergency nursing core curriculum* (6th ed., pp. 781–802). St. Louis, MO: Saunders Elsevier.

Urden, L. D., Stacy, K. M., & Lough, M. E. (2006). Trauma. In *Critical care nursing: Diagnosis and management* (6th ed., pp. 938–976). St. Louis, MO: Elsevier Mosby.

---

67. A patient presents to the emergency department complaining of lower abdominal pain and the inability to void in the past 24 hours. What is the priority intervention the emergency nurse should perform?

A. Obtaining a full set of vital signs
B. Preparing the patient for an abdominal radiograph to assess for bladder calculi
C. Insertion of urinary catheter
D. Administering an intravenous fluid bolus of 500 mL of 0.9% sodium chloride

Rationale

A. Although vital signs are important, relieving bladder pressure is the priority.

B. Bladder calculi is one of several etiologies that may be responsible for urinary retention; however, the priority intervention is to relieve the bladder pressure and prevent bladder rupture.

C. The priority intervention should be to relieve pressure within the bladder and prevent bladder rupture. This is accomplished by the insertion of an indwelling urinary catheter.

D. A lack of urinary output may be related to fluid volume status, however, the patient's absolute inability to void, along with lower abdominal discomfort, strongly suggests that urinary retention, not hypovolemia, is the underlying problem to be addressed.

Category: Gastrointestinal, Genitourinary, Gynecology, and Obstetrical Emergencies/Genitourinary/Urinary retention

Nursing Process: Intervention

Reference

Quallich, S. (2013). Genitourinary emergencies. In B. B. Hammond & P. G. Zimmermann (Eds.), *Sheehy's manual of emergency care* (7th ed., pp. 353–360). St. Louis, MO: Elsevier Mosby.

---

68. A patient who is 32 weeks pregnant is involved in a motor vehicle collision. On arrival to the emergency department, the patient is complaining of severe abdominal pain. Blood is noted on the sheets around the patient's lower extremities, and on assessment, the nurse determines the patient is bleeding vaginally. High-flow oxygen is administered via face mask. The emergency nurse's next action is to perform which of the following?

A. Insert two large-caliber IVs and administer intravenous crystalloid fluids
B. Perform a type and cross-match for a blood transfusion
C. Initiate continuous fetal monitoring
D. Prepare the patient for a cesarean section

Rationale

A. The patient likely has experienced a placental abruption as a result of the motor vehicle collision and requires the immediate administration of intravenous crystalloid fluid to prevent hypovolemia.

B. For patients with suspected placental abruption, a type and screen should be drawn and sent to the laboratory. However, in the case of emergent management, the emergency nurse should anticipate the need to administer type-specific or uncross-matched blood/blood products.

C. Fetal monitoring is important; however, initial interventions are directed toward maintaining the hemodynamic stability of the mother.

D. An emergency cesarean section may be necessary; however, maternal resuscitation is the priority.

Category: Gastrointestinal, Genitourinary, Gynecology, and Obstetrical Emergencies/Obstetrical/Abruptio placenta

Nursing Process: Intervention

References

Criddle, L. (2013). Obstetric trauma. In B. B. Hammond & P. G. Zimmermann (Eds.), *Sheehy's manual of emergency care* (7th ed., pp. 463–468). St. Louis, MO: Elsevier Mosby.

Gaufberg, S. V., & Lo, B. M. (2015, December 29). Emergent management of abruptio placentae. *Medscape*. Retrieved from http://emedicine.medscape.com/article/795514-overview#a9

Repasky, T. M. (2007). Obstetric trauma. In K. S. Hoyt & J. Selfridge-Thomas (Eds.), *Emergency nursing core curriculum* (6th ed., pp. 879–890). St. Louis, MO: Saunders Elsevier.

---

69. A patient who is diagnosed with a *Chlamydia trachomatis* vaginal infection should also be screened for what other associated sexually transmitted disease?

A. Human papillomavirus
B. Bacterial vaginosis
C. Candidiasis
D. Gonorrhea

Rationale

A. Human papillomavirus (HPV) is the most common sexually transmitted disease in the United States. HPV is frequently associated with cervical dysplasia but not with other sexually transmitted diseases.

B. Bacterial vaginosis is not a sexually transmitted disease; rather, it is caused by a disturbance in the normal vaginal flora.

C. Most cases of *Candida* infection are caused by the person's own *Candida* organisms. *Candida* yeasts usually live in the mouth, gastrointestinal tract, and vagina without causing symptoms. However, when an imbalance occurs, such as when the normal acidity of the vagina changes or when hormonal balance changes, *Candida* can multiply and build up. When this occurs, the patient can experience signs and symptoms of candidiasis.

D. Chlamydia is a sexually transmitted infection caused by the *Chlamydia trachomatis* bacterium. Chlamydia and gonorrhea often occur together.

Category: Gastrointestinal, Genitourinary, Gynecology, and Obstetrical Emergencies/Gynecology/Infection

Nursing Process: Assessment

References

Egging, D. (2013). Sexually transmitted infections. In B. B. Hammond & P. G. Zimmermann (Eds.), *Sheehy's manual of emergency care* (7th ed., pp. 361–366). St. Louis, MO: Elsevier Mosby.

Vaginal candidiasis. (2018). *Centers for Disease Control and Prevention*. Retrieved from http://www.cdc.gov/fungal/diseases/candidiasis/genital/index.html

---

70. The emergency nurse is caring for a victim of sexual assault. Which of the following statements made by the victim indicates the need for further education regarding the sexual assault examination process?

A. "Once the exam is finished, I'd like to take a shower."
B. "I am so anxious, I don't know how I will get through all of this."
C. "I really don't want the police in the room with me during the exam."
D. "I will need to be seen again in about 1 week to have more cultures taken."

Rationale

A. Following the examination and collection of evidence, the patient is allowed to shower, and clean clothing should be made available.

B. Being anxious is an expected response to the entire sexual assault experience. The patient may need emotional support, but more education about the actual process will probably not act to lessen the anxiety the patient is experiencing at this time.

C. Unless the patient requests an officer to be present during the examination, it is not done.

D. Sexually transmitted organisms such as chlamydia and gonorrhea that are transmitted during a sexual assault may not be present in sufficient quantity to yield a positive culture result at the time of initial examination. The patient should be instructed to obtain follow-up care within 1 week to obtain additional culture specimens. If the patient received prophylactic treatment, cultures should be obtained if the patient reports having symptoms.

Category: Gastrointestinal, Genitourinary, Gynecology, and Obstetrical Emergencies/Gynecology/Sexual assault/battery

Nursing Process: Evaluation

Reference

Ruiz-Contreras, A. (2010). Abuse and neglect/sexual assault. In P. K. Howard & J. Selfridge-Thomas (Eds.), *Sheehy's emergency nursing: Principles and practice* (6th ed., pp. 51–77). St. Louis, MO: Mosby Elsevier.

---

71. A patient who is 6 days postpartum and breastfeeding presents to the emergency department complaining of fever, with right-sided breast redness and tenderness. The patient is diagnosed with mastitis. In addition to antibiotic therapy, which of the following should be included in the discharge instructions for this patient?

A. Avoid hand-expressing or using a mechanical breast pump
B. Have the baby nurse from the unaffected breast only
C. Stop breastfeeding and supplement feedings with formula until the infection clears
D. Apply a warm compress to the breast before breastfeeding

Rationale

A. Emptying the breast is a important component in the management of mastitis. The use of a hand or mechanical pump is recommended, particularly if the infant is unable to effectively nurse.

B. Breastfeeding should be continued because treatment involves emptying the breast. Mastitis does not change the taste or nutritional value of breast milk.

C. Breastfeeding should be continued because treatment includes emptying the breast.

D. Warm compresses or a hot shower will help alleviate symptoms associated with mastitis and facilitate milk flow.

Category: Gastrointestinal, Genitourinary, Gynecology, and Obstetrical Emergencies/Obstetrical/Postpartum infection

Nursing Process: Intervention

References

Cabou, A., Babineau, S., & St. Anna, L. (2011). What's the best way to relieve mastitis in breastfeeding mothers? *Journal of Family Practice, 60*(9), 551–552.

Wong, A. W., & Lo, B. M. (2015, December 5). Postpartum infections clinical presentation. *Medscape*. Retrieved from http://emedicine.medscape.com/article/796892-clinical#b2

---

72. A patient presents to the emergency department with symptoms of left lower quadrant abdominal cramping with frequent episodes of blood and mucus-containing diarrhea. The symptoms have been present for the past 3 weeks and the patient has noticed a recent weight loss. The emergency nurse anticipates the patient will most likely need further evaluation for which disorder?

A. Ulcerative colitis
B. Colon cancer
C. Salmonella infection
D. Crohn's disease

Rationale

A. Ulcerative colitis is an inflammatory condition that affects the large intestine. Left lower quadrant abdominal pain with bloody diarrhea, a result of the effects of the disease on the lining of the colon, are hallmark signs of the disease. Patients can pass between 10 and 20 liquid stools per day. Additional symptoms include weight loss, fever, and tachycardia.

B. A change in bowel habits and weight loss, which may include constipation and/or diarrhea, are primary symptoms associated with colon-rectal cancers; however, the diarrhea associated with colon cancer is less frequent than that with ulcerative colitis and does not contain mucus. Abdominal cramping with colon cancer is more likely to be associated with a cancerous lesion causing a bowel obstruction.

C. Infectious diarrhea, such as that caused by a salmonella exposure, is characterized by cramping, colicky abdominal pain, and bloody diarrhea. These symptoms usually resolve within 24 hours.

D. Crohns' disease can be characterized by cramping abdominal pain, which is more likely to be in the right lower quadrant. Bloody, mucus-containing stools are not typical for a patient with Crohn's disease.

Category: Gastrointestinal, Genitourinary, Gynecology, and Obstetrical Emergencies/Gastrointestinal/Inflammatory bowel disease

Nursing Process: Assessment

References

Beitz, J. M. (2014). Management of patient with intestinal and rectal disorders. In J. L. Hinkle & K. H. Cheever (Eds.), *Brunner and Suddarth's textbook of medical-surgical nursing* (13th ed., pp. 1285–1333). Philadelphia, PA: Lippincott Williams & Wilkins.

McCance, K. L., & Huether, S. E. (2006). Alterations of digestive function. In *Pathophysiology: The biologic basis for disease in adults and children* (pp. 1385–1445). Philadelphia, PA: Elsevier.

Wolf, L., & Zimmermann, P. G. (2013). Abdominal pain and emergencies. In B. B. Hammond & P. G. Zimmermann (Eds.), *Sheehy's manual of emergency care* (7th ed., pp. 291–301). St. Louis, MO: Elsevier Mosby.

73. A woman who is 10 weeks pregnant presents to the emergency department complaining of vaginal spotting with mild abdominal cramping and is discharged to home after a diagnosis of threatened abortion is made. Which of the following statements, made by the patient, indicates a correct understanding of their discharge instruction?

A. "I will keep a count of the number of tampons I use to determine how much I'm bleeding."
B. "I will need to stay on bed rest for at least a day or two."
C. "I can expect the bleeding to get heavier in a day or two."
D. "While I'm on bed rest, my partner and I can have sexual intercourse as long as it isn't too rough."

Rationale

A. The patient should be instructed to count sanitary pads. Tampon use is discouraged in the presence of a threatened abortion.

B. A patient who is experiencing a threatened abortion will be instructed to maintain bed rest for 24–48 hours or until the bleeding stops.

C. An increase in the amount of bleeding or the passage of tissue may indicate the loss of the pregnancy, and the patient should immediately contact the obstetrician or return to the emergency department.

D. Sexual intercourse should be avoided as long as the bleeding and cramping continue and the patient is on bed rest. Intercourse can worsen cramping and bleeding or introduce infection if the cervical os begins to open.

Category: Gastrointestinal, Genitourinary, Gynecology, and Obstetrical Emergencies/Obstetrical/Threatened/spontaneous abortion

Nursing Process: Evaluation

References

Jordan, K. S. (2007). Obstetric and gynecologic emergencies. In K. S. Hoyt & J. Selfridge-Thomas (Eds.), *Emergency nursing core curriculum* (6th ed., pp. 536–570). St. Louis, MO: Saunders Elsevier.

Mason, D. L. (2010). Obstetric emergencies. In P. K. Howard & R. A. Steinmann (Eds.), *Sheehy's emergency nursing: Principles and practice* (6th ed., pp. 619–629). St. Louis, MO: Saunders Elsevier.

---

74. When suspecting the presence of child maltreatment or neglect in a patient, the emergency nurse is required to:

A. document the names of the suspected abusers in the medical record.
B. inform the parent of the police notification.
C. report the suspected abuse or neglect to the police and child protective services.
D. review the pediatrician or family physician records.

Rationale

A. Documentation of facts is important in the potential child maltreatment or neglect case. The name of the abuser may or may not be known, however, the proper local authorities must be notified of the suspected abuse or neglect.

B. In some cases, this may not be beneficial to the welfare of the child. The parent may attempt to leave the emergency department if notified of the report to police or child protective services.

C. Nurses are mandatory reporters for suspected child maltreatment or neglect. Failure to report may result in possible civil or criminal charges being brought against the nurse.

D. A child's prior pediatrician records or visits may be researched in a case of child maltreatment or neglect, but only after obtaining permission from the provider. Nurses are mandated to report to the police and child protective services in all cases of suspected abuse or neglect.

Category (Pediatric): Psychosocial and Medical Emergencies/Psychosocial/Abuse and neglect

Nursing Process: Analysis

References

Black, A. (2010). Child abuse and neglect. In P. K. Howard & R. A. Steinmann (Eds.), *Sheehy's emergency nursing: Principles and practice* (6th ed., pp. 652–665). St. Louis, MO: Mosby Elsevier.

Black, A. (2012). Child maltreatment. In *Emergency Nursing Pediatric Course: Provider manual* (4th ed., pp. 343–357). Des Plaines, IL: Author. Emergency Nurses Association.

Cohen, S. (2013). Abuse and neglect. In B. B. Hammond & P. G. Zimmermann (Eds.), *Sheehy's manual of emergency care* (7th ed., pp. 521–530). St. Louis, MO: Elsevier Mosby.

---

75. A patient is brought to the emergency department after exhibiting aggressive behavior toward family members. To assess the patient's current mental state, which question would be most important for the emergency nurse to ask the patient?

A. "What are the voices telling you to do?"
B. "What medications are you currently taking?"
C. "What past medical history do you have?"
D. "What brought this behavior on today?"

Rationale

A. Safety is the first priority for patients exhibiting aggressive or violent behavior. Establishing details of the patient's hallucinations yields information into their suicidal or homicidal ideations. It is important to know what auditory hallucinations may be occurring for the patient who is aggressive or violent so that the proper security measures can be initiated.

B. Although determining the patient's current medications is an important question, it would be more important to determine the patient's current mental health status before asking their current medication history.

C. Past medical history is an important question to ask the patient because medical problems can result in psychiatric symptoms in some patients. It is important, however, to quickly establish the patient's current thought processes in relation to their current aggressive behavior.

D. Inquiring about precipitating events leading to the current behavior is important, however, the immediate safety of the patient and others should be uppermost in the mind of the emergency nurse.

Category: Psychosocial and Medical Emergencies/Psychosocial/Aggressive/violent behavior

Nursing Process: Assessment

Reference

Citrome, L. L. (2015) Aggression. *Medscape drugs, diseases, and procedures.* Retrieved from http://emedicine.medscape.com/article/288689-overview#a4

76. A 65-year-old female reports a history of generalized anxiety disorder that is controlled with 0.5 mg of alprazolam (Xanax) three times daily as needed. Which of the following patient statements requires additional follow-up and patient education by the emergency nurse?

A. "I do not take the Xanax every day."
B. "I only take the Xanax before participating in stressful events, such as being in large crowds, in order to prevent anxiety."
C. "I drink several glasses of wine in one setting on a regular basis."
D. "I eat a lot of dairy products frequently and sometimes take the Xanax with milk."

Rationale

A. The medication is prescribed "as needed," so the patient is correct to only take it when needed.

B. Taking Xanax proactively instead of reactively is appropriate use of the medication and may help prevent dependence.

C. Xanax is a benzodiazepine. Alcohol may intensify the effects of benzodiazepines, increasing the risk of falls and respiratory depression. The patient should be cautioned not to drink alcohol with the medication.

D. There is no contraindication to combining dairy products with benzodiazepines.

Category: Psychosocial and Medical Emergencies/Psychosocial/Anxiety/panic
Nursing Process: Evaluation

Reference

DeSelm, T. M. (2016). Mood and anxiety disorders. In J. E. Tintinalli, J. Stapczynski, O. Ma, D. M. Yealy, & G. D. Meckler (Eds.), *Tintinalli's emergency medicine: A comprehensive study guide* (8th ed., pp. 1963–1968). Retrieved from http://accessemergencymedicine.mhmedical.com/content.aspx?bookid=1658&Sectionid=109448311

---

77. Parents arrive to triage with their child, stating that the child has demonstrated recent behavior changes that include extreme anger with family members, no desire to complete required tasks (attend school or do chores), racing thoughts with rapid speech, and impulsive actions. The emergency nurse will be most concerned about which type of psychiatric disorder being demonstrated by the patient?

A. Psychosis
B. Attention-deficit hyperactivity disorder
C. Bipolar disorder
D. Panic disorder

Rationale

A. Psychosis is an altered mental state in which the child experiences a variety of disturbances that affect their perceptions of reality. The presentation includes hallucinations, delusions, and disorganized speech patterns. New-onset psychosis in children is uncommon but may be seen with other psychiatric disorders such as severe anxiety, posttraumatic stress disorder, or depression, or it can be related to an organic cause.

B. Attention-deficit hyperactivity disorder (ADHD) is characterized by symptoms of inattention, hyperactivity, and impulsiveness. The child may frequently interrupt or intrude on others, have trouble completing tasks, or become easily distracted. It is estimated that two children in every classroom have been diagnosed with ADHD.

C. Bipolar disorder is seen in many children who display inability to function in daily life because of frequent mood swings, often going from a depressive state to a manic state (speaking quickly or racing thoughts). Children will lose the ability to complete daily tasks such as going to school and completing chores, and they may experience mood swings with varying severity depending on the age of the child.

D. Panic disorder is a severe form of anxiety. The presentation includes crying, possibly clinging to a parent or loved one, symptoms of chest pain or discomfort, choking sensation, sweating, dizziness, lightheadedness, fear of dying, and a racing pulse.

Category (Pediatric): Psychosocial and Medical Emergencies/Psychosocial/Bipolar disorder
Nursing Process: Assessment

References

Gagnon, L. (2010). Behavioral health emergencies. In P. K. Howard & R. A. Steinmann (Eds.), *Sheehy's emergency nursing: Principles and practice* (6th ed., pp. 677–688). St. Louis, MO: Mosby Elsevier.
Hart, B. (2012). Behavioral emergencies. In *Emergency Nursing Pediatric Course: Provider manual* (4th ed., pp. 317–328). Des Plaines, IL: Emergency Nurses Association.
Manton, A. (2013). Mental health emergencies. In B. B. Hammond & P. G. Zimmermann (Eds.), *Sheehy's manual of emergency care* (7th ed., pp. 505–520). St. Louis, MO: Elsevier Mosby.

---

78. Which diagnostic test should the emergency nurse anticipate to be performed in a patient with bipolar disorder who has been receiving antipsychotic medications for treatment of acute mania?

A. Complete blood count
B. Liver function testing
C. Bladder scan
D. 12-lead electrocardiogram

Rationale

A. Though clozapine (Clozaril), an atypical or second-generation antipsychotic, has the risk of causing neutropenia, this is not associated with all antipsychotics. Performing a complete blood count would not be the most important diagnostic test while in the emergency department.

B. Antipsychotic medications are not commonly associated with hepatic injury. Obtaining a 12-lead electrocardiogram (ECG) and conducting continuous ECG monitoring is more important.

C. Though antipsychotic medications can cause urinary retention and other anticholinergic side effects, this would not be the most important diagnostic test to perform.

D. Most antipsychotic medications can result in prolongation of the QT interval, which can lead to a life-threatening dysrhythmia. Performing a 12-lead ECG and initiating continuous ECG monitoring in a bipolar patient who is exhibiting acute mania is warranted.

Category: Psychosocial and Medical Emergencies/Psychosocial/Bipolar disorder
Nursing Process: Intervention

References

Comes, J. A., Rund, D. A., & Lotfi-Fard, B. (2015). Schizophrenia and bipolar disorder. In Wolfson (Ed.), *Harwood-Nuss' clinical practice of emergency medicine* (6th ed., 806–807). Philadelphia, PA: Wolters Kluwer.
Woo, T. M. (2016). Drugs affecting the central nervous system. In T. M. Woo & M. V. Robinson (Eds.), *Pharmacotherapeutics for advanced practice nurse prescribers* (4th ed., 225–294). Philadelphia, PA: F. A. Davis.

---

79. On review of a patient's current medications, the emergency nurse identifies that the patient has been prescribed an alternative drug for depression. Which of the following is an alternative medication used in the treatment of depression?

A. Bupropion (Wellbutrin)
B. Citalopram (Celexa)
C. Fluoxetine (Prozac)
D. Sertraline (Zoloft)

Rationale

A. Bupropion is considered an alternative drug for treatment of depression. It may also be used to treat attention deficit hyperactivity disorder or to help people quit smoking by decreasing cravings and the effects of nicotine withdrawal. The medication may be used to prevent autumn–winter seasonal depression (seasonal affective disorder). It also may be used with other medications to treat bipolar disorder (depressive phase) and to treat anxiety in people with depression. It is not considered an atypical treatment or frontline drug for depression.

B. Citalopram is a typical antidepressant and is often a frontline treatment for new-onset depression.

C. Fluoxetine is a typical antidepressant and is often a frontline treatment for new-onset depression.

D. Sertraline is a typical antidepressant and is often a frontline treatment for new-onset depression.

Category: Psychosocial and Medical Emergencies/Psychosocial/Depression
Nursing Process: Intervention

References

Gagnon, L. (2010). Behavioral health emergencies. In P. K. Howard & R. A. Steinmann (Eds.), *Sheehy's emergency nursing: Principles and practice* (6th ed., pp. 677–688). St. Louis, MO: Mosby Elsevier.
Manton, A. (2013). Mental health emergencies. In B. B. Hammond & P. G. Zimmermann (Eds.), *Sheehy's manual of emergency care* (7th ed., pp. 505–520). St. Louis, MO: Elsevier Mosby.

---

80. Which of the following interventions would be appropriate for an emergency nurse to perform following the transfer of a patient? The patient has experienced an acute psychotic episode and states, "I'm coming back here when I get released from the hospital, and I am going to kill Jane Smith."

A. Ignore the threat because this is normal behavior in patients who are psychotic
B. Alert proper law enforcement authorities
C. Tell the patient that it is inappropriate to make this statement
D. Request that the hospital chaplain come and talk to the patient

Rationale

A. It would be egregious to ignore something of this nature and not report the threat to both the proper authorities and the individual being named.

B. It is important that proper authorities be notified when patients make statements that are very specific in nature and when they name a particular person. That person should be aware of the threat and should be provided the proper protection.

C. Informing the patient that this is inappropriate will provide no protective care to the individual named and would not be of any benefit to the patient in their current mental state of being.

D. The hospital chaplain would not be an appropriate person to intervene and speak to the patient regarding the threat they have made. This could be an idle threat, or it could be real. It is not appropriate for nonmedical individuals to determine whether the patient's threat is real.

Category: Psychosocial and Medical Emergencies/Psychosocial/Homicidal ideation

Nursing Process: Intervention

References

Citrome, L. L. (2015). Aggression. *Medscape drugs, diseases, and procedures.* Retrieved from http://emedicine.medscape.com/article/288689-overview#a4

Manton, A. (2013). Mental health emergencies. In B. B. Hammond & P. G. Zimmermann (Eds.), *Sheehy's manual of emergency care* (7th ed., pp. 505–520). St. Louis, MO: Elsevier Mosby.

---

81. A homeless patient arrives in the emergency department by emergency medical services after being found wandering on the street and talking to himself. The patient is in possession of proper identification but will not answer to their name. Speech is clear, and the patient displays no signs of aggressive behavior, but will not make eye contact with the emergency nurse or follow simple commands. Which of the following signs and symptoms would alert the emergency nurse to an organic cause for their psychosis?

A. Signs of trauma
B. Normal vital signs
C. Auditory hallucinations
D. Clear speech patterns

Rationale

A. Any signs of trauma, including obvious fractures or contusions, would require further investigation to determine whether the patient's behavior has a psychiatric or an organic basis.

B. Abnormal vital signs may indicate an organic cause of an altered mental response—for example, hypoxia or hypotension.

C. Nonauditory hallucinations may be caused hypoxia or hypoglycemia.

D. Impaired speech may be a sign of an organic cause of a possible traumatic brain injury or a cerebral vascular incident.

Category: Psychosocial and Medical Emergencies/Psychosocial/Psychosis

Nursing Process: Analysis

Reference

Deal, N., & Matorin, A. (2015). Stabilization and management of the acutely agitated or psychotic patient. *Emergency Medicine Clinics of North America, 33*, 739–752. https://doi.org/10.1016/j.emc.2015.07.003

---

82. A patient presents to triage with a complaint of a headache and appears anxious and restless. The patient tells the emergency nurse that the "man at the desk" has followed the patient from Russia, where the patient worked for the Central Intelligence Agency, and that the headache began after the tracking chip implanted in their brain was activated. The nurse observes no one at the desk, and the patient has identification that indicates a local address and that they are a student at a nearby college. There is no indication of recent travel or corroboration of the information. The emergency nurse suspects the cause of the patient's symptoms is related to:

A. an anxiety attack.
B. migraine headache.
C. dementia.
D. psychosis.

Rationale

A. Anxiety attacks are characterized by tachycardia, palpitations, hyperventilation, and diaphoresis. The patient is not demonstrating these symptoms. Although the patient is anxious, it appears they are having other symptoms that do not correspond to anxiety and indicate a more severe mental illness.

B. Other than the report of a headache, there are no other signs or symptoms consistent with migraine, such as a throbbing pain, photophobia, or nausea. Therefore, a migraine headache is not likely the cause of their symptoms.

C. A patient with dementia will appear disoriented, repeat the same information, have difficulty finding the right words to express their thoughts, and not be able to follow a conversation. The patient may be younger than most patients diagnosed with dementia, and although the patient is confused, a dementia diagnosis does not adequately explain the patient's symptoms.

D. Psychosis is a severe mental disorder in which a person loses the ability to recognize reality or relate to others. Symptoms include being paranoid, having false ideas about what is taking place or who one is, and seeing, hearing, or feeling things that are not there. Other associated mental disorders are schizophrenia and bipolar disorder.

Category: Psychosocial and Medical Emergencies/Psychosocial/Psychosis
Nursing Process: Analysis

References

Manton, A. P. (2013). Mental health emergencies. In B. B. Hammond & P. G. Zimmermann (Eds.), *Sheehy's manual of emergency care* (7th ed., pp. 505–520). St. Louis, MO: Elsevier Mosby.
Psychosis. (2015). *PubMed Health.* Retrieved from https://www.ncbi.nlm.nih.gov/pubmedhealth/PMHT0024802/
Rice, K. L., & Albright, M. (2013). Geriatric considerations in emergency nursing. In B. B. Hammond & P. G. Zimmermann (Eds.), *Sheehy's manual of emergency care* (7th ed., pp. 571–592). St. Louis, MO: Elsevier Mosby.
Walsh, R. (2013). Neurologic emergencies. In B. B. Hammond & P. G. Zimmermann (Eds.), *Sheehy's manual of emergency care* (7th ed., pp. 265–274). St. Louis, MO: Elsevier Mosby.

---

83. Ziprasidone (Geodon) is most appropriate for which of the following psychiatric scenarios? The adult patient:

A. who is exhibiting acute depressive disorder and is tearful and sobbing.
B. who is exhibiting acute manic behavior, is in handcuffs, and is being accompanied by police.
C. who is having auditory hallucinations and is being told not to move.
D. who is experiencing extrapyramidal effects related to their psychiatric medications.

Rationale

A. Antimanic drugs are not appropriate in the treatment of depression.

B. Ziprasidone is classified as an antimanic drug that has a rapid onset of action.

C. Auditory hallucinations, without evidence of mania, are not an indication for ziprasidone.

D. This patient would not benefit from receiving an antimanic drug. Extrapyramidal symptoms are treated with benztropine (Cogentin) or diphenhydramine (Benadryl).

Category: Psychosocial and Medical Emergencies/Psychosocial/Situational crisis

Nursing Process: Assessment

Reference

Karch, A. M. (2013). Psychotherapeutic agents. In *Focus on nursing pharmacology* (6th ed., pp. 357–375). Philadelphia, PA: Lippincott Williams & Wilkins.

---

84. A patient presents to the emergency department (ED) voicing thoughts of suicidal ideation. Why is it important to identify and address medical issues before treating the mental health issue?
   A. **Medical problems can mimic mental health problems.**
   B. Mental health problems do not lead to serious illness.
   C. Medical problems can be resolved more quickly than behavioral problems.
   D. Once in the ED, the patient is safe from suicide.

Rationale

A. It is important to rule out potential medical problems that may be life threatening and require immediate correction or patient stabilization. Medical problems can cause behavioral issues and can mimic mental health problems.

B. Mental health problems are true emergencies and may be caused by existing medical health problems.

C. Medical problems may be resolved quickly in some cases, but the reason for medical clearance is to rule out a medical cause for the mental health issue.

D. Patient safety must be ensured at all times during the ED visit. The patient remains at risk for suicide as long as they are having suicidal ideations.

Category: Psychosocial and Medical Emergencies/Psychosocial/Suicidal ideation

Nursing Process: Analysis

Reference

Antai-Otong, D. (2016). What every ED nurse should know about suicide risk assessment. *Journal of Emergency Nursing, 42*(1), 31–36. https://org/10.1016/j.jen.2016.01.001

---

85. A patient presents to the emergency department with sudden onset of lip swelling, facial edema, and throat tightness. Vital signs are BP 90/60 mm Hg, HR 127 beats/minute, RR 22 breaths/minute, T 38.6°C (97.8°F). The emergency nurse anticipates which of the following to be administered to this patient for their signs and symptoms?

A. Epinephrine
B. High-flow oxygen
C. Corticosteroids
D. Aerosol albuterol

Rationale

A. The patient is experiencing an allergic reaction with possible angioedema. The administration of epinephrine promotes peripheral vasoconstriction and bronchodilation and inhibits further release of mediators immediately on entering the bloodstream. The most common causes of an allergic reaction include the administration of antibiotics, bee or wasp stings, and exposure to peanuts.

B. Administration of high-flow oxygen to support oxygenation and treat hypoxia is important but will not act to reverse the signs and symptoms of lip swelling, facial edema, and throat tightness that the patient is experiencing. It is important to treat the patient's allergic reaction symptoms as quickly as possible to minimize the risk of complete airway compromise.

C. Symptoms of an allergic reaction can occur quickly and progress rapidly (anaphylaxis), so prioritizing therapeutic interventions is imperative. Although corticosteroids may be administered to prevent a possible late biphasic reaction, they have no immediate effect in the treatment of an allergic reaction.

D. Administration of albuterol will assist with treating bronchodilation and aid in the patient's breathing and increased gas exchange.

Category: Psychosocial and Medical Emergencies/Medical/Allergic reactions and anaphylaxis
Nursing Process: Intervention

References

Calder, S. A. (2013). Shock. In B. B. Hammond & P. G. Zimmermann (Eds.), *Sheehy's manual of emergency care* (7th ed., pp. 213–222). St. Louis, MO: Elsevier Mosby.

Wade, J., & Barkley, T. W. (2015). Hereditary angioedema: An emergency nursing perspective. *Journal of Emergency Nursing, 41*(5), 391–395. https://doi.org/10.1016/j.jen.2015.02.001

---

86. A patient presents to the emergency department stating they were hunting the previous day in a heavily wooded area. This morning the patient noticed a red, itchy rash with many blisters covering their face, neck, back, and arms. The emergency provider diagnoses the patient with poison ivy. What medication should the emergency nurse anticipate will be prescribed for this patient?

A. A narcotic analgesic
B. An oral antibiotic
C. A topical antifungal agent
D. An oral corticosteroid

Rationale

A. Narcotic pain medications are typically not prescribed in the treatment of poison ivy and may increase the itching the patient is experiencing. Acetaminophen or ibuprofen should be sufficient for the control of any discomfort the patient is experiencing.

B. There are no signs of a bacterial infection at this time, so an antibiotic is not indicated.

C. An antifungal agent would not be the appropriate treatment for poison ivy exposure.

D. The patient's rash is widespread, so it is likely that they will be prescribed an oral corticosteroid such a prednisone.

Category: Psychosocial and Medical Emergencies/Medical/Allergic reactions and anaphylaxis

Nursing Process: Intervention

Reference

Poison ivy rash. (2015). *MayoClinic.org*. Retrieved from http://www.mayoclinic.org/diseases-conditions/poison-ivy/basics/treatment/con-20025866

---

87. Which statement is correct regarding hemophilia disorders?

A. There is an increased incidence of hemophilia in females.
B. Platelet administration is a common treatment in hemophilia.
C. Hemophilia is an inherited sex-linked genetic disorder.
D. Two common triggers of hemophilia are hypoxia and dehydration.

Rationale

A. Hemophilia is a sex-linked genetic disorder and is very rare in females.

B. Treatment for hemophilia may include replacement of factor and administration of plasma or cryoprecipitate. Platelets are administered as part of the treatment for severe thrombocytopenia.

C. Hemophilia is an inherited sex-linked disease that alters factor production and function. The mother is the carrier and passes the trait on to her children. Active disease is most often expressed in males.

D. Hypoxia and dehydration are common triggers of sickle cell episode. Complications from hemophilia are often seen with trauma and invasive procedures.

Category: Psychosocial and Medical Emergencies/Medical/Blood dyscrasias: Hemophilia

Nursing Process: Assessment

References

Hunt, S. (2007). Hematologic/oncologic emergencies. In K. S. Hoyt & J. Selfridge-Thomas (Eds.), *Emergency nursing core curriculum* (6th ed., pp. 409–437). St. Louis, MO: Saunders Elsevier.

Smith, D. (2010). Hematologic and oncologic emergencies. In P. K. Howard & R. A. Steinmann (Eds.), *Sheehy's emergency nursing: Principles and practice* (6th ed., pp. 554–563). St. Louis, MO: Mosby Elsevier.

---

88. An elderly patient arrives to the emergency department following a fall at home. The patient's daily medication includes clopidogrel (Plavix) 300 mg daily. The patient is diagnosed with an intracranial bleed. The emergency nurse anticipates which of the following actions to be taken?

A. Administer vitamin K intravenous (IV) immediately
B. Administer protamine sulfate IV immediately
C. Discontinue the clopidogrel (Plavix) immediately
D. Decrease in the next dose of clopidogrel (Plavix)

Rationale

A. Vitamin K is the antidote for warfarin (Coumadin). There is no antidote for the presence of an excessive amount of clopidogrel in the bloodstream.

B. Protamine sulfate is the antidote for heparin. There is no antidote for the presence of an excessive amount of clopidogrel in the bloodstream.

C. Clopidogrel is an antiplatelet drug given as a 300 mg loading dose and then administered at 75 mg daily. The patient has been taking an excessive amount of the medication, resulting in the intracranial hemorrhage secondary to the fall. There is no chemical antidote or reversal agent for clopidogrel. The clopidogrel should be discontinued immediately.

D. The daily dose of clopidogrel is 75 mg, yet this patient has been taking 300 mg daily. The clopidogrel should be discontinued immediately. However, it can take up to 5 days for platelet aggregation to begin to occur following discontinuation of the medication.

Category (Geriatric): Psychosocial and Medical Emergencies/Medical/Blood dyscrasias: Other coagulopathies

Nursing Process: Intervention

Reference

Wolters Kluwer. (2017). Clopidogrel bisulphate. In *Nursing 2017 drug handbook* (pp. 371–373). Philadelphia, PA: Author.

---

89. A patient with a history of leukemia and who is currently undergoing chemotherapy treatment is being discharged from the emergency department (ED) following a facial laceration repair. Which statement best indicates to the emergency nurse the patient's understanding of the discharge instructions?

A. "I should return to the ED immediately for a temperature of 37.3°C (99.1°F)."
B. "I might not see the common signs of infection."
C. "Because I have a high white blood cell count, I am protected from getting an infection."
D. "Pus will be expected during the healing because of my high white blood cell count."

Rationale

A. A temperature of 37.3°C (99.1°F) is not considered a fever. In most cases, fever is defined as a temperature of 38°C (100.4°F) or greater, in which case the patient should seek medical care.

B. Patients who are immune-compromised are generally neutropenic and are at great risk for infection. Because the body's phagocytic response is impaired, the typical signs of infection, such as redness, swelling, or pus, may not be seen in this patient population.

C. Patients on chemotherapy have low white blood cell counts.

D. Pus is a product of phagocytosis. Patients on chemotherapy are generally neutropenic and may not experience phagocytosis even if they have an infection.

Category: Psychosocial and Medical Emergencies/Medical/Blood dyscrasias: Leukemia

Nursing Process: Evaluation

Reference

Hunt, S. (2007). Hematologic/oncologic emergencies. In K. S. Hoyt & J. Selfridge-Thomas (Eds.), *Emergency nursing core curriculum* (6th ed., pp. 409–437). St. Louis, MO: Saunders Elsevier.

---

90. An African American patient presents to emergency department triage with a complaint of chest pain, shortness of breath, fever, cough, and wheezing. The patient's medications include lisinopril, metformin, and hydroxyurea. The patient is a poor historian and is refusing to answer questions. The emergency nurse should be most concerned about which potential diagnosis for this patient?

A. Acute chest syndrome
B. Acute myocardial infarction
C. Chronic obstructive bronchitis
D. Superior vena cava syndrome

Rationale

A. The patient presentation, in conjunction with their race and current medication history (hydroxyurea), is consistent with a diagnosis of sickle cell disease. Acute chest syndrome (ACS) is one of the leading causes of mortality in patients with sickle cell disease. Symptoms of ACS include chest pain, dyspnea, cough, and hypoxemia, accompanied by wheezing and pulmonary infiltrates on chest radiograph. ACS can quickly progress to acute pulmonary failure. Hydroxyurea stimulates the production of fetal hemoglobin, providing for increased oxygen-carrying hemoglobin in the patient, and is an effective treatment modality for patients with sickle cell disease.

B. Fever, cough, and wheezing are not usually associated with the presence of an acute myocardial infarction.

C. Chronic obstructive bronchitis, a component of chronic obstructive pulmonary disease, does not usually present with chest pain or fever. The adventitious sound that is normally heard with this process is rhonchi. Wheezing can be associated with emphysema, another component of chronic obstructive pulmonary disease.

D. Superior vena cava syndrome is a cancer complication that occurs when a mass obstructs the superior vena cava. An obstruction occurs either inside or outside the vena cava and results in reduced blood flow back to the heart. Symptoms include facial, neck, and arm swelling, chest pain, shortness of breath, and hoarseness. Cerebral edema and airway obstruction can also occur. Fever and wheezing are not symptoms of superior vena cava syndrome.

Category: Psychosocial and Medical Emergencies/Medical/Blood dyscrasias: Sickle cell crisis

Nursing Process: Analysis

References

Carringer, C. J., & Hammond, B. (2013). Hematologic and immunologic emergencies. In B. B. Hammond & P. G. Zimmermann (Eds.), *Sheehy's manual of emergency care* (7th ed., pp. 245–254). St. Louis, MO: Elsevier Mosby.

Smith, D. (2010). Hematologic and oncologic emergencies. In P. K. Howard & R. A. Steinmann (Eds.), *Sheehy's emergency nursing: Principles and practice* (6th ed., pp. 554–563). St. Louis, MO: Mosby Elsevier.

91. Which of the following laboratory test values would alert an emergency nurse that a patient with disseminated intravascular coagulation is beginning to improve?

A. Elevated D-dimer
B. Increased platelet count
C. Prolonged partial thromboplastin time
D. Increased prothrombin

Rationale

A. Disseminated intravascular coagulation (DIC) can cause an elevation in both D-dimer and fibrin degradation factor. A continual D-dimer increase would indicate progression of the disease, not an improvement in the patient's DIC.

B. DIC causes a massive consumption of platelets, which leads to the extensive clotting that occurs; therefore, an increase in the patient's platelet count would indicate that the DIC is lessening and the patient is beginning to improve.

C. The pathophysiology of DIC is one of a prolonged partial thromboplastin time (PTT); therefore, a continued prolonged PTT would not indicate improvement in the patient's condition, but rather that the DIC is continuing.

D. An increase or prolongation of the prothrombin would be a pathophysiological response, not a physiological response, and therefore would not indicate patient improvement.

Category: Psychosocial and Medical Emergencies/Medical/Disseminated intravascular coagulation (DIC)
Nursing Process: Evaluation

References

Levi, M. (2017). Disseminated intravascular coagulation workup. *Medscape*. Retrieved from http://emedicine.medscape.com/article/199627-workup#c6

Smith, D. (2010). Hematologic and oncologic emergencies. In P. K. Howard & R. A. Steinmann (Eds.), *Sheehy's emergency nursing: Principles and practice* (6th ed., pp. 554–563). St. Louis, MO: Mosby Elsevier.

---

92. The emergency nurse anticipates heparin to be administered for the treatment of disseminated intravascular coagulation in which of the following situations?

A. Postpartum bleeding
B. Multiple traumatic injuries
C. Excessive fibrin that has caused digital ischemia
D. Envenomation from a snake bite

Rationale

A. A patient with disseminated intravascular coagulation (DIC) that results in excessive bleeding regardless of the cause (in this case, postpartum bleeding) would not benefit from the use of heparin because of the continued increased risk of bleeding.

B. A patient with DIC that triggers excessive bleeding regardless of the cause (in this case, multiple traumatic injuries) would not benefit from the use of heparin because of the increased risk of bleeding.

C. A patient with DIC and excessive fibrin that has caused acral cyanosis (bluish or purple discoloration) and ischemia in the digits, which may result in a loss of the digit, may benefit from the administration of heparin.

D. A patient with DIC that triggers excessive bleeding regardless of the cause (in this case, a snake bite) would not benefit from the use of heparin because of the increased risk of bleeding.

Category: Psychosocial and Medical Emergencies/Medical/Disseminated intravascular coagulation (DIC)

Nursing Process: Intervention

Reference

Smith, D. (2010). Hematologic and oncologic emergencies. In P. K. Howard & R. A. Steinmann (Eds.), *Sheehy's emergency nursing: Principles and practice* (6th ed., pp. 554–563). St. Louis, MO: Mosby Elsevier.

---

93. A patient complains of transient palpitations and occasional numbness and tingling of their fingers and nose. While vital signs are being obtained, the emergency nurse observes a sudden onset of carpal spasms on the arm on which the blood pressure cuff is being inflated. The nurse recognizes that this finding is consistent with the presence of:

A. hypocalcemia.
B. hypercalcemia.
C. hypokalemia.
D. hyperkalemia.

Rationale

A. Hypocalcemia results in excitation of the nervous system, including tetanic contractions of skeletal muscle. This response is referred to as Trousseau's sign.

B. Hypercalcemia generally presents with muscle weakness and depressed deep tendon reflexes.

C. This particular response is not related to hypokalemia. Hypokalemia may present with hyporeflexia.

D. This particular response is not related to hyperkalemia. Hyperkalemia may present with muscle weakness and flaccid paralysis.

Category: Psychosocial and Medical Emergencies/Medical/Electrolyte/fluid imbalance

Nursing Process: Analysis

References

Kuiper, B. (2010). Fluids and electrolytes In P. K. Howard & R. A. Steinmann (Eds.), *Sheehy's emergency nursing: Principles and practice* (6th ed., pp. 490–498). St. Louis, MO: Mosby Elsevier.

Marett, B. (2013). Metabolic emergencies. In B. B. Hammond & P. G. Zimmermann (Eds.), *Sheehy's manual of emergency care* (7th ed., pp. 303–318). St. Louis, MO: Elsevier Mosby.

---

94. Which of the following conditions caused by an insufficient amount of available antidiuretic hormone results in the patient urinating large amounts of diluted urine?

A. Diabetes insipidus
B. Adrenal crisis
C. Syndrome of inappropriate antidiuretic hormone
D. Cushing's syndrome

Rationale

A. Diabetes insipidus (DI) is a life-threatening condition caused by insufficient production of antidiuretic hormone (ADH) by the hypothalamus, or insufficient ADH being released by the posterior pituitary gland. The patient will excrete large amounts of dilute urine and complain of fatigue and weight loss. Treatment for DI is fluid replacement and ADH replacement with medications such as desmopressin acetate (DDAVP).

B. Adrenal crisis, also known as acute adrenal insufficiency, is a life-threatening condition caused by a decrease in cortisol and aldosterone levels. This results in sodium and water loss from both the kidneys and gastrointestinal tract, causing the patient to become hypotensive and hypovolemic. As the body loses sodium, an increase in potassium occurs, leading to hyperkalemia and the development of fatal dysrhythmias. Treatment includes fluid replacement, correction of hyperkalemia, and hydrocortisone administration.

C. Syndrome of inappropriate antidiuretic hormone (SIADH) is a life-threatening condition in which the pituitary gland releases excessive amounts of ADH. The patient will present with dilutional hyponatremia and water intoxication, which can result in seizures. The patient will also complain of headache, fatigue, and weight gain without the presence of edema. Treatment for SIADH depends on the severity of the patient's hyponatremia. Fluid restriction should be initiated. Severe hyponatremia is treated with hypertonic saline and the administration of furosemide (Lasix).

D. Cushing's syndrome is the result of prolonged exposure to glucocorticoids—either endogenous or exogenous—causing the patient to develop a cushingoid appearance. There is an increased amount of adipose tissue to the face, upper back, and base of the neck.

Category: Psychosocial and Medical Emergencies/Medical/Endocrine conditions
Nursing Process: Assessment

References

Marett, B. E. (2013). Metabolic emergencies. In B. B. Hammond & P. G. Zimmermann. *Sheehy's manual of emergency care* (7th ed., pp. 303–318). St. Louis, MO: Elsevier Mosby.
Morey, C. M. (2010). Endocrine emergencies. In P. K. Howard & R. A. Steinmann (Eds.), *Sheehy's emergency nursing: Principles and practice* (6th ed., pp. 499–512). St. Louis, MO: Mosby Elsevier.
Wall, S. M. (2007). Endocrine emergencies. In K. S. Hoyt & J. Selfridge-Thomas (Eds.), *Emergency nursing core curriculum* (6th ed., pp. 290–309). St. Louis, MO: Saunders Elsevier.

---

95. Which assessment finding in a patient with adrenal crisis would alert the emergency nurse to prepare for an expected complication?

A. Hypokalemia
B. Hypotension
C. Hyperglycemia
D. Bradycardia

Rationale

A. Patients in adrenal crisis are at risk for hyperkalemia, not hypokalemia, because of the presence of insufficient adrenal hormones.

B. Patients in adrenal crisis have significantly low levels of cortisol and aldosterone. The risk of developing hypoglycemia, hyponatremia, hypovolemia/hypotension, and hyperkalemia is significant. The presence of hypotension should alert the nurse to the need for fluid resuscitation and immediate replacement of adrenal hormones.

C. Patients in adrenal crisis are at risk for hypoglycemia, not hyperglycemia, because of the presence of insufficient adrenal hormones.

D. Because of severe hypotension, patients in adrenal crisis are often tachycardic and do not experience bradycardia.

Category: Psychosocial and Medical Emergencies/Medical/Endocrine conditions: Adrenal

Nursing Process: Analysis

References

Cydulka, R. K., & Tagliaferro, J. P. (2015). Adrenal insufficiency. In J. J. Schaider, A. Z. Barkin, P. Shayne, R. E. Wolfe, & S. R. Hayden (Eds.), *Rosen and Barkin's 5-minute emergency medicine consult* (5th ed., pp. 34–35). Philadelphia, PA: Wolters Kluwer.

Field, A. G. (2015). Adrenal and pituitary disorders. In A. B. Wolfson, R. L. Cloutier, G. W. Hendey, L. J. Ling, J. J. Schaider, & C. L. Rosen (Eds.), *Harwood-Nuss' clinical practice of emergency medicine* (6th ed., pp. 1033–1040). Philadelphia, PA: Wolters Kluwer.

---

96. A patient arrives at the emergency department via emergency medical services with sudden onset of altered level of consciousness. The patient was found wandering at the local bus station, is able to answer questions only after much thought, and is unable to recognize that they are currently in a hospital. The patient appears very anxious, is diaphoretic, and has uncontrolled tremors to bilateral arms. Which of the following diagnostic testing would be the first priority for the emergency nurse to obtain in order to assist in proper diagnosis of this problem?

A. Serum creatinine
B. Urinalysis
C. White blood cell count
D. Serum glucose

Rationale

A. A serum creatinine would provide information regarding the patient's renal status, but it takes longer to receive the result; a point-of-care blood glucose value can be obtained much faster.

B. A urinalysis will provide information regarding a urinary tract infection that might lead to the subsequent development of sepsis; however, this diagnostic test requires time and would not provide immediate feedback. Sepsis could present with an altered level of mentation, but hypoglycemia is a more likely cause of the patient's symptoms.

C. A complete blood cell count, which would include a white blood cell count to indicate a possible infectious process, would be appropriate but not a first-line priority in this case; point-of-care blood glucose would provide the most important information.

D. Any patient with an altered level of consciousness should have an immediate blood glucose level performed to rule out the presence of hypoglycemia. This patient is presenting with classic signs of hypoglycemia. Hypoglycemia is one of the most common causes of altered level of consciousness and can be easily treated.

Category: Psychosocial and Medical Emergencies/Medical/Endocrine conditions: Glucose-related disorders

Nursing Process: Intervention

Reference

Morey, C. (2010). Endocrine emergencies. In P. K. Howard & R. A. Steinmann (Eds.), *Sheehy's emergency nursing: Principles and practice* (6th ed., pp. 499–512). St. Louis, MO: Mosby Elsevier.

---

97. When providing discharge instructions to the parents of a child, the nurse is aware that the parents have understood the importance of avoiding products that contain aspirin when they state which of the following?

A. **There is an association between the use of aspirin-containing products in febrile children and the development of Reye's syndrome.**
B. Aspirin is less effective in controlling fevers in the pediatric population because of their immature and developing neurologic system.
C. Aspirin has been shown to increase the risk of febrile seizures given its slower onset of action.
D. There is an association between the use of aspirin in febrile children and the development of asthma.

Rationale

A. Aspirin-containing products should not be given to children with an acute febrile illness because of their association with the development of Reye's syndrome. Reye's syndrome is a rare yet rapidly progressing syndrome that results in encephalopathy. Other factors associated with the syndrome include use of aspirin during a viral illness, after which fatty deposits in the liver lead to altered mental status and altered glucose regulation.

B. The immature pediatric neurologic system increases the risk for febrile seizures. Aspirin is an effective antipyretic but is contraindicated for use in the pediatric population given the potential risk of developing Reye's syndrome.

C. Aspirin has a similar onset of action compared to other antipyretics but is contraindicated because of the risk of developing Reye's syndrome. The immature neurologic system in the younger child increases the risk for febrile seizures.

D. Aspirin is a known trigger for asthma in some patients but has not been shown to increase the incidence of asthma. The use of aspirin is contraindicated given the risk of Reye's syndrome in febrile children.

Category (Pediatric): Psychosocial and Medical Emergencies/Medical/Fever

Nursing Process: Evaluation

References

Balamuth, F., Henretig, F. M., & Alpern, E. R. (2016). Fever. In K. N. Shaw & R. G. Bachur (Eds.), *Fleisher and Ludwig's textbook of pediatric emergency medicine* (7th ed., pp. 176–185). Philadelphia, PA: Wolters Kluwer.

Lazear, S. E., & Roberts, A. (2007). Medical emergencies. In K. S. Hoyt & J. Selfridge-Thomas (Eds.), *Emergency nursing core curriculum* (6th ed., pp. 483–509). St. Louis, MO: Saunders Elsevier.

---

98. Which of the following may be a subtle sign of sepsis that should be considered by the triage nurse during the initial assessment of a patient presenting to the emergency department?

A. Systolic blood pressure greater than 90 mm Hg
B. Respiratory rate greater than 22 breaths/minute
C. Temperature of 37°C (98.6°F)
D. Capillary refill less than 2 seconds

Rationale

A. Systolic blood pressure less than 90 mm Hg is considered a subtle sign of sepsis.

B. A cough, dyspnea, tachypnea, and a respiratory rate of 22 breaths/minute have been found to be subtle signs of sepsis that should be considered during the assessment of a patient in triage.

C. Temperature > 38.3°C (100.94°F) or < 36°C (96.8°F) may be a subtle sign of sepsis.

D. Capillary refill greater than 2 seconds may be a subtle sign of sepsis.

Category: Psychosocial and Medical Emergencies/Medical/Sepsis and septic shock

Nursing Process: Assessment

References

Buck, K. (2014). Developing and early sepsis alert program. *Journal of Nursing Care Quarterly, 29*(20), 124–132.

Doble, M. (2017). Making sense of the updated sepsis definitions. *Nursing Center.* Retrieved from http://www.nursingcenter.com/ncblog/march-2016/making-sense-of-the-updated-sepsis-definitions

Keegan, J., & Wira, C. (2014). Early identification and management of patients with severe sepsis and septic shock in the emergency department. *Emergency Medicine Clinics of North America, 32,* 759–776.

Miller, J. (2014). Surviving sepsis: A review of the latest guidelines. *Nursing 2017, 44*(4), 24–30.

Rhoades, C., Holleran, R. S., Carpenter, L., & Grissom, C. (2010). Management of the critical care patient in the emergency department. In P. K. Howard & R. A. Steinmann (Eds.), *Sheehy's emergency nursing: Principles and practice* (6th ed., pp. 211–230). St. Louis, MO: Mosby Elsevier.

Schorr, C. (2016). Nurses can help improve outcomes in severe sepsis. *American Nurse Today, 11*(3), 20–25.

---

99. A patient presents to the emergency department with possible signs and symptoms of compartment syndrome 2 days following surgery for a fractured left tibia/fibula. Which of the following would alert the emergency nurse that this patient may be experiencing possible organ failure?

A. Rales
B. Jaundice
C. Dark, scanty urine
D. Generalized edema

Rationale

A. Rales are an indication of fluid collecting in the lungs. Compartment syndrome does not result in the presence of rales.

B. Jaundice is caused by the presence of an excessive amount bilirubin in the blood. Compartment syndrome results in poor skin color (pallor) and cool temperature, indicating poor perfusion and possible organ failure. Delayed capillary refill may also indicate decreased perfusion in the affected extremity.

C. Significant muscle damage and cellular destruction releases myoglobin, a muscle protein, into the bloodstream. As the myoglobin enters the kidneys, it causes the appearance of dark red or brown urine. The myoglobin can also clog the renal glomerulus, resulting in an acute renal injury. If the myoglobin is not flushed from the kidneys with large amounts of fluid, permanent renal impairment or injury can result.

D. The compartment or limb of the affected extremity will feel tight or tense on palpation. The skin may appear taut and shiny as the skin stretches. This edema is localized to the effected extremity and is not generalized.

Category: Maxillofacial, Ocular, Orthopedic, and Wound Emergencies/Orthopedic/Compartment syndrome

Nursing Process: Analysis

Reference

Bratcher, C. M. (2014). Musculoskeletal trauma. In D. Gurney (Ed.), *Trauma Nursing Core Course: Provider manual* (7th ed., pp. 193–204). Des Plaines, IL: Emergency Nurses Association.

---

100. A patient presents to triage with a complaint of continuous chest pain for the past 3 days. Vital signs are BP 108/70 mm Hg, HR 68 beats/minute, RR 18 breaths/minute, SpO_2 99% on room air, T 37°C (98.6°F). The patient describes the pain as sharp, located on the right side of the chest, and made worse by breathing and arm movement. The patient denies shortness of breath and any trauma or recent surgeries but does report having an upper respiratory infection the previous week. The emergency nurse anticipates the cause of the patient's symptoms is which of the following?

A. Pericarditis
B. Pulmonary contusion
C. Anxiety
D. Costochondritis

Rationale

A. Pericarditis can be caused by bacterial, fungal, or viral infections, but sometimes the cause is unknown. With pericarditis, the pain can also be sharp and increase with movement, but pain is usually worse when the patient is lying down. In addition, the patient may have fever, fatigue, and possibly weight loss.

B. Pulmonary contusions are often the result of blunt force trauma and may develop over several days. Pulmonary contusions are characterized by blood moving into the lung tissue following blunt trauma to the chest, which can result in tissue edema. There may be point tenderness over the site, and the patient may appear to be short of breath or working hard to breathe.

C. Anxiety can be a cause of chest pain and result in a patient being short of breath. Although this can be on the diagnosis differential, it is important to obtain a good social history, recent stressors, and a history of previous episodes of similar pain.

D. Costochondritis is an inflammation of the costal cartilage and can present as sharp pain that is worse on breathing in or with movement. Because the pain is reproducible, it is most likely related to costochondritis, which can occur following upper respiratory infections, particularly when patients have been persistently coughing.

Category: Maxillofacial, Ocular, Orthopedic, and Wound Emergencies/Orthopedic/Costochondritis

Nursing Process: Assessment

Reference

Cerepani, M. J., & Ramponi D. R. (2007). Orthopedic emergencies. In K. S. Hoyt & J. Selfridge-Thomas. *Emergency nursing core curriculum* (6th ed., pp. 585–603). St. Louis, MO: Saunders Elsevier.

---

101. A young mother presents to triage with her toddler, stating the child fell while walking and now will not move their left arm. However, the child fell on their right side. What should the emergency triage nurse do next?

A. Order a radiograph of the right arm per standing orders
B. Suspect child maltreatment because the story does not match the injury
C. Ask the mother if she attempted to prevent the child from falling by holding onto the opposite arm
D. Assess the injured left arm by using passive range of motion

Rationale

A. A radiograph study is frequently unwarranted in radial subluxation. The diagnosis of radial subluxation can be made by physical examination. The subluxation can be easily relocated with good return of function. It is not necessary to immobilize the extremity following relocation of the subluxation.

B. In this case, the concern of child maltreatment may or may not match the history of the event. The nurse should further assess the situation to determine if the concern for maltreatment is warranted. However, the first priority is to assess for the presence of possible radial head subluxation injury (nursemaid's elbow).

C. Assess for the presence of possible radial head subluxation injury (nursemaid's elbow) caused by pulling on the child's arm to prevent them from falling. Subluxation is partial joint disruption (partial dislocation) that maintains some contact with the articulating surfaces. In children under the age of 5, radial head subluxation is present in approximately 20% of upper extremity injuries.

D. If the arm is fractured, it is not best practice to use passive range of motion to assess the extremity. If a radial head subluxation is present, the patient reduction of the partial dislocation should be performed by the emergency care provider. Reduction of the subluxation is not within the scope of practice for an emergency nurse.

Category (Pediatric): Maxillofacial, Ocular, Orthopedic, and Wound Emergencies/Orthopedic/Fractures/dislocations

Nursing Process: Intervention

Reference

Cerepani, M. J. (2010). Orthopedic and neurovascular trauma. In P. K. Howard & R. A. Steinmann (Eds.), *Sheehy's emergency nursing: Principles and practice* (6th ed., pp. 321–339). St. Louis, MO: Mosby Elsevier.

---

102. A patient presents to triage complaining of pain in the right distal forearm after falling onto their outstretched arm. There is an obvious deformity above the patient's right wrist. Right radial pulse is present and color and sensation are intact distally, however, the patient is unable to sustain a wrist grip. The emergency nurse is aware that it is best to immobilize the right forearm using a(n):

A. traction splint.
B. padded rigid long arm splint.
C. soft splint.
D. ice application.

Rationale

A. Traction splints are used for actual or potential femur or proximal tibial fractures and would not be indicated for an upper extremity injury.

B. Splinting of the extremity is indicated when there is evidence of deformity, pain, bony crepitus, edema, ecchymosis, open soft tissue injury, paralysis, or paresthesia. Always immobilize joints above and below a suspected fracture site.

C. Soft splints include pillows and slings and could be an option if a rigid splint is not available. The presence of an obvious deformity makes the use of a rigid splint the best choice of treatment for this patient.

D. Application of ice and elevation are indicated to reduce swelling and pain but will not provide immobilization of the extremity. A rigid splint is the best choice for the immediate treatment of this patient.

Category: Maxillofacial, Ocular, Orthopedic, and Wound Emergencies/Orthopedic/Fractures/dislocations

Nursing Process: Intervention

References

Bratcher, C. M. (2014). Musculoskeletal trauma. In D. Gurney (Ed.), *Trauma Nursing Core Course: Provider manual* (7th ed., pp. 193–204). Des Plaines, IL: Emergency Nurses Association.

Halpern, J. S. (2013). Musculoskeletal trauma. In B. B. Hammond & P. G. Zimmermann (Eds.), *Sheehy's manual of emergency care* (7th ed., pp. 427–438). St. Louis, MO: Elsevier Mosby.

103. The emergency nurse is preparing to discharge a female geriatric patient who presented to the emergency department for severe "heartburn." Medication reconciliation reveals the patient is on alendronate (Fosamax). What information should the emergency nurse provide to the patient with the discharge instructions?

A. Always take alendronate with food
B. Sit or stand upright for 30 minutes after taking alendronate
C. Have calcium blood levels monitored monthly
D. Take alendronate at bedtime

Rationale

A. The patient should be instructed to take the medication on an empty stomach with a full glass of water to promote absorption of the drug and to avoid eating and drinking for 30 minutes after taking it.

B. A side effect of alendronate is esophageal irritation, so the patient must remain upright 30 minutes after taking the medication. In severe cases, the esophageal irritation can result in esophageal erosion.

C. Alendronate is a bisphosphonate that works by inhibiting the resorption of the bone and increasing bone mass. Calcium levels need to be monitored in patients taking hormones such as calcitonin and teriparatide.

D. Alendronate is to be taken 30 minutes before meals and should not be taken at bedtime. A side effect of alendronate is esophageal irritation, so the patient must remain upright for 30 minutes after taking the medication.

Category (Geriatric): Maxillofacial, Ocular, Orthopedic, and Wound Emergencies/Orthopedic/Inflammatory conditions

Nursing Process: Intervention

Reference

Abel, L. E. (2013). Metabolic bone conditions. In Nation Association Orthopaedic Nurses. *Core curriculum for orthopaedic nursing* (7th ed., pp. 377–390). Chicago, IL: National Association of Orthopaedic Nurses.

---

104. A patient is observed walking into the emergency department with a severely increased thoracic curve, or "humpback." The emergency nurse knows that this condition is referred to as:

A. scoliosis.
B. lordosis.
C. genu varum.
D. kyphosis.

Rationale

A. Scoliosis is a lateral deformity, or curvature of the spine.

B. Lordosis is an increase in the lumbar curve, or swayback.

C. Genu varum is a bow-legged appearance of the legs in children.

D. Kyphosis refers to an increased thoracic curvature of the spine, or "humpback." Kyphosis (dowager's hump) is a collapse of the spine that produces the appearance of a shortened trunk.

Category (Geriatric): Maxillofacial, Ocular, Orthopedic, and Wound Emergencies/Orthopedic/Low back pain

Nursing Process: Assessment

Reference

Cerepani, M. J., & Ramponi, D. R. (2007). Orthopedic emergencies. In K. S. Hoyt & J. Selfridge-Thomas. *Emergency nursing core curriculum* (6th ed., pp. 585–603). St. Louis, MO: Saunders Elsevier.

---

105. A motorcyclist arrives to the emergency department via emergency medical services following a collision with a motor vehicle. The motorcyclist, who was thrown across the hood of the car, was helmeted and wearing leather clothing. The patient's primary survey is within normal limits. The secondary survey reveals pain and paresthesia to the right arm and hand, with pronounced weakness but no swelling, pallor, or coolness in the extremity. The emergency nurse anticipates the patient has the signs and symptoms of which of the following?

A. Brachial plexus injury
B. Compartment syndrome
C. Fracture of the humerus
D. Brachial artery dissection

Rationale

A. The brachial plexus arises from the C5 to T1 spinal nerves. These nerves are responsible for supplying motor control and sensation to the arm, wrist, and hand. Injury to these spinal nerves will result in pain and paresthesia to the arm and wrist and hand weakness.

B. Compartment syndrome occurs when pressure increases within a fascial compartment. Signs and symptoms include pain out of proportion to the injury, pallor, decreased pulse, paresthesia, and paralysis, and the area feels firm to palpation.

C. Fractures must be ruled out. A fractured humerus would likely include deformity, ecchymosis, swelling, and inability to raise the arm.

D. Signs and symptoms of an arterial dissection may be similar to compartment syndrome with decreased radial pulses. It would be reasonable to rule out this injury with arteriogram, but this patient does not have the key symptoms, such as swelling, pallor, or coolness of the extremity.

Category: Maxillofacial, Ocular, Orthopedic, and Wound Emergencies/Orthopedic/Trauma

Nursing Process: Analysis

Reference

Crowley, M. (2014). Spinal cord and vertebral column trauma. In D. Gurney (Ed.), *Trauma Nursing Core Course: Provider manual* (7th ed., pp. 173–192). Des Plaines, IL: Emergency Nurses Association.

---

106. A construction worker is brought to the emergency department by their coworkers. The patient reports that while descending from a ladder, they unintentionally fired a nail gun into their right thigh. Immediately following, the patient was unable to straighten their leg, and their coworkers had to cut the patient's jeans off from around the nail head. A radiograph reveals the presence of a foreign body embedded in the patient's right femur. The nurse anticipates that this injury will be managed as a(n):

A. foreign body.
B. open fracture.
C. comminuted fracture.
D. high-pressure grease injury.

Rationale

A. The presence of a retained foreign body may provide a nucleus of infection. Wound incision and drainage and foreign body removal are critical for healing to occur without the occurrence of infection.

B. An injury is classified as an open fracture if a penetrating foreign body enters the bone or creates an opening in the tissue directly over the bone.

C. Comminuted fractures occur from severe direct trauma to the bone and result in more than two bone fragments.

D. High-pressure injection injuries from a paint or grease gun can result in the substance traveling down the fascial plane or tendon sheath, causing severe infection or permanent impairment. Immediate surgical intervention is necessary to drain the foreign substance from the tissue and preserve function.

Category: Maxillofacial, Ocular, Orthopedic, and Wound Emergencies/Orthopedic/Fractures/dislocations

Nursing Process: Analysis

References

Halpern, J. S. (2013). Musculoskeletal trauma. In B. B. Hammond & P. G. Zimmermann, *Sheehy's manual of emergency care* (7th ed., pp. 427–438). St. Louis, MO: Elsevier Mosby.

Herr, R. D. (2013). Wound management. In *Sheehy's manual of emergency care* (7th ed., pp. 147–160). St. Louis, MO: Elsevier Mosby.

---

107. The emergency nurse is preparing to discharge a patient who has received treatment to close a facial laceration. The nurse recognizes the patient's understanding of the discharge instructions when stating the following:

A. "I will be sure to call my doctor in the morning for a prescription for an antibiotic."
B. "I need to place a thin layer of antibiotic ointment over the sutures daily."
C. "I will be sure to have my staples removed after 3 weeks."
D. "I will return to the emergency department in 14 days for suture removal."

Rationale

A. Uncomplicated wounds in a healthy individual do not usually require systemic antibiotics.

B. The application of antibiotic ointment will help to prevent wound infection.

C. Staple wound closures are limited to areas where a scar will not be apparent, and therefore are not indicated for facial wounds.

D. Facial sutures are typically removed in 3–5 days. Sutures over joints require 14 days to heal before removal.

Category: Maxillofacial, Ocular, Orthopedic, and Wound Emergencies/Wound/Infections
Nursing Process: Evaluation

Reference

Denke, N. J. (2010). Wound management. In P. K. Howard & R. A. Steinmann (Eds.), *Sheehy's emergency nursing: Principles and practice* (6th ed., pp. 111–126). St. Louis, MO: Mosby Elsevier.

---

108. The emergency nurse is caring for a patient who was found lying on the floor for 2 days, unable to get up following a fall. The patient's skin assessment reveals an area of purple discoloration along the patient's greater trochanter, which is boggy and warm to the touch. The emergency nurse recognizes this wound as a(n):

A. stage 1 pressure ulcer.
B. area of bruising.
C. potential deep tissue injury.
D. stage 4 pressure ulcer.

Rationale

A. A stage 1 pressure ulcer is described as intact skin with nonblanchable redness of a localized area, usually over a bony prominence. This is inconsistent with a wound that is boggy and warm to the touch.

B. A bruise is the extravasation of blood in the tissues as a result of blunt force impact to the body. This is not the most accurate description relating to the etiology of this wound.

C. A deep tissue injury is described as a purple or maroon localized area of discolored intact skin or blood-filled blister resulting from damage of underlying soft tissue from pressure and/or shear. This injury results from intense and/or prolonged pressure and shear forces at the bone–muscle interface, which is consistent with the patient's history of lying on the floor for 2 days.

D. A stage 4 pressure ulcer is described as full thickness tissue loss with exposed bone, tendon, or muscle. This is inconsistent with an area of purple discoloration that is boggy and warm to the touch.

Category: Maxillofacial, Ocular, Orthopedic, and Wound Emergencies/Wound/Trauma
Nursing Process: Assessment

Reference

National Pressure Ulcer Advisory Panel. (n.d.). *Deep tissue injury* [White paper]. Retrieved from http://www.npuap.org/wp-content/uploads/2012/01/DTI-White-Paper.pdf

National Pressure Ulcer Advisory Panel. (n.d.). *NPUAP pressure injury stages.* Retrieved from http://www.npuap.org/resources/educational-and-clinical-resources/npuap-pressure-injury-stages/

---

109. Which wound is the highest risk for development of osteomyelitis?

A. Laceration to the palmar surface of the hand resulting from a carving knife
B. Stage 1 pressure injury to the heel
C. Laceration to the elbow from breaking glass
D. Deep puncture wound in the foot from stepping on a nail

Rationale

A. This is not a high-risk wound for developing osteomyelitis.

B. A stage 1 pressure wound on a heel is not at high risk for developing osteomyelitis.

C. A laceration from breaking glass is not a high-risk wound for the development of osteomyelitis.

D. A puncture wound of the foot is associated with deep penetration resulting from weight bearing on a sharp object with frequent penetration of a metatarsal bone. The patient will complain of pain, redness, and swelling within 4–7 days following injury as the infection begins to develop.

Category: Maxillofacial, Ocular, Orthopedic, and Wound Emergencies/Wound/Puncture wounds

Nursing Process: Assessment

Reference

Herr, R. D. (2013). Wound management. In B. B. Hammond & P. G. Zimmermann (Eds.), *Sheehy's manual of emergency care* (7th ed., pp. 147–160). St. Louis, MO: Elsevier Mosby.

---

110. What is the priority assessment for a patient who has sustained a traumatic laceration to the upper arm?

A. Range of motion in the fingers
B. The presence of a distal or radial pulse
C. Capillary refill
D. Skin color and temperature

Rationale

A. Finger range of motion will indicate whether there is tendon involvement; however, this is not the priority assessment.

B. Lack of distal pulse indicates vascular compromise to the arm and requires immediate intervention to preserve limb function.

C. The presence of capillary refill will indicate adequate or decreased perfusion to the arm, but the presence of a radial pulse is a more reliable indicator of adequate tissue perfusion.

D. Skin color, temperature, and moisture will indicate adequate or decreased perfusion to the arm, but the presence of a radial pulse is a more reliable indicator of adequate tissue perfusion.

Category: Maxillofacial, Ocular, Orthopedic, and Wound Emergencies/Wound/Lacerations

Nursing Process: Assessment

Reference

Herr, R. D. (2013). Wound management. In B. B. Hammond & P. G. Zimmermann (Eds.), *Sheehy's manual of emergency care* (7th ed., pp. 147–160). St. Louis, MO: Elsevier Mosby.

111. An elderly patient arrives to the emergency department via emergency medical services with profuse epistaxis that has persisted for over an hour. After initiating universal precautions, the next priority intervention for the emergency nurse to perform is which of the following?

A. Obtain blood pressure
B. Initiate intravenous access
C. Maintain airway patency
D. Initiate direct pressure by instructing the patient to pinch their nostrils

Rationale

A. Although vital signs are important to obtain, they should never take priority over assessing airway patency.

B. This patient will need intravenous hydration because of the duration of the bleeding and suspected blood loss, but assessing and maintaining airway patency is always the first priority.

C. Posterior nasal bleeding can interfere with a patient's airway patency. Posterior bleeding can be chronic and is most common in elderly patients who may have a history hypertension and who take an anticoagulation-type medication.

D. This maneuver is effective with anterior nasal bleeds but will not act to minimize the amount of bleeding in a posterior nasal bleed. Anterior nasal bleeds usually arise from the area of the Kiesselbach plexus. This patient is demonstrating signs and symptoms of a posterior bleed.

Category: Maxillofacial, Ocular, Orthopedic, and Wound Emergencies/Maxillofacial/Epistaxis
Nursing Process: Intervention

Reference

Egging, D. (2013). Facial, ENT, and dental emergencies. In B. B. Hammond & P. G. Zimmermann (Eds.), *Sheehy's manual of emergency care* (7th ed., pp. 275–284). St. Louis, MO: Elsevier Mosby.

---

112. A patient presents to emergency triage and tells the emergency nurse that they are experiencing a severe throbbing-type headache pain located over the frontal left region. The patient has a history of polymyalgia rheumatica. The emergency nurse suspects the patient's current discomfort is related to the presence of which of the following?

A. Temporomandibular joint dislocation
B. Temporal arteritis
C. Cluster headache
D. Sinusitis

Rationale

A. Temporomandibular joint dislocation (TMJ) is a joint dislocation at the anterior and superior joint that results in spasms and muscle contraction of the jaw muscles, leading to the condyles not being able to return to their normal position. TMJ can be the result of trauma or from simply opening the mouth too wide, such as during dental work.

B. Temporal arteritis is also referred to as systemic arterial vasculitis and produces a severe frontal throbbing type of pain. Palpation over the temporal region results in severe discomfort for the patient. Patients who experience temporal arteritis have a history of polymyalgia rheumatica and are usually over the age of 50.

C. Cluster headaches occur commonly in men and are related to a dysfunction of the trigeminal nerve. The headache is characterized by an intense unilateral pain in the orbital or temporal region lasting from 15 minutes to 3 hours.

D. Sinusitis results from the blockage of drainage from the paranasal sinuses. It can be caused by a recent upper respiratory infection or allergic rhinitis. The patient experiences dull achy discomfort over the affected sinus.

Category: Maxillofacial, Ocular, Orthopedic, and Wound Emergencies/Maxillofacial

Nursing Process: Assessment

References

Baxter, C. S. (2007). Neurological emergencies. In K. S. Hoyt & J. Selfridge-Thomas (Eds.), *Emergency nursing core curriculum* (6th ed., pp. 510–535). St. Louis, MO: Saunders Elsevier.

Nolan, E. G. (2010). Dental, ear, nose, throat, and facial emergencies. In P. K. Howard & R. A. Steinmann (Eds.), *Sheehy's emergency nursing* (6th ed., pp. 590–601). St. Louis, MO: Mosby Elsevier.

Walsh, R. (2013). Neurologic emergencies. In B. B. Hammond & P. G. Zimmermann (Eds.), *Sheehy's manual of emergency care* (7th ed., pp. 265–274). St. Louis, MO: Elsevier Mosby.

---

113. A patient with a history of diabetes presents to the emergency department complaining of increasing swelling and severe pain in the left eye with movement of the eye. On assessment, the patient demonstrates decreased visual acuity, decreased pupillary reflexes, and the presence of erythema and edema of the upper and lower eyelids and of the left cheek area. The emergency nurse anticipates the patient has signs and symptoms of:

A. conjunctivitis.
B. anterior uveitis.
C. iritis.
D. orbital cellulitis.

Rationale

A. Conjunctivitis involves the eyelid and conjunctiva and results in redness, some edema, and drainage. Conjunctivitis does not affect the patient's visual acuity. The patient will usually not experience pain with eye movement.

B. Anterior uveitis is the inflammation of the upper eyelid. It is associated with the presence of excessive tearing, redness of the eye, and decreased visual acuity. Pain will not be present with eye movement.

C. Iritis is the inflammation of the iris, resulting in pain, edema, tearing, and sensitivity to light, with some decrease in visual acuity. Pain is not present with eye movement.

D. Orbital cellulitis is a serious emergency that involves the eye itself, resulting in painful movement, reduced visual acuity, and severe swelling and redness of the orbital area. Patients who are immunocompromised or who have a history of diabetes are more susceptible to complicating infections. Orbital cellulitis is be considered a life-threatening infection process because of the potential for the infection to enter the brain, resulting in meningitis.

Category: Maxillofacial, Ocular, Orthopedic, and Wound Emergencies/Maxillofacial/Infections

Nursing Process: Analysis

Reference

Gerhart, A. E. (2007). Ocular emergencies. In K. S. Hoyt & J. Selfridge-Thomas (Eds.), *Emergency nursing core curriculum* (6th ed., pp. 571–584). St. Louis, MO: Saunders Elsevier.

---

114. An unresponsive patient involved in a high-speed motor vehicle collision with multiple facial injuries arrives in the emergency department via emergency medical services. Because of the presence of numerous facial injuries, it is determined that the patient is at risk for an upper airway obstruction. Which of the following maneuvers is best to initiate to prevent an upper airway obstruction?

A. Maintain the patient in semi-Fowler's position at a 45-degree angle to maintain airway patency
B. Place airway adjunct into the patient
C. Place patient in a left lateral "recovery" position to maintain an open airway
D. Assist the emergency provider to control facial bleeding using vessel ligation to prevent the occlusion of the upper airway as the result of significant bleeding

Rationale

A. Up to 10% of patients with significant blunt force facial injuries will also have the presence of a corresponding cervical spine injury; therefore, cervical spine immobilization should be maintained until the presence of a cervical injury can be determined by radiographic studies.

B. A nasopharyngeal airway can be placed in patients who are either conscious or unconscious. An oropharyngeal airway is only used in patients who have an absent gag reflex. These devices can maintain an open airway until further interventions can be performed, such as endotracheal intubation or cricothyroidotomy to maintain airway patency.

C. Placing the patient into a left lateral position should not be performed until the presence or absence of a cervical spine injury can be determined. Up to 10% of patients with significant blunt facial injuries will also have corresponding cervical spine injury; therefore, spinal immobilization should be maintained.

D. Vessel ligation should only be performed under direct visualization after careful identification of the bleeding vessel.

Category: Maxillofacial, Ocular, Orthopedic, and Wound Emergencies/Maxillofacial/Trauma

Nursing Process: Intervention

References

Gurney, D., & Westergard, A. M. (2014). Initial assessment. In D. Gurney (Ed.), *Trauma Nursing Core Course: Provider manual* (7th ed., pp. 39–54). Des Plaines, IL: Emergency Nurses Association.

O'Neal, J. (2013). Airway management. (2013). In B. B. Hammond & P. G. Zimmermann (Eds.), *Sheehy's manual of emergency care* (7th ed., pp. 77–88). St. Louis, MO: Elsevier Mosby.

---

115. A patient presents to the emergency department after being splashed in the both eyes with a cleaning solution. During assessment, the emergency nurse notes the presence of bilateral corneal clouding and prepares to irrigate the eyes. The emergency nurse knows the irrigation may be discontinued when:

A. the ocular pH reaches 7.0 in each eye.
B. 1 hour has passed.
C. the pain in each eye has been relieved.
D. 1000 mL of irrigation solution has been used.

Rationale

A. Normal ocular pH is 7.0–7.3. Irrigation is performed until the ocular pH is within normal range.

B. The duration of irrigation is determined by a resulting normal pH, not the length of the irrigation. Depending on the chemical substance, irrigation may take more or less time before reaching normal ocular pH.

C. Relief of pain is not a determining factor in discontinuation of irrigation. Irrigation will continue until normal ocular pH has been achieved.

D. Volume of the irrigating solution is not a determining factor in discontinuation of irrigation. Irrigation will continue until normal ocular pH has been achieved.

Category: Maxillofacial, Ocular, Orthopedic, and Wound Emergencies/Ocular/Burns
Nursing Process: Evaluation

Reference

Shea, S. S. (2007). Ocular and maxillofacial trauma. In K. S. Hoyt & J. Selfridge-Thomas (Eds.), *Emergency nursing core curriculum* (6th ed., pp. 848–878). St. Louis, MO: Saunders Elsevier.

---

116. An elderly patient presents to the emergency department complaining of a severe boring type pain of the right eye. The patient reports nausea, seeing halos around objects, and the presence of a headache behind the right eye. The patient has been diagnosed with acute angle-closure glaucoma and has received both 500 mg of acetazolamide (Diamox) intravenously and a 500 mg dose orally. Timolol (Timoptic) was instilled topically into the right eye. The emergency nurse identifies that this therapy has been effective when which of the following occurs?

A. The patient's intraocular pressure (IOP) is 35 mm Hg.
B. The patient's IOP is 20 mm Hg.
C. The patient's nausea has been alleviated.
D. The patient no longer complains of pain in their right eye.

Rationale

A. Normal intraocular pressure is 12–22 mm Hg, and eye pressure of greater than 22 mm Hg is considered higher than normal.

B. Acute angle-closure is defined as at least two of the following symptoms: ocular pain, nausea/vomiting, and a history of intermittent blurring of vision with halos; and at least three of the following signs: IOP greater than 21 mm Hg, conjunctival injection, corneal epithelial edema, mid-dilated nonreactive pupil, and shallower chamber in the presence of occlusion. Acetazolamide and topical beta-blockers are administered to decrease intraocular pressure.

C. Nausea often accompanies acute angle-closure glaucoma. Antiemetics should be administered because vomiting increases intraocular pressure.

D. Acetazolamide and topical beta-blockers both work to decrease intraocular pressure, which may lessen the patient's eye pain. However, the primary action is to lower the intraocular pressure.

Category: Maxillofacial, Ocular, Orthopedic, and Wound Emergencies/Ocular/Glaucoma
Nursing Process: Evaluation

References

Egging, D. (2010). Ocular emergencies. In P. K. Howard & R. A Steinmann (Eds.), *Sheehy's emergency nursing: Principles and practice* (6th ed., pp. 602–615). St. Louis, MO: Mosby Elsevier.

Freedman, J. (2017). Acute angle-closure glaucoma in emergency medicine. *Medscape*. Retrieved from http://emedicine.medscape.com/article/798811-overview

---

117. You are discharging a 3-year-old patient who has been diagnosed and treated for conjunctivitis. You ask the parent to repeat the instructions for care and determine the child will receive the appropriate care for when the parent states:

A. "My child may return to daycare when there is no crusting around the eyes upon awakening in the morning."
B. "Everyone must practice good handwashing techniques, and my child may not attend daycare until the eye infection has resolved."
C. "My child may continue to sleep in the same bed with his brother."
D. "My child may return to school tomorrow because it is only viral conjunctivitis."

Rationale

A. The child should not return to daycare until the redness and burning are resolved and there is no crusty discharge around the eyes upon awakening in the morning.

B. Bacterial and viral conjunctivitis are severely contagious. Strategies to reduce transmission are rigorous handwashing, not sharing towels and washcloths or pillows, and keeping the child out of the swimming pool.

C. Strategies to avoid spread of the disease include not sharing pillows, washcloths, or towels and by performing vigorous handwashing.

D. Bacterial and viral conjunctivitis are both severely contagious. The child should stay home until the redness and burning are resolved and there is no morning crusty discharge.

Category (Pediatric): Maxillofacial, Ocular, Orthopedic, and Wound Emergencies/Ocular/Infections
Nursing Process: Evaluation

Reference

Egging, D. (2013). Ocular emergencies. In B. B. Hammond & P. G. Zimmermann (Eds.), *Sheehy's manual of emergency care* (7th ed., pp. 285–290). St. Louis, MO: Elsevier Mosby.

---

118. An elderly patient presents to the emergency department complaining of blindness in the left eye. The patient reports a history of two prior episodes that resolved after a few seconds and denies pain or recent trauma. The emergency nurse anticipates the patient has experienced which of the following?

A. Retinal detachment
B. Acute angle-closure glaucoma
C. Anterior uveitis
D. Central retinal artery occlusion

Rationale

A. Retinal detachment may be distinguished by the patient's visual complaint, such as the presence of "floaters," a "veil" or "curtain," or flashes of light that affect their field of vision. A tear in the retina affects the eye's ability to perceive light.

B. Acute angle-closure glaucoma is described as a severe, sudden, painful onset; vision is described as blurred, or seeing halos around lights, with photophobia. Visual acuity is decreased, and, if left untreated, it can result in permanent blindness.

C. Anterior uveitis is a painful inflammation affecting the uveal or middle layer of the eye. The affected eye is reddened with excessive tearing, and the patient will complain of photophobia. The eyelid will also appear edematous.

D. Central retinal artery occlusion is the sudden painless unilateral loss of vision caused by an embolus or thrombus; it may be preceded by sudden temporary vision losses lasting seconds to minutes, which is referred to as amaurosis fugax.

Category (Geriatric): Maxillofacial, Ocular, Orthopedic and Wound Emergencies/Ocular/Retinal artery occlusion

Nursing Process: Analysis

References

Egging, D. (2003). Ocular emergencies. In L. Newberry (Ed.), *Sheehy's emergency nursing: Principles and practice* (5th ed., pp. 691–706). St. Louis, MO: Mosby.

Gerhart, A. E. (2007). Ocular emergencies. In K. S. Hoyt & J. Selfridge-Thomas (Eds.), *Emergency nursing core curriculum* (6th ed., pp. 571–584). St. Louis, MO: Saunders Elsevier.

---

119. A patient presents to triage stating that they were hit in the eye with a ball while playing softball. A Snellen visual acuity is performed and determines the patient has no loss of vision. While awaiting to be seen by the emergency provider, the patient begins to complain of "an aching" eye pain that is associated with sudden onset of blurred vision. Which statement made by the patient would cause the emergency nurse the greatest concern?

A. The patient complains of increased lacrimation.
B. A decreased ability for the patient to look upward.
C. The patient reports that everything is looking red.
D. The cornea appears cloudy.

Rationale

A. The presence of a hyphema is not associated with excessive tearing, exudates, or discharge from the eye.

B. The decreased ability to look upward with the affected eye is a symptom of entrapment of extraocular muscles associated with an orbital fracture and not the presence of a hyphema.

C. In the presence of a hyphema (blood in the anterior chamber of the eye), some patients may report "seeing red," or blood-tinged vision from viewing the world through the layer of blood in the anterior chamber of the eye. Excessive coughing, sneezing, or continually leaning forward can result in the bleeding to resume, filling the entire anterior chamber of the eye with blood. As the outflow tracts clog with blood, anterior chamber pressure increases, which can lead to glaucoma and permanent vision loss. Secondary bleeding can occur 3–5 days following the initial injury, leading to an increased risk of vision loss.

D. Glaucoma will present with a cloudy or hazy cornea. A cloudy-appearing cornea is not associated with the presence of a hyphema.

Category: Maxillofacial, Ocular, Orthopedic, and Wound Emergencies/Ocular/Trauma
Nursing Process: Analysis

References

Shea, S. S. (2007). Ocular and maxillofacial trauma. In K. S. Hoyt & J. Selfridge-Thomas (Eds.), *Emergency nursing core curriculum* (6th ed., pp. 848–878). St. Louis, MO: Saunders Elsevier.

Solheim, J. (2013). Facial, ocular, ENT, and dental trauma. In B. B. Hammond & P. G. Zimmermann (Eds.), *Sheehy's manual of emergency care* (7th ed., pp. 439–452). St. Louis, MO: Elsevier Mosby.

---

120. An adult patient presents to the emergency department with a thermal burn to the right forearm. The burn is very painful and sensitive to air. The patient's forearm area is red, involving the first few layers of the dermis, with a large fluid-filled blister. The nurse would appropriately classify the burn as a:

A. superficial partial-thickness burn.
B. fourth-degree burn.
C. deep partial-thickness burn.
D. full thickness burn.

Rationale

A. Only the epidermis is involved with superficial burns. The skin is red and painful. Superficial burns do not have blistering.

B. Fourth-degree burns involve underlying tissues, including muscles and tendons.

C. Deep partial-thickness burns are very painful and involve only the first few layers of the dermis. Blistering is common with deep partial-thickness burns.

D. Full thickness burns involve subcutaneous tissue and do not include blistering. These burns may be surrounded by deep partial or superficial partial burns.

Category: Environment and Toxicology Emergencies, and Communicable Diseases/Environment/Burns
Nursing Process: Assessment

Reference

Ribbens, K. A., & DeVries, M. (2013). Burns. In B. B. Hammond & P. G. Zimmermann (Eds.), *Sheehy's manual of emergency care* (7th ed., pp. 453–462). St. Louis, MO: Elsevier Mosby.

---

121. Which of the following patients should receive rabies prophylaxis?

A. The patient with a bite from a pet cat
B. The patient with a bite from a pet dog
C. The patient who may or may not have been bitten by a bat in the house
D. The patient who may or may not have been bitten by a guinea pig

Rationale

A. Domestic cats are usually vaccinated against rabies. Bites from any animal that can be observed for 2 weeks usually do not require rabies prophylaxis.

B. Domestic dogs are usually vaccinated against rabies. Bites from any animal that can be observed for 2 weeks usually do not require rabies prophylaxis.

C. Bats are a common carrier of rabies. Rabies prophylaxis is recommended when someone has been either exposed to a bat or bitten by a bat.

D. Rodent transmission of rabies is unusual. Bites from any animal that can be observed for 2 weeks usually do not require rabies prophylaxis.

Category: Environment and Toxicology Emergencies, and Communicable Diseases/Environment/Vector-borne illnesses: Rabies
Nursing Process: Analysis

Reference

Herr, R. D. (2013). Wound management. In B. B. Hammond & P. G. Zimmermann (Eds.), *Sheehy's manual of emergency care* (7th ed., pp. 147–160). St. Louis, MO: Elsevier.

---

122. Which of the following is considered an appropriate treatment for a patient with a venomous snake bite?

A. Immobilize the involved area at or below the level of the heart
B. Administer hepatitis B vaccine as soon as possible and continue recommended dosing
C. Immediately apply ice packs and elevate the extremity
D. Contact poison control to have a specific antivenin prepared from the individual snake

Rationale

A. Providing immobilization and maintaining the extremity at the level of the heart is considered appropriate therapy following a venomous snake bite. Ice application, tourniquets, and wound suction have been shown to worsen patient outcomes.

B. Updating tetanus vaccination is recommended for the presence of venomous snake bites but not hepatitis B vaccinations. Venomous snakes have not been proved to carry the hepatitis B virus.

C. Ice application has been proved to worsen patient outcomes following venomous snake bites because of tissue vasoconstriction. The extremity should be maintained at or below the level of the heart to minimize the risk of the snake venom entering the central circulation.

D. There are universal antivenins available in most emergency departments for common venomous pit viper snake bites. Bites from snakes not localized to the United States may require use of poison control. The antivenin should be administered as directed within 4 hours of the bite. Antivenin has been shown to be effective for up to 24 hours following envenomation.

Category: Environment and Toxicology Emergencies, and Communicable Diseases/Environment/ Envenomation emergencies

Nursing Process: Intervention

Reference

Sedlak, S. K. (2013). Bite and sting emergencies. In B. B. Hammond & P. G. Zimmermann (Eds.), *Sheehy's manual of emergency care* (7th ed., pp. 345–352). St. Louis, MO: Elsevier Mosby.

---

123. A patient is being discharged following treatment for excessive vomiting and diarrhea from a possible foodborne illness. You know the patient understands the discharge instructions when the patient states:

A. "I will drink clear liquids, such as sports drinks, for the next 24 hours."
B. "I am OK to eat my regular diet when I leave here."
C. "Drinking milk will settle my stomach."
D. "I will drink clear liquids, such as orange juice and milk, for the next 24 hours."

Rationale

A. Once vomiting has been controlled, oral hydration should begin with the use of fluids that contain glucose, sodium, and potassium, such as sport or electrolyte replacement drinks.

B. Institution of a regular diet following vomiting and diarrhea may induce the vomiting and diarrhea again. Patients should be instructed to gradually increase their diet as tolerated.

C. Milk or milk products are not recommended following vomiting and diarrhea.

D. Clear liquids are defined as liquids that a person can see through, such as water, fruit juice without pulp, broth, clear sodas (7 UP, ginger ale), Jell-O, and popsicles. Milk and orange juice are not defined as clear liquids.

Category: Environment and Toxicology Emergencies, and Communicable Diseases/ Environment/Food poisoning

Nursing Process: Evaluation

Reference

Rossoll, L. W. (2007). Abdominal emergencies. In K. S. Hoyt & J. Selfridge-Thomas (Eds.), *Emergency nursing core curriculum* (6th ed., pp. 159–186). St. Louis, MO: Saunders Elsevier.

124. The nurse is providing discharge education for an adult patient diagnosed with an infestation of *Sarcoptes scabiei* (scabies). Which of the following patient statements indicates that the patient understands the discharge instructions?

A. "I should not go to work or school for 7 days following treatment."
B. "I must discard all of my clothing and linens prior to treatment."
C. "It is normal to continue to experience itching for up to 7 days following treatment."
D. "It is not necessary to treat my family members."

Rationale

A. Patients may return to work or school after the first treatment for scabies.

B. Discarding clothing and linens is an option, but washing the items in hot water and then placing them in a hot clothes dryer is also acceptable.

C. It is common for patients to continue to have an itching sensation for up to 1 week following treatment. Patients should not be retreated without consulting their provider.

D. Scabies is highly contagious, and members of the household may also require treatment.

Category: Environment and Toxicology Emergencies, and Communicable Diseases/Environment/Parasite and fungal infestations

Nursing Process: Evaluation

Reference

Short, W. R., Kemper, M., & Jackson, J. (2013). Infectious diseases. In B. B. Hammond & P. G. Zimmermann (Eds.), *Sheehy's manual of emergency care* (7th ed., pp. 232–244). St. Louis, MO: Elsevier Mosby.

---

125. There are four classifications of radiation particles that can affect life: alpha particles, beta particles, gamma radiation, and neutrons. Of these four, which one is able to penetrate the most objects (paper, wood, concrete) and is therefore more dangerous to life?

A. Gamma radiation
B. Beta particles
C. Neutrons
D. Alpha particles

Rationale

A. Gamma radiation can be absorbed by paper and wood but cannot be absorbed by concrete.

B. Beta particles can only be absorbed by paper, not by wood or concrete. Their radioactive particles are capable of producing long-term health effects depending on the degree of exposure.

C. Neutrons can be absorbed by all three objects—paper, wood, and concrete—and are therefore more dangerous to life.

D. Alpha particles cannot be absorbed by paper, wood, or concrete. However, their radioactive particles can have long-term health effects based on the amount of Exposure.

Category: Environment and Toxicology Emergencies, and Communicable Diseases/Environment/Radiation exposure

Nursing Process: Analysis

Reference

Stopford, B. M., & Colon, W. L. (2007). Weapons of mass destruction. In K. S. Hoyt & J. Selfridge-Thomas (Eds.), *Emergency nursing core curriculum* (6th ed., pp. 970–996). St. Louis, MO: Saunders Elsevier.

---

126. A child is brought to the emergency department after falling through the ice while skating on a lake. On arrival, the patient's core temperature is 26.8°C (80.2°F). The nurse would anticipate this patient to exhibit which signs or symptoms?

A. Slow or slurred speech
B. An increased respiratory rate and effort
C. An increased urinary output
D. A decreased medication effect

Rationale

A. The basal metabolic rate decreases by two to three times the normal rate in the hypothermic patient. The most evident response is seen in the central nervous system.

B. In the hypothermic patient, it is expected to see a respiratory rate and effort that is decreased. This can lead to carbon dioxide retention, hypoxia, and acidosis.

C. Renal blood flow decreases, and the glomerular filtration rate declines in the hypothermic patient. Therefore, a decrease in urine output would be expected.

D. Metabolism in the liver slows, so medications may last longer in the hypothermic patient. Therefore, an increased medication effect would be expected.

Category (Pediatric): Environment and Toxicology Emergencies, and Communicable Diseases/Environment/Temperature-related emergencies

Nursing Process: Assessment

Reference

Flarity, K. (2012). Environmental emergencies. In Emergency Nursing Association, *Emergency Nursing Pediatric Course: Provider manual* (4th ed., pp. 329–341). Des Plaines, IL: Emergency Nursing Association.

---

127. A patient presents with fever and a small, flat, pink, nonpruritic maculular rash on the palms of their hands and soles of their feet. The patient describes removing a tick from their forearm several days ago. Which tickborne disease would you suspect this patient has?

A. Tularemia
B. Rocky Mountain spotted fever
C. Lyme disease
D. Colorado tick fever

Rationale

A. Patients with tularemia typically present with a skin lesion at the site of the bite, which may ulcerate in 2–3 days. Mild edema may be observed with regional adenopathy.

B. Patients with Rocky Mountain spotted fever typically have a fever along with a flat, pink, macular nonpruritic rash. Occurring within the first 10 days following the bite, the rash is generally on the palms, forearms, soles, and ankles. The rash will initially blanche and then becomes raised bumps. Nausea with vomiting can also occur as a result of the disease process.

C. Lyme disease may present with a target or bull's eye rash with bright borders and a fading center. Patients present with malaise, viral syndrome, lymphadenopathy, and headache.

D. Patients with Colorado tick fever present with flulike illness, including fever, chills, malaise, myalgia, and lethargy. No rash is typically identified.

Category: Environment and Toxicology Emergencies, and Communicable Diseases/Environment/Vector-borne illnesses: Tick-borne illness

Nursing Process: Analysis

Reference

Sedlak, S. K. (2013). Bite and sting emergencies. In B. B. Hammond & P. G. Zimmermann (Eds.), *Sheehy's manual of emergency care* (7th ed., pp. 345–352). St. Louis, MO: Elsevier Mosby.

---

128. A patient is being discharged from the emergency department (ED) for treatment of carbon monoxide poisoning. The emergency nurse knows that the patient understands their discharge instructions when the patient states:

A. "I will use the space heater in the bedroom sometimes."
B. "I will not use a space heater."
C. "I can continue to use the space heater with the door closed."
D. "I will return to the ED the next time I get a headache and feel tired."

Rationale

A. Carbon monoxide poisoning from faulty heaters or inadequate ventilation in the winter is the most frequent source of poisoning in the United States.

B. The use of space heaters in small enclosed spaces can contribute to carbon monoxide poisoning.

C. Many severe cases of carbon monoxide poisonings are caused by faulty heating systems and poor ventilation.

D. Causes of headache can be numerous, and while it can accompany the presence of carbon monoxide poisoning, it is not the only symptom the patient will exhibit. Accompanying symptoms of carbon monoxide poisoning include loss of memory and concentration, personality changes, irritability, and extreme fatigue.

Category: Environment and Toxicology Emergencies, and Communicable Diseases/Toxicology/Carbon monoxide

Nursing Process: Evaluation

Reference

Flarity, K. (2010). Environmental emergencies. In P. K. Howard & R. A. Steinmann (Eds.), *Sheehy's emergency nursing: Principles and practice* (6th ed., pp. 535–553). St. Louis, MO: Elsevier Mosby.

---

129. The emergency nurse is aware that a potential sign associated with the presence of cyanide poisoning is:

A. cherry-red skin.
B. symmetrical descending muscular weakness.
C. excessive secretions.
D. the odor of bitter almonds.

Rationale

A. The appearance of cherry-red skin is associated with carbon monoxide poisoning. Patients will also exhibit headache, nausea, and shortness of breath.

B. Botulism results in the patient experiencing symmetrical descending muscular weakness. The patient may also experience blurred vision as a result of botulism.

C. Patients with organophosphate poisoning will experience excessive secretions, in addition to feelings of confusion. The patient may also experience crackles in bilateral lung fields.

D. Cyanide has the odor of bitter almonds. Cyanide interferes with cellular respiration and decreases use of oxygen, resulting in feelings of dizziness, bradycardia, and labored respirations.

Category: Environment and Toxicology Emergencies, and Communicable Diseases/Toxicology/Cyanide

Nursing Process: Assessment

References

Phillips, M. (2007). Toxicologic emergencies. In K. S. Hoyt & J. Selfridge-Thomas (Eds.), *Emergency nursing core curriculum* (6th ed., pp. 604–658). St. Louis, MO: Saunders Elsevier.
Stopford, B., & Colon, W. (2007). Weapons of mass destruction. In K. S. Hoyt & J. Selfridge-Thomas (Eds.), *Emergency nursing core curriculum* (6th ed., pp. 970–996). St. Louis MO: Saunders Elsevier.

---

130. An adolescent is brought in to the emergency department by ambulance. The patient was at a "rave" party and experienced a seizure. The patient is confused and agitated. Vital signs are BP 180/98 mm Hg, HR 136 beats/minute, RR 26 breaths/minute, SpO_2 97%, T 39.6°C (103.2°F). Which of the following would be the first nursing intervention for this patient?

A. Initiate an intravenous line with a large-caliber catheter
B. Obtain a urine sample for analysis
C. Place the patient in seizure precautions
D. Administer a short-acting benzodiazepine medication

Rationale

A. This patient will need an intravenous line, but ensuring a safe environment is the first action the nurse should take.

B. A urine analysis is indicated for this patient to determine the cause of the patient's signs and symptoms, but it is not a priority intervention.

C. This first action should always be patient safety. The patient should be in a padded bed with side rails up and the bed placed in the lowest position.

D. Short-acting benzodiazepines may be indicated for this patient, but it would not be the first intervention that the nurse should complete.

Category (Pediatric): Environment and Toxicology Emergencies, and Communicable Diseases/ Toxicology/Substance abuse

Nursing Process: Intervention

References

Hahn, I. H. (2016). MDMA toxicity treatment and management. *Medscape*. Retrieved from http://emedicine.medscape.com/article/821572-treatment

Stout-Demps, L., & Williams, D. A. (2013). Substance abuse. In B. B. Hammond & P. G. Zimmermann (Eds.), *Sheehy's manual of emergency care* (7th ed., pp. 131–136). St. Louis, MO: Elsevier Mosby.

---

131. An adolescent patient was brought in by ambulance from a party at a friend's house. Paramedics report that the patient was drinking an unknown amount of alcohol at the party. The patient is lethargic and only responds to painful stimuli by moaning. Vital signs are BP 110/60 mm Hg, HR 122 beats/minute, RR 14 breaths/minute, SpO_2 94%, T 36.2°C (97.1°F). Which of the following diagnostic studies has the highest priority for this patient?

A. Serum glucose level

B. Computed tomography of the head

C. Blood alcohol level

D. Urine analysis for drugs of abuse

Rationale

A. Obtaining a serum glucose level is a priority to determine if hypoglycemia is present. Hypoglycemia is a common occurrence in alcohol toxicity, and it could also be the cause of the patient's altered level of consciousness. Severe hypoglycemia can be fatal.

B. Computed tomography of the head is an appropriate diagnostic study, but it is not the highest priority.

C. A blood alcohol level will help to determine if alcohol abuse is the cause of the patient's signs and symptoms, but it has limited value in patient management; therefore, it is not the priority diagnostic study.

D. Obtaining a urine analysis to determine if the patient has used substances that may be causing the altered level of consciousness is appropriate but not the highest priority for this patient.

Category (Pediatric): Environment and Toxicology Emergencies, and Communicable Diseases/ Toxicology/Substance abuse

Nursing Process: Intervention

References

Levine, M. D., & Barker, T. D. (2016). Alcohol toxicity. *Medscape*. Retrieved from http://emedicine.medscape.com /article/812411-overview

Stout-Demps, L., & Williams, D. A. (2013). Substance abuse. In B. B. Hammond & P. G. Zimmermann (Eds.), *Sheehy's manual of emergency care* (7th ed., pp. 131–136). St. Louis, MO: Elsevier Mosby.

---

132. The emergency nurse is caring for an adult patient who was brought in by ambulance after having a tonic–clonic seizure. The patient is confused, appears anxious, and has obvious hand tremors. The patient's vital signs are BP 140/90 mm Hg, HR 128 beats/minute, RR 26 breaths/minute, SpO_2 98%, T 37.4°C (99.3°F). The patient reports that they consume alcohol on a daily basis but stopped drinking alcohol about 2 days ago. What is the priority concern for this patient?

A. The patient is at risk for dehydration.
B. The patient is at risk for decreased cardiac output.
C. The patient is at risk for experiencing hallucinations.
D. The patient is at great risk for injury.

Rationale

A. This patient is at risk for dehydration and will likely require fluid and electrolyte replacement; however, protecting the patient from injury is the highest priority.

B. The patient is at risk for decreased cardiac output if not treated for the alcohol withdrawal, but there are no signs and symptoms indicating an altered cardiac output.

C. This is an appropriate concern for a patient experiencing alcohol withdrawal, but ensuring patient safety is a higher priority for the plan of care.

D. This patient is at risk for injury because of the potential for seizures, falls, confusion, and other alcoholic withdrawal complications. The first priority should always be patient safety.

Category: Environment and Toxicology Emergencies, and Communicable Diseases/Toxicology/ Withdrawal syndrome

Nursing Process: Analysis

References

Phillips, M. (2007). Toxicologic emergencies. In K. S. Hoyt & J. Selfridge-Thomas (Eds.), *Emergency nursing core curriculum* (6th ed., pp. 604–658). St. Louis, MO: Saunders Elsevier.

Stout-Demps, L., & Williams, D. A. (2013). Substance abuse. In B. B. Hammond & P. G. Zimmermann (Eds.), *Sheehy's manual of emergency care* (7th ed., pp. 131–136). St. Louis, MO: Elsevier Mosby.

---

133. A patient presents with a 24-hour history of abdominal pain, fever, nausea, and watery diarrhea. On further questioning, the patient states that they have been prescribed sulfamethoxazole/trimethoprim (Bactrim) for a urinary tract infection. What would your primary intervention be for this patient?

A. Request a stool sample from the patient
B. Place the patient in a private room on contact isolation
C. Prepare to infuse a isotonic crystalloid solution bolus
D. Prepare to administer antibiotics

Rationale

A. Obtaining a stool sample to send for culture is common. However, these results take 48–96 hours, so the higher priority would be to isolate the patient.

B. Patients with known or suspected *Clostridium difficile* **(***C. difficile)* **infections should be immediately placed on contact isolation to prevent spread to other patients and staff.** *C. difficile* **is a highly contagious bacterium causing colitis in the large intestine. The bacteria may colonize or grow when a patient is on antibiotics and normal intestinal flora are disrupted. Patients are capable of shedding the bacteria for several days after symptom resolution. Stool is highly contagious, and contact precautions should be implemented.**

C. A normal saline bolus may be indicated based on the patient's hydration status. The higher priority would be to immediately isolate the patient.

D. Antibiotics are the standard treatment for *C. difficile*; however, getting the patient to a private room and isolation would be a higher priority.

Category: Environment and Toxicology Emergencies, and Communicable Diseases/Communicable Diseases/*C. difficile*

Nursing Process: Intervention

References

Centers for Disease Control and Prevention. (2012). *Frequently asked questions about clostridium difficile for health-care providers.* Retrieved from http://www.cdc.gov/HAI/organisms/cdiff/Cdiff_faqs_HCP.html
Mayo Clinic. (2015). *Urinary tract infection (UTI).* Retrieved from http://www.mayoclinic.org/diseases-conditions/urinary-tract-infection/basics/treatment/con-20037892
Mayo Clinic. (2016). *C. difficile infection.* Retrieved from http://www.mayoclinic.org/diseases-conditions/c-difficile/diagnosis-treatment/treatment/txc-20202426

---

134. You answer a call from a primary care provider who is sending a 14-year-old patient to be evaluated. The provider tells you the patient is experiencing extreme fatigue, fever, sore throat, body aches, and rash, and there is a "knot" in the left axilla. You suspect the patient may have:

A. abscess to left axilla.
B. infectious mononucleosis.
C. strep throat.
D. meningitis.

Rationale

A. The presence of an isolated abscess to the left axilla would not cause the other associated symptoms the patient is experiencing. An abscess could be the cause of the swelling to the left axilla and fever but would not cause a sore throat, rash, enlarged liver, or enlarged spleen.

B. Symptoms of infectious mononucleosis include extreme fatigue, fever, sore throat, head and body aches, swollen lymph nodes in the neck and axilla, enlarged liver, enlarged spleen, and the presence of a fine red macular rash.

C. A beta-hemolytic streptococci infection results in the symptoms associated with strep throat, which include fever, sore throat, and difficulty swallowing or talking, and would cause swelling to the cervical lymph nodes in the neck, not in the axilla.

D. Patients with meningitis may have symptoms of fatigue, fever, rash, body aches, and headache. Meningitis generally does not cause the patient to experience a sore throat or swollen lymph nodes in the axilla.

Category (Pediatric): Environment and Toxicology Emergencies, and Communicable Diseases/ Communicable Diseases/Mononucleosis

Nursing Process: Assessment

References

Centers for Disease Control and Prevention. (2016). *Epstein-Barr virus and infectious mononucleosis: About infectious mononucleosis*. Retrieved from http://www.cdc.gov/epstein-barr/about-mono.html

Centers for Disease Control and Prevention. (2016). *Worried your sore throat may be strep?* Retrieved from http://www.cdc.gov/Features/strepthroat/

---

135. The key to safe and effective care of the trauma patient is associated with which of the following?

A. Identified roles and responsibilities of the team members
B. Group diversity
C. Individual mental processes and individual leadership
D. Engage in individual member review of performance activities

Rationale

A. Clear and defined roles of each of the team members are key components to the safe and effective delivery of trauma care.

B. The trauma team needs to be able to communicate effectively with one another to minimize errors and to improve patient outcomes.

C. The trauma team needs one identified leader from which all members of the team receive direction. This will lead to minimal errors, better team organization, and the development of clear goals.

D. A well-organized trauma team will conduct a review of the entire trauma resuscitation and critique how they can improve their communication for optimal patient outcomes.

Category: Professional Issues/Nurse/Evidence-based practice

Cognitive Level: Application

Reference

Hohenhaus, S. M., & Nierstedt, P. (2014). Teamwork and trauma care. In D. Gurney (Ed.), *Trauma Nursing Core Course: Provider manual* (7th ed., pp. 5–8). Des Plaines, IL: Emergency Nurses Association.

---

136. The child of a hospital employee has died in the emergency department. The emergency staff and hospital employees are visibly upset and are having difficulty coping with the child's death. Hospital administration decides to conduct a critical incident stress management (CISM) debriefing for the staff. Ideally the CISM debriefing should take place within what time frame?

A. As soon as possible
B. Within 24–72 hours
C. Within 3–5 days
D. Within 1 week

Rationale

A. The emergency department nurse manager will be unable to schedule a CISM debriefing immediately following the incident. The social work department, CISM team, and chaplain will schedule the formal debriefing within 1–3 days.

B. A formal debriefing should be scheduled within 24–72 hours (1–3 days) of the incident to allow the involved staff to debrief and to openly discuss their feelings.

C. The sooner involved staff members are able to discuss their feelings, the sooner they can begin their grieving and healing process to cope with the events of the incident.

D. If the CISM debriefing takes place after more than 72 hours have passed, those involved may have forgotten key elements they wish to discuss surrounding the event. This delay can actually cause staff members to be unable to understand their feelings surrounding the event. Staff members may be unable to return to work in a timely fashion because of their continued stress relating to the event.

Category: Professional Issues/Nurse/Critical Incident Stress Management

Cognitive Level: Application

References

Healy, M. M., & Gurney, D. (2014). Psychosocial aspects of trauma care. In D. Gurney (Ed.), *Trauma Nursing Core Course: Provider manual* (7th ed., pp. 295–310). Des Plaines, IL: Emergency Nurses Association.

Maloney, C. (2012). Critical incident stress debriefing and pediatric nurses: An approach to support the work environment and mitigate negative consequences. *Pediatric Nursing, 38*(2), 110–113.

---

137. The emergency nurse is aware that the practice of lifelong learning is an essential element leading to the achievement of which of the following?

A. Professional expertise
B. Promotion to a management position
C. Academic success
D. Personal fulfillment

Rationale

A. As evidenced in the nursing theory text *From Novice to Expert* by Patricia Benner, participation in lifelong learning is an essential element in the transition from a novice to an expert professional.

B. Depending on the specific qualifications of the management position, a program of lifelong learning may or may not be a requirement.

C. Lifelong learning can contribute to academic success; however, lifelong learning often occurs outside the classroom with coaches or mentors who have no direct relation to an academic program.

D. Lifelong learning may contribute to a nurse's personal fulfillment, but it is not an essential component in the transition from novice to expert.

Category: Professional Issues/Nurse/Lifelong learning

Cognitive Level: Knowledge/Recall

Reference

Emergency Nurses Association. (2012). *Nurse leaders in emergency care.* Des Plains, IL: Author.

---

138. In preparing the body of an organ donor for eye tissue donation, the emergency nurse should perform which of the following?

A. Close the eyes and cover the eyelids with dry, sterile gauze
B. Apply warm compresses to the eyelids to promote circulation
C. Elevate the head of the bed 20 degrees
D. Prepare the patient for transfer to the operating room

Rationale

A. The eyelids should be taped shut with paper tape. Artificial tears may be instilled, but it is not required.

B. Cool compresses or ice should be applied to the eyelids to prevent swelling.

C. When corneas are to be donated, the head of the bed should be elevated at 20 degrees, and the eyelids should be taped shut with paper tape. Artificial tears may be instilled into the eyes, but it is not required.

D. Eye enucleation is a clean procedure, using sterile technique, that can be performed in any area of the hospital or at an outside mortuary.

Category: Professional Issues/Patient/End-of-life issues: Organ and tissue donation

Cognitive Level: Application

References

Bonalumi, N. (2010). Organ and tissue donation. In P. K. Howard & R. A. Steinmann (Eds.), *Sheehy's emergency nursing: Principles and practice* (6th ed., pp. 155–163). St. Louis, MO: Mosby Elsevier.

Cronin, T. D. (2013). End-of-life issues for emergency nurses. In B. B. Hammond & P. G. Zimmermann (Eds.), *Sheehy's manual of emergency care* (7th ed., pp. 175–182). St. Louis, MO: Elsevier Mosby.

---

139. Accurate documentation of the "chain of custody" in the handling of forensic evidence is necessary to ensure which of the following?

A. Validating the competency of the individual who collected the evidence
B. Safeguarding the integrity of the evidence
C. Providing law enforcement with evidence needed to convict the suspected criminal
D. Limiting the number of individuals who handle the evidence

Rationale

A. Documentation of a chain of custody does not validate the competence of the evidence collector; it only provides a detailed account of when the evidence was collected, secured, and properly transferred without interference, potential contamination, or loss.

B. Accurate documentation of the chain of custody when handling forensic evidence establishes the integrity of the evidence and ensures that it was not subjected to contamination or tampering.

C. Emergency nurses do not collect evidence to show proof that a crime was committed. The chain of custody validates the authenticity of the evidence so that it can be accepted in a court proceeding.

D. The best practice in forensic evidence collection is to limit the number of individuals who handle the evidence. However, the chain of custody documentation only identifies the individuals who handled the evidence; it does not limit the number.

Category: Professional Issues/Patient/Forensic evidence collection

Cognitive Level: Recall

Reference

Sheridan, D., Nash, K. R., & Bresee, H. (2010). Forensic nursing in the emergency department. In P. K. Howard & R. A. Steinmann (Eds.), *Sheehy's emergency nursing: Principles and practice* (6th ed., pp. 174–186). St. Louis, MO: Mosby Elsevier.

---

140. The nurse is aware that the most reliable method of assessing a patient's pain is which of the following?

A. Utilizing a nurse-initiated pain management protocol
B. Observing specific pain-associated behaviors such as grimacing or crying
C. Asking the patient to describe what pain-relieving medications have been effective for them in the past
D. Acknowledging the patient's self-report of pain

Rationale

A. Nurse-initiated pain management protocols can shorten the time that the patient must wait before receiving pain medication. However, the protocol is a nursing intervention that must be based on an accurate pain assessment.

B. The behaviors and attitudes exhibited by an individual who is experiencing pain (i.e., stoicism versus emotive) may be driven by familial, ethnic, or cultural norms; therefore, observing specific behaviors is not a valid means of measuring an individual's level of pain.

C. The pain experienced by the patient may not be related to the current pain experience. Pain medication is an intervention that must be based on an accurate and valid assessment of the patient's current level of pain.

D. The most reliable means of assessing a patient's pain is based on the patient's self-report of pain. The various pain scales available provide the patient with a tool that can objectively measure the intensity of the pain experience.

Category: Professional Issues/Patient//Pain management and procedural sedation

Cognitive Level: Application

References

Campbell, C. M., & Edwards, R. R. (2012). Ethnic differences in pain and pain management. *Pain Management, 2*(3), 219–230. https://doi.org/10.2217/pmt.12.7

Meyer, D. (2013). Care of the patient with pain. In B. B. Hammond & P. G. Zimmermann (Eds.), *Sheehy's manual of emergency care* (7th ed., pp. 121–130). St. Louis, MO: Elsevier Mosby.

Tanabe, P., Holleran, R. S., & Reddin, C. J. (2010). Pain. In P. K. Howard & R.A. Steinmann (Eds.), *Sheehy's emergency nursing: Principles and practice* (6th ed., pp. 127–147). St. Louis, MO: Mosby Elsevier.

---

141. A 5-year-old patient presents to a general emergency department. The patient requires a dose of oral medication for the illness. The nurse understands that this patient is at increased risk for medication errors because of which of the following?

A. Inability to swallow medications
B. Parent being a poor historian
C. Patient having no known allergies
D. Weight-based dosing

Rationale

A. A patient's inability to swallow is of concern, and precautions or a change in the route of administration should be considered. However, the primary cause for medication errors in children is the failure to administer medications per weight-based dosing.

B. A parent who is unable to provide an adequate health history is not the primary cause for medication errors in children. For mediations to be administered in the appropriate dose, the child's weight must be obtained and the medication dose properly calculated.

C. It is important to be aware of any drug allergies a patient may have before the administration of medication. However, for mediations to be administered in the appropriate dose, the child's weight must be obtained and the medication dose properly calculated.

D. Children pose a risk for emergency care because most emergency departments are built around adult needs. Children are at increased risk of medication errors because of weight-based dosing, medicine dilution, and the inability to communicate their needs or responses.

Category: Professional Issues/Patient/Patient safety

Cognitive Level: Application

Reference

Hohenhas, S. (2013). Patient safety in the emergency department. In B. B. Hammond & P. G. Zimmermann (Eds.), *Sheehy's manual of emergency care* (7th ed., pp. 37–42). St. Louis, MO: Elsevier Mosby.

---

142. A patient with an acute myocardial infarction is being prepared for transport by ground ambulance to the nearby medical center. The patient is stable but is receiving multiple intravenous vasoactive medications. The emergency nurse should be most concerned regarding which of the following?

A. The patient's spouse is insisting that they ride along in the ambulance.
B. The patient is being transferred via ground ambulance rather than helicopter.
C. The transport team comprises individuals with extensive training in basic life support.
D. The patient experiences motion sickness when flying or riding in a vehicle.

Rationale

A. It is understandable that a family member would want to ride along in the ambulance, and their presence can be comforting for the patient, especially a child, but the practice is not always wise or possible. Transport companies have specific policies regarding family members accompanying patients in the ambulance.

B. Although it is desirable to transport this patient as quickly as possible, factors such as weather and patient size and weight may influence the choice of vehicle for patient transport. The Emergency Medical Treatment and Active Labor Act requires only that a transfer be carried out by qualified personnel using equipment required by the patient's condition.

C. Members of the transport team must have the necessary knowledge and skills to care for the patient. The management of intravenous vasoactive medication is beyond the scope of a basic life support provider. The nurse should not allow the transport to proceed until an advanced life support provider is available to accompany the patient.

D. The patient who experiences motion sickness should be prophylactically premedicated to prevent nausea and vomiting. Motion sickness is not a reason to abort or delay the transfer.

Category: Professional Issues/Patient/Transfer and stabilization

Cognitive Level: Analysis

References

Holleran, R. S. (2010). Air and surface patient transport. In P. K. Howard & R. A. Steinmann (Eds.), *Sheehy's emergency nursing: Principles and practice* (6th ed., pp. 83–98). St. Louis, MO: Mosby Elsevier.

Robinson, K. (2007). Emergency patient transfer and transport. In K. S. Hoyt & J. Selfridge-Thomas (Eds.), *Emergency nursing core curriculum* (6th ed., pp. 1011–1024). St. Louis, MO: Saunders Elsevier.

143. A non–English-speaking patient presents to the triage nurse. The best method for the emergency triage nurse to effectively communicate with the patient is to use which of the following?

A. A member of the healthcare staff who speaks the patient's native language
B. A member of the patient's family or friend
C. An illustrated chart for the patient to point at descriptors of the symptoms
D. A certified translator fluent in the patient's native language

Rationale

A. Fluency in a language does not guarantee that an individual is a qualified interpreter. A certified interpreter or designated interpretation service is a better alternative.

B. Using a family member or friend of the patient to provide interpretive services would be a violation of the patient's right to privacy.

C. The use of an illustrated chart may be helpful in some situations, however, use of the illustrations alone does not comply with Title VI of the Civil Rights Act.

D. Title VI of the Civil Rights Act requires interpreter services for all patients with limited English proficiency. The patient must be afforded the ability to ask questions and understand the answers to their questions and participate in their plan of care. A certified interpreter or language interpretation service should be used.

Category: Professional Issues/Patient/Cultural considerations

Cognitive Level: Application

References

Hinkle, J. L., & Cheever, K. H. (2014). Adult health and nutritional assessment. In *Brunner & Suddarth's textbook of medical-surgical nursing* (13th ed., pp. 56–74). Philadelphia, PA: Lippincott Williams & Wilkins.

Juckett. G., & Unger, K. (2014). Appropriate use of medical interpreters. *American Family Physician, 90*(7), 476–480. Retrieved from http://www.aafp.org/afp/2014/1001/p476.html

Rice, S. (2014, August 30). Hospitals often ignore policies on using qualified medical interpreters. *Modern Healthcare.* Retrieved from http://www.modernhealthcare.com/article/20140830/MAGAZINE/308309945

---

144. The emergency nurse caring for an elderly patient delegates hourly vital signs to unlicensed assistive personnel. The unlicensed assistive staff member does not report a hypotensive blood pressure to the registered nurse and only documents it on the patient's chart. The patient suffers a poor outcome. Who is at fault for not reporting the hypotensive blood pressure to the emergency department provider?

A. The registered nurse who delegated the task of vital signs
B. The assistive staff member who took the patient's vital signs
C. The charge nurse
D. The physician assistant

Rationale

A. The registered nurse (RN) holds the unlicensed assistive personnel responsible for the completion of the delegated task and for reporting any changes in the patient's condition. However, the RN is responsible for the delegation decision, the process, and the ongoing monitoring of the outcomes of the patient's nursing care.

B. The RN holds the unlicensed assistive personnel responsible for the completion of the delegated task and for reporting any changes in the patient's condition. However, the RN is accountable for the delegation decision, the process, and the ongoing monitoring of the outcomes of the patient's nursing care.

C. The RN holds the unlicensed assistive personnel responsible for the completion of the delegated task and for reporting any changes in the patient's condition. However, the RN is accountable for the delegation decision, the process and the ongoing monitoring of the outcomes of the patient's nursing care.

D. The RN holds the unlicensed assistive personnel responsible for the completion of the delegated task and for reporting any changes in the patient's condition. However, the RN is accountable for the delegation decision, the process, and the ongoing monitoring of the outcomes of the patient's nursing care.

Category: Professional Issues/System/Delegation of tasks to assistive personnel

Cognitive Level: Application

Reference

Bonalumi, N. M., & King, D. (2007). In K. S. Hoyt & J. Selfridge-Thomas, *Emergency nursing core curriculum* (6th ed., pp. 1046–1056). St. Louis, MO: Saunders Elsevier.

---

145. Using the mass casualty START triage system for adults, which of the following patients would be classified as a yellow (delayed) patient?

A. A patient who is able to stand and walk to a designated area as instructed
B. A patient who is unable to ambulate, with a respiratory rate of 32 breaths/minute
C. A patient who is unable to ambulate, has no spontaneous respirations even with repositioning airway, has absent central pulse, and does not follow commands
D. A patient who is unable to ambulate and who can follow commands, with a respiratory rate under 30 breaths/minute

Rationale

A. Patients who are able to ambulate unassisted and walk to a designated area are classified as "walking wounded," or the green simple triage and rapid treatment (START) triage category.

B. This patient is classified as red in the START triage category because of a respiratory rate over 30 breaths/minute and being unable to ambulate.

C. Patients who do not have spontaneous respirations after repositioning of their airway are classified as black (expectant). Additional classifying criteria do not matter because this patient is not breathing and is considered expectant; attempting resuscitative measures in a mass casualty incident would require more resources than are potentially available.

D. Patients who are unable to ambulate but meet the START triage criteria of respiratory rate less than 30, capillary refill of less than 2 seconds, and are able to follow commands fall into the yellow START triage category.

Category: Professional Issues/System/Disaster management

Cognitive Level: Application

Reference

Assid, P. A. (2014). Disaster management. In D. Gurney (Ed.), *Trauma Nursing Core Course: Provider manual* (7th ed., pp. 311–324). Des Plaines, IL: Emergency Nurses Association.

---

146. The National Incident Management System requires that hospitals have plans and procedures in place to be prepared for emergency management situations, such as mass casualty incidents and disasters. One system that helps hospitals to be prepared and creates a command structure is the:

A. Federal Emergency Management Agency
B. National Response Framework
C. Hospital Incident Command System
D. Disaster Medical Assistance Team

Rationale

A. Federal Emergency Management Agency (FEMA) is one of the federal agencies that trains and assists the country during disasters. FEMA may be involved in disaster management at the hospital level depending on the size of the event. However, Hospital Incident Command System (HICS) is the system that is specific to hospital command in a disaster or mass casualty incident.

B. National Response Framework is a plan for how the United States as a nation responds to disasters. This can be from the local level all the way up to the national level for disasters that require federal support. HICS is the hospital command structure that is used within hospitals to plan, prepare, and implement a command structure for disasters and mass casualty incidents.

C. HICS is a National Incident Management System approved for hospitals to use in their response to mass casualty incidents and disaster management. The HICS provides a command structure for hospitals with specific job functions under each command level to assist a hospital in managing emergency response situations.

D. A Disaster Medical Assistance Team (DMAT) is a trained medical team that responds to disasters when needed. Although a DMAT may assist a hospital when a mass casualty event or disaster happens, it is not a system used by hospitals to respond in a disaster. HICS is the hospital command structure that is used within hospitals to plan, prepare, and implement a command structure for disasters and mass casualty incidents.

Category: Professional Issues/System/Disaster management

Cognitive Level: Recall

Reference

Andress, K. (2010). Nuclear, biologic, and chemical agents of mass destruction. In P. K. Howard & R. A. Steinmann (Eds.), *Sheehy's emergency nursing: Principles and practice* (6th ed., pp. 198–210). St. Louis, MO: Mosby Elsevier.

---

147. To be compliant with the United States Emergency Medical Treatment and Active Labor Act, all patients presenting to the emergency department must have had which of the following performed?

A. Triage assessment by a registered nurse
B. Emergency Severity Index acuity level assigned
C. Medical screening exam
D. At least one set of vital signs

Rationale

A. Triage is not a medical screening exam (MSE). Triage assessment and assignment of an acuity rating do not fulfill the legal requirement of the patient receiving an MSE.

B. Completing triage and assigning an Emergency Severity Index acuity level are not equivalent to performing an MSE. Triage assessment and assignment of an acuity rating do not fulfill the legal requirement of the patient receiving an MSE.

C. An MSE is performed by a physician or physician extender as identified by the hospital bylaws.

D. One set of vitals would be a component of an MSE but does not entail the complete MSE process.

Category: Professional Issues/System/Federal regulations
Cognitive Level: Recall

Reference

Gilroy, N., & Travers, D. (2007). Triage. In K. S. Hoyt & J. Selfridge-Thomas (Eds.), *Emergency nursing core curriculum* (6th ed., pp. 28–50). St. Louis, MO: Saunders.

---

148. An unresponsive trauma patient is brought to the emergency department (ED) by ambulance. There are no family members present, and no contact information is available for the patient's family. It is appropriate for ED personnel to treat this patient based on which type of consent?

A. Implied consent
B. Expressed consent
C. Involuntary consent
D. Informed consent

Rationale

A. When a patient is unconscious or unable to provide verbal consent, no family members are present to provide consent for treatment, and immediate interventions are necessary to save the patient's life and/or limb, the physician is obligated to act on the patient's behalf. The action is referred to as implied consent.

B. If the patient was alert and orientated, they could have provided expressed consent. Expressed consent occurs when a patient voluntarily consents to medical treatment and is predicated on the patient's mental capacity. Because the patient is unresponsive and in a life-threatening situation, treatment for this patient is based on implied consent.

C. Involuntary consent is indicated when an incompetent individual refuses necessary medical treatment, and the patient requires immediate intervention to save life or limb.

D. Provided by the physician, informed consent describes the procedure being performed, the alternatives to the procedure, and the risks and benefits associated with the procedure. Informed consent is based on the patient's understanding of the risks, benefits, and alternatives to any therapy or procedures. Because the patient is unresponsive, they cannot be provided with the description, alternatives, risks, and benefits of any therapy or procedures.

Category: Professional Issues/System/Patient consent for treatment

Cognitive Level: Application

Reference

Jagim, M. (2007). Legal and regulatory issues. In K. S. Hoyt & J. Selfridge Thomas (Eds.), *Emergency nursing core curriculum* (6th ed., pp. 1033–1045). St. Louis, MO: Saunders Elsevier.

---

149. According to The Joint Commission, the overwhelming majority of serious medical errors that occur during patient handoff can be attributed to which type of mechanism?

A. Equipment failure
B. Inappropriate staffing mix at the receiving facility
C. Communication breakdown
D. Use of unapproved abbreviations

Rationale

A. Equipment failure, especially when it involves a monitoring device, can impact patient safety during medication administration, but it is usually not a concern at the time of patient handoff/transfer.

B. Communication at the time of patient handoff/transfer should occur between caregivers of equal or higher level of knowledge, skill, and critical thinking ability, so the staffing mix at the time of transfer would not be relevant.

C. The Joint Commission requires accredited organizations to use a standardized approach to handoff communications, citing research suggesting that approximately 80% of serious medical errors occur because of miscommunication rates during patient handoffs/transfers.

D. The use of unapproved abbreviations contributes to medication errors. However, their use is only part of the communication process that takes place at the time of patient handoff/transfer.

Category: Professional Issues/System/Risk management

Cognitive Level: Analysis

References

Emergency Nurses Association. (2013). *Patient handoff/transfer*. Des Plains, IL: Author. Retrieved from https://www.ena.org/practice-research/Practice/Position/Pages/PositStmts.aspx

Friesen, M., White, S., & Byers, J. (2008). Handoffs: Implications for nurses. In R. Hughes, *Patient safety and quality: An evidence-based handbook for nurses* (Chapter 34). Rockville, MD: Agency for Healthcare Research and Quality.

---

150. A patient who recently returned from a trip to East Africa presents to triage complaining of fever, abdominal pain, bloody diarrhea, and weakness. The triage nurse recognizes that this patient is most at risk for which of the following?

A. Ebola virus
B. Chickenpox
C. Gastroenteritis
D. Influenza

Rationale

A. Fever, abdominal pain, weakness, muscle pain, diarrhea, fatigue, vomiting, and unexplained hemorrhage and bruising with known recent travel to East Africa put this patient most at risk for having the Ebola virus.

B. Chickenpox presents with a vesicular rash, fever, loss of appetite, fatigue, and headache. Recent travel to Africa would be less likely to result in contracting chickenpox as compared with contracting the Ebola virus.

C. Diarrhea, vomiting, abdominal pain, fever, and fatigue are all signs and symptoms of gastroenteritis. Gastroenteritis is contagious and caused by a virus, but with the patient's recent travel to Africa and the unexplained bleeding and bruising, the nurse should be more concerned that the patient may have contracted the Ebola virus.

D. Influenza is another viral illness, but patients will typically present with fever, cough, sore throat, runny nose, muscle or body aches, fatigue, and headache. The recent travel to Africa and unexplained bleeding should cause the nurse to be more concerned regarding the possibility of the Ebola virus rather than the presence of influenza.

Category: Professional Issues/System/Symptom surveillance: Recognizing symptom clusters

Cognitive Level: Analysis

Reference

Stopford, B. M., & Dolon, W. L. (2007). Weapons of mass destruction. In K. S. Hoyt & J. Selfridge-Thomas (Eds.), *Emergency nursing core curriculum* (6th ed., pp. 970–996). St. Louis, MO: Saunders Elsevier.

SELF-DIAGNOSTIC PROFILE

How to Use the Self-Assessment Worksheet

1. Indicate on your answer sheet whether your answers are correct or incorrect.
2. Note the items you answered incorrectly.
3. Count the total number of items you answered incorrectly in each category.
4. Compare the total number of items you answered incorrectly in each category with the total number of items per category. This information will give you an idea of where you will need to focus your continued study.

Content Category	Questions Answered Incorrectly	Total Number of Questions Answered Incorrectly in Each Category	Total Number of Questions in Each CEN Content Category
Cardiovascular Emergencies			20
Respiratory Emergencies			16
Neurological Emergencies			16
Gastrointestinal, Genitourinary, Gynecology, and Obstetrical Emergencies			21
Psychosocial and Medical Emergencies			25
Maxillofacial, Ocular, Orthopedic, and Wound Emergencies			21
Environment and Toxicology Emergencies, and Communicable Diseases			15
Professional Issues			16

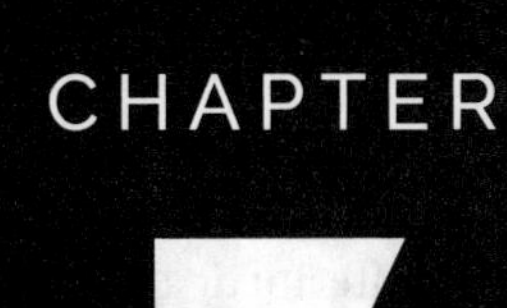

CHAPTER 7

Practice Examination 2

PART 1

1. A patient presents to the emergency department complaining of a 2-day history of a dull substernal ache that has continued to increase in intensity. The patient states that they had some relief after taking a nitroglycerin tablet yesterday. Vital signs are: BP 114/68 mm Hg; HR 68 beats/minute; RR 22 breaths/minute. The electrocardiogram demonstrates a new onset left bundle branch block. The priority intervention for this patient is:
   A. continuous monitoring for development of ST segment elevation.
   B. serial cardiac markers.
   C. preparing the patient for transport to interventional cardiology.
   D. admission to a telemetry unit for observation.

2. During the completion of a 12-lead electrocardiogram, the nurse identifies excessive artifact in lead II and lead III. To resolve this technical difficulty, the nurse should:
   A. change the right arm electrode.
   B. check for cable movement.
   C. change the left leg electrode.
   D. instruct the patient to momentarily hold their breath.

3. When determining the presence of ST segment elevation on an electrocardiogram (ECG), the ST segment is compared to which interval or segment of the ECG?
   A. P-R interval
   B. T-P interval
   C. Q-T interval
   D. P-R segment

4. A middle-aged patient presents to the emergency department via emergency medical services. The patient states that they were awoken from sleep with midsternal chest pain approximately 4–5 hours ago. In the presence of an acute myocardial infarction (AMI), the initial elevation of the troponin cardiac biomarkers occurs within:
   A. 1–2 hours after onset of an AMI.
   B. 4–8 hours after onset of an AMI.
   C. 24–30 hours after onset of an AMI.
   D. 10–24 hours after onset of an AMI.

5. The nurse suspects a patient may have an acute aortic dissection when, during the history-taking process, the patient describes the pain as:
   A. squeezing, burning epigastric pain that may radiate to the middle back area.
   B. right upper quadrant pain referred to right scapula and shoulder.
   C. sudden, severe tearing or ripping chest, interscapular, or back pain.
   D. sharp, stabbing chest pain radiating to neck, arms, or left shoulder.

6. You are assisting in the resuscitation of an elderly patient in cardiac arrest. A waveform capnography is in place, and high-quality cardiopulmonary resuscitation is being performed. A sudden increase in the level of the end-tidal carbon dioxide indicates the:
   A. need for deeper and faster chest compressions.
   B. need for an additional dose of a vasopressor, such as intravenous bolus epinephrine.
   C. presence of an irreversible cardiac arrest.
   D. return of spontaneous circulation.

7. A patient in cardiac arrest presents to the emergency department receiving cardiopulmonary resuscitation by emergency medical services personnel. The cardiac monitor displays sinus rhythm, but no palpable pulse can be detected. The most likely cause of this pulseless electrical activity is:
   A. glucose level of 145 mg/dL.
   B. potassium value of 1.3 mmol/L (1.3 mEq/L).
   C. arterial pH of 7.36.
   D. magnesium level of 3.0 mg/dL.

8. Which of the following physiological conditions would result in the loss of ventricular capture for a patient being transcutaneously paced?
   A. Lactic acidosis
   B. Hypomagnesemia
   C. Metabolic alkalosis
   D. Hypokalemia

9. A patient arrives to the emergency department by emergency medical services with a complaint of weakness and near syncope. The patient's HR is 24 beats/minute, and BP is 80/60 mm Hg. The patient underwent a heart transplant 6 months ago, and the cardiac monitor displays third-degree heart block. The emergency nurse is aware the patient will immediately require which medication to increase the patient's heart rate?
   A. Atropine sulfate (Atropine)
   B. Isoproterenol (Isuprel)
   C. Digoxin (Lanoxin)
   D. Amiodarone (Cordarone)

10. On examination of a febrile patient presenting to the emergency department with a chief complaint of "flulike symptoms" and a history of intravenous drug use, the nurse notes a cardiac murmur, crackles in bilateral lung bases, subungual hemorrhages, nontender erythematous macules on the palms of the hand and soles of the feet, and painful erythematous nodules on the tips of the fingers and toes. Which is the most important initial intervention for this patient?
    A. Echocardiogram
    B. Chest radiography
    C. Surgery
    D. Antibiotics

11. A patient presents with an episode of acute worsening of chronic systolic congestive heart failure. Blood pressure is 150/70 mm Hg. The patient complains of dyspnea, and rales are heard bilaterally. The patient is not hypoxic, nor does the electrocardiogram demonstrate evidence of an acute myocardial ischemia or infarction. Which of the following medications would be harmful to administer to the patient at this time?
    A. Vasodilators
    B. Vasopressor agents
    C. Diuretics
    D. Opiates

12. A patient presents to the emergency department complaining of a severe headache. Vital signs reveal a BP of 270/170 mm Hg; HR 80 beats/minute; and RR 20 breaths/minute. The patient is alert and describes being recently diagnosed with high blood pressure. A priority intervention for this patient would be to:
    A. initiate intravenous medication to lower the patient's BP immediately.
    B. obtain baseline laboratory data.
    C. consider emergency cardioversion for BP control.
    D. evaluate BP cuff size for accuracy.

13. Administration of nitroprusside (Nipride) to a patient in hypertensive crisis is considered effective when the patient demonstrates which of the following?
    A. The patient responds to verbal stimuli.
    B. The systolic blood pressure reaches 160 mm Hg.
    C. The systolic blood pressure reaches 120 mm Hg.
    D. The patient reports relief of chest pain.

14. Signs and symptoms of cardiac tamponade include:
    A. widening pulse pressure.
    B. muffled heart tones.
    C. jugular vein flattening.
    D. jugular vein distention, narrowing pulse pressure, and tracheal deviation.

15. The parent of a toddler tells the nurse that the child was recently diagnosed with "hand, foot, and mouth disease." Today the child began to complain of chest pain that hurts more while coughing and "when taking a deep breath." The nurse notes that the child is sitting upright on the mother's lap and is leaning forward. Based on the patient's most recent illness history, the nurse knows this patient is at risk for developing:
    A. pneumonia.
    B. pericarditis.
    C. respiratory syncytial virus.
    D. commotio cordis.

16. Which of the following would further enhance the symptoms of peripheral vascular disease, causing the patient increased discomfort?
    A. Narcotics
    B. Calcium channel blockers
    C. Alcohol use
    D. Smoking

17. A patient presents to the emergency department complaining of pain in their left leg that began suddenly while they were sitting in their car. The patient denies any recent trauma. Which of the following elements of the patient's history is most concerning?
    A. The patient is a noninsulin-dependent diabetic with an $HgbA_{1C}$ of 6.8% at their last physician appointment.
    B. The patient had a myocardial infarction 4 years ago that was successfully treated with stent placement, and now they take 162 mg of aspirin daily.
    C. The patient is a regional sales representative who spends much of their time driving and smokes two packs of cigarettes a day.
    D. The patient has poorly controlled hypertension and takes a "blood pressure pill" and a "water pill" most days.

18. Assessment of a patient from a motor vehicle collision reveals a seat belt sign on the patient's chest, premature ventricular contractions, chest pain, and hypotension. Oxygen, intravenous fluids, and pain medication have been administered. Which of the following reevaluation criteria would cause the nurse to be concerned?
    A. Lactic acid of 3 mmol/L
    B. Heart tones of S1, S2
    C. Breath sounds with crackles
    D. Oxygen saturation of 95%

19. Patient assessment findings after a motor vehicle collision reveal decreased cardiac contractility and output without volume loss. Goal-directed therapy includes fluid boluses and inotropic support. Which of the following will the nurse monitor for in this patient?
    A. Fluid overload
    B. Urinary output
    C. Tension pneumothorax
    D. Hemorrhage

20. Which of the following interventions decreases the amount of a patient's preload?
    A. Administration of a beta-blocker
    B. Successful cardioversion of new onset atrial fibrillation to sinus rhythm
    C. Placing the patient in a supine position with legs elevated
    D. Administration of morphine sulfate 2–4 mg intravenous

21. A parent presents to the triage area with an infant, stating, "My baby hasn't been breathing right since last night and won't take a bottle." The infant's respiratory rate is 72 breaths/minute, and they appear pale. The emergency nurse is aware this presentation indicates:
    A. that the infant is experiencing a rapid decline in their cardiopulmonary status.
    B. a respiratory rate that is within normal parameters for an infant.
    C. that infants are normally more tachypnic.
    D. that there are multiple reasons for an increased respiratory rate in infants.

22. A characteristic sign associated with the presence of chronic obstructive pulmonary disease is:
    A. pink frothy sputum.
    B. fever.
    C. decreased breath sounds on one side of the chest.
    D. pursed lip breathing.

23. A main goal of treatment for patients with chronic obstructive pulmonary disease is to:
  A. avoid hospitalizations.
  B. cure the disease and return lung function to normal.
  C. prevent further lung damage.
  D. avoid increasing the use of medications.

24. A critically ill emergency department patient with an exacerbation of their chronic obstructive pulmonary disease is diagnosed with respiratory acidosis. The priority medication that should be administered and that would be most beneficial to this patient is a(n):
  A. bronchodilator.
  B. corticosteroid.
  C. diuretic.
  D. antibiotic.

25. A patient arrives via emergency medical services and is extremely confused, febrile, and tachypnic, with the presence of crackles in the right lower lobe on auscultation of the lung fields. The provider diagnoses the patient with pneumonia. As the emergency nurse caring for the patient, you would anticipate the arterial blood gases to show which abnormality?
  A. pH: 7.25, $PaCO_2$: 65 mm Hg, HCO_3: 22 mEq/L
  B. pH: 7.35, $PaCO_2$: 40 mm Hg, HCO_3: 22 mEq/L
  C. pH: 7.30, $PaCO_2$: 35 mm Hg, HCO_3: 16 mEq/L
  D. pH: 7.5, $PaCO_2$: 40 mm Hg, HCO_3: 38 mEq/L

26. A motorcyclist who was not wearing a helmet is involved in a collision. On arrival to the emergency department, the patient is assessed to have sustained significant facial injuries, and audible gurgling is heard. The priority intervention for this patient is to:
  A. prepare for endotracheal intubation.
  B. control facial venous bleeding.
  C. place the patient in the high-Fowler's position.
  D. suction the oropharynx.

27. An emergency patient is being treated for carbon monoxide poisoning. The patient's response to treatment is best evaluated by:
  A. obtaining a pulse oximetry reading.
  B. obtaining a Glasgow Coma Scale score.
  C. obtaining an arterial blood gas measurement.
  D. obtaining a peak flow reading.

28. In assessing a patient for the presence of a suspected tracheobronchial injury, the emergency nurse can expect to auscultate which of the following?
  A. Bowel sounds heard in the thoracic cavity
  B. Pleural friction rub auscultated over the axilla
  C. Rales auscultated at the bilateral lung bases
  D. Crunching or bubbling sound heard over the precordium that is synchronous with the heartbeat

29. A patient arrives at the emergency department complaining of progressively worsening chest pain. They said they were involved in a motor vehicle collision 3 days ago. The patient is hemodynamically stable, and assessment reveals the presence of dullness on percussion over the left lung fields. The emergency nurse anticipates that the dullness on percussion is the result of:

A. pneumothorax.
B. pulmonary contusion.
C. pleural effusion.
D. pericardial effusion.

30. A patient presents to the emergency department complaining of chest pain and dyspnea. A chest radiograph is obtained and shows a visible lung margin with air filling the pleural space. Supplemental oxygen has been administered, and intravenous access has been established. Which intervention should the emergency nurse anticipate next?

A. Endotracheal intubation
B. Needle thoracostomy
C. Bilevel positive airway pressure
D. Chest tube thoracostomy

31. A patient presents pale and diaphoretic with initial vital signs as follows: BP 130/85 mm Hg; HR 135 beats/minute; RR 40 breaths/minute; SpO_2 48% room air; T 37.2°C (99.0°F). Lung sounds are diminished bilaterally throughout, with crackles at the bases. The patient has been visiting from Florida for the past 4 days, and the current the elevation is 9500 feet. The priority intervention for the emergency nurse to perform is to:

A. obtain an electrocardiogram.
B. place the patient on a nonrebreather mask.
C. establish intravenous access.
D. obtain a chest radiograph.

32. A patient arrives complaining of dyspnea and mild right-sided chest pain that began the previous evening and increases in intensity with exertion. Initial vital signs are: BP 108/56 mm Hg; HR 115 beats/minute; RR 28 breaths/minute; SpO_2 87% room air; T 36.6°C (97.8°F). Lung sounds have fine scattered crackles bilaterally. The patient states that 3 days ago, they sustained an injury to their right leg while playing tennis. Based on this information, the emergency nurse suspects the patient has a:

A. pneumothorax.
B. pneumonia.
C. pleural effusion.
D. pulmonary embolism.

33. A patient with severe acute respiratory distress syndrome will have critical levels of hypoxemia. The nurse can potentially improve the patient's oxygenation by placing the patient into which position?

A. High-Fowler's position
B. Prone position
C. On left side with head elevated
D. Reverse Trendelenburg position

34. A pneumothorax can be classified as a simple, open, or tension pneumothorax. In a tension pneumothorax, assessment findings may include which of the following?
   A. Symmetrical chest wall movement
   B. Tracheal deviation
   C. Muffled heart tones
   D. Sucking chest wound

35. The primary cause of mortality in the advanced stages of chronic obstructive pulmonary disease is which of the following?
   A. Cardiac-related event
   B. Pneumonia
   C. Pneumothorax
   D. Blood clot

36. To auscultate vesicular breath sounds, it is best to listen over the:
   A. trachea/thorax region.
   B. major bronchi.
   C. peripheral lung fields.
   D. scapular region.

37. The emergency nurse is conducting a confusion assessment method assessment in a patient. Which of the following assessments would indicate the patient is confused?
   A. The patient engages in a conversation.
   B. The patient has abnormal vital signs.
   C. The patient is unable to complete a simple task.
   D. The patient has a decreased level of consciousness.

38. A patient presents to triage complaining of a 2-week history of fatigue and tingling in their hands, and has experienced several falls recently. Vital signs are: BP 116/72 mm Hg; HR 86 beats/minute; RR 16 breaths/minute; T 37.0°C (98.6°F). The emergency nurse anticipates that which of the following will provide the most information regarding the patient's symptoms?
   A. Magnetic resonance imaging of the brain and spinal cord
   B. Serum lactate
   C. Spinal computed tomography scan of the brain and spinal cord
   D. Complete blood count

39. A patient who has been evaluated for a right facial droop is being discharged with instructions related to their diagnosis of Bell's palsy. The patient asks if their facial paralysis is permanent. The most appropriate response from the emergency nurse is:
   A. "The damage from the virus will not resolve but over time, but you will become accustomed to the facial droop."
   B. "All of your facial weakness will resolve, just be patient with the recovery."
   C. "This is difficult to predict, but most patients have a complete recovery within 3 to 6 months following the onset of their symptoms."
   D. "Your facial weakness will come and go."

40. A patient presents to triage complaining of a headache that feels as though someone is squeezing their head in a tight grip. The patient states they experience these headaches every month, and they complain of no other signs or symptoms. The emergency nurse is aware that the patient is describing the which type of headache?

A. Migraine headache
B. Subcortical headache
C. Tension headache
D. Hydronephrosis headache

41. Each of the following patients presents to the emergency department with a chief complaint of headache. Which patient would most likely require intracranial imaging?

A. A patient diagnosed with small cell lung cancer who complains of a new-onset headache
B. A patient with a history of migraines who presents with their typical symptom complex
C. A 25-year-old patient who presents with a new-onset tension-type headache
D. A patient with a headache accompanied by a fever, elevated erythrocyte sedimentation rate, and no leukocytosis.

42. A patient presents to the emergency department after being found unresponsive at home. The patient's family member states that the patient regularly abuses alcohol. There was noted bruising to the patient's face and head. The emergency nurse notes the patient has a fixed and dilated left pupil, has increased deep respirations with periods of apnea, is bradycardic, and is experiencing a continual rise in only the systolic blood pressure. The emergency nurse is most concerned regarding which of the following?

A. Presence of a subdural hematoma
B. An absence seizure
C. An ischemic stroke
D. A narcotic overdose

43. A patient with a previously diagnosed brain tumor arrives at the emergency department unresponsive. Following the patient's initial assessment and interventions, an osmotic diuretic is administered. Which of the following findings indicates to the emergency nurse an effective response to this medication?

A. Urinary output 30 mL/hour
B. Widening pulse pressures
C. Absence of pulsus paradoxus
D. Glasgow Coma Score of 13

44. The emergency nurse is a caring for a patient who has sustained a subdural hematoma. The provider has ordered that the patient be placed in a semi-Fowler's position to facilitate blood return to the heart. The emergency nurse is aware that this intervention has been successful when the patient has a:

A. PaO_2 of 55 mm Hg.
B. mean arterial pressure of 70 mm Hg.
C. systolic blood pressure of 80 mm Hg.
D. $PaCO_2$ 50 mm Hg.

45. The emergency nurse is aware that the most common symptom of bacterial meningitis is the presence of a:

A. seizure.
B. stiff neck.
C. high fever.
D. petechial rash.

46. On assessing a patient with complaint of severe headache and fever, the nurse observes that when the patient's head is flexed forward, their knees and hips also flex. Based on this assessment finding, the emergency nurse anticipates that this patient has which of the following?

A. Spinal cord injury
B. Cervical spine fracture
C. Trapezius muscle injury
D. Meningitis

47. An elderly patient presents to triage with a history of a near syncope event. The patient has no known prior medical history, currently takes no medications, and has a blood glucose level of 133. The patient suddenly has a tonic–clonic seizure. Their airway is being properly maintained. The emergency nurse is aware that the priority assessment for this patient is to:

A. assess for the presence of a pulse.
B. assess the patient's blood pressure.
C. assess for the presence of bowel sounds.
D. assess the patient's extraocular movement.

48. A patient presents to the emergency department with a free phenytoin (Dilantin) level of 22 mcg/mL. The emergency nurse would anticipate which of the following assessment findings?

A. Nystagmus
B. Ataxia
C. Confusion
D. Hypotension

49. A patient presents to the emergency department after a motor vehicle collision. Neurogenic shock is suspected secondary to a spinal cord injury. Which of the following hemodynamic parameters is most consistent with neurogenic shock?

A. Hypertension
B. Increased central venous pressure
C. Bradycardia
D. Decreased SvO_2

50. The emergency nurse is monitoring the blood pressure of a patient with a subarachnoid hemorrhage. The patient's blood pressure is currently 180/98. The nurse anticipates that the provider will order which medication for this patient?

A. Hypertonic saline
B. Intropin (Dopamine)
C. Labetalol (Trandate)
D. Propofol (Diprivan)

51. When performing the motor portion of the Glasgow Coma Scale assessment on a patient, the emergency nurse observes that the patient does not follow commands, but they do move their right arm in an attempt to remove the source of pressure that is being applied to their left arm. The patient is noted to cross the midline to get to the source of the applied pressure to their arm. Based on this observation, the emergency nurse will document a motor score of:

A. 5: localization.
B. 6: localization.
C. 4: withdrawal.
D. 5: withdrawal.

52. The emergency nurse would determine an unconscious patient's Glasgow Coma Score by:
   A. speaking loudly to the patient.
   B. monitoring for spontaneous movement.
   C. assessing the patient's Babinski reflex.
   D. applying a painful stimulus.

53. An adult patient presents to the emergency department stating that they have been retching and vomiting for the past 12 hours and now has started vomiting bright red blood. The emergency nurse anticipates that the patient may have which of the following conditions?
   A. Mallory–Weiss syndrome
   B. Peptic ulcer disease
   C. Ruptured esophageal varices
   D. Esophageal stricture

54. A patient is being prepared for discharge after being diagnosed with cholecystitis. Which statement made by the patient to the emergency nurse indicates their understanding of the dietary discharge instructions?
   A. "It is important to eat foods rich in potassium."
   B. "I need to stay away from foods with seeds and nuts."
   C. "I should eat small, frequent meals rather than three large meals each day."
   D. "I should avoid high-fat and fried foods."

55. A 60-year-old patient presents to the emergency department complaining of left lower quadrant abdominal pain, nausea, constipation, and anorexia that began 2 days ago. Vital signs: BP 118/78 mm Hg; HR 98 beats/minute; RR 18 breaths/minute; T 38.2°C (100.8°F). Assessment findings include abdominal distention, left-sided abdominal tenderness, and a palpable mass in the left lower quadrant. Bowel sounds are hyperactive in all four quadrants. The nurse suspects the patient may have:
   A. appendicitis.
   B. diverticulitis.
   C. cholecystitis.
   D. pancreatitis.

56. When caring for a patient with bleeding esophageal varices, the emergency nurse would anticipate an order to initially administer which of the following medications?
   A. Pantoprazole (Protonix)
   B. Sulfasalazine (Azulfidine)
   C. Somatostatin (Octreotide)
   D. Sucralfate (Carafate)

57. The emergency nurse is preparing discharge instructions for a patient with abdominal pain and anticipates a prescription for a proton pump inhibitor as treatment for the patient's new diagnosis of:
   A. cholecystitis.
   B. hepatitis.
   C. diverticulitis.
   D. esophagitis.

58. The parents of a young child state their child may have swallowed a coin-sized lithium battery. The child has a patent airway but is drooling. Radiographs confirm that the battery is lodged in the child's esophagus. The emergency nurse should perform which of the following interventions?

A. Prepare the patient for immediate endoscopy to remove the battery
B. Provide the patient with popsicles and repeat the radiograph in 1 hour
C. Discharge the patient to home and provide parent with instructions to examine stool for the battery
D. Administer intravenous glucagon

59. A 9-month-old presents to the emergency department (ED) with a 24-hour history of vomiting and diarrhea. The child's lips are dry and cracked, and tears are noted when the child cries. The parents state that the last wet diaper was 2 hours before arrival at the ED. The emergency nurse would be most concerned with what additional assessment finding?

A. Capillary refill 3 seconds
B. Systolic blood pressure 84 mm Hg
C. Apical heart rate 150 beats/minute
D. Respiratory rate 48 breaths/minute

60. An 18-month-old child with a 3-day history of diarrhea is brought to the emergency department by the parents. The child is irritable, mucus membranes are dry, and capillary refill is less than 3 seconds. The parents state that the child has had only one wet diaper in the past 8 hours. The emergency nurse anticipates the priority intervention for this patient is to:

A. obtain intravenous access and infuse a 0.9% sodium chloride bolus at 20 mL/kg.
B. obtain a stool culture.
C. administer an antiemetic medication.
D. offer small, frequent sips of an oral rehydration solution.

61. While examining a patient who presents with nausea, vomiting, and abdominal pain, a firm and tender mass is palpated in the lower right abdominal quadrant. The emergency nurse suspects that the patient may have of which of the following?

A. Diverticulitis
B. Crohn's disease
C. Appendicitis
D. Incarcerated hernia

62. Which statement made by a patient with a history of inflammatory bowel disease is most consistent with a diagnosis of Crohn's disease?

A. "I keep getting these sores in my rectal area."
B. "I keep having flare-ups of my disease and have lost a lot of weight recently."
C. "One of my doctors told me that I might be able to have surgery on my colon that can cure this disease."
D. "Last time I was here, I had to have steroids and intravenous fluids."

63. An infant is brought to the emergency department by their parents, who state that the infant has been irritable and vomiting, and has a change in the color and consistency of their stools. The infant is diagnosed with intussusception. The parents tell the nurse they do not understand what is wrong with their child. The best explanation by the nurse to the parents is to say:
   A. "Intussusception occurs when the muscle that controls how the stomach empties is too tight, so the stomach contents back up."
   B. "These changes in the stool can happen when a child is transitioned from breastmilk to formula and cereal."
   C. "This happens when one portion of the bowel slides into the next. It's similar to a telescope and results in a blockage within the bowel."
   D. "This can happen when the bowel pushes through the abdominal muscles. As long as the blood supply isn't cut off, surgery isn't needed."

64. A patient with a large stab wound to the abdomen is received in the emergency department. On assessment, the patient has a loop of small bowel protruding from the wound. The emergency nurse should immediately cover the exposed bowel with which of the following?
   A. A semipermeable transparent dressing
   B. Dry, sterile dressings
   C. Saline-soaked gauze
   D. Nonstick gauze and an abdominal binder

65. A 40-year-old male presents with complaints of a painful penile erection for the past several hours that is not associated with sexual stimulation. The patient has a history of chronic back pain, schizophrenia, and hepatitis C. The prolonged erection is most likely due to the patient's use of:
   A. risperidone (Risperdal).
   B. ribavirin (Virazole).
   C. celecoxib (Celebrex).
   D. buprenorphine/naloxone (Buprenex).

66. A patient with a diagnosis of renal calculi is being prepared for discharge from the emergency department. Which of the following statements made by the patient demonstrates their understanding of the discharge instructions?
   A. "I will eliminate all calcium-containing foods from my diet."
   B. "I should increase the amount of water I drink during the day."
   C. "Once the pain resolves, I will no longer need to strain my urine."
   D. "I can expect to run a fever until the stone passes."

67. A 28-year-old female presents to the emergency department with complaints of heavy, bright red vaginal bleeding for the past 1 month. She complains of feeling tired but is alert and oriented and denies feelings of dizziness or lightheadedness. The patient states that she has not been sexually active for the past 3 months. Vital signs: BP 116/74 mm Hg; HR 86 beats/minute; RR 18 breaths/minute; T 36.8°C (98.4°F). The patient's hemoglobin is 9.4 g/dL, and the urine pregnancy test is negative. The nurse should prepare the patient for a(n):
   A. immediate exploratory laparotomy.
   B. transfusion with 1 unit of packed red blood cells.
   C. vaginal examination.
   D. STAT administration of levonorgestrel (Plan B).

68. A patient diagnosed with chlamydia verbalizes understanding of the disease process when they state:
   A. "Symptoms of a chlamydia infection include a vaginal discharge with a 'fishy' odor."
   B. "Men who have sex with other men are not at risk to contract chlamydia infection."
   C. "Most patients with chlamydia do not have symptoms."
   D. "Once treated, a patient develops immunity against future chlamydia infections."

69. A 26-week-pregnant female presents with bright red vaginal bleeding. The patient states she has saturated one feminine pad every hour for the past 3 hours. On examination by the care provider, the uterus is painful and tender to palpation and fetal heart tones are 160 beats/minute. Vital signs: BP 124/80 mm Hg; HR 110 beats/minute; RR 20 breaths/minute; SpO_2 98% on room air; T 37°C (98.9°F). The emergency nurse should anticipate which of the following interventions to be performed next?
   A. Admission for fetal monitoring
   B. Emergent caesarean section
   C. Immediate blood transfusion
   D. Discharge to home on bedrest with physician follow-up

70. A 26-year-old female presents to triage with a sudden onset of right lower abdominal pain, followed by a syncopal episode and heavy vaginal bleeding. Based on the presenting symptoms, which of the following conditions would the emergency nurse most likely suspect?
   A. Ruptured ectopic pregnancy
   B. Pelvic inflammatory disease
   C. Ruptured ovarian cyst
   D. Acute exacerbation of endometriosis

71. Approximately 10 minutes following the vaginal delivery of a full-term neonate in the emergency department, the emergency nurse observes a sudden gush of blood from the mother's vagina. The nurse suspects which of the following?
   A. Uterine rupture has occurred.
   B. The patient has sustained a cervical tear during delivery.
   C. The placenta has separated from the uterine wall.
   D. Delivery of an unanticipated second neonate is imminent.

72. A 28-week-pregnant female arrives to the emergency department with chief complaint of shortness of breath and right upper abdominal pain. Which of the following laboratory results would suggest to the emergency nurse that the patient is developing HELLP syndrome?
   A. Platelet count 90,000/mm^3
   B. Glycosuria
   C. Serum potassium 5.8 mEq/L
   D. Serum magnesium 1.7 mEq/L

73. A patient who is 32 weeks pregnant presents to the emergency department complaining of severe abdominal pain. Which of the following assessment findings would place the patient at risk for preterm labor?
   A. Having a long interval between pregnancies
   B. Smoking during pregnancy
   C. Having a previous full-term birth
   D. Maternal age between 30 and 35 years

74. A young mother presents to triage with a 2 1/2-year-old toddler who sustained a lip laceration related to a fall while playing in the yard. The mother tells the triage nurse that her daughter is "very clumsy." The child has numerous bruises in various stages of healing on bilateral knees and a healing abrasion on one elbow, but no other apparent injuries. Which of the following statements about assessment for potential child maltreatment is most accurate for this situation?

A. Unintentional injuries tend to occur on bony prominences, which may be normal for a toddler.
B. The bruises in various stages of healing are a clear sign of potential abuse and should be evaluated.
C. Multiple areas of injury are indicative of potential abuse, especially in the toddler population.
D. Intentional injuries are easily spotted because they are generally inflicted in patterns.

75. A patient with a history of depression and bipolar disorder presents to the emergency department with suicidal ideation and auditory hallucinations. While awaiting a mental health bed to become available, the patient becomes increasingly agitated, begins to pace about the treatment area, and threatens staff members. The nurse actively listens and speaks in clear, concise language while ensuring the patient's safety. Which of the following demonstrates a desired response to the interventions?

A. The patient states that they do not need to be in restraints any longer.
B. The patient is able to verbalize their feelings.
C. The patient accepted their medication.
D. The patient's suicidal ideation has ceased.

76. A patient reports experiencing short episodes of intense fear accompanied by chest pain, shortness of breath, lightheadedness, and numbness. Which of the following statements made by the patient indicate an understanding of the treatment options for this experience?

A. "I should call for an ambulance as soon as the symptoms start."
B. "I should first try to determine what made me feel anxious."
C. "Breathing in and out into a paper bag may help the symptoms initially subside."
D. "I should take some over-the-counter pain medication when I experience these symptoms."

77. A combat veteran is brought to the emergency department by their social worker. The patient has a history of depression, increasing angry outbursts and nightmares since returning from combat. The patient appears anxious, is tearful, and tells the triage nurse, "I can't take this anymore. Please help me." Vital signs: BP 134/80 mm Hg; HR 89 beats/minute; RR 18 breaths/minute; T 36.7° C (98.2°F). The emergency nurse escorts the patient to a quiet room and suspects that their symptoms are suggestive of which condition?

A. Alcohol withdrawal syndrome
B. Posttraumatic stress disorder
C. Acute psychosis
D. Panic attack

78. A patient who received an injection of an antipsychotic medication to manage acute mania is now experiencing an acute dystonic reaction. Which of the following medications would the emergency nurse expect to administer to treat this medication side effect?

A. Diazepam (Valium)
B. Naloxone (Narcan)
C. Flumazenil (Romazicon)
D. Diphenhydramine (Benadryl)

79. A patient presents to the emergency department following the recent loss of both their job and significant other. The patient appears despondent, with a flat affect. Which of the following is the highest priority intervention for the emergency nurse to perform in the case of this patient?

A. Inform the patient about possible grief counseling groups
B. Assess if the patient plans to harm themself
C. Refer the patient to their primary care physician
D. Assist the patient with resources to find a new job

80. A patient presents to triage dressed in a robe and carrying a staff, stating that they "are Jesus Christ" and "are going to save the world." Which of the following interventions should be considered for this patient?

A. Speaking calmly to the patient
B. Restraining the patient
C. Telling the patient they are not "Jesus Christ"
D. Administering intravenous haloperidol

81. Law enforcement arrives to the emergency department with a patient who was found wandering around a local neighborhood. The patient is alert, oriented, and cooperative but appears agitated. They are pacing in circles and mumbling to themself. Vital signs are within normal limits. The officer tells you that the patient has a psychiatric and seizure history and is well-known to local law enforcement. The patient complains of headache, nausea, and vertigo and states they've been having nightmares. The most likely cause of the patient's current condition is which of the following?

A. Abrupt discontinuation from phenytoin
B. Withdrawal from benzodiazepines medication
C. Overdose on selective serotonin inhibitor medication
D. Overdose on tricyclic antidepressants medication

82. Which Emergency Severity Index classification level will be designated for a patient with an isolated complaint of suicidal ideation and no medical health problems?

A. Level 1: immediate life-saving interventions
B. Level 2: high risk
C. Level 3: many resources
D. Level 5: no resources

83. A patient arrives to the emergency department after sustaining multiple bee stings while working on a roof. The patient complains of chest pains, lightheadedness, and difficulty breathing. Prior medical history includes hypertension and "heart problems." Vital signs: BP 70/40 mm Hg; HR 122 beats/minute; RR 24 breaths/minute; SpO_2 88% on room air; T 37.7°C (100.0°F). Which intervention would be the highest priority the emergency nurse should initiate for this patient?

A. Obtain a 12-lead electrocardiogram
B. Administer epinephrine
C. Administer high-flow oxygen via nonrebreather face mask
D. Obtain intravenous access

84. A patient presents to the emergency department complaining of a red rash covering their face, chest, and back. The emergency nurse recognizes the patient, who was treated several days earlier for an ear infection. The emergency nurse anticipates that the cause of the patient's rash is which of the following?

A. Allergic reaction to the prescribed antibiotics
B. Impetigo
C. Scabies
D. Shingles (herpes zoster)

85. A mother arrives to triage with her 5-year-old son, stating that her child recently had a viral illness and now has developed a generalized nonitching rash and is bruising easily. The child's vital signs are within normal limits for age. The child is diagnosed with idiopathic thrombocytopenic purpura (ITP), and intravenous immune globulin (IVIG) has been administered. The emergency nurse can expect which of the following outcomes from the administration of the IVIG?

A. Resolution of the infection that caused ITP
B. Increase in the prothrombin time and partial prothrombin time levels
C. Rapid increase in platelet count
D. Increase in white blood cell count

86. Which of the following patients, each with a history of hemophilia A would have the highest priority for care by the emergency nurse?

A. Patient with bleeding gums following a tooth extraction
B. Patient who presents with an epistaxis (nosebleed)
C. Patient with severe swelling into the knee joint following a fall
D. Patient with a headache following a fall

87. A patient with a history of leukemia presents to triage with a complaint of increasing dyspnea over the past several days. The patient is pale and has multiple bruises on all their extremities. Which of the following is the most likely cause of the patient's bruising?

A. Generalized lymphadenopathy
B. Immaturity of white blood cells
C. Thrombocytopenia
D. Malignant cells within the dermis

88. The emergency nurse is providing discharge teaching to a patient with sickle cell disease. Which of the following instructions is most appropriate for this patient?

A. "Be sure to exercise vigorously."
B. "Apply ice to the painful, swollen areas to reduce swelling and discomfort."
C. "Apply moist heat to the sore areas to reduce swelling and pain."
D. "Decrease your fluid intake until you are feeling better."

89. Which disease process is most commonly associated with a patient developing disseminated intravascular coagulation?

A. Cardiac tamponade
B. Renal failure
C. Intracerebral hemorrhage
D. Sepsis

90. A patient with renal failure, abdominal cramping, diarrhea, and a potassium level of 6.8 mEq/L is being treated in the emergency department for hyperkalemia. Tall peaked T-waves are noted on the electrocardiogram. Priority interventions, in addition to cardiac monitoring, include the administration of:

A. intravenous (IV) dextrose solution followed by regular insulin.
B. sodium polystyrene (Kayexalate) via nasogastric tube.
C. a potassium-sparing diuretic, such as spironolactone.
D. 0.9% sodium chloride IV bolus.

91. Which of the following conditions caused by a decrease in both cortisol and aldosterone levels is considered a life-threatening condition?

A. Cushing's syndrome
B. Diabetes insipidus
C. Myxedema coma
D. Adrenal crisis

92. A patient is being discharged from the emergency department following evaluation for Cushing's syndrome. The patient is currently taking dexamethasone (Prednisone) for their Cushing's syndrome, but the emergency provider prescribes a different medication for the patient's joint inflammation. Which of the following instructions would the emergency nurse provide regarding the dexamethasone?

A. Continue with both medications
B. Decrease the dose to one tablet a week for 2 weeks and discontinue
C. Immediately discontinue medication
D. Discontinue with tapering doses over period of time

93. Symptoms that are associated with hypoglycemia can be attributed to the release of catecholamines when blood glucose levels decrease. Which of the following symptoms would be caused by this pathophysiological response?

A. Diaphoresis
B. Pupillary constriction
C. Dry skin
D. Abdominal cramping

94. A patient has been diagnosed with diabetic ketoacidosis. Laboratory values include a blood glucose level of 525 mg/dL, an arterial pH of 7.30, a potassium level of 4.8 mEq/L, and elevated levels of blood urea nitrogen, creatinine, and hematocrit. Which of the following orders written by the provider would be *most* correct in the treatment of this patient?

A. Furosemide 40 mg intravenous (IV) push
B. Sodium bicarbonate 1 amp IV bolus
C. Potassium hydrochloride 40 mEq over 1 hour
D. Regular insulin 0.15 units/kg IV bolus

95. An adult patient presents to the emergency department with palpitations, agitation, high fever, hot, dry skin, and exophthalmoses. Vital signs: BP 172/48 mm Hg; HR 174 beats/minute; RR 24 breaths/minute; T 40.1°C (104.3°F). The emergency nurse would anticipate orders from the provider based on which clinical condition this patient is experiencing?

A. Syndrome of inappropriate antidiuretic hormone secretion
B. Hypothyroid coma or myxedema coma
C. Acute adrenal insufficiency
D. Thyroid storm/hyperthyroid crisis

96. Which of the following questions asked by the triage nurse would provide the best information regarding possible causes of a febrile illness in a child?

A. "Has your child been in contact with anyone who is ill?"
B. "Does your child attend daycare?"
C. "Is your child up to date on immunizations?"
D. "When did your child start having a fever?"

97. A patient presents to emergency department triage complaining of increasing shortness of breath, dysphagia, and hoarseness. The patient reports being diagnosed with HIV several years ago but has never received treatment for this condition. The emergency nurse observes numerous purple and black nodules located on the hard palate inside the patient's mouth. Based on the patient's history, the emergency nurse suspects which condition?

A. Staining from cigarette smoking
B. Dental decay
C. Kaposi's sarcoma
D. Benign lesions

98. A patient presents to the emergency department with a productive cough, fever of 40°C (104°F), and RR 22 breaths/minute. The patient's chest radiograph reveals a right lower lobe pneumonia. Antibiotics are being administered. The patient's RR increases to 30 breaths/minute, and they become agitated and confused. The emergency nurse identifies that these signs indicate the patient is now experiencing:

A. a response to the elevated temperature.
B. life-threatening organ dysfunction.
C. an allergic reaction to the intravenous antibiotic.
D. the presence of a pulmonary embolus.

99. A patient with a history of heroin abuse arrives to the emergency department by ambulance. The patient was found lying on their left side with their head positioned on their forearm for an unknown period of time. The patient is now responsive following an appropriate dose of naloxone (Narcan) and is complaining of severe pain in their left forearm. The extremity is swollen, and skin is taut and cool to touch. The emergency nurse assesses that the patient's left radial pulse is weaker than the right radial pulse, and the patient is unable to rotate the left upper extremity. The emergency nurse anticipates that the patient is exhibiting signs and symptoms of:

A. ecchymosis.
B. upper extremity fracture.
C. rhabdomyolysis.
D. compartment syndrome.

100. A patient is referred for care from an urgent care center to the emergency department for possible costochondritis. On patient assessment, the emergency nurse anticipates this patient will have which of the following findings?

A. The presence of ectopy on electrocardiogram
B. Atelectasis on chest radiograph film
C. Muffled heart sounds
D. Tenderness of the midsternal area

101. A patient arrives to the emergency department after falling out of their wheelchair, injuring their hip. The emergency nurse anticipates that the patient has fractured their hip based on which of the following assessment findings?

A. Absence of pedal pulses
B. Ligamentous instability in the lower leg
C. Misalignment of the extremity
D. Cool extremity

102. A child presents to the emergency department with a suspected "nursemaid's" elbow. The emergency nurse is aware that the correct terminology for this type of injury is which of the following?

A. Radial head subluxation
B. Radial head fracture
C. Olecranon fracture
D. Olecranon dislocation

103. Before discharging a patient with a lower extremity fracture home with crutches, the emergency nurse is aware that the patient understands the proper use of the crutches when they demonstrate which of the following actions?

A. The patient's elbows remain at a 90-degree angle when using the handgrips.
B. The patient's elbows are slightly bent when using the handgrips.
C. The crutches are placed approximately 3 inches from either side of the patient.
D. The crutches are placed close to the body on either side of the patient.

104. An elderly male presents to triage complaining of stiff knees every morning, joint pain with movement, and swelling for the past several months. He has not seen his family doctor in over 10 years. The emergency nurse suspects that this patient has the symptoms of:

A. osteoporosis.
B. osteoarthritis.
C. osteomyelitis.
D. osteomalacia.

105. A patient arrives to triage with a complaint of joint pain that began the previous day in the small joints of both hands. The joints of the fingers in both hands are swollen, red, and tender to touch. The emergency provider orders a complete blood count and erythrocyte sedimentation rate (ESR). The emergency nurse is aware that the ESR is used as a(n):

A. predictor for the severity of sepsis.
B. definitive diagnosis for the presence of rheumatoid arthritis.
C. indicator of a nonspecific inflammatory process.
D. indicator of tissue damage within the body.

106. A patient presents to the emergency department with lower back pain related to muscle spasms following an acute lumbosacral strain. On providing discharge instructions, the emergency nurse should instruct the patient to do which of the following?

A. Twist gently from side to side to maintain range of motion in the spine.
B. Keep the head elevated slightly and flex the knees when resting in bed.
C. Lying flat, place a small pillow under the upper back to flex the lumbar spine gently.
D. Avoid the use of ice because it will exacerbate the muscle spasms.

107. In caring for a patient who has been diagnosed with an ankle sprain, the patient asks, "What is a grade II ankle sprain?" The most appropriate answer for the emergency nurse to provide is:

A. "A sprain involves injury to the tendon or muscle. There is a partial tear to the tendon or muscle, but the joint is still stable."
B. "A sprain involves injury to the ligaments. With a grade II sprain, there is a partial tear to the ligament, but the ankle joint is still stable."
C. "A sprain involves injury to the ligaments. There is a remarkable tear to the ligament, and the joint is not stable."
D. "A sprain involves injury to the tendon or muscle. The muscle or tendon has ruptured, and the joint is not stable."

108. An elderly woman is admitted to the emergency department by ambulance after being found lying on the floor at home for the past 6 hours. The patient is alert and states that she tripped and fell. She did not lose consciousness, but she was unable to get up to call for help. The emergency nurse knows that the most common initial finding in the patient with possible rhabdomyolysis is the presence of:

A. pain out of proportion to the injury.
B. a petechial chest rash.
C. tea- or cola-colored urine.
D. shortness of breath at rest.

109. A patient presents to the emergency department complaining of pain around their Achilles tendon after walking several miles earlier in the day. The patient denies any recent injury to the ankle or foot. On reviewing the patient's current medication list, the emergency nurse identifies which of the following medications that places the patient at risk for a tendon rupture?

A. Losartan (Cozaar)
B. Levothyroxine (Synthroid)
C. Levofloxacin (Levaquin)
D. Lisinopril (Zestril)

110. What should the emergency nurse anticipate in the care of a patient with an avulsed injury to their scalp?

A. Trimming edges of the wound that are gray or dusky in appearance
B. Preparing the wound for local injection of lidocaine with epinephrine before suturing the wound
C. Cleaning and debridement of the devitalized tissue
D. Applying wet-to-dry dressing

111. An emergency nurse is evaluating a wound that was irrigated with saline via a syringe and attached 18-gauge catheter. The nurse identifies that the wound has been properly irrigated when they observe which of the following?

A. There is the presence of white tissue around the wound without debris.
B. There is no obvious presence of debris.
C. There is no redness surrounding the wound.
D. The wound is no longer actively bleeding.

112. A dose of LET (lidocaine, epinephrine and tetracaine) gel has been applied to a child in preparation for wound closure. The emergency nurse is aware this preparation has been effective when:

A. redness is observed around wound.
B. 10 minutes have passed.
C. blanching is observed around the wound.
D. 20 minutes have passed and the child is now sleepy.

113. A patient receives sutures to repair a facial laceration. The emergency nurse provides discharge instructions to the patient. The patient acknowledges understanding of their discharge instructions when the patient states the following:

A. "I will return in 3–5 days to have the sutures removed."
B. "I will return in 6–7 days to have the sutures removed."
C. "I will return in 10–14 days to have the sutures removed."
D. "I will return in 7–10 days to have the sutures removed."

114. In caring for a patient who has repeatedly been placed on BiPAP for severe respiratory distress, the emergency nurse observes the presence of a deep open wound across the bridge of the patient's nose under the mask. This wound should be documented as a:

A. stage 1 pressure injury.
B. stage 2 pressure injury.
C. stage 4 pressure injury.
D. unstageable pressure injury.

115. A patient presents to the emergency department with a canine bite to the hand. What is the emergency nurse's priority assessment?

A. The source of the bite
B. Presence of any active bleeding or exudate
C. When the bite occurred
D. Treatment of the bite prior to arrival

116. A patient presents to the triage nurse with a tooth in their hand. The patient states that they were involved in an altercation approximately 4 hours ago and that the tooth was knocked out at that time. Which of the following is the most appropriate action for the emergency nurse to take?

A. Determine if the patient has sustained any other injuries and advise that it is likely not possible that the tooth be implanted back into the dental socket.
B. Inspect and irrigate the dental socket with normal saline sprayed through an 18-gauge bore needle.
C. Place the tooth in milk or Save-a-Tooth solution.
D. Dispose of the tooth.

117. A patient presents to triage with epistaxis (nosebleed). The patient is coughing and spitting blood into a towel. The patient informs the emergency nurse that they are currently taking warfarin (Coumadin). The priority intervention for this patient is to:

A. perform oropharyngeal suction.
B. administer Vitamin K (phytonadione).
C. provide supplemental oxygen.
D. apply direct pressure to the patient's nostrils.

118. A patient arrives at the emergency department in full cervical spine precautions following an all-terrain vehicle collision. Initial assessment reveals the presence of rhinorrhea and otorrhea, which tests positive for the presence of glucose. The emergency nurse anticipates that the patient has sustained which type of fracture?

A. Depressed skull fracture
B. Le Fort I fracture
C. Mandibular fracture
D. Cribriform plate fracture

119. A child arrives to the emergency department by emergency medical services, who report that the patient was tackled while playing football and is now complaining of difficulty breathing. Patient assessment reveals swelling and ecchymosis of the neck, subcutaneous emphysema, inspiratory stridor, and a hoarse voice. The emergency nurse anticipates this patient has sustained a:

A. cardiac tamponade.
B. tension pneumothorax.
C. fractured larynx.
D. pulmonary contusion.

120. An adult patient weighing 65 kg presents to the emergency department with full thickness burns to the head, chest, and bilateral arms. Using the rule of nines to determine total body surface area burned, how much fluid replacement should the emergency nurse plan to administer based on the Parkland formula?

A. 5850 mL in the first 8 hours and another 5850 mL in the following 16 hours, for a total of 11,700 mL in the first 24 hours
B. 2925 mL in the first 8 hours and another 5850 mL in the following 16 hours, for a total of 8775 mL in the first 24 hours
C. 5850 mL every 8 hours, for a total of 17,550 mL in 24 hours
D. 8775 mL in the first 8 hours and another 5850 mL in the following 16 hours, for a total of 14,625 mL in 24 hours

121. A 3-year-old is brought to the emergency department after having hydrofluoric acid spilled on their upper legs. In addition to extensive irrigation to decontaminate the area and prevent hypothermia, the nurse needs to monitor:

A. the patient's glucose levels.
B. the pH of the patient's skin where the exposure took place.
C. the need for ongoing pain medication administration.
D. the patient's serum calcium levels.

122. A clinical symptom highly characteristic of human scabies is:

A. macular red lesions and vesicular lesions that do not cross the midline.
B. vesicular lesions on the extremities.
C. ring-shaped lesions with central clearing.
D. nocturnal pruritis.

123. Which form of radiation exposure is considered to have an expectant or fatal outcome?

A. Central nervous system syndrome
B. Hematopoietic (bone marrow) syndrome
C. Gastrointestinal syndrome
D. Cutaneous radiation injury

124. Following several hours of observation, a drowning victim is being prepared for discharge home. Which of the following statements by the parent indicates understanding of the discharge instructions?

A. "I will wake my child hourly to make sure they knows where they are."
B. "I will observe my child for any trouble breathing or confusion."
C. "I will provide plenty of liquids that will aid in recovery."
D. "I will have my child lie down with their feet elevated to help promote water drainage from the lungs."

125. A 4-year-old is brought to the emergency department after being found locked in a car on a hot day. The patient is agitated and confused, their skin is hot to touch, and their lips are parched. The recommended intervention for this patient is to:

A. prepare to administer a Ringer's lactate solution.
B. immerse the patient in an ice water bath.
C. initiate core temperature monitoring.
D. encourage increased water intake.

126. Which of the following statements made by the child's parent during a heat advisory indicates understanding of discharge instructions to prevent heat injury to their child?

A. "I can briefly leave my child inside my automobile while I run in to the market."
B. "I will provide frequent drink breaks."
C. "I can maintain my child's soccer and sports activity schedule between 11:00 a.m. and 2:00 p.m."
D. "I will keep my child dressed in dark-colored clothing."

127. Which of the following patients must receive the series of rabies prophylaxis?

A. The patient who may or may not have been bitten by a guinea pig.
B. The patient with a bite from a pet cat.
C. The patient with a bite from a pet dog.
D. The patient who may or may not have been bitten by a bat.

128. The nurse is caring for a patient who complains of muscle weakness on the right side of their face, malaise, headache, and fatigue. The patient has a red bull's-eye-shaped rash on their leg, which presented after removing a tick. The patient's vital signs are: BP 132/76 mm Hg; HR 88 beats/minute; RR 22 breaths/minute; SpO_2 98%; T 37.0°C (98.6°F). Which of the following diagnoses should the nurse suspect?

A. Rocky Mountain spotted fever
B. Lyme disease
C. Cellulitis
D. Tularemia

129. A patient presents to the emergency department after ingesting a full bottle of oxycodone (Oxycontin). Which of the following signs and symptoms is associated with an overdose of oxycodone?

A. Dilated pupils
B. Bradycardia
C. Hypertension
D. Tachypnea

130. An unaccompanied patient suddenly appears in the ambulance entry area of the emergency department. The patient is unresponsive to stimuli. Skin is pale, cool, and dry. The nurse notes bilateral pupil constriction. There are no signs of injury observed. Vital signs are: BP 84/58 mm Hg; HR 52 beats/minute; RR 6 breaths/minute; SpO_2 88%; T 35.4°C (95.7°F). Which of the following is the highest priority intervention for this patient?

A. Open the airway and provide bag-mask device respirations
B. Obtain a serum glucose level to evaluate for hypoglycemia
C. Administer 0.4 to 2 mg of naloxone (Narcan) intravenously
D. Initiate intravenous (IV) access with a large-caliber IV catheter and begin an infusion of normal saline

131. The emergency nurse is preparing to admit a patient to the hospital. After asking the patient a series of alcohol screening questions, the nurse has determined that the patient drinks 6–8 alcoholic drinks every day. How long after the last drink of alcohol would the nurse expect the patient to begin demonstrating early signs and symptoms of acute alcohol withdrawal?

A. 2–3 hours
B. 4–5 hours
C. 6–8 hours
D. 12–72 hours

132. A patient with suspected alcohol intoxication presents to the emergency department. To prevent the onset of Wernicke-Korsakoff syndrome, the nurse should anticipate the administration of which medication to the patient?

A. Thiamine (Vitamin B1)
B. Dextrose 50%
C. Lorazepam (Ativan)
D. Magnesium

133. You are assessing a patient who has arrived to the emergency department with a 2-day history of watery diarrhea, low-grade fever, loss of appetite, nausea, and abdominal tenderness. On reviewing their medication history, you find the patient just began taking pantoprazole (Protonix) for gastroesophageal reflux disease. What could be the cause of the symptoms the patient is now experiencing?

A. *Escherichia coli*
B. Norovirus
C. *Clostridium difficile*
D. Salmonella

134. You are caring for a 15-year-old female who is being discharged after being diagnosed with infectious mononucleosis. Which of the statements made by the patient shows an understanding of the discharge instructions?

A. "I should remember to always cover my mouth when sneezing or coughing until my doctor says I'm no longer infectious."
B. "I should not shake hands or hug anyone until my doctor says I'm no longer infectious."
C. "I can't kiss my boyfriend for at least the next 2–4 weeks or until my doctor says I'm no longer infectious."
D. "I can go back to school and participate in soccer practice tomorrow."

135. Several emergency department staff members were involved in the care of a 10-year-old trauma victim, and resuscitation efforts were not successful. Knowing this will have a significant emotional impact on staff members, it is most important that the nurse manager do which of the following?

A. Mandate that all emergency department staff attend a debriefing session within 24 hours of the event
B. Schedule a formal debriefing session within 24–72 hours of the event
C. Meet individually with the involved staff members to discuss their perception of the critical event
D. Arrange for the affected staff to care only for adult patients for the next 2–3 days

136. The emergency department nurse recognizes that a sentinel event may require the staff directly involved in the event to complete a(n):

A. root cause analysis.
B. incident report.
C. investigation.
D. patient safety report.

137. Which of the following is most important to consider when developing evidence-based practice guidelines for the emergency department?

A. Findings from relevant research, combined with practitioner expertise and patient preferences
B. Findings obtained from the results of well-conducted randomized controlled trial research studies alone
C. The availability of published clinical practice guidelines to direct the change in practice
D. The availability of advanced practice nurses or nursing researchers to identify an appropriate clinical research question

138. A patient diagnosed with gastroesophageal reflux disease is being discharged and prescribed a proton pump inhibitor. The instructions provided by the emergency nurse should instruct the patient to take the medication at which time?

A. At bedtime
B. 20–30 minutes before a meal
C. At the first indication of stomach pain
D. 2 hours before or after bismuth subsalicylate

139. While awaiting the determination of brain death for a patient who has sustained multiple traumatic injuries and is a potential organ donor, the emergency nurse should anticipate which of the following interventions to maintain organ perfusion?

A. Administer intravenous fluids
B. Administer vasoactive agents
C. Administer norepinephrine to avoid hypotension
D. Administer atropine to treat bradydysrhythmias

140. A patient who has sustained a self-inflicted gunshot wound is brought to the emergency department. Which of the following interventions describes the appropriate collection and handling of forensic evidence?

A. Projectiles such as bullets or BBs should be secured in a sterile plastic container using a metal instrument.
B. Place the patient's clothing in a plastic bag.
C. Place paper bags over both hands of the patient.
D. Document any personal items that have been returned to the family.

141. An employee from the hospital's nuclear medicine department arrives at the emergency department stating that they may have been exposed to radioactive material. The patient is pale and diaphoretic and is complaining of a sudden onset of midsternal chest pain that radiates to the jaw. The priority action for the emergency nurse is to:

A. don personal protective equipment.
B. prepare the patient to obtain a 12-lead electrocardiogram.
C. secure intravenous (IV) access and administer atropine 1 mg IV STAT.
D. accompany the patient to the decontamination shower.

142. Hand-off communication between providers is most effective when patient information is shared using which type of communication tool?

A. Suitable for use by a care provider with a lower level of knowledge or skill
B. Adaptable to a format for an audiotaped report
C. Standardized
D. Focused solely on the patient and the plan of care

143. Which of the following is most likely to be related to inadequate communication?

A. Medication errors
B. Blood transfusion hypersensitivity reaction
C. Emergency department overcrowding
D. Improper delegation of nursing tasks

144. Which of the following actions would work best to propose a solution to the problem of emergency department (ED) overcrowding?

A. Petition the nursing administration to hire additional transporters to assist with patient flow
B. Serve on a hospital-wide committee to discuss patient flow
C. Participate in a strategic planning session to expand the number of telemetry beds
D. Contribute to the development of ED protocols to divert overflow patients to neighboring hospitals

145. A non-English-speaking patient presents to emergency department triage. To best communicate with the patient, the triage nurse should use which of the following methods?

A. A hospital employee who speaks the patient's native language
B. A member of the patient's family who speaks English
C. A certified translator employed by the hospital
D. A picture-based communication board

146. The registered nurse instructs the assistive personnel to reassess the patient's pain level following the administration of pain medications. Is this an appropriate task to delegate to the assistive personnel to perform?

A. Yes
B. No
C. Only if the assistive personnel has been trained in pain scales
D. Only if the assistive personnel feels comfortable doing so

147. The JumpSTART pediatric triage for mass casualty events uses the same criteria for triage as the adult START triage, with respiratory rate, capillary refill, and mental status; however, JumpSTART triage includes which additional intervention?

A. Rescue breaths
B. Warming
C. Intravenous fluids
D. Glucose

148. A patient presents to the emergency department with chest pain, but the hospital does not accept their medical insurance plan. To be compliant with the Emergency Medical Treatment and Active Labor Act, what must be a component of the medical screening exam for a patient complaining of chest pain?

A. Electrocardiogram
B. Basic laboratory studies, including a troponin level
C. Vital signs
D. Assessment by a physician or physician assistant

149. An unaccompanied 16-year-old female arrives at triage seeking treatment for a sexually transmitted disease. The patient's request for treatment is:

A. permitted.
B. not permitted.
C. granted only if her parents provide consent.
D. granted only if the patient can provide documentation that she is emancipated.

150. There are five fundamental principles for customer service in the emergency department setting. The acronym for those five principles is AIDET, which stands for Acknowledge, Introduce, Duration, Explanation, and:

A. Trauma.
B. Treatment.
C. Time.
D. Thank You.

PART 2

1. A patient presents to the emergency department complaining of a 2-day history of a dull substernal ache that has continued to increase in intensity. The patient states that they had some relief after taking a nitroglycerin tablet yesterday. Vital signs are: BP 114/68 mm Hg; HR 68 beats/minute; RR 22 breaths/minute. The electrocardiogram demonstrates a new onset left bundle branch block. The priority intervention for this patient is:

   A. continuous monitoring for development of ST segment elevation.
   B. serial cardiac markers.
   C. preparing the patient for transport to interventional cardiology.
   D. admission to a telemetry unit for observation.

Rationale

A. A left bundle branch block can obscure ST segment elevation. Continued monitoring for suspected ST segment elevation would delay the patient's transport to interventional radiology and myocardial reperfusion of tissue.

B. Preparing the patient for transport to interventional radiology should not be delayed for the results of serum serial cardiac markers.

C. New onset of a left bundle branch block is treated as a ST segment elevation myocardial infarction. The patient should be prepared for a percutaneous transluminal coronary angioplasty and early reperfusion of the myocardium.

D. The patient will require hospitalization, but admission should not take priority over preparing the patient for transfer to interventional radiology. Delay in reestablishing myocardial perfusion in the presence of new onset left bundle branch block is associated with a high degree of mortality.

Category: Cardiovascular Emergencies/Acute coronary syndrome

Nursing Process: Intervention

Reference

Hammond, B. B. (2013). Cardiovascular emergencies. In Hammond, B. B., Zimmermann, P. G., & Sheehy, S. B. (Eds.), *Sheehy's manual of emergency care* (pp. 201–212). St. Louis, MO: Elsevier/Mosby.

---

2. During the completion of a 12-lead electrocardiogram, the nurse identifies excessive artifact in lead II and lead III. To resolve this technical difficulty, the nurse should:

   A. change the right arm electrode.
   B. check for cable movement.
   C. change the left leg electrode.
   D. instruct the patient to momentarily hold their breath.

Rationale

A. The left leg electrode is common to both lead II and lead III. Changing the right arm electrode would not affect the appearance of lead III.

B. Cable movement could be the reason for excessive artifact; however, it would result in movement also being detected in other leads.

C. The left leg electrode is common to both lead II and lead III. The development of artifact and decreased conductivity results when the conducting gel in the electrode becomes dry.

D. Interference from respiration tends to reflect a wandering baseline and not generalized artifact in lead II and lead III. Lead II and lead III are limb leads, which are less affected by respiration.

Category: Cardiovascular Emergencies/Acute coronary syndrome

Nursing Process: Intervention

Reference

Williams, D. (2010). Cardiovascular emergencies. In P. K. Howard & R. A. Steinmann (Eds.), *Sheehy's emergency nursing: Principles and practice* (6th ed., pp. 411–444). St. Louis, MO: Mosby Elsevier.

3. When determining the presence of ST segment elevation on an electrocardiogram (ECG), the ST segment is compared to which interval or segment of the ECG?

A. P-R interval
B. T-P interval
C. Q-T interval
D. P-R segment

Rationale

A. The P-R interval represents atrial depolarization and repolarization but does not represent an isoelectric interval.

B. T-P interval represents the interval between the end of ventricular repolarization and the beginning of atrial depolarization. This interval represents an absence of electrical heart activity and therefore is used as the isoelectric reference for the presence of ST segment elevation or ST segment depression.

C. The Q-T interval encompasses the QRS complex, ST segment, and T wave and does not present with an isoelectric reference for ST segment elevation or ST segment depression.

D. The P-R segment may present as an isoelectric line; there are conditions that may cause this segment to appear depressed.

Category: Cardiovascular Emergencies/Acute coronary syndrome

Nursing Process: Assessment

Reference

Garcia, T. B., & Miller, G. T. (2004). Vectors and the basic beat. In *Arrhythmia recognition: The art of interpretation* (pp. 27–39). Sudbury, MA: Jones and Bartlett.

4. A middle-aged patient presents to the emergency department via emergency medical services. The patient states that they were awoken from sleep with midsternal chest pain approximately 4–5 hours ago. In the presence of an acute myocardial infarction (AMI), the initial elevation of the troponin cardiac biomarkers occurs within:

A. 1–2 hours after onset of an AMI.
B. 4–8 hours after onset of an AMI.
C. 24–30 hours after onset of an AMI.
D. 10–24 hours after onset of an AMI.

Rationale

A. 1–2 hours following onset of an AMI is too early to detect any rise in the troponin cardiac biomarkers.

B. Troponin I cardiac biomarkers provide a bioassay to measure proteins found in the myofibrils of the heart muscle. Troponins are detectable based on assay 4–8 hours after the AMI. Troponin levels will peak at 18–24 hours following AMI.

C. The troponin levels are beginning to fall within 24 hours of an AMI.

D. 10–24 hours following onset of an AMI is the mean peak time range for troponin levels.

Category: Cardiovascular Emergencies/Acute coronary syndrome
Nursing Process: Assessment

References

Schreiber, D., & Miller, S. M. (2017). Cardiac markers. *Medscape*. Retrieved from http://emedicine.medscape.com/article/811905-overview

Williams, D. (2010). Cardiovascular emergencies. In P. K. Howard & R. A. Steinmann (Eds.), *Sheehy's emergency nursing: Principles and practice* (6th ed., pp. 411–444). St. Louis, MO: Mosby Elsevier.

---

5. The nurse suspects a patient may have an acute aortic dissection when, during the history-taking process, the patient describes the pain as:

A. squeezing, burning epigastric pain that may radiate to the middle back area.
B. right upper quadrant pain referred to right scapula and shoulder.
C. sudden, severe tearing or ripping chest, interscapular, or back pain.
D. sharp, stabbing chest pain radiating to neck, arms, or left shoulder.

Rationale

A. Squeezing, burning epigastric pain that may radiate to the midback is characteristic of discomfort associated with the presence of a gastric ulcer.

B. Right upper quadrant pain referred to right scapula and shoulder is characteristic of cholecystitis.

C. Sudden, severe tearing or ripping chest, interscapular, or back pain is classic presentation of an aortic dissection.

D. Sharp, stabbing chest pain radiating to the neck, arms, or left shoulder is characteristic of acute pericarditis.

Category: Cardiovascular Emergencies/Aneurysm/dissection

Nursing Process: Assessment

References

Criddle, L. M. (2007). Cardiovascular emergencies. In K. S. Hoyt & J. Selfridge-Thomas (Eds.), *Emergency nursing core curriculum* (6th ed., pp. 187–248). St. Louis, MO: Saunders Elsevier.

Rossoll, L. W. (2007). Abdominal emergencies. In K. S. Hoyt & J. Selfridge-Thomas (Eds.), *Emergency nursing core curriculum* (6th ed., pp. 178–181). St. Louis, MO: Saunders Elsevier.

---

6. You are assisting in the resuscitation of an elderly patient in cardiac arrest. A waveform capnography is in place, and high-quality cardiopulmonary resuscitation is being performed. A sudden increase in the level of the end-tidal carbon dioxide indicates the:

A. need for deeper and faster chest compressions.
B. need for an additional dose of a vasopressor, such as intravenous bolus epinephrine.
C. presence of an irreversible cardiac arrest.
D. return of spontaneous circulation.

Rationale

A. A decrease in the end-tidal carbon dioxide ($ETCO_2$) waveform would indicate the possible need for deeper and faster compressions.

B. A decrease in the $ETCO_2$ waveform would indicate the possible need for a dose of a vasopressor such as epinephrine.

C. A sudden increase in the $ETCO_2$ level indicates a return of spontaneous circulation. A continued decrease in the level of $ETCO_2$ would be an indicator of failure to resuscitate or respiratory compromise/misplaced endotracheal tube.

D. Although no clinical study has examined whether titrating resuscitative efforts to physiologic parameters during cardiopulmonary resuscitation (CPR) improves outcome, it may be reasonable to use physiologic parameters (quantitative waveform capnography, arterial relaxation diastolic pressure, arterial pressure monitoring, and central venous oxygen saturation) when feasible to monitor and optimize CPR quality, guide vasopressor therapy, and detect return of spontaneous circulation.

Category (Geriatric): Cardiovascular Emergencies/Cardiopulmonary arrest

Nursing Process: Evaluation

Reference

Criddle, L. M. (2007). Cardiovascular emergencies. In K. S. Hoyt & J. Selfridge-Thomas (Eds.), *Emergency nursing core curriculum* (6th ed., pp. 187–248). St. Louis, MO: Saunders Elsevier.

Link, M. S., Berkow, L. C., Kudenchuk, P. J., Halperin, H. R., Hess, E. P., Moitra, V. K., . . . Donnino, M. W. (2015). Part 7: adult advanced cardiovascular life support: 2015 American Heart Association guidelines update for cardiopulmonary resuscitation and emergency cardiovascular care. *Circulation, 132*(Suppl. 2), S444–S464.

---

7. A patient in cardiac arrest presents to the emergency department receiving cardiopulmonary resuscitation by emergency medical services personnel. The cardiac monitor displays sinus rhythm, but no palpable pulse can be detected. The most likely cause of this pulseless electrical activity is:

A. glucose level of 145 mg/dL.
B. potassium value of 1.3 mmol/L (1.3 mEq/L).
C. arterial pH of 7.36.
D. magnesium level of 3.0 mg/dL.

Rationale

A. A normal glucose level ranges from 80 mg/dL to 120 mg/dL. Although a reading of 145 mg/dL is elevated, this would not be the cause of pulseless electrical activity (PEA).

B. Hypokalemia, or decreased potassium level, may be a cause of PEA in the cardiac arrest patient. Electrical activity may be present in the heart muscle with absence of contractility. A normal potassium level is 3.5 mmol/L to 5.0 mmol/L (3.5 mEq/L to 5.0 mEq/L). A potassium level of 1.3 mmol/L is severe hypokalemia and is considered a critical or life-threatening value.

C. A pH of 7.36 is within the normal pH range of 7.35–7.45 and would not be a cause of PEA.

D. A normal magnesium level is in the range of 1.7–2.1 mg/dL. Hypomagnesemia (level less than 1.7 mg/dL) can cause ventricular dysrhythmias. A level of 3.0 mg/dL would be considered elevated or hypermagnesemic.

Category: Cardiovascular Emergencies/Cardiopulmonary arrest

Nursing Process: Assessment

Reference

American Heart Association. (2016). The ACLS cases: Cardiac arrest, pulseless electrical activity. In: *Advanced cardiac life support* (16th ed., pp. 110–113). Dallas, TX: Author.

Marett, B. (2013). Metabolic emergencies. In B. B. Hammond & P. G. Zimmermann (Eds.), *Sheehy's manual of emergency care* (7th ed., pp. 303–318). St. Louis, MO: Elsevier Mosby.

---

8. Which of the following physiological conditions would result in the loss of ventricular capture for a patient being transcutaneously paced?

A. Lactic acidosis
B. Hypomagnesemia
C. Metabolic alkalosis
D. Hypokalemia

Rationale

A. The presence of lactic acidosis resulting from decreased tissue oxygenation alters myocardial contractility, leading to a decreased ability to achieve ventricular capture.

B. Hypomagnesemia may present with torsade de pointes, ventricular tachycardia, and ventricular fibrillation. Hypomagnesemia does not cause a lack of ventricular capture with transcutaneous pacing.

C. Metabolic alkalosis may present with atrial tachycardia, but it would not be responsible for the lack of ventricular capture with transcutaneous pacing.

D. Hypokalemia presents with U waves on the electrocardiogram, ventricular dysrhythmias, or pulseless electrical activity. Hypokalemia does not prevent ventricular capture with transcutaneous pacing.

Category: Cardiovascular Emergencies/Dysrhythmias

Nursing Process: Analysis

References

Poole-Wilson, P. A. (1982). Acidosis and contractility of heart muscle. *Ciba Foundation Symposium, 87*, 58–76. Retrieved from https://www.ncbi.nlm.nih.gov/pubmed/6804193

Williams, D. Cardiovascular emergencies. (2010). In P. K. Howard & R. A. Steinmann (Eds.), *Sheehy's emergency nursing: Principles and practice* (6th ed., pp. 411–444). St. Louis, MO: Mosby Elsevier.

---

9. A patient arrives at the emergency department by emergency medical services with a complaint of weakness and near syncope. The patient's HR is 24 beats/minute, and BP is 80/60 mm Hg. The patient underwent a heart transplant 6 months ago, and the cardiac monitor displays third-degree heart block. The emergency nurse is aware the patient will immediately require which medication to increase the patient's heart rate?

A. Atropine sulfate (Atropine)
B. Isoproterenol (Isuprel)
C. Digoxin (Lanoxin)
D. Amiodarone (Cordarone)

Rationale

A. Atropine sulfate (Atropine) acts to increase the heart rate by blocking the parasympathetic system. The parasympathetic connections were severed during this patient's heart transplant surgery. Atropine would not affect the patient's bradycardia.

B. A transplanted heart will not respond to drugs that act to block parasympathetic tone. The parasympathetic connections were cut during the transplant surgery. Isoproterenol (Isuprel), glucagon, or epinephrine would increase heart rate, but they do not act to block parasympathetic tone. Isoproterenol is the most commonly used drug to increase heart rate following heart transplant surgery.

C. Digoxin (Lanoxin) would not be indicated to increase the patient's heart rate because it is used to slow the heart rate and improve contractility of the myocardium.

D. Amiodarone (Cordarone) is used in the presence of ventricular and other dysrhythmias, not to increase heart rate.

Category: Cardiovascular Emergencies/Dysrhythmias

Nursing Process: Intervention

References

Barash, P. G., Cullen, B. F., & Stoelting, R. K. (Eds.). (2006). *Clinical anesthesia* (5th ed., pp. 311–318). Philadelphia, PA: Lippincott.

Wolters Kluwer. *Nursing 2016 Drug Handbook*. Philadelphia, PA: Author.

10. On examination of a febrile patient presenting to the emergency department with a chief complaint of "flulike symptoms" and a history of intravenous drug use, the nurse notes a cardiac murmur, crackles in bilateral lung bases, subungual hemorrhages, nontender erythematous macules on the palms of the hand and soles of the feet, and painful erythematous nodules on the tips of the fingers and toes. Which is the most important initial intervention for this patient?

A. Echocardiogram
B. Chest radiography
C. Surgery
D. Antibiotics

Rationale

A. An echocardiogram is helpful in the diagnosis of infective endocarditis, but prompt initiation of antibiotic therapy is a crucial intervention. It is recommended that three sets of blood cultures should be obtained before initiation of antibiotic therapy.

B. A chest radiograph may be helpful in ruling out pneumonia and determining the status of the lungs and heart size, but prompt initiation of antibiotic therapy is a crucial intervention for a patient with infective endocarditis.

C. Surgery may be indicated for a patient with infective endocarditis, but not before prompt initiation of antibiotic therapy. There is also a higher risk if surgery is performed on patients during the active phase of infective endocarditis.

D. Patients with a history of intravenous drug use are at risk for infective endocarditis. The impurities in the injectable substance can attach to and invade the heart valve leaflets, causing a murmur. Bacteria or fungi colonize (vegetations); these vegetations may embolize and be "showered" throughout the cardiovascular system, causing splinter hemorrhages under the fingernails, nontender nodules on the palms and soles (Janeway lesions) and fingers and toes (Osler nodes). Empirical therapy for infective endocarditis includes prompt initiation of antibiotics.

Category: Cardiovascular Emergencies/Endocarditis

Nursing Process: Intervention

Reference

Habib, G., Lancellotti, P., Antunes, M. J., Bongiorni, M. G., Casalta, J., Del Zotti, F., Dulgheru, R., . . . Zamorano, J. L. (2015). 2015 ESC guidelines for the management of infective endocarditis: The Task Force for the Management of Infective Endocarditis of the European Society of Cardiology (ESC). *European Heart Journal, 36*, 3075–3123. http://doi.org/10.1093/eurheartj/ehv319

---

11. A patient presents with an episode of acute worsening of chronic systolic congestive heart failure. Blood pressure is 150/70 mm Hg. The patient complains of dyspnea, and rales are heard bilaterally. The patient is not hypoxic, nor does the electrocardiogram demonstrate evidence of an acute myocardial ischemia or infarction. Which of the following medications would be harmful to administer to the patient at this time?

A. Vasodilators
B. Vasopressor agents
C. Diuretics
D. Opiates

Rationale

A. If hypotension is absent, a vasodilator may be considered as an adjunct to diuretic therapy in acute congestive heart failure (CHF).

B. The patient is not currently hypotensive and does not need treatment with vasopressor agents.

C. Guidelines recommend diuretic therapy as the cornerstone of therapy for acute CHF.

D. Intravenous opiates should be considered in patients with CHF who exhibit anxiousness or restlessness.

Category: Cardiovascular Emergencies/Heart failure

Nursing Process: Analysis

Reference

Lewis, T. (2014). Current guidelines for the management of heart failure. *EM Practice Guidelines Update, 6*(1), 1–16.

---

12. A patient presents to the emergency department complaining of a severe headache. Vital signs reveal a BP of 270/170 mm Hg; HR 80 beats/minute; and RR 20 breaths/minute. The patient is alert and describes being recently diagnosed with high blood pressure. A priority intervention for this patient would be to:

A. initiate intravenous medication to lower the patient's BP immediately.
B. obtain baseline laboratory data.
C. consider emergency cardioversion for BP control.
D. evaluate BP cuff size for accuracy.

Rationale

A. Although lowering the patient's BP is a priority, the BP should be lowered slowly, over several hours.

B. Baseline laboratory data is important for patient evaluation but is not a priority in treating the patient's severe hypertension.

C. Cardioversion is used for emergency treatment for various cardiac dysrhythmias, including tachycardia. This patient has a heart rate of 80. Cardioversion is not indicated for the presence of hypertension.

D. Accurate BP values must be ensured before instituting BP-lowering measures. Appropriate size cuffs should be available and used for all patients. Using a blood pressure cuff that is too large will result in a blood pressure reading that is lower than the patient's actual blood pressure and using a cuff that is too small will result in a blood pressure reading that is higher than the patient's actual blood pressure.

Category: Cardiovascular Emergencies/Hypertension

Nursing Process: Intervention

References

Hammond, B. B. (2013). Cardiovascular emergencies. In B. B. Hammond & P. G. Zimmermann (Eds.), *Sheehy's manual of emergency care* (7th ed., pp. 201–211). St. Louis, MO: Elsevier Mosby.

Wofford, M., Harkins, K. G., King, D. S., Habeeb, G. E., Wyatt, S. B., & Jones, D. W. (2002). Accurate cuff size in blood pressure measurement. *American Journal of Hypertension, 15*(S3), 92.

---

13. Administration of nitroprusside (Nipride) to a patient in hypertensive crisis is considered effective when the patient demonstrates which of the following?

A. The patient responds to verbal stimuli.
B. The systolic blood pressure reaches 160 mm Hg.
C. The systolic blood pressure reaches 120 mm Hg.
D. The patient reports relief of chest pain.

Rationale

A. The patient in hypertensive crisis may present with altered mental status and other neurological findings. This finding is not consistent with evidence of effective treatment of a patient in hypertensive crisis.

B. Evidence has shown that the systolic blood pressure (SBP) should be lowered to 160 mm Hg; a lower SBP can compromise cerebral blood flow and cause organ hypoperfusion and tissue ischemia.

C. Evidence has shown that the SBP should be lowered to about 160 mm Hg; a lower SBP can compromise cerebral blood flow and cause organ hypoperfusion and tissue ischemia.

D. The patient in hypertensive crisis may present with chest pain and other cardiovascular manifestations. The relief of chest pain is not consistent with effective treatment of a patient in hypertensive crisis.

Category: Cardiovascular Emergencies/Hypertension

Nursing Process: Evaluation

References

Criddle, L. (2007). Cardiovascular emergencies. In K. S. Hoyt & J. Selfridge-Thomas (Eds.), *Emergency nursing core curriculum* (6th ed., pp. 187–248). St. Louis, MO: Saunders Elsevier.

Williams, D. (2010). Cardiovascular emergencies. In P. K. Howard & R. A. Steinmann (Eds.), *Sheehy's emergency nursing: Principles and practice* (6th ed., pp. 411–444). St. Louis, MO: Mosby Elsevier.

---

14. Signs and symptoms of cardiac tamponade include:

A. widening pulse pressure.
B. muffled heart tones.
C. jugular vein flattening.
D. jugular vein distention, narrowing pulse pressure, and tracheal deviation.

Rationale

A. Jugular venous distention occurs when blood is unable to enter and fill the chambers, resulting in decreased cardiac output and hypotension; as the blood pressure drops, the pulse pressure will narrow, not widen.

B. Cardiac tamponade is the result of blood accumulation within the pericardial sac. As the heart is compressed within the pericardial sac, blood is prevented from filling the heart, resulting in muffled heart sounds, a narrowing pulse pressure related to decreased cardiac output, and decreased blood pressure.

C. Because of increased pressure within the heart, the patient will demonstrate jugular neck vein distention.

D. Tracheal deviation occurs as a late sign in the presence of tension pneumothorax; it is not associated with cardiac tamponade.

Category: Cardiovascular Emergencies/Pericardial tamponade

Nursing Process: Assessment

Reference

Day, M. W. (2014). Thoracic and neck trauma. In D. Gurney (Ed.), *Trauma Nursing Core Course: Provider manual* (7th ed., pp. 137–149). Des Plaines, IL: Emergency Nurses Association.

---

15. The parent of a toddler tells the nurse that the child was recently diagnosed with "hand, foot, and mouth disease." Today the child began to complain of chest pain that hurts more while coughing and "when taking a deep breath." The nurse notes that the child is sitting upright on the mother's lap and is leaning forward. Based on the patient's most recent illness history, the nurse knows this patient is at risk for developing:

A. pneumonia.
B. pericarditis.
C. respiratory syncytial virus.
D. commotio cordis.

Rationale

A. Pneumonia may cause pleuritic chest pain symptoms, but the patient's symptoms and recent illness history indicate the presence of pericarditis.

B. Coxsackie virus (otherwise known as "hand, foot, and mouth disease") is the most common cause of viral pericarditis. The common symptoms of pericarditis include sharp, pleuritic chest pain that improves when sitting up and leaning forward and is made worse with coughing or inspiration. Tuberculosis is the most common cause of pericarditis worldwide.

C. Symptoms of respiratory syncytial virus include cough, congestion, and fever.

D. Commotio cordis is not related to any preexisting illness. Commotio cordis is the result of a direct blow to the chest directly over the heart, which often causes a lethal disruption in the cardiac rhythm; the patient would present in cardiac arrest.

Category: Cardiovascular Emergencies/Pericarditis

Nursing Process: Analysis

References

Mattu, A., & Martinez, J. P. (2013). Pericarditis, pericardial tamponade, and myocarditis. In J. G. Adams, E. D. Barton, J. L. Collins, P. M. C. DeBlieux, M. A. Gisondi, & E. S. Nadel (Eds.), *Emergency medicine clinical essentials* (2nd ed., pp. 514–523). Philadelphia, PA: Elsevier Saunders.

PEPID LLC. (2016). PEPID Emergency Medicine Platinum (version 17.1.1) [Mobile application software]. Retrieved from http://pepid.com

16. Which of the following would further enhance the symptoms of peripheral vascular disease, causing the patient increased discomfort?

A. Narcotics
B. Calcium channel blockers
C. Alcohol use
D. Smoking

Rationale

A. Narcotics may be used to treat pain caused by vasospasms or decreased blood flow, but narcotics will not contribute to worsening of the patient's symptoms.

B. Calcium channel blockers may be used as a therapy for peripheral vascular disease to decrease the presence of vasospasms.

C. Although alcohol use may cause disorientation and increase the patient's risk for falling, the consumption of alcohol is not associated with development of peripheral vascular disease.

D. Smoking has been proved to further enhance peripheral vascular disease because of the vasoconstrictive effect of nicotine. If a patient continues to smoke, the peripheral vascular disease may worsen.

Category: Cardiovascular Emergencies/Peripheral vascular disease
Nursing Process: Analysis

Reference

Criddle, L. (2007). Cardiovascular emergencies. In K. S. Hoyt & J. Selfridge-Thomas (Eds.), *Emergency nursing core curriculum* (6th ed., pp. 187–248). St. Louis, MO: Saunders Elsevier.

---

17. A patient presents to the emergency department complaining of pain in their left leg that began suddenly while they were sitting in their car. The patient denies any recent trauma. Which of the following elements of the patient's history is most concerning?

A. The patient is a noninsulin-dependent diabetic with an $HgbA_{1C}$ of 6.8% at their last physician appointment.
B. The patient had a myocardial infarction 4 years ago that was successfully treated with stent placement, and now they take 162 mg of aspirin daily.
C. The patient is a regional sales representative who spends much of their time driving and smokes two packs of cigarettes a day.
D. The patient has poorly controlled hypertension and takes a "blood pressure pill" and a "water pill" most days.

Rationale

A. Although being a diabetic does increase their risk, smoking is a much greater risk factor for developing peripheral arterial disease (PAD).

B. A prior myocardial infarction establishes the presence of PAD, and taking a daily aspirin may be beneficial for someone with PAD.

C. Smoking and a sedentary lifestyle are the two greatest risk factors for PAD. These two factors put this patient at a very high risk for developing arterial occlusions—in this case, in their left leg.

D. Hypertension is a risk factor for PAD but is not the most concerning of this patient's risk factors.

Category: Cardiovascular Emergencies/Thromboembolic disease

Nursing Process: Analysis

Reference

Selvin, E., & Erlinger, T. P. (2004, August 10). Prevalence of and risk factors for peripheral arterial disease in the United States: Results from the National Health and Nutrition Examination Survey, 1999–2000. *Circulation, 110*(6), 738–743.

---

18. Assessment of a patient from a motor vehicle collision reveals a seat belt sign on the patient's chest, premature ventricular contractions, chest pain, and hypotension. Oxygen, intravenous fluids, and pain medication have been administered. Which of the following reevaluation criteria would cause the nurse to be concerned?
    - A. Lactic acid of 3 mmol/L
    - B. Heart tones of S1, S2
    - **C. Breath sounds with crackles**
    - D. Oxygen saturation of 95%

Rationale

A. Lactic acid of 3 mmol/L is within normal limits.

B. Heart tones of S1, S2 are normal.

C. This patient has a cardiac contusion, and cardiac function may be severely depressed. The right ventricle is at greatest risk for cardiac contusion because of its prominence; thus, volume replacement must proceed cautiously. Cell injury and bruising lead to decreased contractility, so the cautious use of fluid is recommended.

D. Oxygen saturation of 95% is within acceptable range of 94–98%

Category: Cardiovascular Emergencies/Trauma

Nursing Process: Evaluation

Reference

Day, M. W. (2014). Thoracic and neck trauma. In D. Gurney (Ed.), *Trauma Nursing Core Course: Provider manual* (7th ed., pp. 137–149). Des Plaines, IL: Emergency Nurses Association.

---

19. Patient assessment findings after a motor vehicle collision reveal decreased cardiac contractility and output without volume loss. Goal-directed therapy includes fluid boluses and inotropic support. Which of the following will the nurse monitor for in this patient?
    - **A. Fluid overload**
    - B. Urinary output
    - C. Tension pneumothorax
    - D. Hemorrhage

Rationale

A. This patient is demonstrating signs and symptoms of cardiogenic shock. Successful emergent stabilization includes administering judicious fluid boluses to improve preload and inotropic support to improve contractility. An excess of volume administration or an increase in afterload can result in pulmonary edema and increased myocardial ischemia.

B. Monitoring urinary output is important when the patient has volume loss associated with hypovolemic shock. However, this patient is in cardiogenic shock, so the priority is to evaluate for the presence of fluid overload.

C. Mediastinal shift with obstruction to atrial filling is the pathology underlying a tension pneumothorax and is associated with the presence of obstructive shock, not cardiogenic shock.

D. Hemorrhage is associated with volume loss and hypovolemic shock, not cardiogenic shock.

Category: Cardiovascular Emergencies/Shock (cardiogenic and obstructive)

Nursing Process: Evaluation

Reference

Pentecost, D. A. (2014). Shock. In D. Gurney (Ed.), *Trauma Nursing Core Course: Provider manual* (7th ed., pp. 73–90). Des Plaines, IL: Emergency Nurses Association.

---

20. Which of the following interventions decreases the amount of a patient's preload?

A. Administration of a beta-blocker
B. Successful cardioversion of new onset atrial fibrillation to sinus rhythm
C. Placing the patient in a supine position with legs elevated
D. Administration of morphine sulfate 2–4 mg intravenous

Rationale

A. Beta blockade will increase preload by slowing the heart rate, therefore allowing for an increased ventricular filling time.

B. Successful cardioversion and returning the patient to sinus rhythm will work to increase, not decrease, preload.

C. Placing the patient in a supine position with legs elevated will act to increase the patient's preload.

D. Morphine sulfate will act to decrease or limit the amount of blood returning to the heart and therefore would decrease preload.

Category: Cardiovascular Emergencies/Shock (cardiogenic and obstructive)

Nursing Process: Intervention

Reference

Klabunde, R. E. (2014). *Cardiovascular physiology concepts*. Retrieved from http://www.cvphysiology.com

21. A parent presents to the triage area with an infant, stating, "My baby hasn't been breathing right since last night and won't take a bottle." The infant's respiratory rate is 72 breaths/minute, and they appear pale. The emergency nurse is aware this presentation indicates:

A. that the infant is experiencing a rapid decline in their cardiopulmonary status.
B. a respiratory rate that is within normal parameters for an infant.
C. that infants are normally more tachypnic.
D. that there are multiple reasons for an increased respiratory rate in infants.

Rationale

A. Children with sustained respiratory rates of greater than 60 breaths/minute are at risk for respiratory failure because of compensatory mechanisms that fail faster than those of an adult.

B. A respiratory rate of 72 breaths/minute is not within the parameters of respiratory rates for infants. Respiratory rates greater than 60 breaths/minute in an infant require immediate interventions.

C. A respiratory rate of 72 breaths/minute is outside of the normal parameters for an infant. The infant is also pale, indicating that tissue is not receiving adequate oxygenation. This requires immediate intervention.

D. Increased respiratory rate can be caused by fever, pain, or an infection. The infant's pale skin indicates a decline in their respiratory status and inadequate tissue oxygenation.

Category (Pediatric): Respiratory Emergencies/Respiratory distress syndrome
Nursing Process: Analysis

Reference

Hohenhaus, S. M. (2012). Focused assessment, triage and decision making. In Emergency Nurses Association (Ed.), *Emergency Nursing Pediatric Course: Provider manual* (4th ed., pp. 51–61). Des Plaines, IL: Emergency Nurses Association.

---

22. A characteristic sign associated with the presence of chronic obstructive pulmonary disease is:

A. pink frothy sputum.
B. fever.
C. decreased breath sounds on one side of the chest.
D. pursed lip breathing.

Rationale

A. Blood-tinged or pink frothy sputum is a sign of pulmonary edema.

B. Fever accompanied by purulent sputum and can be a sign of pneumonia.

C. Sudden increased shortness of breath and the presence of decreased or absent breath sounds in one lung indicates a pneumothorax.

D. Chronic hyperinflation and enlargement of the lungs results in changes in the shape of the chest. Pursed lip breathing is an effort to prevent airways from collapsing during expiration. It prolongs expiration and slows the rate of breathing.

Category: Respiratory Emergencies/Chronic obstructive pulmonary disease (COPD)
Nursing Process: Assessment

References

The Cleveland Clinic Foundation. (2014). *Pursed lip breathing.* Retrieved from http://my.clevelandclinic.org/health/diseases_conditions/hic_Understanding_COPD/hic_Pulmonary_Rehabilitation_Is_it_for_You/hic_Pursed_Lip_Breathing

Walsh, R. (2013). Respiratory emergencies. In B. B. Hammond & P. G. Zimmermann (Eds.), *Sheehy's manual of emergency care* (7th ed., pp. 185–199). St. Louis, MO: Elsevier Mosby.

---

23. A main goal of treatment for patients with chronic obstructive pulmonary disease is to:

A. avoid hospitalizations.
B. cure the disease and return lung function to normal.
C. prevent further lung damage.
D. avoid increasing the use of medications.

Rationale

A. Early hospitalization may decrease the severity and duration of a chronic obstructive pulmonary disease (COPD) exacerbation.

B. COPD is a progressive illness that advances with each exacerbation. Currently there is no cure for COPD.

C. COPD is a lung disease that progressively worsens with each exacerbation. To decrease the frequency of exacerbations, patients should avoid risk factors such as smoking, environmental pollution, and exposure to chemicals and dust.

D. As the disease progresses, adjusting the medication regimen may assist in reducing symptoms and limit the occurrence of acute exacerbations.

Category: Respiratory Emergencies/Chronic obstructive pulmonary disease (COPD)

Nursing Process: Evaluation

Reference

Hanania, N. A., & Sharafkhaneh, A. (2016). Chronic obstructive pulmonary disease. In E. T. Bope & R. D. Kellerman (Eds.), *Conn's current therapy 2016* (pp. 385–389). Philadelphia, PA: Elsevier.

---

24. A critically ill emergency department patient with an exacerbation of their chronic obstructive pulmonary disease is diagnosed with respiratory acidosis. The priority medication that should be administered and that would be most beneficial to this patient is a(n):

A. bronchodilator.
B. corticosteroid.
C. diuretic.
D. antibiotic.

Rationale

A. Respiratory acidosis is an indication of retained carbon dioxide in the lungs. Bronchodilators, given by nebulizer or single-metered-dose inhaler, work through direct action on the smooth muscle cells of the airway, thereby dilating airway passages and increasing oxygen and carbon dioxide exchange in the lungs. Bronchodilator use is an important therapy in the initial treatment of an acute exacerbation of chronic obstructive pulmonary disease (COPD).

B. Corticosteroids work to decrease inflammation and to enhance the action of the bronchodilator during an acute exacerbation of COPD, but they do not have the same immediate effects that bronchodilators exert on lung tissue.

C. Diuretics are prescribed for heart failure and are not indicated in the immediate treatment of an exacerbation of COPD.

D. Antibiotics have been shown to improve outcomes from COPD exacerbations, especially if the patient has recent changes in sputum production and/or sputum consistency or is currently febrile. However, the immediate treatment for a COPD patient in respiratory acidosis is to administer a bronchodilator.

Category: Respiratory Emergencies/Chronic obstructive pulmonary disease (COPD)

Nursing Process: Intervention

Reference

Tashkin, D. P., & Fergunson, G. T. (2013). Combination bronchodilator therapy in the management of chronic obstructive pulmonary disease. *Respiratory Research, 14*(1), 49.

---

25. A patient arrives via emergency medical services and is extremely confused, febrile, and tachypnic, with the presence of crackles in the right lower lobe on auscultation of the lung fields. The provider diagnoses the patient with pneumonia. As the emergency nurse caring for the patient, you would anticipate the arterial blood gases to show which abnormality?

A. pH: 7.25, $PaCO_2$: 65 mm Hg, HCO_3: 22 mEq/L

B. pH: 7.35, $PaCO_2$: 40 mm Hg, HCO_3: 22 mEq/L

C. pH: 7.30, $PaCO_2$: 35 mm Hg, HCO_3: 16 mEq/L

D. pH: 7.5, $PaCO_2$: 40 mm Hg, HCO_3: 38 mEq/L

Rationale

A. This blood gas shows an uncompensated respiratory acidosis, which is expected in a patient with poor gas exchange, resulting in CO_2 retention and confusion from CO_2 narcosis.

B. These are normal blood gas values.

C. This blood gas reveals the presence of metabolic acidosis. This abnormality would be found in a patient with diabetic ketoacidosis or renal disease.

D. This blood gas reveals the presence of metabolic alkalosis. This abnormality would be found in a patient who is vomiting or who has consumed a large amount of sodium bicarbonate.

Category: Respiratory Emergencies/Infection

Nursing Process: Evaluation

Reference

Maiden, J. M. (2014). Pulmonary diagnostic procedures. In L. Urden, K. Stacy, & M. Lough (Eds.), *Critical care nursing* (7th ed., pp. 502–513). Philadelphia, PA: Mosby.

26. A motorcyclist who was not wearing a helmet is involved in a collision. On arrival to the emergency department, the patient is assessed to have sustained significant facial injuries, and audible gurgling is heard. The priority intervention for this patient is to:

A. prepare for endotracheal intubation.
B. control facial venous bleeding.
C. place the patient in the high-Fowler's position.
D. suction the oropharynx.

Rationale

A. Although endotracheal intubation is an appropriate intervention, it is not the immediate priority. Ensuring a patent airway by suctioning the oropharynx is the priority intervention. Once the airway is patent and cervical spine protection has been established, breathing with endotracheal intubation is the next component of the trauma primary assessment.

B. Although controlling venous bleeding is an appropriate intervention, it is not the priority. Ensuring a patent airway is the initial priority intervention. Controlling facial venous bleeding would be initiated in the secondary assessment.

C. Ensuring a patent airway by suctioning the oropharynx is the initial priority intervention for this patient. Cervical spinal precautions should be in place in the trauma primary assessment. Placing the patient in the high-Fowler's position is not indicated and may be harmful.

D. Ensuring a patent airway by suctioning the oropharynx is the priority intervention in this scenario. Airway is the first component of the trauma primary assessment, along with cervical spine stabilization.

Category: Respiratory Emergencies/Trauma

Nursing Process: Intervention

Reference

Gurney, D., & Westergard, A. M. (2014). Initial assessment. In D. Gurney (Ed.), *Trauma Nursing Core Course: Provider manual* (7th ed., pp. 39–54). Des Plaines, IL: Emergency Nurses Association.

---

27. An emergency patient is being treated for carbon monoxide poisoning. The patient's response to treatment is best evaluated by:

A. obtaining a pulse oximetry reading.
B. obtaining a Glasgow Coma Scale score.
C. obtaining an arterial blood gas measurement.
D. obtaining a peak flow reading.

Rationale

A. The pulse oximeter cannot differentiate between hemoglobin being bound to oxygen or carbon monoxide. An arterial blood gas measurement is necessary to differentiate between blood that is saturated with oxygen and blood that is saturated with carbon monoxide.

B. The Glasgow Coma Scale will evaluate the patient's level of consciousness but will not evaluate for the presence of carbon monoxide poisoning.

C. A patient with carbon monoxide poisoning is treated with oxygen until the carboxyhemoglobin levels drop below 10%.

D. A peak flow reading is used to evaluate a patient's response in the treatment of asthma but is not indicated in the treatment of carbon monoxide poisoning.

Category: Respiratory Emergencies/Inhalation injuries

Nursing Process: Analysis

Reference

Churbock, C. P. (2014). Surface and burn trauma. In D. Gurney (Ed.), *Trauma Nursing Core Course: Provider manual* (7th ed., pp. 205–224). Des Plaines, IL: Emergency Nurses Association.

---

28. In assessing a patient for the presence of a suspected tracheobronchial injury, the emergency nurse can expect to auscultate which of the following?

A. Bowel sounds heard in the thoracic cavity
B. Pleural friction rub auscultated over the axilla
C. Rales auscultated at the bilateral lung bases
D. Crunching or bubbling sound heard over the precordium that is synchronous with the heartbeat

Rationale

A. The presence of bowel sounds in the thoracic cavity is consistent with the presence of a diaphragm rupture, not a suspected tracheobronchial injury.

B. A pleural friction rub is a low-pitched, dry grating sound heard on both inspiration and expiration and can indicate the presence of pleurisy.

C. Rales is an assessment finding consistent with fluid in the lungs.

D. Disruption of the tracheobronchial tree is usually the result of blunt force trauma. This results in air leakage into the mediastinum, resulting in a crunching or bubbling sound that is produced by the heart beating against air-filled tissues.

Category: Respiratory Emergencies/Obstruction

Nursing Process: Assessment

Reference

Everson, F. (2013). Chest trauma. In B. B. Hammond & P. G. Zimmermann (Eds.), *Sheehy's manual of emergency care* (7th ed., pp. 407–418). St. Louis, MO: Elsevier Mosby.

---

29. A patient arrives at the emergency department complaining of progressively worsening chest pain. They patient said they were involved in a motor vehicle collision 3 days ago. The patient is hemodynamically stable, and assessment reveals the presence of dullness on percussion over the left lung fields. The emergency nurse anticipates that the dullness on percussion is the result of:

A. pneumothorax.
B. pulmonary contusion.
C. pleural effusion.
D. pericardial effusion.

Rationale

A. Pneumothorax is an accumulation of air in the pleural space that may be spontaneous or the result of trauma. A pneumothorax will produce pleuritic chest pain, dyspnea, cough, and decreased breath sounds but typically has a sudden onset and is hyperresonant to percussion. Depending on the size of the pneumothorax, symptoms may be mild to severe.

B. Pulmonary contusion is a potentially-life threatening injury caused by chest trauma. Respiratory failure may develop hours after the injury due to alveolar damage. Decreased breath sounds, crackles, and wheezes will be present due to alveolar edema and hemorrhage and can cause hemodynamic instability.

C. Inflammation from blunt chest trauma causes an increase in capillary permeability, allowing fluid to leak into the pleural space. Pleural effusions may have a delayed and gradual onset and are often mild. These do not often require intervention because symptoms are typically minor and do not cause hemodynamic instability.

D. Pericardial effusion is the abnormal accumulation of fluid in the pericardial sac. As the fluid accumulates, pressure on the heart increases, limiting ventricular filling and decreasing cardiac output. This is known as a cardiac tamponade. The patient will exhibit muffled heart sounds and hemodynamic instability.

Category: Respiratory Emergencies/Pleural effusion

Nursing Process: Analysis

References

Everson, F. P. (2013). Chest trauma. In B. B. Hammond & P. G. Zimmermann (Eds.), *Sheehy's manual of emergency care* (7th ed., pp. 407–418). St. Louis, MO: Elsevier Mosby.

Walsh, R. (2013). Respiratory emergencies. In B. B. Hammond & P. G. Zimmermann (Eds.), *Sheehy's manual of emergency care* (7th ed., pp. 185–199). St. Louis, MO: Elsevier Mosby.

---

30. A patient presents to the emergency department complaining of chest pain and dyspnea. A chest radiograph is obtained and shows a visible lung margin with air filling the pleural space. Supplemental oxygen has been administered, and intravenous access has been established. Which intervention should the emergency nurse anticipate next?

A. Endotracheal intubation
B. Needle thoracostomy
C. Bilevel positive airway pressure
D. Chest tube thoracostomy

Rationale

A. Supplemental oxygen must be administered to improve hypoxia in a pneumothorax. However, mechanical ventilation through endotracheal intubation will not improve ventilation until the trapped air is relieved and negative pressure in the pleural space is restored, allowing the lung to re-expand. Furthermore, in the presence of a pneumothorax, the positive pressure of mechanical ventilation may cause the development of a tension pneumothorax, a medical emergency.

B. Needle thoracostomy is indicated only for the emergent treatment of a tension pneumothorax. In this scenario, a chest tube would be appropriate.

C. Supplemental oxygen must be administered to improve hypoxia in a pneumothorax. However, positive airway pressure will not improve ventilation until the trapped air is relieved and negative pressure in the pleural space is restored, allowing the lung to re-expand. Furthermore, in the presence of a pneumothorax, the positive pressure may cause the development of a tension pneumothorax, a medical emergency.

D. The chest radiograph indicates a pneumothorax; the margin of the collapsed lung is visible, with air filling the space outside the lung. The appropriate treatment would be to release the trapped air through placement of a chest tube to water seal.

Category: Respiratory Emergencies/Pneumothorax

Nursing Process: Intervention

References

Everson, F. P. (2013). Chest trauma. In B. B. Hammond & P. G. Zimmermann (Eds.), *Sheehy's manual of emergency care* (7th ed., pp. 407–418). St. Louis, MO: Elsevier Mosby.

Walsh, R. (2013). Respiratory emergencies. In B. B. Hammond & P. G. Zimmerman (Eds.), *Sheehy's manual of emergency care* (7th ed., pp. 185–199). St. Louis, MO: Elsevier Mosby.

---

31. A patient presents pale and diaphoretic with initial vital signs as follows: BP 130/85 mm Hg; HR 135 beats/minute; RR 40 breaths/minute; SpO_2 48% room air; T 37.2°C (99.0°F). Lung sounds are diminished bilaterally throughout, with crackles at the bases. The patient has been visiting from Florida for the past 4 days, and the current the elevation is 9500 feet. The priority intervention for the emergency nurse to perform is to:

A. obtain an electrocardiogram.
B. place the patient on a nonrebreather mask.
C. establish intravenous access.
D. obtain a chest radiograph.

Rationale

A. After correcting the patient's oxygenation and breathing, evaluation of the effects to their cardiovascular system will be necessary. An electrocardiogram (ECG) should be obtained and evaluated for possible myocardial injury.

B. Placing the patient on supplemental oxygen is the priority. The use of a nonrebreather mask will increase the level of inspired oxygen to the patient. The patient may require an ECG and intravenous (IV) access, but the first priority is to maintain airway, breathing, and circulation along with the correction of oxygenation.

C. The first priority is to provide supplemental oxygen to the patient because their initial oxygen saturation indicates 48%. Establishing IV access is not the first priority.

D. A chest radiograph will need to be completed on this patient. However, because of the emergent nature of the patient's complaint, maintaining airway, breathing, and circulation, followed by supplemental oxygenation, is the priority intervention.

Category: Respiratory Emergencies/Pulmonary edema, noncardiac

Nursing Process: Intervention

Reference

Walsh, R. (2013). Respiratory emergencies. In B. B. Hammond & P. G. Zimmermann (Eds.), *Sheehy's manual of emergency care* (7th ed., pp. 185–199). St. Louis, MO: Elsevier Mosby.

---

32. A patient arrives complaining of dyspnea and mild right-sided chest pain that began the previous evening and increases in intensity with exertion. Initial vital signs are: BP 108/56 mm Hg; HR 115 beats/minute; RR 28 breaths/minute; SpO_2 87% room air; T 36.6°C (97.8°F). Lung sounds have fine scattered crackles bilaterally. The patient states that 3 days ago, they sustained an injury to their right leg while playing tennis. Based on this information, the emergency nurse suspects the patient has a:

A. pneumothorax.
B. pneumonia.
C. pleural effusion.
D. pulmonary embolism.

Rationale

A. On assessment, the patient demonstrates bilateral lung sounds that are inconsistent with a pneumothorax. A patient with a pneumothorax would have absent or diminished breath sounds on the affected side.

B. The patient is afebrile, with fine scattered crackles bilaterally. A patient with pneumonia would present with course crackles on auscultation and bronchial breath sounds over the affected area.

C. A patient with a pleural effusion would have diminished or absent breath sounds over the area of the effusion.

D. Risk factors for a pulmonary embolism include venous stasis, recent trauma, obesity, pregnancy, and a history of thrombosis. The patient is tachycardic and tachypneic, with a room air SpO_2 of 87%. In addition, the patient had a recent trauma to their right leg, indicating a possible deep vein thrombus with possible dislodgement, resulting in a pulmonary embolus.

Category: Respiratory Emergencies/Pulmonary embolus

Nursing Process: Analysis

Reference

Walsh, R. (2013). Respiratory emergencies. In B. B. Hammond & P. G. Zimmermann (Eds.), *Sheehy's manual of emergency care* (7th ed., pp. 185–199). St. Louis, MO: Elsevier Mosby.

---

33. A patient with severe acute respiratory distress syndrome will have critical levels of hypoxemia. The nurse can potentially improve the patient's oxygenation by placing the patient into which position?

A. High-Fowler's position
B. Prone position
C. On left side with head elevated
D. Reverse Trendelenburg position

Rationale

A. Sitting the patient upright encourages edema to settle in dependent areas in the lungs.

B. Prone positioning allows recruitment of alveoli in dependent parts of the lungs, potentially increasing oxygenation. Postural drainage may allow more secretions to be suctioned from the airway. Pressure from the heart and abdominal organs resting on the lungs may also be relieved.

C. A side-lying position does not improve oxygenation in acute respiratory distress syndrome.

D. Reverse Trendelenburg position does not improve dependent edema; however, it may help relieve the pressure of abdominal organs on the lungs and can be combined with a prone position for this purpose.

Category: Respiratory Emergencies/Respiratory distress syndrome

Nursing Process: Intervention

References

Drahnak, D. M., & Custer, N. (2015). Prone positioning of patients with acute respiratory distress syndrome. *Critical Care Nurse, 35*(6), 29–37.

Gibbons, C. (2015). Acute respiratory distress syndrome. *Radiologic Technology, 86*(4), 419–436.

---

34. A pneumothorax can be classified as a simple, open, or tension pneumothorax. In a tension pneumothorax, assessment findings may include which of the following?

A. Symmetrical chest wall movement
B. Tracheal deviation
C. Muffled heart tones
D. Sucking chest wound

Rationale

A. Asymmetrical chest wall movement, not symmetrical chest wall movement, is an assessment finding with tension pneumothorax.

B. Tracheal deviation is an assessment finding in a patient with a tension pneumothorax when air enters the interpleural space but cannot escape on expiration.

C. Muffled heart tones is an assessment finding consistent with a pericardial tamponade; it is not typically an assessment finding with tension pneumothorax.

D. Sucking chest wound is an assessment finding consistent with the presence of an open pneumothorax.

Category: Respiratory Emergencies/Trauma

Nursing Process: Assessment

Reference

Day, M. W. (2014). Thoracic and neck trauma. In D. Gurney (Ed.), *Trauma Nursing Core Course: Provider manual* (7th ed., pp. 137–149). Des Plaines, IL: Emergency Nurses Association.

---

35. The primary cause of mortality in the advanced stages of chronic obstructive pulmonary disease is which of the following?

A. Cardiac-related event
B. Pneumonia
C. Pneumothorax
D. Blood clot

Rationale

A. Ischemic heart disease, heart failure, and dysrhythmias are more common in chronic obstructive pulmonary disease (COPD) patients due in part to chronic systemic and pulmonary inflammation. Heart disease and COPD also share similar risk factors such as smoking, genetic factors, and age.

B. Although patients with COPD are more susceptible to pneumonia and can be acutely ill than a healthy person with a similar pneumonia, it is not the number one cause of death in patients with COPD.

C. A spontaneous pneumothorax is a serious complication of COPD that typically occurs because of a rupture of a subpleural apical emphysematous bleb, smoking history, or in patients with an increased body height.

D. COPD can lead to an increased risk of deep vein thrombosis, pulmonary embolism, and stroke due to hypercoagulability secondary to systemic inflammation and erythrocytosis.

Category: Respiratory Emergencies/Chronic obstructive pulmonary disease (COPD)

Nursing Process: Analysis

Reference

Rastogi, S., Jain, A., Basu, S. K., & Rastogi, D. (2015). Current overview of COPD with special reference to emphysema. In M. Glass (Ed.), *Chronic obstructive pulmonary disease* (pp. 105–140). New York, NY: Hayle Medical.

---

36. To auscultate vesicular breath sounds, it is best to listen over the:

A. trachea/thorax region.
B. major bronchi.
C. peripheral lung fields.
D. scapular region.

Rationale

A. Bronchial breath sounds are auscultated over the trachea and thorax and are noted for their high pitch, loud amplitude, and short duration on inspiration, and long duration on expiration.

B. Bronchovesicular breath sounds are auscultated over the major bronchi, between the scapulae, and around the sternum in the first and second intercostal spaces. Bronchovesicular sounds are noted to have a moderate pitch, moderate amplitude, and the same duration on inspiration and expiration.

C. There are three types of normal breath sounds: that include bronchial, bronchovesicular, and vesicular. Vesicular breath sounds are auscultated over the peripheral lung fields and are noted for their low pitch, soft amplitude, and long duration on inspiration, and short duration on expiration.

D. It is very difficult to auscultate breath sounds directly over the scapula. Vesicular breath sounds are auscultated over the peripheral lung fields and are noted for their low pitch, soft amplitude, and long duration on inspiration, and short duration on expiration.

Category: Respiratory Emergencies

Nursing Process: Assessment

Reference

Weber, J. R., & Kelley, J. H. (2014). *Health assessment in nursing.* (5th ed.) Philadelphia, PA: Wolters Kluwer Health.

---

37. The emergency nurse is conducting a confusion assessment method assessment in a patient. Which of the following assessments would indicate the patient is confused?

A. The patient engages in a conversation.
B. The patient has abnormal vital signs.
C. The patient is unable to complete a simple task.
D. The patient has a decreased level of consciousness.

Rationale

A. The confused patient makes abrupt and inconsistent changes in a conversation and has difficulty engaging is a conversation.

B. Vital sign assessment is not a component of the confusion assessment method (CAM), although it is an important assessment parameter.

C. Asking the patient to complete a simple task, such saying the days of the week backward, can be used to determine their level of alertness. The CAM has four areas of assessment: (1) acute onset and fluctuating course, (2) inattention, (3) disorganized thinking, and (4) altered level of consciousness. The diagnosis of delirium requires the presence of both criteria 1 and 2 in combination with either criteria 3 or 4.

D. A decreased level of consciousness is a finding in many different conditions and is not specific to a confusion assessment.

Category: Neurological Emergencies/Alzheimer's disease/dementia
Nursing Process: Assessment

Reference

Haugh, K. (2015). Head to toe: Organizing your baseline patient physical assessment. *Nursing, 45*(12), 58–61. http://doi.org/10.1097/01.nurse.0000473396.43930.9d

---

38. A patient presents to triage complaining of a 2-week history of fatigue and tingling in their hands, and has experienced several falls recently. Vital signs are: BP 116/72 mm Hg; HR 86 beats/minute; RR 16 breaths/minute; T 37.0°C (98.6°F). The emergency nurse anticipates that which of the following will provide the most information regarding the patient's symptoms?

A. Magnetic resonance imaging of the brain and spinal cord
B. Serum lactate
C. Spinal computed tomography scan of the brain and spinal cord
D. Complete blood count

Rationale

A. This patient is exhibiting signs and symptoms that are highly suspicious for the presence of multiple sclerosis (MS). The 2015 Consortium of Multiple Sclerosis Centers recommends magnetic resonance imaging (MRI) to provide a better diagnosis for patients with suspected signs and symptoms. MRI is approximately 75% accurate in making the diagnosis of MS.

B. Serum lactate is a diagnostic test to predict the presence and severity of lactic acid in the blood and is used in the diagnosis of sepsis. Serum lactate will not provide any information regarding the presence of a neurological disorder.

C. This test may be ordered to rule out infection or structural abnormality; however, it does not aid in the diagnosis of a neurological disorder such as MS.

D. This test can rule out infections (viral/bacterial) but is generally not helpful in making the diagnosis of MS.

Category: Neurological Emergencies/Chronic neurological disorders

Nursing Process: Analysis

References

Faguy, K. (2016). Multiple sclerosis: An update. *Radiologic Technology, 87*(5), 529–553.

Niccolai, C., Portaccio, E., Goretti, B., Hakiki, B., Giannini, M., Pastò, L., . . . Viterbo, R. G. (2015). A comparison of the brief international cognitive assessment for multiple sclerosis and the brief repeatable battery in multiple sclerosis patients. *BMC Neurology, 151*(5), 204. http://doi.org/10.1186/s12883-015-0460-8

39. A patient who has been evaluated for a right facial droop is being discharged with instructions related to their diagnosis of Bell's palsy. The patient asks if their facial paralysis is permanent. The most appropriate response from the emergency nurse is:

A. "The damage from the virus will not resolve but over time, but you will become accustomed to the facial droop."

B. "All of your facial weakness will resolve, just be patient with the recovery."

C. "This is difficult to predict, but most patients have a complete recovery within 3 to 6 months following the onset of their symptoms."

D. "Your facial weakness will come and go."

Rationale

A. A majority of patients with Bell's palsy recover totally without treatment. If symptoms have not resolved within 6 months, a referral to neurologist may be required.

B. A majority of patients with Bell's palsy recover totally without treatment. If symptoms have not resolved within 6 months, a referral to neurologist may be required.

C. A majority of patients with Bell's palsy recover totally without treatment. If symptoms have not resolved within 6 months, a referral to neurologist may be required.

D. Weakness and paralysis associated with Bell's palsy are the result of decreased lower motor neuron function from viral pathogens. Patients with Bell's palsy are not expected to have recurrent episodes of remission and relapse of their symptoms.

Category: Neurological Emergencies/Chronic neurological disorders

Nursing Process: Intervention

Reference

Dunphy, L., Winland-Brown, J., Porter, B., & Thomas, D. (2015). *Primary care: The art and science of advanced practice nursing* (4th ed.). Philadelphia, PA: F. A. Davis.

40. A patient presents to triage complaining of a headache that feels as though someone is squeezing their head in a tight grip. The patient states they experience these headaches every month, and they complain of no other signs or symptoms. The emergency nurse is aware that the patient is describing the which type of headache?

A. Migraine headache
B. Subcortical headache
C. Tension headache
D. Hydronephrosis headache

Rationale

A. A migraine headache can occur with or without an aura. Migraine headache without aura is usually unilateral in nature, can have a pulsating quality, and is aggravated by physical activity. Migraine headache with aura is commonly localized to the cerebral cortex or brain stem. It commonly develops over 20 minutes and can last up to 72 hours, with the patient experiencing photophobia and nausea.

B. Subcortical refers to the area below the cortex of the brain and is not a type of headache.

C. A tension headache is associated with a report of tightening- or squeezing-type pain. A tension headache usually starts at the occipital area and moves around to the front area as if a band is squeezing the head. This type of headache can last up to 7 days.

D. Hydronephrosis refers to alterations within the kidney that are related to ischemic tissue changes. Hydronephrosis is not a type of headache.

Category: Neurological Emergencies/Headache

Nursing Process: Assessment

References

Baxter, C. S. (2007). Neurological emergencies. In K. S. Hoyt & J. Selfridge-Thomas (Eds.), *Emergency nursing core curriculum* (6th ed., pp. 510–535). St. Louis, MO: Saunders Elsevier.

Brown, A., & King, D. (2010). Neurological emergencies. In P. K. Howard & R. A. Steinmann. (Eds.). *Sheehy's emergency nursing: Principles and practice* (6th ed., pp. 457–466). St. Louis, MO: Mosby Elsevier.

---

41. Each of the following patients presents to the emergency department with a chief complaint of headache. Which patient would most likely require intracranial imaging?

A. A patient diagnosed with small cell lung cancer who complains of a new-onset headache
B. A patient with a history of migraines who presents with their typical symptom complex
C. A 25-year-old patient who presents with a new-onset tension-type headache
D. A patient with a headache accompanied by a fever, elevated erythrocyte sedimentation rate, and no leukocytosis.

Rationale

A. A patient who presents with new onset of headache and who has secondary headache risk factors should be imaged regardless of other neurological findings or deficits. Secondary headache is caused by an underlying disorder. Examples of secondary headache risk factors are (1) human immunodeficiency virus, (2) uncontrolled hypertension, (3) malignancy, and (4) recent head injury. A secondary type of headache must be ruled out in these circumstances.

B. A patient with a chronic primary headache diagnosis and a presentation that is typical based on their history does not require intracranial imaging. Any change in the onset and/or characteristics of the headache or accompanying neurological deficits would require intracranial imaging.

C. Any patient younger than 5 and older than 50 who presents with a headache has a higher risk of secondary headaches and would require intracranial imaging to rule out potential risk factors.

D. A headache accompanied by fever and elevated erythrocyte sedimentation rate but without the presence of leukocytosis is most likely temporal arteritis. In addition, physical examination findings may include an increase in pain with palpation of the temporal artery. This diagnosis would require a temporal artery biopsy and would not have a strong indication for intracranial imaging.

Category: Neurological Emergencies/Headache
Nursing Process: Analysis

References

Andelova, M., Borsook, D., & Sprenger, T. (2015). Imaging of migraine. *Headache*, 117–136. https://doi.org/10.1007/978-3-319-15621-7_6

Miller, S., & Matharu, M. S. (2015). Imaging of other primary headaches. *Headache*, 137–153. https://doi.org/10.1007/978-3-319-15621-7_7

---

42. A patient presents to the emergency department after being found unresponsive at home. The patient's family member states that the patient regularly abuses alcohol. There was noted bruising to the patient's face and head. The emergency nurse notes the patient has a fixed and dilated left pupil, has increased deep respirations with periods of apnea, is bradycardic, and is experiencing a continual rise in only the systolic blood pressure. The emergency nurse is most concerned regarding which of the following?

A. **Presence of a subdural hematoma**
B. An absence seizure
C. An ischemic stroke
D. A narcotic overdose

Rationale

A. The patient is known to abuse alcohol and has signs of a possible traumatic brain injury, which increases the patient's risk for a subdural hematoma. A subdural hematoma is a slow-growing intracranial venous bleed that, left untreated, can result in coma and death from brain herniation. Signs of brain herniation include Cushing's triad: (1) bradycardia, (2) abnormal or apneic respirations, and (3) a widening pulse pressure secondary to a rising systolic blood pressure. In this case, the patient has Cheyne–Stokes respirations (increased deep respirations with periods of apnea), bradycardia, and a rising systolic blood pressure.

B. An absence seizure causes a short period of "blanking out" or staring into space but does not cause unconsciousness; there should be no changes in breathing pattern, heart rate, or systolic blood pressure.

C. Classic pupillary changes that result with stroke reveal sluggishness of pupils. A fixed dilated pupil is most likely associated with a intracranial hemorrhage.

D. A narcotic overdose may cause bradycardia and irregular or apneic respirations but does not present with a widening pulse pressure. There is also no information to suggest a possible overdose or narcotic use. Pupils would be pinpoint bilaterally with a narcotic overdose.

Category: Neurological Emergencies/Increased intracranial pressure

Nursing Process: Analysis

References

Belcastro, V., Giordano, L., Pruna, D., Peruzzi, C., Madeddu, F., Accorsi, P., . . . Striano, P. (2015). Do pure absence seizures occur in myoclonic epilepsy of infancy? A case series. *Seizure*, *24*(1), 8–11. https://doi.org/10.1016/j.seizure.2014.11.002

McLaughlin, J. C. (2014). Brain, cranial, and maxillofacial trauma. In D. Gurney (Ed.), *Trauma Nursing Core Course: Provider manual* (7th ed., pp. 105–122). Des Plaines, IL: Emergency Nurses Association.

---

43. A patient with a previously diagnosed brain tumor arrives at the emergency department unresponsive. Following the patient's initial assessment and interventions, an osmotic diuretic is administered. Which of the following findings indicates to the emergency nurse an effective response to this medication?

A. Urinary output 30 mL/hour
B. Widening pulse pressures
C. Absence of pulsus paradoxus
D. Glasgow Coma Score of 13

Rationale

A. Osmotic diuresis decreases intracranial pressure by pulling fluid from the brain and excreting it in the urine. Although this output is a desirable effect of therapy, its presence is not indicative of improvement.

B. Widening pulse pressures occur as systolic blood pressures rise and diastolic pressures decrease. This is an indication of increasing intracranial pressure. In combination with bradycardia and irregular respirations, it is also known as Cushing's response as the body attempts to compensate rising intracranial pressure.

C. Pulsus paradoxus is a symptom of cardiac tamponade. As the heart is compressed by fluid in the pericardial sac, the left and right sides compete for filling volume, resulting in a drop in blood pressure.

D. An unresponsive patient receives a score of 1 on the eye-opening portion of the Glasgow Coma Score. The maximum score for verbal response is 5 and for motor response is 6. The maximum score on initial presentation cannot exceed 12. An improving score indicates improvement in neurological status.

Category: Neurological Emergencies/Increased intracranial pressure

Nursing Process: Evaluation

References

Bolaug, B. A. (2016). Pulsus paradoxus in pericardial disease. *UpToDate*. Retrieved from http://www.uptodate.com/contents/pulsus-paradoxus-in-pericardial-disease

Brown, A., & King, D. (2009). Neurological emergencies. In P. K. Howard & R. A. Steinmann (Eds.), *Sheehy's emergency nursing principles & practice* (6th ed., pp. 457–466). St. Louis: Mosby Elsevier.

Criddle, L. M. (2007). Cardiovascular emergencies. In K. S. Hoyt & J. Selfridge-Thomas (Eds.), *Emergency nursing core curriculum* (6th ed., pp. 187–248). St. Louis, MO: Saunders Elsevier.

March, K. S., & Hickey, J. V. (2013). Intracranial hypertension: Theory and management of increased intracranial pressure. In J. V. Hickey (Ed.), *The clinical practice of neurological and neurosurgical nursing* (7th ed.). Philadelphia, PA: Lippincott Williams & Wilkins.

44. The emergency nurse is a caring for a patient who has sustained a subdural hematoma. The provider has ordered that the patient be placed in a semi-Fowler's position to facilitate blood return to the heart. The emergency nurse is aware that this intervention has been successful when the patient has a:

A. PaO_2 of 55 mm Hg.
B. mean arterial pressure of 70 mm Hg.
C. systolic blood pressure of 80 mm Hg.
D. $PaCO_2$ 50 mm Hg.

Rationale

A. A single episode of hypoxemia indicated by a PaO_2 of less than 60 mm Hg is considered detrimental to the patient.

B. It is recommended that mean arterial pressure be kept between 50 mm Hg and 150 mm Hg.

C. The brain that does not receive adequate blood flow becomes ischemic; the patient can sustain irreversible damage, as evidenced by increasing confusion, dizziness, and, eventually, unresponsiveness.

D. $PaCO_2$ greater than 45 mm Hg results in vasodilatation and an increase in the patient's intracranial pressure.

Category: Neurological Emergencies/Increased intracranial pressure

Nursing Process: Evaluation

References

Bajsarowicz, P., Prakash, I., Lamoureux, J., Saluja, R. S., Feyz, M., Maleki, M., & Marcoux, J. (2015). Nonsurgical acute traumatic subdural hematoma: What is the risk? *Journal of Neurosurgery, 123*(5), 1176–1183. https://doi.org/10.3171/2014.10.jns141728

McLaughlin, J. C. (2014). Brain, cranial, and maxillofacial trauma. In D. Gurney (Ed.), *Trauma Nursing Core Course: Provider manual* (7th ed., pp. 105–122). Des Plaines, IL: Emergency Nurses Association.

---

45. The emergency nurse is aware that the most common symptom of bacterial meningitis is the presence of a:

A. seizure.
B. stiff neck.
C. high fever.
D. petechial rash.

Rationale

A. Seizure may result from a high fever, but it is a nonspecific symptom of bacterial meningitis. The most common symptoms are headache and high fever.

B. Stiff neck, or nuchal rigidity, is a common symptom associated with bacterial meningitis, but it is not always present.

C. The most common symptoms associated with bacterial meningitis are headache and high fever.

D. Petechial rash is associated with the presence of meningococcemia, but it is not always visible in the populations with darker skin coloration.

Category: Neurological Emergencies/Meningitis

Nursing Process: Assessment

References

Cole, B. (2014). Identifying and treating a life-threatening disease. *Emergency Nurse, 21*(9), 18–21.

Richard, G. C., & Lepe, M. (2013). Meningitis in children: Diagnosis and treatment for the emergency clinician. *Clinical Pediatric Emergency Medicine, 14*(2), 146–156. https://doi.org/10.1016/j.cpem.2013.04.008

Stockdale, A., Weekes, M., & Aliyu, S. (2011). An audit of acute bacterial meningitis in a large teaching hospital 2005–10. *Quarterly Journal of Medicine, 104*(12), 1055–1063. https://doi.org/10.1093/qjmed/hcr123

Viale, P., Scudeller, L., Pea, F., Tedeschi, S., Lewis, R., Bartoletti, M., Sbrojavacca, R., . . . Giannella, M. (2015). Implementation of a meningitis care bundle in the emergency room reduces mortality associated with acute bacterial meningitis. *Annals of Pharmacotherapy, 49*(9), 978–985. https://doi.org/10.1177/1060028015586012

---

46. On assessing a patient with complaint of severe headache and fever, the nurse observes that when the patient's head is flexed forward, their knees and hips also flex. Based on this assessment finding, the emergency nurse anticipates that this patient has which of the following?

A. Spinal cord injury
B. Cervical spine fracture
C. Trapezius muscle injury
D. Meningitis

Rationale

A. Spinal cord injury typically results in loss of movement and or sensation.

B. Fractures typically present with pain and may have an associated spinal cord injury.

C. The pain would typically be limited to the shoulder area and not involve the leg.

D. The patient is experiencing signs of possible meningitis. The involuntary flexion of the hips and/or the knees when the neck is flexed, also known as Brudzinski's sign, is an indication of meningeal irritation.

Category: Neurological Emergencies/Meningitis
Nursing Process: Analysis

References

Baxter, C. S. (2007). Neurological emergencies. In K. S. Hoyt & J. Selfridge-Thomas (Eds.), *Emergency nursing core curriculum* (6th ed., pp. 510–535). St. Louis, MO: Saunders Elsevier.

Schuh, S., Lindner, G., Exadaktylos, K., Mühlemann, K., & Täuber, M. (2013). Determinants of timely management of acute bacterial meningitis in the ED. *American Journal of Emergency Medicine, 31*(7), 1056–1061. https://doi.org/10.1016/j.ajem.2013.03.042

---

47. An elderly patient presents to triage with a history of a near syncope event. The patient has no known prior medical history, currently takes no medications, and has a blood glucose level of 133. The patient suddenly has a tonic–clonic seizure. Their airway is being properly maintained. The emergency nurse is aware that the priority assessment for this patient is to:

A. assess for the presence of a pulse.
B. assess the patient's blood pressure.
C. assess for the presence of bowel sounds.
D. assess the patient's extraocular movement.

Rationale

A. Circulation assessment is a priority. Assessing for the presence of a pulse, along with the quality, amplitude, and rhythm of the pulse, is a priority for this patient. The presence of ventricular rhythms can lead to syncope and seizures because of decreased cardiac output and tissue perfusion.

B. Obtaining the patient's blood pressure is not a priority at this time. Assessing for the presence of a pulse is the priority for this patient.

C. Assessing the presence of bowel sounds is part of the secondary assessment, not the primary assessment.

D. Extraocular movement may not be assessed at this time. The presence of active seizures precludes this assessment because the patient is unable to respond to verbal direction.

Category (Geriatric): Neurological Emergencies/Seizure disorders

Nursing Process: Intervention

Reference

Yamamoto, L., Olaes, E., & Lopez, A. (2004). Challenges in seizure management: Neurologic versus cardiac emergencies. *Topics in Emergency Medicine, 26*(3), 212–224.

---

48. A patient presents to the emergency department with a free phenytoin (Dilantin) level of 22 mcg/mL. The emergency nurse would anticipate which of the following assessment findings?

A. Nystagmus
B. Ataxia
C. Confusion
D. Hypotension

Rationale

A. A normal free (also known as unbound) phenytoin (Dilantin) level is 1–2 mcg/mL. Levels > 15 mcg/mL are most commonly associated with nystagmus, whereas levels > 30 mcg/mL are most commonly associated with ataxia, confusion, and frank motor movement disorders.

B. A normal free (also known as unbound) phenytoin (Dilantin) level is 1–2 mcg/mL. Levels > 15 mcg/mL are most commonly associated with nystagmus, whereas levels > 30 mcg/mL are most commonly associated with ataxia, confusion, and frank motor movement disorders.

C. A normal free (also known as unbound) phenytoin (Dilantin) level is 1–2 mcg/mL. Levels > 15 mcg/mL are most commonly associated with nystagmus, whereas levels > 30 mcg/mL are most commonly associated with ataxia, confusion, and frank motor movement disorders.

D. A normal free (also known as unbound) phenytoin (Dilantin) level is 1–2 mcg/mL. Levels > 15 mcg/mL are most commonly associated with nystagmus, whereas levels > 30 mcg/mL are most commonly associated with ataxia, confusion, and frank motor movement disorders. Rapid intravenous infusion can lead to hypotension and bradycardia.

Category: Neurological Emergencies/Seizure disorders

Nursing Process: Analysis

Reference

Wyte, C. D., & Berk, W. A. (2001). Severe phenytoin overdose does not cause cardiovascular morbidity. *Annuals of Emergency Medicine, 20*(5), 508–512.

---

49. A patient presents to the emergency department after a motor vehicle collision. Neurogenic shock is suspected secondary to a spinal cord injury. Which of the following hemodynamic parameters is most consistent with neurogenic shock?

A. Hypertension
B. Increased central venous pressure
C. Bradycardia
D. Decreased SvO_2

Rationale

A. Hypertension is not an assessment finding in the presence of neurogenic shock

B. Increased intracranial pressure is not an assessment finding in the presence of neurogenic shock.

C. Neurogenic shock is a type of distributive shock related to spinal trauma and results in a complete loss of vasomotor tone. As a result of a loss of sympathetic and vasomotor tone, the hemodynamic findings include hypotension, bradycardia, decreased pulmonary occlusion pressure, decreased cardiac index, decreased systemic vascular resistance, decreased central venous pressure, and decreased SvO_2.

D. An increased SvO_2 is not an assessment finding in the presence of neurogenic shock.

Category: Neurological Emergencies/Spinal cord injuries

Nursing Process: Assessment

Reference

Marino, P. (2013). *The ICU book.* Philadelphia, PA: Lippincott Williams & Wilkins.

---

50. The emergency nurse is monitoring the blood pressure of a patient with a subarachnoid hemorrhage. The patient's blood pressure is currently 180/98. The nurse anticipates that the provider will order which medication for this patient?

A. Hypertonic saline
B. Intropin (Dopamine)
C. Labetalol (Trandate)
D. Propofol (Diprivan)

Rationale

A. Hypertonic saline is indicated for the management of increased intracranial pressure but is not indicated in the management of blood pressure.

B. Dopamine will increase the patient's blood pressure, not reduce their blood pressure. The patient's blood pressure in a subarachnoid hemorrhage (SAH) should be kept below 160 mm Hg systolic, but hypotension must be avoided.

C. The patient with a SAH should have their systolic blood pressure kept below 160 mm Hg to avoid further risk of hemorrhage, but hypotension must be avoided. Nicardipine may also be used to lower the patient's systolic blood pressure.

D. Propofol may be ordered for sedation, but it is not for blood pressure management. Propofol has a hypotensive effect but is not used to lower a patient's blood pressure.

Category: Neurological Emergencies/Stroke

Nursing Process: Intervention

Reference

Grimm, J. (2015). Aneurysmal subarachnoid hemorrhage: A potentially lethal neurological disease. *Journal of Emergency Nursing, 41*(4), 281–284.

---

51. When performing the motor portion of the Glasgow Coma Scale assessment on a patient, the emergency nurse observes that the patient does not follow commands, but they do move their right arm in an attempt to remove the source of pressure that is being applied to their left arm. The patient is noted to cross the midline to get to the source of the applied pressure to their arm. Based on this observation, the emergency nurse will document a motor score of:

A. 5: localization.
B. 6: localization.
C. 4: withdrawal.
D. 5: withdrawal.

Rationale

A. The motor scale scoring for the Glasgow Coma Scale (GCS) is: 6: follows commands; 5: localizes (crosses midline); 4: withdraws; 3: decorticates; 2: decerebrates; and 1: no response to pain.

B. A score of 6 indicates that the patient follows commands. This patient is not following commands. The motor scale scoring for the GCS is: 6: follows commands; 5: localizes (crosses midline); 4: withdraws; 3: decorticates; 2: decerebrates; and 1: no response to pain.

C. Withdrawal does not involve the purposeful attempt to remove a pain source. The motor scale scoring for the GCS is: 6: follows commands; 5: localizes (crosses midline); 4: withdraws; 3: decorticates; 2: decerebrates; and 1: no response to pain.

D. A score of 5 represents localization, an effort to remove the source of a painful stimuli. The motor scale scoring for the GCS is: 6: follows commands; 5: localizes (crosses midline); 4: withdraws; 3: decorticates; 2: decerebrates; and 1: no response to pain.

Category: Neurological Emergencies/Trauma

Nursing Process: Evaluation

References

Broering, B. (2010). Head trauma. In P. K. Howard & R. A. Steinmann (Eds.), *Sheehy's emergency nursing: Principles and practice* (6th ed., pp. 254–271). St. Louis, MO: Mosby Elsevier.

McLaughlin, J. C. (2014). Brain, cranial, and maxillofacial trauma. In D. Gurney (Ed.), *Trauma Nursing Core Course: Provider manual* (7th ed., pp. 105–122). Des Plaines, IL: Emergency Nurses Association.

52. The emergency nurse would determine an unconscious patient's Glasgow Coma Score by:
A. speaking loudly to the patient.
B. monitoring for spontaneous movement.
C. assessing the patient's Babinski reflex.
D. applying a painful stimulus.

Rationale

A. The unconscious patient is unable to follow verbal commands and will require the use of a painful stimulus to determine their motor response.

B. Spontaneous movement assessment does not evaluate the patient's ability for eye opening, verbal stimuli, or motor function.

C. Babinski reflex is present in patients with upper motor neuron disease and is not a component of the Glasgow Coma Scale.

D. The unconscious patient is unable to follow commands and will require the use of pain to determine if the patient is able to move away from the painful stimulus, has abnormal posturing, or has no response to the painful stimulus.

Category: Neurological Emergencies/Trauma
Nursing Process: Intervention

References

Broering, B. (2010). Head trauma. In P. K. Howard & R. A. Steinmann (Eds.), *Sheehy's emergency nursing: Principles and practice* (6th ed., pp. 254–271). St. Louis, MO: Mosby Elsevier.
Hickey, J. (2013). *The clinical practice of neurological and neurosurgical nursing* (7th ed.). Philadelphia, PA: Lippincott.
McLaughlin, J. C. (2014). Brain, cranial, and maxillofacial trauma. In D. Gurney (Ed.), *Trauma Nursing Core Course: Provider manual* (7th ed., pp. 105–122). Des Plaines, IL: Emergency Nurses Association.

53. An adult patient presents to the emergency department stating that they have been retching and vomiting for the past 12 hours and now has started vomiting bright red blood. The emergency nurse anticipates that the patient may have which of the following conditions?
A. Mallory–Weiss syndrome
B. Peptic ulcer disease
C. Ruptured esophageal varices
D. Esophageal stricture

Rationale

A. Vomiting and retching normal stomach contents before the onset of bleeding is suggestive of a Mallory–Weiss tear of the esophagus.

B. Peptic ulcer disease is characterized by an onset of a gnawing and burning pain that progressively worsens and may or may not be relieved by eating. Upper gastrointestinal bleeding may occur with peptic ulcer disease, but the initial vomitus would be bright red or the color of coffee grounds.

C. Esophageal varices are the result of dilated esophageal veins formed when the portal veins are under pressure, secondary to severe liver disease. Bleeding from ruptured esophageal varices is hemorrhagic in nature, leading to hypovolemic shock and even death.

D. The patient with an esophageal stricture will usually present with the chief complaint of trouble swallowing, or dysphagia.

Category: Gastrointestinal, Genitourinary, Gynecology, and Obstetrical Emergencies/Gastrointestinal/Bleeding

Nursing Process: Analysis

References

Ansari, P. (2018). Overview of GI bleeding. *Merck Manual Online* Retrieved from http://www.merckmanuals.com/professional/gastrointestinal-disorders/gi-bleeding/overview-of-gi-bleeding

Wolf, L., & Zimmermann, P. G. (2013). Abdominal pain and emergencies. In B. B. Hammond & P. G. Zimmermann (Eds.), *Sheehy's manual of emergency care* (7th ed., pp. 291–301). St. Louis, MO: Elsevier Mosby.

---

54. A patient is being prepared for discharge after being diagnosed with cholecystitis. Which statement made by the patient to the emergency nurse indicates their understanding of the dietary discharge instructions?

A. "It is important to eat foods rich in potassium."
B. "I need to stay away from foods with seeds and nuts."
C. "I should eat small, frequent meals rather than three large meals each day."
D. "I should avoid high-fat and fried foods."

Rationale

A. Serum potassium levels are not altered by an inflamed gallbladder.

B. Patients with diverticular disease are often counseled to avoid foods with seeds and nuts, but this is not a dietary instruction that applies to the patient with gallbladder disease.

C. Small, frequent meals will help to rest an irritated digestive system, but it is more important that the patient be aware of the foods that cause gallbladder pain and know to avoid them.

D. The symptoms associated with cholecystitis usually occur after consuming a meal high in fat content.

Category: Gastrointestinal, Genitourinary, Gynecology, and Obstetrical Emergencies/Gastrointestinal/Cholecystitis

Nursing Process: Evaluation

Reference

Rossoll, L. W. (2007). Abdominal emergencies. In K. S. Hoyt & J. Selfridge-Thomas (Eds.), *Emergency nursing core curriculum* (6th ed., pp. 178–181). St. Louis, MO: Saunders Elsevier.

---

55. A 60-year-old patient presents to the emergency department complaining of left lower quadrant abdominal pain, nausea, constipation, and anorexia that began 2 days ago. Vital signs: BP 118/78 mm Hg; HR 98 beats/minute; RR 18 breaths/minute; T 38.2°C (100.8°F). Assessment findings include abdominal distention, left-sided abdominal tenderness, and a palpable mass in the left lower quadrant. Bowel sounds are hyperactive in all four quadrants. The nurse suspects the patient may have:

A. appendicitis.
B. diverticulitis.
C. cholecystitis.
D. pancreatitis.

Rationale

A. The pain associated with appendicitis occurs in the right lower abdominal quadrant and is accompanied by nausea, vomiting, and rebound tenderness over the appendix. If perforation of the appendix has occurred, abdominal rigidity can result.

B. Diverticulitis is often referred to as the "left-sided appendicitis." Patients typically present with constant pain that is localized in the left lower quadrant. A low-grade fever, nausea, constipation, and anorexia are symptoms frequently associated with diverticulitis.

C. The discomfort associated with cholecystitis typically presents in the right upper quadrant, radiating to the back or right shoulder, and most often occurs after eating a meal high in fat content.

D. Patients with pancreatitis experience a sudden onset of severe left upper quadrant abdominal pain that may radiate to the back. Nausea, vomiting, tachycardia, and fever are commonly associated with the presence of pancreatitis.

Category: Gastrointestinal, Genitourinary, Gynecology, and Obstetrical Emergencies/Gastrointestinal/ Diverticulitis

Nursing Process: Analysis

References

Cartwright, S. L., & Knudson, M. P. (2008). Evaluation of acute abdominal pain in adults. *American Family Physicians, 77*(7), 971–978.

Wilkins, T., Embry, K., & George, R. (2013). Diagnosis and management of acute diverticulitis. *American Family Physicians, 87*(9), 612–620.

Wolf, L., & Zimmermann, P. G. (2013). Abdominal pain and emergencies. In B. B. Hammond & P. G. Zimmermann (Eds.), *Sheehy's manual of emergency care* (7th ed., pp. 291–301). St. Louis, MO: Elsevier Mosby.

---

56. When caring for a patient with bleeding esophageal varices, the emergency nurse would anticipate an order to initially administer which of the following medications?

A. Pantoprazole (Protonix)
B. Sulfasalazine (Azulfidine)
C. Somatostatin (Octreotide)
D. Sucralfate (Carafate)

Rationale

A. Proton pump inhibitors, such as pantoprazole (Protonix), are indicated in the treatment of upper gastrointestinal bleeding *not* caused by bleeding varices.

B. Sulfasalazine (Azulfidine) is an anticholinergic agent that is indicated in the treatment of irritable bowel disease.

C. Vasopressors such as somatostatin (Octreotide) reduce pressure in the portal circulation, which will slow bleeding from esophageal varices. This is an important first step as the patient is prepared for an endoscopy.

D. Sucralfate (Carafate) produces a thick, gel-like substance that coats the base of peptic ulcers and protects the mucosa from further damage from stomach acids. Sucralfate is not indicated in the treatment of esophageal varices.

Category: Gastrointestinal, Genitourinary, Gynecology, and Obstetrical Emergencies/Gastrointestinal/ Esophageal varices

Nursing Process: Intervention

References

Herrington, A. (2010). Gastrointestinal emergencies. In P. K. Howard & R. A. Steinmann (Eds.), *Sheehy's emergency nursing: Principles and practice* (6th ed., pp. 467–477). St. Louis, MO: Mosby Elsevier.

Wolf, L., & Zimmermann, P. G. (2013). Abdominal pain and emergencies. In B. B. Hammond & P. G. Zimmermann (Eds.), *Sheehy's manual of emergency care* (7th ed., pp. 291–301). St. Louis, MO: Elsevier Mosby.

---

57. The emergency nurse is preparing discharge instructions for a patient with abdominal pain and anticipates a prescription for a proton pump inhibitor as treatment for the patient's new diagnosis of:

A. cholecystitis.
B. hepatitis.
C. diverticulitis.
D. esophagitis.

Rationale

A. Mild cases of cholecystitis can be treated with low-fat dietary restrictions and analgesics. More severe cases will require hospitalization, intravenous hydration, and surgery to remove the gallbladder.

B. Hepatitis is a viral infection that is treated with antiviral medications; several available vaccines can protect against acquiring the disease.

C. The recommended treatment for diverticulitis includes a clear liquid diet. Additionally, if an infection is suspected, antibiotics will be prescribed for the patient. Diverticulitis is not normally treated with the administration of a proton pump inhibitor

D. Esophagitis is most commonly associated with gastroesophageal reflux disease due to an excess of stomach acid. A proton pump inhibitor medication is indicated for this patient to reduce gastric acid secretion.

Category: Gastrointestinal, Genitourinary, Gynecology, and Obstetrical Emergencies/Gastrointestinal/ Esophagitis

Nursing Process: Assessment

Reference

Herrington, A. (2010). Gastrointestinal emergencies. In P. K. Howard & R. A. Steinmann (Eds.), *Sheehy's emergency nursing: Principles and practice* (6th ed., pp. 467–477). St. Louis, MO: Mosby Elsevier.

---

58. The parents of a young child state their child may have swallowed a coin-sized lithium battery. The child has a patent airway but is drooling. Radiographs confirm that the battery is lodged in the child's esophagus. The emergency nurse should perform which of the following interventions?

A. Prepare the patient for immediate endoscopy to remove the battery
B. Provide the patient with popsicles and repeat the radiograph in 1 hour
C. Discharge the patient to home and provide parent with instructions to examine stool for the battery
D. Administer intravenous glucagon

Rationale

A. Button batteries that are lodged in the esophagus for more than 2 hours can cause esophageal burns and erosion of tissue, leading to possible perforation of the esophagus. The battery must be removed before it results in tissue damage.

B. The patient should not be permitted to eat or drink prior to the removal of the battery as this may cause the battery to enter the stomach and potentially cause damage to the stomach. The priority is to remove the battery from the child's esophagus before it causes esophageal burns.

C. The patient should not be discharged prior to the removal of the battery. Allowing the battery to travel through the gastrointestinal tract can lead to further damage and injury to the child. The priority is to remove the battery from the child's esophagus before it causes esophageal burns.

D. Intravenous glucagon is indicated for the adult patient who has a food bolus in the esophagus. The priority is to remove the battery from the child's esophagus before it causes esophageal burns.

Category (Pediatric): Gastrointestinal, Genitourinary, Gynecology, and Obstetrical Emergencies/Gastrointestinal/Foreign bodies

Nursing Process: Intervention

References

Reilly, J. S. (2013, April 29). *Coin-size lithium batteries can cause serious injury, death in a matter of hours if swallowed.* American Academy of Pediatrics. Retrieved from http://www.aappublications.org/content/34/5/13

Wolf, L., & Zimmermann, P. G. (2013). Abdominal pain and emergencies. In B. B. Hammond & P. G. Zimmermann (Eds.), *Sheehy's manual of emergency care* (7th ed., pp. 291–301). St. Louis, MO: Elsevier Mosby.

---

59. A 9-month-old presents to the emergency department (ED) with a 24-hour history of vomiting and diarrhea. The child's lips are dry and cracked, and tears are noted when the child cries. The parents state that the last wet diaper was 2 hours before arrival at the ED. The emergency nurse would be most concerned with what additional assessment finding?

A. Capillary refill 3 seconds
B. Systolic blood pressure 84 mm Hg
C. Apical heart rate 150 beats/minute
D. Respiratory rate 48 breaths/minute

Rationale

A. Normal capillary refill should be < 2 seconds. Prolonged capillary refill suggests hypoperfusion in this child.

B. The minimum systolic blood pressure for a child is calculated by using the following formula: Systolic blood pressure $= 70 +$ (age in years $\times$ 2). The minimum blood pressure for this child is 72 mm Hg.

C. The normal apical heart rate for a 9-month-old is 100–160 beats/minute.

D. The normal respiratory rate for a 9-month-old is 30–60 breaths/minute.

Category (Pediatric): Gastrointestinal, Genitourinary, Gynecology, and Obstetrical Emergencies/Gastrointestinal/Gastritis

Nursing Process: Assessment

References

Andreoni, C. (2013). Pediatric considerations in emergency nursing. In B. B. Hammond & P. G. Zimmermann (Eds.), *Sheehy's manual of emergency care* (7th ed., pp. 547–570). St. Louis, MO: Elsevier Mosby.

Mecham, N. L. (2010). Pediatric emergencies. In P. K. Howard & R. A. Steinmann (Eds.), *Sheehy's emergency nursing: Principles and practice* (6th ed., pp. 630–651). St. Louis, MO: Mosby Elsevier.

O'Leary, R., Campbell, K., Kruger, M., & Barbarossa, S. (2012). Neonatal resuscitation. In *Emergency Nursing Pediatric Course: Provider manual* (4th ed., pp. 141–159). Des Plaines, IL: Emergency Nurses Association.

---

60. An 18-month-old child with a 3-day history of diarrhea is brought to the emergency department by the parents. The child is irritable, mucus membranes are dry, and capillary refill is less than 3 seconds. The parents state that the child has had only one wet diaper in the past 8 hours. The emergency nurse anticipates the priority intervention for this patient is to:

A. obtain intravenous access and infuse a 0.9% sodium chloride bolus at 20 mL/kg.
B. obtain a stool culture.
C. administer an antiemetic medication.
D. offer small, frequent sips of an oral rehydration solution.

Rationale

A. Based on various dehydration scales, this patient is not identified to have severe dehydration symptoms (lethargic, sunken eyes, absent tear production, prolonged cap refill, increased work of breathing, minimal urine output). Therefore, the urgency for intravenous hydration may be deferred until oral rehydration is unsuccessful or the patient presentation worsens.

B. A stool culture can be considered in patients who have had symptoms longer than 7 days, who have blood in the stool, who are younger than 3 months, who have been exposed to an infectious pathogen, who are immunocompromised, or who appear toxic.

C. An antiemetic medication would be indicated in a patient who is vomiting. It is not effective as an intervention for diarrhea.

D. Based on various clinical dehydration scales, this child has mild to moderate dehydration. The management should focus on oral rehydration therapy, with an emphasis on replacing the deficits and preventing ongoing fluid losses.

Category (Pediatric): Gastrointestinal, Genitourinary, Gynecology, and Obstetrical Emergencies/Gastrointestinal/Gastroenteritis

Nursing Process: Intervention

References

Andreoni, C. (2013). Pediatric considerations in emergency nursing. In B. B. Hammond & P. G. Zimmermann (Eds.), *Sheehy's manual of emergency care* (7th ed., pp. 547–570). St. Louis, MO: Elsevier Mosby.

Carson, R. A., Mudd, S. S., & Madati, P. J. (2016). Clinical practice guideline for the treatment of pediatric acute gastroenteritis in the outpatient setting. *Journal of Pediatric Health Care, 30*(6), 610–616.

61. While examining a patient who presents with nausea, vomiting, and abdominal pain, a firm and tender mass is palpated in the lower right abdominal quadrant. The emergency nurse suspects that the patient may have of which of the following?

A. Diverticulitis
B. Crohn's disease
C. Appendicitis
D. Incarcerated hernia

Rationale

A. The patient with diverticulitis will usually present with anorexia, nausea, and vomiting. The pain associated with diverticulitis is located in the left lower abdominal quadrant.

B. The pain associated with Crohn's disease may be felt in the right lower quadrant or periumbilical area. A palpable mass would not be present.

C. A patient with appendicitis typically presents with right lower abdominal pain, anorexia, and vomiting and a low-grade fever. Rebound tenderness is elicited over McBurney's point in the right lower quadrant, but there is not a palpable mass.

D. An inguinal hernia typically presents as a firm, tender mass in the inguinal canal or femoral area.

Category: Gastrointestinal, Genitourinary, Gynecology, and Obstetrical Emergencies/Gastrointestinal/Hernia

Nursing Process: Assessment

Reference

Wolf, L., & Zimmermann, P. G. (2013). Abdominal pain and emergencies. In B. B. Hammond & P. G. Zimmermann (Eds.), *Sheehy's manual of emergency care* (7th ed., pp. 291–301). St. Louis, MO: Elsevier Mosby.

---

62. Which statement made by a patient with a history of inflammatory bowel disease is most consistent with a diagnosis of Crohn's disease?

A. "I keep getting these sores in my rectal area."
B. "I keep having flare-ups of my disease and have lost a lot of weight recently."
C. "One of my doctors told me that I might be able to have surgery on my colon that can cure this disease."
D. "Last time I was here, I had to have steroids and intravenous fluids."

Rationale

A. Symptoms such as anal fissures, perianal fistulae, and abscesses are signs of Crohn's disease.

B. Exacerbation of symptoms and weight loss are associated with both ulcerative colitis and Crohn's disease.

C. This statement suggests that the patient may have ulcerative colitis; this disease only affects the colon, and surgery may be curative. Crohn's disease affects the entire gastrointestinal tract, from the mouth to the anus, and surgery is only indicated for control of symptoms; it is not a curative measure for Crohn's disease.

D. Symptom management and treatment for both ulcerative colitis and Crohn's disease include corticosteroids, anti-inflammatory and antidiarrheal medications, bowel rest, and intravenous rehydration.

Category: Gastrointestinal, Genitourinary, Gynecology, and Obstetrical Emergencies/Gastrointestinal/Inflammatory bowel disease

Nursing Process: Assessment

Reference

Wolf, L., & Zimmermann, P. G. (2013). Abdominal pain and emergencies. In B. B. Hammond & P. G. Zimmermann (Eds.), *Sheehy's manual of emergency care* (7th ed., pp. 291–301). St. Louis, MO: Elsevier Mosby.

---

63. An infant is brought to the emergency department by their parents, who state that the infant has been irritable and vomiting, and has a change in the color and consistency of their stools. The infant is diagnosed with intussusception. The parents tell the nurse they do not understand what is wrong with their child. The best explanation by the nurse to the parents is to say:

A. "Intussusception occurs when the muscle that controls how the stomach empties is too tight, so the stomach contents back up."
B. "These changes in the stool can happen when a child is transitioned from breastmilk to formula and cereal."
C. "This happens when one portion of the bowel slides into the next. It's similar to a telescope and results in a blockage within the bowel."
D. "This can happen when the bowel pushes through the abdominal muscles. As long as the blood supply isn't cut off, surgery isn't needed."

Rationale

A. Constriction of the gastric outlet is usually due to pyloric stenosis. Pyloric stenosis usually occurs within the first weeks of life and is characterized by projectile vomiting; it usually does not cause pain.

B. Abdominal pain, vomiting, and red "currant jellylike" stools are the classic symptoms associated with intussusception.

C. Intussusception occurs when a portion of the bowel telescopes into itself, resulting in an obstruction.

D. A hernia occurs when a loop of bowel protrudes through the abdominal muscle, most commonly in the inguinal and umbilical areas. Unless incarcerated, it is not a surgical emergency.

Category (Pediatric): Gastrointestinal, Genitourinary, Gynecology, and Obstetrical Emergencies/Gastrointestinal/Intussusception

Nursing Process: Intervention

References

Golder, D. (2013). Childhood illness. In *Emergency Nursing Pediatric Course: Provider manual* (4th ed., pp. 147–169). Des Plaines, IL: Emergency Nurses Association.
Mecham, N. L. (2010). Pediatric emergencies. In P. K. Howard & R. A. Steinmann (Eds.), *Sheehy's emergency nursing: Principles and practice* (6th ed., pp. 630–651). St. Louis, MO: Mosby Elsevier.
Wolf, L., & Zimmermann, P. G. (2013). Abdominal pain and emergencies. In B. B. Hammond & P. G. Zimmermann (Eds.), *Sheehy's manual of emergency care* (7th ed., pp. 291–301). St. Louis, MO: Elsevier Mosby.

---

64. A patient with a large stab wound to the abdomen is received in the emergency department. On assessment, the patient has a loop of small bowel protruding from the wound. The emergency nurse should immediately cover the exposed bowel with which of the following?

A. A semipermeable transparent dressing
B. Dry, sterile dressings
C. Saline-soaked gauze
D. Nonstick gauze and an abdominal binder

Rationale

A. It is important to keep the exposed bowel moist in order to keep it viable for replacement into the abdominal cavity. A semipermeable transparent dressing will allow moisture to move away from the bowel, allowing it to dry out.

B. Eviscerated abdominal organs should be kept moist to keep them viable for surgical replacement into the abdominal cavity. Placing a dry, sterile dressing over the exposed bowel will impair the viability of the exposed organ and decrease likelihood of surgical replacement of the exposed bowel back into the abdominal cavity.

C. Eviscerated abdominal organs should be kept moist to keep them viable for surgical replacement into the abdominal cavity.

D. The exposed bowel must be kept moist. The nurse should not attempt to push the exposed organs back into the abdominal cavity because this may further injure the tissue.

Category: Gastrointestinal, Genitourinary, Gynecology, and Obstetrical Emergencies/Gastrointestinal/Trauma

Nursing Process: Intervention

Reference

Bacidore, V. (2010). Abdominal and genitourinary trauma. In P. K. Howard & R. A. Steinmann (Eds.), *Sheehy's emergency nursing: Principles and practice* (6th ed., pp. 301–312). St. Louis, MO: Mosby Elsevier.

---

65. A 40-year-old male presents with complaints of a painful penile erection for the past several hours that is not associated with sexual stimulation. The patient has a history of chronic back pain, schizophrenia, and hepatitis C. The prolonged erection is most likely due to the patient's use of:

A. risperidone (Risperdal).
B. ribavirin (Virazole).
C. celecoxib (Celebrex).
D. buprenorphine/naloxone (Buprenex).

Rationale

A. Risperidone is an antipsychotic used to treat schizophrenia. A side effect associated with the administration of risperidone is the presence of priapism.

B. Ribavirin is an antiviral used in the treatment of hepatitis C, but priapism is not a known side effect of this medication.

C. Celecoxib is a nonsteroidal anti-inflammatory agent used for the management of pain. Priapism is not a known side effect of this medication.

D. Buprenorphine is used for treatment of opioid dependence, but priapism is not a known side effect of this medication.

Category: Gastrointestinal, Genitourinary, Gynecology, and Obstetrical Emergencies/Genitourinary/Priapism

Nursing Process: Analysis

References

Baxter, C. S. (2010). Renal and genitourinary emergencies. In P. K. Howard & R. A. Steinmann (Eds.), *Sheehy's emergency nursing: Principles and practice* (6th ed., pp. 478–489). St. Louis, MO: Mosby Elsevier.

Vallerand, A. H., & Sanoski, C. (2014). *Davis's drug guide for nurses* (14th ed.). Philadelphia, PA: F. A. Davis.

---

66. A patient with a diagnosis of renal calculi is being prepared for discharge from the emergency department. Which of the following statements made by the patient demonstrates their understanding of the discharge instructions?

A. "I will eliminate all calcium-containing foods from my diet."
B. "I should increase the amount of water I drink during the day."
C. "Once the pain resolves, I will no longer need to strain my urine."
D. "I can expect to run a fever until the stone passes."

Rationale

A. Renal calculi consist of 80% calcium, but calcium is a necessary nutrient, and eliminating it from the diet may result in a nutritional deficit. The patient should be encouraged to avoid consuming large amounts of calcium-containing food, including milk, but should not totally eliminate calcium from their diet.

B. Increasing the amount of fluid intake, especially water, will dilute the urine and discourage the collection of stone-forming crystals.

C. The acute pain related to a renal calculi is the result of the stone descending from the renal pelvis through the ureter. There is often little to no discomfort as the stone passes from the bladder through the urethra. The patient should continue to strain the urine for up to 72 hours after the pain is relieved in order to retrieve the stone for chemical analysis.

D. Fever is not a symptom associated with renal calculi unless an infection is present. The patient should be advised to return to the emergency department if fever is present, because hospital admission is generally indicated.

Category: Gastrointestinal, Genitourinary, Gynecology, and Obstetrical Emergencies/Genitourinary/Renal calculi

Nursing Process: Evaluation

References

Baxter, C. S. (2010). Renal and genitourinary emergencies. In P. K. Howard & R. A. Steinmann (Eds.), *Sheehy's emergency nursing: Principles and practice* (6th ed., pp. 478–489). St. Louis, MO: Mosby Elsevier.

Jordan, K. S. (2007). Genitourinary emergencies. In K. S. Hoyt & J. Selfridge-Thomas (Eds.), *Emergency nursing core curriculum* (6th ed., pp. 387–408). St. Louis, MO: Saunders Elsevier.

National Kidney Foundation. (2016). *Calcium oxalate stones.* Retrieved from https://www.kidney.org/atoz/content/calcium-oxalate-stone

67. A 28-year-old female presents to the emergency department with complaints of heavy, bright red vaginal bleeding for the past 1 month. She complains of feeling tired but is alert and oriented and denies feelings of dizziness or lightheadedness. The patient states that she has not been sexually active for the past 3 months. Vital signs: BP 116/74 mm Hg; HR 86 beats/minute; RR 18 breaths/minute; T 36.8°C (98.4°F). The patient's hemoglobin is 9.4 g/dL, and the urine pregnancy test is negative. The nurse should prepare the patient for a(n):

A. immediate exploratory laparotomy.
B. transfusion with 1 unit of packed red blood cells.
C. vaginal examination.
D. STAT administration of levonorgestrel (Plan B).

Rationale

A. A uterine dilation and curettage (D and C) may eventually be indicated, but the patient's hemodynamic status does not suggest there is an immediate threat to her well-being.

B. Although anemic, this patient is hemodynamically stable and does not require a blood transfusion.

C. Because the patient is not pregnant, a vaginal exam should be performed.

D. Abnormal vaginal bleeding frequently occurs after levonorgestrel (Plan B) is taken for emergency contraception within 72 hours of unprotected sexual intercourse. The patient denies recent sexual activity, and the medication is not indicated as a therapy for dysfunctional vaginal bleeding.

Category: Gastrointestinal, Genitourinary, Gynecology, and Obstetrical Emergencies/Gynecology/Bleeding/dysfunction (vaginal)

Nursing Process: Intervention

References

Jordan, K. S. (2010). Gynecologic emergencies. In P. K. Howard & R. A. Steinmann (Eds.), *Sheehy's emergency nursing: Principles and practice* (6th ed., pp. 578–589). St. Louis, MO: Mosby Elsevier.

Kelly, L. (2013). Gynecological emergencies. In B. B. Hammond & P. G. Zimmermann (Eds.), *Sheehy's manual of emergency care* (7th ed., pp. 497–503). St. Louis, MO: Elsevier Mosby.

---

68. A patient diagnosed with chlamydia verbalizes understanding of the disease process when they state:

A. "Symptoms of a chlamydia infection include a vaginal discharge with a 'fishy' odor."
B. "Men who have sex with other men are not at risk to contract chlamydia infection."
C. "Most patients with chlamydia do not have symptoms."
D. "Once treated, a patient develops immunity against future chlamydia infections."

Rationale

A. A vaginal discharge with a "fishy" odor is a symptom associated with a *trichomonas vaginalis* infection.

B. Chlamydia can be transmitted through oral and anal sexual contact, so homosexual men are at risk to develop a chlamydia infection.

C. It is estimated that up to 75% of patients with a chlamydia infection are asymptomatic.

D. A patient who has been treated for chlamydia can become infected again if they have unprotected sex with a partner who is infected with chlamydia.

Category: Gastrointestinal, Genitourinary, Gynecology, and Obstetrical Emergencies/Gynecology/Infection

Nursing Process: Evaluation

References

Centers for Disease Control and Prevention. (2017). *Chlamydia fact sheet.* Retrieved from https://www.cdc.gov/std/chlamydia/stdfact-chlamydia.htm

Egging, D. (2013). Sexually transmitted infections. In B. B. Hammond & P. G. Zimmermann (Eds.), *Sheehy's manual of emergency care* (7th ed., pp. 361–366). St. Louis, MO: Elsevier Mosby.

---

69. A 26-week-pregnant female presents with bright red vaginal bleeding. The patient states she has saturated one feminine pad every hour for the past 3 hours. On examination by the care provider, the uterus is painful and tender to palpation and fetal heart tones are 160 beats/minute. Vital signs: BP 124/80 mm Hg; HR 110 beats/minute; RR 20 breaths/minute; SpO_2 98% on room air; T 37°C (98.9°F). The emergency nurse should anticipate which of the following interventions to be performed next?

A. Admission for fetal monitoring
B. Emergent caesarean section
C. Immediate blood transfusion
D. Discharge to home on bedrest with physician follow-up

Rationale

A. This patient is most likely experiencing placental abruption. Because her vital signs are stable and fetal heart tones (FHT) are within normal limits, she would most likely be admitted for a trial of fetal monitoring and modified bedrest before determining her disposition.

B. Although emergent caesarean section may be indicated in placental abruption, the patient's VS and the FHT are stable at this time. Because she is not near term in her pregnancy (< 36 weeks), monitoring would definitely be the first choice in the stable patient.

C. With stable VS and FHT, immediate blood transfusion is not indicated at this time, although blood work ordered would probably include blood and Rh typing.

D. Although the patient appears stable at this time, fetal monitoring is indicated to ensure maintained stability of both the patient and the fetus.

Category: Gastrointestinal, Genitourinary, Gynecology, and Obstetrical Emergencies/Obstetrical/Abruptio placenta

Nursing Process: Analysis

References

Antonette, D. (2017). Abrtuptio placentae. *Merck Manual Online.* Retrieved from http://www.merckmanuals.com/professional/gynecology-and-obstetrics/abnormalities-of-pregnancy/abruptio-placentae

Poole, J. H., & Thompson, J. E. (2013). Obstetric emergencies. In B. B. Hammond & P. G. Zimmermann (Eds.), *Sheehy's manual of emergency care* (7th ed., pp. 483–495). St. Louis, MO: Elsevier Mosby.

70. A 26-year-old female presents to triage with a sudden onset of right lower abdominal pain, followed by a syncopal episode and heavy vaginal bleeding. Based on the presenting symptoms, which of the following conditions would the emergency nurse most likely suspect?

A. Ruptured ectopic pregnancy
B. Pelvic inflammatory disease
C. Ruptured ovarian cyst
D. Acute exacerbation of endometriosis

Rationale

A. Early symptoms and signs of ectopic pregnancy include pelvic pain, vaginal bleeding, and cervical motion tenderness. Syncope or hemorrhagic shock can occur with rupture. This is a high-risk condition and, when suspected in triage, should be given a high priority.

B. Symptoms of pelvic inflammatory disease (PID) include lower abdominal pain, cervical discharge, and irregular vaginal bleeding. An associated history of a syncopal episode is unlikely in a patient with PID.

C. Most ovarian cysts are asymptomatic. Blood-filled corpus luteum cysts may rupture, resulting in abdominal pain and intraperitoneal bleeding. Although these symptoms may be confused with those of a ruptured ectopic pregnancy, the bleeding is intraperitoneal, not vaginal.

D. The symptoms of endometriosis are dependent on the location of the endometrial tissue implanted outside the uterine cavity. Symptoms may include dysmenorrhea, dyspareunia, infertility, dysuria, and pain during defecation. Pain is the most common symptom to this triage patient, but the other symptoms most likely would not be present.

Category: Gastrointestinal, Genitourinary, Gynecology, and Obstetrical Emergencies/Obstetrical/Ectopic pregnancy

Nursing Process: Analysis

References

Dulay, A. (2017). Ectopic pregnancy. *Merck Manual Online.* Retrieved from http://www.merckmanuals.com/professional/gynecology-and-obstetrics/abnormalities-of-pregnancy/ectopic-pregnancy

Jordan, K. S. (2010). Gynecologic emergencies. In P. K. Howard & R. A. Steinmann (Eds.), *Sheehy's emergency nursing: Principles and practice* (6th ed., pp. 578–589). St. Louis, MO: Mosby Elsevier.

Liu, J., & Bill, A. H. (2017). Endometriosis. *Merck Manual Online.* Retrieved from http://www.merckmanuals.com/professional/gynecology-and-obstetrics/endometriosis/endometriosis

McNeeley, S. G. (2017). Benign ovarian masses. *Merck Manual Online.* Retrieved from http://www.merckmanuals.com/professional/gynecology-and-obstetrics/benign-gynecologic-lesions/benign-ovarian-masses

Soper, D. E. (2015). Pelvic inflammatory disease (PID). *Merck Manual Online.* Retrieved from http://www.merckmanuals.com/professional/gynecology-and-obstetrics/vaginitis,-cervicitis,-and-pelvic-inflammatory-disease-pid/pelvic-inflammatory-disease-pid

71. Approximately 10 minutes following the vaginal delivery of a full-term neonate in the emergency department, the emergency nurse observes a sudden gush of blood from the mother's vagina. The nurse suspects which of the following?

A. Uterine rupture has occurred.
B. The patient has sustained a cervical tear during delivery.
C. The placenta has separated from the uterine wall.
D. Delivery of an unanticipated second neonate is imminent.

Rationale

A. Uterine rupture is a rare obstetrical emergency that occurs before delivery. It is typically the result of blunt force, deceleration, or compression injury.

B. Following delivery of the placenta, vaginal bleeding should lessen. A cervical tear can be the cause of significant postpartum bleeding, but the bleeding is characterized by a steadier flow rather than a single gush.

C. Approximately 10 minutes after the birth of the infant, the patient enters the third stage of labor, placental delivery. This stage is preceded by a sudden gush of blood from the vagina as the placenta separates from the uterine wall.

D. Signs of an imminent delivery include a bulging of the perineum or visualization or palpation of the presenting fetal parts. A second neonate often has intact membranes, so a gush of amniotic fluid may occur, but not blood.

Category: Gastrointestinal, Genitourinary, Gynecology, and Obstetrical Emergencies/Obstetrical/Emergent delivery

Nursing Process: Evaluation

References

Jordan, K. S. (2007). Obstetric and gynecologic emergencies. In K. S. Hoyt & J. Selfridge-Thomas (Eds.), *Emergency nursing core curriculum* (6th ed., pp. 536–570). St. Louis, MO: Saunders Elsevier.

Mason, D. (2010). Obstetric emergencies. In P. K. Howard & R. A. Steinmann (Eds.), *Sheehy's emergency nursing: Principles and practice* (6th ed., pp. 619–629). St. Louis, MO: Mosby Elsevier.

Poole, J. H., & Thompson, J. E. (2013). Obstetric emergencies. In B. B. Hammond & P. G. Zimmermann (Eds.), *Sheehy's manual of emergency care* (7th ed., pp. 488–495). St. Louis, MO: Elsevier Mosby.

---

72. A 28-week-pregnant female arrives to the emergency department with chief complaint of shortness of breath and right upper abdominal pain. Which of the following laboratory results would suggest to the emergency nurse that the patient is developing HELLP syndrome?

A. **Platelet count 90,000/mm^3**
B. Glycosuria
C. Serum potassium 5.8 mEq/L
D. Serum magnesium 1.7 mEq/L

Rationale

A. HELLP is a life-threatening complication of pregnancy whose defining characteristics are hemolysis (H); elevated liver enzymes (EL); and low platelet count (LP). The development of hemolysis leads to the activation of the coagulation cascade, causing consumption of the patient's platelets.

B. Unless the patient is known to have diabetes mellitus (DM) or is developing gestational DM, she should not have the presence of glucose in her urine with HELLP syndrome.

C. HELLP does not cause a rise in serum potassium or affect other serum electrolytes values.

D. The magnesium value is within the normal range. HELLP does not affect serum electrolytes.

Category: Gastrointestinal, Genitourinary, Gynecology, and Obstetrical Emergencies/Obstetrical/Preeclampsia, eclampsia, HELLP syndrome

Nursing Process: Analysis

References

Jordan, K. S. (2007). Obstetric and gynecologic emergencies. In K. S. Hoyt & J. Selfridge-Thomas (Eds.), *Emergency nursing core curriculum* (6th ed., pp. 536–570). St. Louis, MO: Saunders Elsevier.

Mason, D. (2010). Obstetric emergencies. In P. K. Howard & R. A. Steinmann (Eds.), *Sheehy's emergency nursing: Principles and practice* (6th ed., pp. 619–629). St. Louis, MO: Mosby Elsevier.

---

73. A patient who is 32 weeks pregnant presents to the emergency department complaining of severe abdominal pain. Which of the following assessment findings would place the patient at risk for preterm labor?

A. Having a long interval between pregnancies
B. Smoking during pregnancy
C. Having a previous full-term birth
D. Maternal age between 30 and 35 years

Rationale

A. Women who become pregnant soon after a previous delivery are at greater risk to experience preterm labor.

B. Smoking during pregnancy is a common risk factor associated with premature birth and poor fetal outcomes.

C. Mothers who have had a previous preterm birth are at greater risk to experience preterm labor during subsequent pregnancies.

D. Women younger than 17 years and older than 40 years are more likely to experience premature labor

Category: Gastrointestinal, Genitourinary, Gynecology, and Obstetrical Emergencies/Obstetrical/Preterm labor

Nursing Process: Assessment

References

O'Connor, C., & Gennaro, S. (2015). Prenatal and intrapartum strategies to prevent prematurity: A case study. *March of Dimes*. Retrieved from https://www.marchofdimes.org/nursing/modnemedia/othermedia/articles/art04_strategies_prev_prematurity.pdf

Ross, M. G., & Smith, C. V. (2016, December 9). Preterm labor. *Medscape*. Retrieved from http://emedicine.medscape.com/article/260998-overview#a3

---

74. A young mother presents to triage with a 2 1/2-year-old toddler who sustained a lip laceration related to a fall while playing in the yard. The mother tells the triage nurse that her daughter is "very clumsy." The child has numerous bruises in various stages of healing on bilateral knees and a healing abrasion on one elbow, but no other apparent injuries. Which of the following statements about assessment for potential child maltreatment is most accurate for this situation?

A. Unintentional injuries tend to occur on bony prominences, which may be normal for a toddler.
B. The bruises in various stages of healing are a clear sign of potential abuse and should be evaluated.
C. Multiple areas of injury are indicative of potential abuse, especially in the toddler population.
D. Intentional injuries are easily spotted because they are generally inflicted in patterns.

Rationale

A. As toddlers are learning to walk and run, it is not uncommon to see bruises on bony prominences such as knees and elbows.

B. Although bruises in various stages of healing may be signs of abuse and should be evaluated, they are not necessarily *clear* signs.

C. Multiple areas of injury may be signs of abuse; however, the nurse must consider the developmental age of the patient.

D. Intentional injuries are not necessarily easily spotted. Abusers may cover intentional injures with clothing. Pattern injuries could be associated with intentional injury and should be evaluated.

Category (Pediatric): Psychosocial and Medical Emergencies/Psychosocial/Abuse and neglect

Nursing Process: Assessment

References

Black, A. (2010). Child abuse and neglect. In P. K. Howard & R. A. Steinmann (Eds.), *Sheehy's emergency nursing: Principles and practice* (6th ed., pp. 652–665). St. Louis, MO: Mosby Elsevier.

Black, A. (2012). Child maltreatment. In *Emergency Nursing Pediatric Course: Provider manual* (4th ed., pp. 343–357). Des Plaines, IL: Emergency Nurses Association.

---

75. A patient with a history of depression and bipolar disorder presents to the emergency department with suicidal ideation and auditory hallucinations. While awaiting a mental health bed to become available, the patient becomes increasingly agitated, begins to pace about the treatment area, and threatens staff members. The nurse actively listens and speaks in clear, concise language while ensuring the patient's safety. Which of the following demonstrates a desired response to the interventions?

A. The patient states that they do not need to be in restraints any longer.
B. The patient is able to verbalize their feelings.
C. The patient accepted their medication.
D. The patient's suicidal ideation has ceased.

Rationale

A. Restraints indicate that the patient did not respond to the verbal interventions attempted by the nurse.

B. An appropriate response to establishing rapport by active listening and speaking in clear and concise sentences is the patient being able to verbalize their feelings.

C. Medication may have had to be administered, but an initial appropriate response to therapeutic communication is that the patient can communicate back to the nurse.

D. Resolution of suicidal ideations is a desired response to treatment, but an initial response to therapeutic communication is that the patient is able to communicate back to the nurse. Restraint may be appropriate for a physically assaultive patient, but it is not the most therapeutic action while the patient is escalating.

Category: Psychosocial and Medical Emergencies/Psychosocial/Aggressive/violent behavior

Nursing Process: Evaluation

References

Manton, A. (2013). Mental health emergencies. In B. B. Hammond & P. G. Zimmermann (Eds.), *Sheehy's manual of emergency care* (7th ed., pp. 505–519). St. Louis, MO: Elsevier Mosby.

Tan, M. F., Lopez, V., & Cleary, M. (2015). Nursing management of aggression in a Singapore emergency department: A qualitative study. *Nursing & Health Sciences, 17*(3), 307–312. https://doi.org/10.1111/nhs.12188

---

76. A patient reports experiencing short episodes of intense fear accompanied by chest pain, shortness of breath, lightheadedness, and numbness. Which of the following statements made by the patient indicate an understanding of the treatment options for this experience?

A. "I should call for an ambulance as soon as the symptoms start."
B. "I should first try to determine what made me feel anxious."
C. "Breathing in and out into a paper bag may help the symptoms initially subside."
D. "I should take some over-the-counter pain medication when I experience these symptoms."

Rationale

A. The patient should try to alleviate symptoms temporarily and, if unable to do so, proceed to seeking care from a medical provider.

B. Determining the cause of the onset of the panic attack is a realistic expectation, but initially the patient should try to get symptoms to subside. Focusing on the cause may not alleviate the symptoms.

C. Panic attacks are short-lived episodes of anxiety or intense fear accompanied by a range of somatic symptoms (common cardiac, gastrointestinal, or neurologic). These symptoms often mimic symptoms of life-threatening conditions. Having the patient rebreathe their own carbon dioxide using a paper bag may result in temporary subsiding of symptoms.

D. The physical signs and symptoms originated because of an intense fear or anxiety reaction. A decrease in carbon dioxide (CO_2) results in the continuation and progression of symptoms. Rebreathing CO_2 may help decrease or eliminate the somatic symptoms, and analgesics are not necessary.

Category: Psychosocial and Medical Emergencies/Psychosocial/Anxiety/panic
Nursing Process: Evaluation

References

DeSelm, T. M. (2016). Mood and anxiety disorders. In *Tintinalli's emergency medicine: A comprehensive study guide* (8th ed.). Retrieved from http://accessemergencymedicine.mhmedical.com/content.aspx?bookid=1658&Sectionid=109448311

Huecker, M. R., & O'Brien, D. J. (2011). Chest pain. In C. Stone & R. L. Humphries (Eds.), *Current diagnosis & treatment: Emergency medicine* (7th ed.). Retrieved from http://accessemergencymedicine.mhmedical.com/content.aspx?bookid=385&Sectionid=40357228

Potts, K. (2012). Assessment of a patient presenting with suspected pulmonary embolism, *British Journal of Cardiac Nursing, 7*(10), 483–489.

Sucu, M., Ozer, O., Davutoglu, V., Ercan, S., Yuce, M., Coskun, F. Y. (2015). Relationship between neurocardiogenic syncope and ventricular repolarization. *Pacing & Clinical Electrophysiology, 38*(5), 625–629. https://doi.org/10.1111/pace.12599

Sule, H. (2014). Pulmonary embolism. In S. C. Sherman, J. M. Weber, M. A. Schindlbeck, & G. P. Rahul (Eds.), *Clinical emergency medicine.* Retrieved from http://accessemergencymedicine.mhmedical.com/content.aspx?bookid=991&Sectionid=57307762

Tompkins, O. (2010). Panic attacks. *American Association of Occupational Health Nurses Journal, 58*(6), 268. https://doi.org/10.3928/08910162-20100526-07

Wisniewski, A. (2006). Taking a closer look at costochondritis. *Nursing, 36*(11), 64.

77. A combat veteran is brought to the emergency department by their social worker. The patient has a history of depression, increasing angry outbursts and nightmares since returning from combat. The patient appears anxious, is tearful, and tells the triage nurse, "I can't take this anymore. Please help me." Vital signs: BP 134/80 mm Hg; HR 89 beats/minute; RR 18 breaths/minute; T 36.7° C (98.2°F). The emergency nurse escorts the patient to a quiet room and suspects that their symptoms are suggestive of which condition?

A. Alcohol withdrawal syndrome
B. Posttraumatic stress disorder
C. Acute psychosis
D. Panic attack

Rationale

A. Alcohol withdrawal syndrome is a potentially life-threatening emergency characterized by shaking, fever, and elevated heart rate. The patient is not trembling, and vital signs are within normal limits. There is no information indicating the patient's alcohol intake.

B. Posttraumatic stress disorder is defined as an anxiety disorder in response to an extremely traumatic event. Given the patient's history of being a combat veteran, coupled with a history of depression, the patient is most likely exhibiting signs of posttraumatic stress disorder, including nightmares, flashbacks, feeling emotionally numb, and loss of interest in previously enjoyed activities.

C. Signs and symptoms of acute psychosis present quickly and are short lived. The patient may experience hallucinations, delusions, and disorganized speech. The patient in this scenario has experienced a gradual onset of symptoms, and there is no report of hallucinations or delusions.

D. Although the patient could be experiencing a panic attack, the signs and symptoms presented gradually. A panic attack is typically an acute onset, characterized by a pounding heart rate, hyperventilation, diaphoresis, and intense anxiety.

Category: Psychosocial and Medical Emergencies/Psychosocial/Anxiety/panic

Nursing Process: Analysis

Reference

Manton, A. (2013). Mental health emergencies. In B. B. Hammond & P. G. Zimmermann (Eds.), *Sheehy's manual of emergency care* (7th ed., pp. 505–519). St. Louis, MO: Elsevier Mosby.

---

78. A patient who received an injection of an antipsychotic medication to manage acute mania is now experiencing an acute dystonic reaction. Which of the following medications would the emergency nurse expect to administer to treat this medication side effect?

A. Diazepam (Valium)
B. Naloxone (Narcan)
C. Flumazenil (Romazicon)
D. Diphenhydramine (Benadryl)

Rationale

A. Benzodiazepines, such as diazepam, are often used concurrently with antipsychotics to manage acute mania. The combination of both medications increases the level of sedation. Benzodiazepines have no benefit in treating acute dystonia.

B. Naloxone is the reversal agent for opioid overdoses and has no benefit in treating acute dystonia.

C. Flumazenil is the reversal agent for benzodiazepine overdoses and has no benefit in treating acute dystonia.

D. Diphenhydramine, an anticholinergic and antihistamine, is the drug of choice for treating acute dystonia, which is a known side effect of antipsychotics.

Category: Psychosocial and Medical Emergencies/Psychosocial/Bipolar disorder
Nursing Process: Intervention

References

Gagnon, L. (2010). Behavioral health emergencies. In P. K. Howard & R. A. Steinmann (Eds.), *Sheehy's emergency nursing: Principles and practice* (6th ed., pp. 677–688). St. Louis, MO: Mosby Elsevier.

Woo, T. M. (2016). Drugs affecting the central nervous system. In T. M. Woo & M. V. Robinson (Eds.), *Pharmacotherapeutics for advanced practice nurse prescribers* (4th ed., pp. 225–294). Philadelphia, PA: F. A. Davis.

---

79. A patient presents to the emergency department following the recent loss of both their job and significant other. The patient appears despondent, with a flat affect. Which of the following is the highest priority intervention for the emergency nurse to perform in the case of this patient?

A. Inform the patient about possible grief counseling groups
B. Assess if the patient plans to harm themself
C. Refer the patient to their primary care physician
D. Assist the patient with resources to find a new job

Rationale

A. Grief counseling may assist the patient with their depression, but securing their immediate safety and security is the most important.

B. Ensuring the patient's safety and security is the highest priority and the most important aspect in the initial phases of care of the acutely depressed patient. The emergency nurse needs to ensure that the patient's immediate environment is safe from objects that they could potentially harm themself with and that the patient feels safe and secure in the emergency department (ED) setting.

C. This patient may require follow-up with their primary care physician after their immediate care needs have been met. The emergency nurse should provide comfort, safety, and security in response to the patient's decision to seek medical management in the ED.

D. The role of the emergency nurse is to provide a sense of safety and security. Referral to a social worker may be indicated to assist with the patient's immediate social care needs.

Category: Psychosocial and Medical Emergencies/Psychosocial/Depression
Nursing Process: Intervention

References

Gagnon, L. (2010). Behavioral health emergencies. In P. K. Howard & R. A. Steinmann (Eds.), *Sheehy's emergency nursing: Principles and practice* (6th ed., pp. 677–688). St. Louis, MO: Mosby Elsevier.

Manton, A. (2013). Mental health emergencies. In B. B. Hammond & P. G. Zimmermann (Eds.), *Sheehy's manual of emergency care* (7th ed., pp. 505–519). St. Louis, MO: Elsevier Mosby.

80. A patient presents to triage dressed in a robe and carrying a staff, stating that they "are Jesus Christ" and "are going to save the world." Which of the following interventions should be considered for this patient?

A. Speaking calmly to the patient
B. Restraining the patient
C. Telling the patient they are not "Jesus Christ"
D. Administering intravenous haloperidol

Rationale

A. When a patient is experiencing a possible psychotic episode, behavioral approaches should be used initially. De-escalation techniques should be employed, including establishing a rapport with the patient; speaking calmly; and recognizing patient needs, such as for food, water, and safety. At times, the patient may be in physical pain and in need of pain management.

B. Attempting to restrain the patient could result in further agitation and could escalate to violence, resulting in injury to the patient and staff.

C. Challenging or arguing with the patient may agitate them further and cause them to escalate to violent behavior.

D. Medication may be indicated, but de-escalation techniques should be attempted first, especially if the patient is cooperative with the staff. Development of a trusting relationship between the patient and staff is an important intervention.

Category: Psychosocial and Medical Emergencies/Psychosocial/Psychosis

Nursing Process: Intervention

References

Deal, N., & Matorin, A. (2015). Stabilization and management of the acutely agitated or psychotic patient. *Emergency Medicine Clinics of North America, 33*, 739–752.
Wheat, S., & Taleri, M. (2016). Psychiatric emergencies. *Primary Care: Clinics in Office Practice, 43*(2), 341–354.

---

81. Law enforcement arrives to the emergency department with a patient who was found wandering around a local neighborhood. The patient is alert, oriented, and cooperative but appears agitated. They are pacing in circles and mumbling to themself. Vital signs are within normal limits. The officer tells you that the patient has a psychiatric and seizure history and is well-known to local law enforcement. The patient complains of headache, nausea, and vertigo and states they've been having nightmares. The most likely cause of the patient's current condition is which of the following?

A. Abrupt discontinuation from phenytoin
B. Withdrawal from benzodiazepines medication
C. Overdose on selective serotonin inhibitor medication
D. Overdose on tricyclic antidepressants medication

Rationale

A. Sudden cessation of phenytoin may result in increased seizure activity or frequency of seizures, not the symptoms being exhibited by this patient.

B. Benzodiazepines, often used to treat anxiety, alcohol withdrawal, and seizures, may cause physical dependence. Sudden withdrawal from benzodiazepines is likely to cause the symptoms being exhibited by this patient: agitation, anxiety, and hallucinations.

C. Signs and symptoms of selective serotonin inhibitor overdose include altered level of consciousness, respiratory depression, and hyperthermia. This patient's vital signs are within normal limits, and they are oriented.

D. Signs and symptoms of tricyclic antidepressants overdose include altered level of consciousness, dysrhythmias, and hypotension. This patient is not exhibiting these symptoms.

Category: Psychosocial and Medical Emergencies/Psychosocial/Situational crisis

Nursing Process: Evaluation

References

Karch, A. M. (2013). *Focus on nursing pharmacology* (6th ed.). Philadelphia, PA: Wolters Kluwer/Lippincott Williams & Wilkins.

Phillips, M. (2007). Toxicologic emergencies. In K. S. Hoyt & J. Selfridge-Thomas (Eds.), *Emergency Nursing Core Curriculum*. (6th ed., pp. 604–658). St. Louis, MO: Saunders Elsevier.

---

82. Which Emergency Severity Index classification level will be designated for a patient with an isolated complaint of suicidal ideation and no medical health problems?

A. Level 1: immediate life-saving interventions
B. Level 2: high risk
C. Level 3: many resources
D. Level 5: no resources

Rationale

A. The level 1 designation is reserved for those who are unstable and need immediate life-saving interventions. The patient is high risk and should be evaluated immediately but does not require life-saving interventions at this time.

B. The patient is high risk and should be evaluated immediately. The patient will require resources such as a psychiatric consult and diagnostic testing (serum blood test, urine test, etc.).

C. The patient with suicidal ideation is considered high risk and should be evaluated immediately. Designating this patient as a level 3 is a common example of undertriage and not considering the possible patient safety risk.

D. Resources such as a psychiatric consult and diagnostic testing (serum blood test, urine test) will be required.

Category: Psychosocial and Medical Emergencies/Psychosocial/Suicidal ideation

Nursing Process: Assessment

Reference

Brosinski, C., & Riddell, A. (2015). Mitigating nursing biases in management of intoxicated and suicidal patients. *Journal of Emergency Nursing, 4*(4), 296–299. https://doi.org/10.1016/j.jen.2014.11.002

83. A patient arrives to the emergency department after sustaining multiple bee stings while working on a roof. The patient complains of chest pains, lightheadedness, and difficulty breathing. Prior medical history includes hypertension and "heart problems." Vital signs: BP 70/40 mm Hg; HR 122 beats/minute; RR 24 breaths/minute; SpO_2 88% on room air; T 37.7°C (100.0°F). Which intervention would be the highest priority the emergency nurse should initiate for this patient?

A. Obtain a 12-lead electrocardiogram
B. Administer epinephrine
C. Administer high-flow oxygen via nonrebreather face mask
D. Obtain intravenous access

Rationale

A. Assessing the patient's airway patency and administering oxygen is the priority for this patient. Obtaining an electrocardiogram is indicated to rule acute myocardial infarction secondary to the bee sting, also known as Kounis syndrome, but the first priority is oxygenation. Kounis syndrome is characterized by the concurrence of acute coronary syndrome and a mast cell degranulation induced by allergic or hypersensitivity reactions.

B. Counteracting the anaphylactic reaction with epinephrine is an important part of the treatment regimen for anaphylaxis. However, airway and breathing should be the first priority of care.

C. The patient is likely experiencing an anaphylactic reaction to a bee sting. Therefore, initial management should be to ensure airway patency and adequate oxygenation. The patient's SpO_2 should be kept greater than 90%.

D. Obtaining intravenous access for medication administration is important; however, maintaining a patent airway and performing the patient's breathing assessment is the priority.

Category: Psychosocial and Medical Emergencies/Medical/Allergic reactions and anaphylaxis

Nursing Process: Intervention

References

Aribas, A., Akilli, H., Aribas, F. Z., Kayrak, M., & Turan, Y. (2013). Acute myocardial infarction triggered by bee sting. *Emergency Medicine Australasia, 25*(3), 282–283. https://doi.org/10.1111/1742-6723.12069

Calder. S. A. (2013). Shock. In B. B. Hammond & P. G. Zimmermann (Eds.), *Sheehy's manual of emergency care* (7th ed., pp. 213–221). St. Louis, MO: Elsevier Mosby.

Sedlak, S. K. (2013). Bite and sting emergencies. In B. B. Hammond & P. G. Zimmermann (Eds.), *Sheehy's manual of emergency care* (7th ed., pp. 345–352). St. Louis, MO: Elsevier Mosby.

---

84. A patient presents to the emergency department complaining of a red rash covering their face, chest, and back. The emergency nurse recognizes the patient, who was treated several days earlier for an ear infection. The emergency nurse anticipates that the cause of the patient's rash is which of the following?

A. Allergic reaction to the prescribed antibiotics
B. Impetigo
C. Scabies
D. Shingles (herpes zoster)

Rationale

A. A rash may occur as a side effect or as an allergic reaction to antibiotics. The patient was treated for an ear infection and started on antibiotics a few days ago, so this should be considered as a possible cause of the rash. The rash usually starts within the first week of taking a new medication. It often starts as red spots that spread and merge, eventually covering large areas of the body. If the drug is stopped, the rash will typically clear within few days or weeks.

B. Impetigo is a bacterial infection, usually caused by either a streptococcus or a staphylococcus infection. It manifests as discreet pustules that crust into honey-colored lesions. Impetigo is highly contagious and requires either topical or systemic antibiotic treatment.

C. Scabies is due to infestation of mites and results in pruritic erythematous papules, vesicles, and crusted pinpoint lesions. The rash is often located in the creases of the skin.

D. Shingles is a viral infection that manifests in erythematous vesicles that rupture along the sensory nerve ganglia, most commonly along the ribs, but can occur anywhere. The vesicles will open and then crust. The patient will complain of severe itching, burning, tingling, or pain until the lesions have healed completely.

Category: Psychosocial and Medical Emergencies/Medical/Allergic reactions and anaphylaxis
Nursing Process: Analysis

Reference

Mayo Clinic. (2016). *Common skin rashes.* Retrieved from http://www.mayoclinic.org/skin-rash/sls-20077087?s=4

---

85. A mother arrives to triage with her 5-year-old son, stating that her child recently had a viral illness and now has developed a generalized nonitching rash and is bruising easily. The child's vital signs are within normal limits for age. The child is diagnosed with idiopathic thrombocytopenic purpura (ITP), and intravenous immune globulin (IVIG) has been administered. The emergency nurse can expect which of the following outcomes from the administration of the IVIG?

A. Resolution of the infection that caused ITP
B. Increase in the prothrombin time and partial prothrombin time levels
C. Rapid increase in platelet count
D. Increase in white blood cell count

Rationale

A. ITP is a decrease in platelet count (< 150,000) that may occur because of a recent viral illness, or it can be associated with vaccinations. IVIG is not given to treat the infection but has been found to increase platelet count.

B. ITP results in a decrease in the patient's platelet count (< 150,000). Prothrombin time and partial prothrombin time levels usually remain constant in the presence of thrombocytopenia. IVIG is given to increase the patient's platelet count.

C. ITP is a decrease in platelet count (< 150,000) that may occur as a result of a recent viral illness, or it can be associated with vaccinations and results in petechial rash and ecchymosis. ITP is usually self-limiting, but some patients have a more severe response requiring immunoglobulin, corticosteroids, and possibly splenectomy.

D. The presence of ITP results in a decrease in the patient's platelet count (< 150,000). White blood cell count may be elevated because of the presence of an infection; however, IVIG is given to increase the patient's platelet count.

Category (Pediatric): Psychosocial and Medical Emergencies/Medical/Blood dyscrasias
Nursing Process: Evaluation

Reference

Mecham, N. L. (2010). Pediatric emergencies. In P. K. Howard & R. A. Steinmann (Eds.), *Sheehy's emergency nursing: Principles and practice* (6th ed., pp. 630–651). St. Louis, MO: Mosby Elsevier.
Smith, D. (2010). Hematologic and oncologic emergencies. In P. K. Howard & R. A. Steinmann (Eds.), *Sheehy's emergency nursing: Principles and practice* (6th ed., pp. 554–563). St. Louis, MO: Mosby Elsevier.

---

86. Which of the following patients, each with a history of hemophilia A would have the highest priority for care by the emergency nurse?

A. Patient with bleeding gums following a tooth extraction
B. Patient who presents with an epistaxis (nosebleed)
C. Patient with severe swelling into the knee joint following a fall
D. Patient with a headache following a fall

Rationale

A. Hemophilia patients with loss of a tooth may have bleeding gums on presentation. The patient should be instructed to bite down on gauze to minimize and control the bleeding.

B. The presence of a prolonged nosebleed may be serious in a patient with hemophilia. The prolonged bleeding is related to decreased factor VIII. Direct pressure to the area of bleeding via nose-packing may be required to stop the bleeding.

C. Severe swelling into joints with decreased movement of the joint can be common after an injury to the joint space. Elevation of the extremity, immobilization, application of ice, and compression dressing will assist in decreasing swelling and bleeding into the joint.

D. A headache or a change in mental status following a fall would have the highest priority for care because of the risk for the presence of an intracranial bleed. This patient would require an emergent computed tomography scan. The presence of an intracranial bleed is often the cause of death in patients with hemophilia.

Category: Psychosocial and Medical Emergencies/Medical/Blood dyscrasias: Hemophilia
Nursing Process: Analysis

References

Carringer, C. J., & Hammond, B. B. (2013). Hematologic and immunologic emergencies. In B. B. Hammond & P. G. Zimmermann (Eds.), *Sheehy's manual of emergency care* (7th ed., pp. 245–253). St. Louis, MO: Elsevier Mosby.
Golder, D. (2013). Childhood illness. In Emergency Nurses Association (Ed.), *Emergency Nursing Pediatric Course: Provider manual* (4th ed., pp. 147–169). Des Plaines, IL: Emergency Nurses Association.
Smith, D. A. (2010). Hematologic and oncologic emergencies. In P. K. Howard & R. A. Steinmann (Eds.), *Sheehy's emergency nursing: Principles and practice* (6th ed., pp. 554– 563). St. Louis, MO: Mosby Elsevier.

---

87. A patient with a history of leukemia presents to triage with a complaint of increasing dyspnea over the past several days. The patient is pale and has multiple bruises on all their extremities. Which of the following is the most likely cause of the patient's bruising?

A. Generalized lymphadenopathy
B. Immaturity of white blood cells
C. Thrombocytopenia
D. Malignant cells within the dermis

Rationale

A. Lymphadenopathy in leukemia is caused by infiltration of cancerous blood cells. It is not directly related to the appearance of bruising.

B. Proliferation of immature white blood cells results in increased vulnerability to infection. It is not directly related to the appearance of bruising.

C. Decreased number of thrombocytes, or platelets, is a result of bone marrow depression. Without adequate platelets to activate the clotting cascade, petechiae, ecchymoses, and gingival bleeding may be present.

D. Leukemia is a malignant neoplasm arising from hematopoietic stem cells. Typically, malignant cells do not deposit within the dermis.

Category: Psychosocial and Medical Emergencies/Medical/Blood dyscrasias: Leukemia

Nursing Process: Analysis

Reference

Grossman, S. C., & Porth, C. M. (2014). Disorders of white blood cells and lymphoid tissues pages. In *Porth's pathophysiology: Concepts of altered health states* (9th ed., 688–710). Philadelphia, PA: Wolters Kluwer/Lippincott Williams & Wilkins.

---

88. The emergency nurse is providing discharge teaching to a patient with sickle cell disease. Which of the following instructions is most appropriate for this patient?

A. "Be sure to exercise vigorously."
B. "Apply ice to the painful, swollen areas to reduce swelling and discomfort."
C. "Apply moist heat to the sore areas to reduce swelling and pain."
D. "Decrease your fluid intake until you are feeling better."

Rationale

A. Rest should be encouraged to avoid triggering a sickle cell crisis. Strenuous exercise could trigger a sickle cell crisis.

B. The application of ice to an area of pain in treatment for sickle cell disease can actually worsen the patient's pain. In sickle cell disease, red blood cells (RBCs) contain abnormal hemoglobin (HbS) that precipitates into long crystals, causing RBCs to assume a sickle shape when exposed to cold temperatures, low oxygen levels, dehydration, infection, or strenuous exercise.

C. The application of heat to areas of soreness assists in reducing swelling and pain, symptoms associated with sickle cell disease and crisis. Heat promotes vasodilatation, decreasing the painful vascular occlusion caused by clumps of sickled cells.

D. Patients should be encouraged to maintain adequate hydration to avoid triggering a sickle cell crisis.

Category: Psychosocial and Medical Emergencies/Medical/Blood dyscrasias: Sickle cell crisis
Nursing Process: Intervention

References

Reddin, C., Cerrentano, E., & Tanabe, P. (2011). Sickle cell disease management in the emergency department: What every emergency nurse should know. *Journal of Emergency Nursing, 37*(4), 341–345. https://doi.org/10.1016/j.jen.2010.04.014

Smith, D. A. (2010). Hematologic and oncologic emergencies. In P. K. Howard & R. A. Steinmann (Eds.), *Sheehy's emergency nursing: Principles and practice* (6th ed., pp. 554–563). St. Louis, MO: Mosby Elsevier.

---

89. Which disease process is most commonly associated with a patient developing disseminated intravascular coagulation?

A. Cardiac tamponade
B. Renal failure
C. Intracerebral hemorrhage
D. Sepsis

Rationale

A. Cardiac tamponade may result from the clotting problems that disseminated intravascular coagulation (DIC) causes, but cardiac tamponade is not a cause of DIC.

B. Renal failure may result from a patient having DIC but is generally not a cause of DIC.

C. Intracerebral hematoma leading to hemorrhage may result from the clotting problems that DIC causes, but intracerebral hematoma is not a cause of DIC.

D. Patients who develop sepsis have a 30–50% chance of developing DIC.

Category: Psychosocial and Medical Emergencies/Medical/Disseminated intravascular coagulation (DIC)
Nursing Process: Assessment

Reference

Smith, D. A. (2010). Hematologic and oncologic emergencies. In P. K. Howard & R. A. Steinmann (Eds.), *Sheehy's emergency nursing: Principles and practice* (6th ed., pp. 554–563). St. Louis, MO: Mosby Elsevier.

---

90. A patient with renal failure, abdominal cramping, diarrhea, and a potassium level of 6.8 mEq/L is being treated in the emergency department for hyperkalemia. Tall peaked T-waves are noted on the electrocardiogram. Priority interventions, in addition to cardiac monitoring, include the administration of:

A. intravenous (IV) dextrose solution followed by regular insulin.
B. sodium polystyrene (Kayexalate) via nasogastric tube.
C. a potassium-sparing diuretic, such as spironolactone.
D. 0.9% sodium chloride IV bolus.

Rationale

A. This therapy is a temporary measure to correct hyperkalemia. Insulin facilitates the transport of glucose and potassium back into cells. Other measures may be implemented, such as administration of sodium polystyrene or hemodialysis to lower the patient's potassium level.

B. Although sodium polystyrene might be part of the treatment regimen in the presence of hyperkalemia, it would not be a priority intervention. The administration of IV dextrose solution followed by regular insulin is the priority intervention.

C. This would not be a treatment option because potassium-sparing diuretics cause the retention of potassium.

D. 0.9% sodium chloride alone will not correct the patient's elevated potassium level quickly. This patient needs to have their potassium levels quickly lowered to avoid cardiac arrest.

Category: Psychosocial and Medical Emergencies/Medical/Electrolyte/fluid balance

Nursing Process: Intervention

Reference

Marett, B. E. (2013). Metabolic emergencies. In B. B. Hammond & P. G. Zimmermann (Eds.), *Sheehy's manual of emergency care* (7th ed., pp. 303–318). St. Louis, MO: Elsevier Mosby.

---

91. Which of the following conditions caused by a decrease in both cortisol and aldosterone levels is considered a life-threatening condition?

A. Cushing's syndrome
B. Diabetes insipidus
C. Myxedema coma
D. Adrenal crisis

Rationale

A. Cushing's syndrome is the result of a prolonged exposure to glucocorticoids (either endogenous or exogenous), causing the patient to develop a cushinoid appearance. There is an increased amount of adipose tissue to the face upper back and base of the neck.

B. Diabetes insipidus is a life-threatening condition in which insufficient antidiuretic hormone (ADH) is produced by the hypothalamus, or is not released by the posterior pituitary gland. The patient will excrete large amounts of dilute urine and complain of fatigue and weight loss. Treatment is fluid replacement and ADH replacement with medications such as desmopressin acetate (DDAVP).

C. Myxedema coma is a rare, life-threatening, and serious complication of hypothyroidism that affects older patients with pulmonary or vascular disease. Patients complain of fatigue, shortness of breath, and weight gain and may experience tongue swelling. Treatment includes support of the patient's airway, breathing, and circulation (ABCs) as well as thyroid hormone replacement.

D. Adrenal crisis, also known as acute adrenal insufficiency, is a life-threatening condition caused by a decrease in cortisol and aldosterone levels. This result is sodium and water loss from both the kidneys and gastrointestinal tract, causing the patient to become hypotensive and hypovolemic. As the body loses sodium, there is an increase in potassium, leading to hyperkalemia and the development of fatal dysrhythmias. Treatment includes fluid replacement, correction of hyperkalemia, and hydrocortisone administration.

Category: Psychosocial and Medical Emergencies/Medical/Endocrine conditions

Nursing Process: Assessment

References

Marett, B. (2013). Metabolic emergencies. In B. B. Hammond & P. G. Zimmermann (Eds.), *Sheehy's manual of emergency care* (7th ed., pp. 303–317). St. Louis, MO: Elsevier Mosby.

Morey, D. M. (2010). Endocrine emergencies. In P. K. Howard & R. A. Steinmann (Eds.), *Sheehy's emergency nursing: Principles and practice* (6th ed., pp. 499–512). St. Louis, MO: Mosby Elsevier.

Wall, S. M. (2007). Endocrine emergencies. In K. S Hoyt & J. Selfridge-Thomas (Eds.), *Emergency nursing core curriculum* (6th ed., pp. 290–309). St. Louis, MO: Saunders Elsevier.

---

92. A patient is being discharged from the emergency department following evaluation for Cushing's syndrome. The patient is currently taking dexamethasone (Prednisone) for their Cushing's syndrome, but the emergency provider prescribes a different medication for the patient's joint inflammation. Which of the following instructions would the emergency nurse provide regarding the dexamethasone?

A. Continue with both medications
B. Decrease the dose to one tablet a week for 2 weeks and discontinue
C. Immediately discontinue medication
D. Discontinue with tapering doses over period of time

Rationale

A. The dexamethasone may be causing an increase in Cushing's syndrome symptoms and is probably the causative agent for the syndrome. The medication should be decreased, with a tapering dose over a period of time until discontinued.

B. Abruptly discontinuing the dexamethasone may cause acute adrenal insufficiency. The medication should be tapered, decreasing the dose over a period of time until discontinued.

C. Abruptly discontinuing the dexamethasone may cause acute adrenal crisis with the absence of the steroid.

D. Prolonged use of steroids such as dexamethasone may cause Cushing's syndrome. The medication should be discontinued with a tapering dose over a period of time. Abrupt discontinuing of the medication may cause acute adrenal insufficiency or adrenal crisis.

Category: Psychosocial and Medical Emergencies/Medical/Endocrine conditions: Adrenal
Nursing Process: Intervention

Reference

Marett, B. (2013). Metabolic emergencies. In B. B. Hammond & P. G. Zimmermann (Eds.), *Sheehy's manual of emergency care* (7th ed., pp. 303–318). St. Louis, MO: Elsevier Mosby.

---

93. Symptoms that are associated with hypoglycemia can be attributed to the release of catecholamines when blood glucose levels decrease. Which of the following symptoms would be caused by this pathophysiological response?

A. Diaphoresis
B. Pupillary constriction
C. Dry skin
D. Abdominal cramping

Rationale

A. The release of epinephrine during an episode of hypoglycemia can cause diaphoresis, anxiety, dry mouth, mydriasis (papillary dilation), and tremors. The release of epinephrine can also interfere with the manner in which the body uses the glucose that is present for the duration of these episodes.

B. The release of epinephrine is part of the "fight or flight" response, which is part of the sympathetic nervous system. Mydriasis, or papillary dilation, is part of the sympathetic response. Pupillary constriction is a parasympathetic response.

C. Although dry mouth can be part of the process of hypoglycemia, patients tend to experience diaphoresis, not dry skin, during a hypoglycemic event.

D. Hunger can be one of the autonomic responses when patients become hypoglycemic, however, abdominal cramping would most likely be associated with the parasympathetic response in an individual.

Category: Psychosocial and Medical Emergencies/Medical/Endocrine conditions: Glucose-related conditions

Nursing Process: Analysis

References

Chawla, J. (2016). Autonomic nervous system anatomy. *Medscape*. Retrieved from http://emedicine.medscape.com/article/1922943-overview#a5

Marett, B. (2013). Metabolic emergencies. In B. B. Hammond & P. G. Zimmermann (Eds.), *Sheehy's manual of emergency care* (7th ed., pp. 303–318). St. Louis, MO: Elsevier Mosby.

Morey, C. M. (2010). Endocrine emergencies. In P. K. Howard & R. A. Steinmann (Eds.), *Sheehy's emergency nursing: Principles and practice* (6th ed., pp. 499–512). St. Louis, MO: Mosby Elsevier.

---

94. A patient has been diagnosed with diabetic ketoacidosis. Laboratory values include a blood glucose level of 525 mg/dL, an arterial pH of 7.30, a potassium level of 4.8 mEq/L, and elevated levels of blood urea nitrogen, creatinine, and hematocrit. Which of the following orders written by the provider would be *most* correct in the treatment of this patient?

A. Furosemide 40 mg intravenous (IV) push
B. Sodium bicarbonate 1 amp IV bolus
C. Potassium hydrochloride 40 mEq over 1 hour
D. Regular insulin 0.15 units/kg IV bolus

Rationale

A. This patient's creatinine is already increased, which would most likely preclude the use of furosemide. The patient with diabetic ketoacidosis (DKA) is already dehydrated, which would also create a situation in which a medication to encourage dieresis would not be applicable.

B. The pH for this patient is decreased, indicating an acidotic state. However, unless the pH is dramatically low, the administration of sodium bicarbonate is not indicated. As the serum glucose lowers, the pH will return to normal. The routine use of sodium bicarbonate is discouraged because it can cause an alkalosis to occur; it also can cause a decrease in potassium and elevate the potential for the development of cerebral edema.

C. This patient's potassium level is at the high end of normal. Providing a dose of intravenous IV potassium at this time could be dangerous. It is important to watch the potassium level because it can decrease as the serum glucose level returns to a normal state as a result of the administration of fluids and insulin and the correction of the acidotic state. Potassium replacements may occur but more as maintenance rather than a bolus type of dosing.

D. This is the correct dosing of insulin for patients who have developed DKA. An IV bolus should be provided, followed by an insulin drip at 0.1 units/kg/hour. Only regular insulin should be given by IV.

Category: Psychosocial and Medical Emergencies/Medical/Endocrine conditions: Glucose-related disorders

Nursing Process: Intervention

References

Marett, B. (2013). Metabolic emergencies. In B. B. Hammond & P. G. Zimmermann (Eds.), *Sheehy's manual of emergency care* (7th ed., pp. 303–318). St. Louis, MO: Elsevier Mosby.

Morey, C. M. (2010). Endocrine emergencies. In P. K. Howard & R. A. Steinmann (Eds.), *Sheehy's emergency nursing: Principles and practice* (6th ed., pp. 499–512). St. Louis, MO: Mosby Elsevier.

---

95. An adult patient presents to the emergency department with palpitations, agitation, high fever, hot, dry skin, and exophthalmoses. Vital signs: BP 172/48 mm Hg; HR 174 beats/minute; RR 24 breaths/minute; T 40.1°C (104.3°F). The emergency nurse would anticipate orders from the provider based on which clinical condition this patient is experiencing?

A. Syndrome of inappropriate antidiuretic hormone secretion
B. Hypothyroid coma or myxedema coma
C. Acute adrenal insufficiency
D. Thyroid storm/hyperthyroid crisis

Rationale

A. Signs and symptoms of syndrome of inappropriate antidiuretic hormone secretion include headache, fatigue, and confusion with decreased level of consciousness, nausea, vomiting, and weight gain without edema.

B. Hypothyroid coma, or myxedema coma, is characterized by signs of a decreased metabolism experienced by the patient. The patient exhibits bradycardia and bradypnea, and often skin is cool and pale. Body temperatures can be as low as 35.5°C (96°F).

C. Acute adrenal insufficiency, or adrenal crisis, is a rare, life-threatening condition characterized by depletion of adrenal glucocorticoids and can be seen as a complication of Addison's disease. Patients may present with tachycardia at rest, orthostatic hypotension, and signs of severe dehydration. Classic presentation involves peaked T-waves secondary to severe hyperkalemia as a result of aldosterone deficiency.

D. Thyroid storm, or hyperthyroid crisis, is a life-threatening complication of hyperthyroidism and is due to a rapid rise in thyroid hormone, resulting in severe tachycardia (heart rates may be greater than beats/minute) and respiratory distress. Blood pressure will often exhibit a high systolic and low diastolic wide pulse pressure, and extreme agitation and short attention span may be common. Exophthalmos occurs as the eyes become more protuberant.

Category: Psychosocial and Medical Emergencies/Medical/Endocrine conditions: Thyroid

Nursing Process: Analysis

References

Marett, B. (2013). Metabolic emergencies. In B. B. Hammond & P. G. Zimmermann (Eds.), *Sheehy's manual of emergency care* (7th ed., pp. 303–318). St. Louis, MO: Elsevier Mosby.

Morey, C. M. (2010). Endocrine emergencies. In P. K. Howard & R. A. Steinmann (Eds.), *Sheehy's emergency nursing: Principles and practice* (6th ed., pp. 499–512). St. Louis, MO: Mosby Elsevier.

---

96. Which of the following questions asked by the triage nurse would provide the best information regarding possible causes of a febrile illness in a child?

A. "Has your child been in contact with anyone who is ill?"
B. "Does your child attend daycare?"
C. "Is your child up to date on immunizations?"
D. "When did your child start having a fever?"

Rationale

A. Asking about sick contacts is a valid question, but this knowledge is not as helpful in identifying possible causes of the fever. Questions regarding immunization status should always be asked when assessing a febrile patient.

B. Children in daycare do have an increased risk for contracting infections due to close contact, but this knowledge is not as helpful in identifying possible causes of the fever. Questions regarding immunization status should always be asked when assessing a febrile patient.

C. Unimmunized or underimmunized children are at an increased risk for contracting serious infections. Their immunization status should be assessed during any visit to the emergency department. Children who are up to date on their immunizations have a reduced incidence of contracting a preventable disease.

D. Knowing the onset of the fever may be helpful in identifying certain causes, but questions regarding immunization status will assist with evaluating for specific etiologies and should always be asked when assessing a febrile patient.

Category (Pediatric): Psychosocial and Medical Emergencies/Medical/Fever

Nursing Process: Assessment

References

Lazear, S. E., & Roberts, A. (2007). Medical emergencies. In K. S. Hoyt & J. Selfridge-Thomas (Eds.), *Emergency nursing core curriculum* (6th ed., pp. 483–509). St. Louis, MO: Saunders Elsevier.

Sterling, S. A., & Jones, A. E. (2015). Fever. In A. B. Wolfson & R. L. Cloutier (Eds.), *Harwood-Nuss' clinical practice of emergency medicine* (6th ed., pp. 74–79). Philadelphia, PA: Wolters Kluwer.

97. A patient presents to emergency department triage complaining of increasing shortness of breath, dysphagia, and hoarseness. The patient reports being diagnosed with HIV several years ago but has never received treatment for this condition. The emergency nurse observes numerous purple and black nodules located on the hard palate inside the patient's mouth. Based on the patient's history, the emergency nurse suspects which condition?

A. Staining from cigarette smoking
B. Dental decay
C. Kaposi's sarcoma
D. Benign lesions

Rationale

A. Tobacco use may lead to staining of teeth and fingers. However, the lesions on the hard palate are consistent with Kaposi's sarcoma (KS).

B. The lesions described are consistent with KS, not dental decay.

C. KS is a rare form of skin cancer that occurs in immunosuppressed individuals. The disease usually manifests as nodules or blotches that may be purple, red, black, or brown and may be found on the skin, mouth, gastrointestinal tract, and respiratory tract. Within the oral cavity, the hard palate is most commonly affected. Patients with KS associated with the presence of immunodeficiency or immunosuppression show a decrease in progression of KS when the immune system dysfunction is treated.

D. The description of the lesions, coupled with the patient's history and presenting illness, is consistent with KS.

Category: Psychosocial and Medical Emergencies/Medical/Immunocompromise
Nursing Process: Assessment

Reference

Kadar, S. Q. M. A., Nah, A. A. S., Yunus, M. R. M., Vivekanandan, A., & Ismail, F. (2015). Kaposi sarcoma of the tonsils and pulmonary tuberculosis secondary to HIV infection. *International Medical Journal, 22*(6), 558–559.

---

98. A patient presents to the emergency department with a productive cough, fever of 40°C (104°F), and RR 22 breaths/minute. The patient's chest radiograph reveals a right lower lobe pneumonia. Antibiotics are being administered. The patient's RR increases to 30 breaths/minute, and they become agitated and confused. The emergency nurse identifies that these signs indicate the patient is now experiencing:

A. a response to the elevated temperature.
B. life-threatening organ dysfunction.
C. an allergic reaction to the intravenous antibiotic.
D. the presence of a pulmonary embolus.

Rationale

A. A patient with an elevated temperature may have an altered mental status and increased respiratory rate, but in the presence of a known infection, the patient is at increased risk of life-threatening organ dysfunction.

B. The Sequential (sepsis-related) Organ Failure Assessment (SOFA) tool was developed to assess for signs of life-threatening organ dysfunction in a patient who has a diagnosed infection and is at risk for septic shock. This tool has been adapted to qSOFA, or the quick SOFA. The qSOFA can identify a patient at risk of life-threatening organ dysfunction based on the following: RR of 22 or greater; an altered mental status (GSC $<$ 15); and a systolic blood pressure of 100 or less. If two of these criteria are present in a patient with an infection, the risk of organ dysfunction is increased, and appropriate interventions should be rapidly initiated.

C. Generally, an allergic reaction to an antibiotic would include a rash, oral swelling, wheezing, and an increase in the patient's respiratory rate.

D. Symptoms of a pulmonary embolus include chest pain, along with shortness of breath. Pulmonary embolus does not typically result in the presence of a fever.

Category: Psychosocial and Medical Emergencies/Medical/Sepsis and septic shock

Nursing Process: Analysis

References

Buck, K. (2014). Developing an early sepsis alert program. *Journal of Nursing Care Quarterly, 29*(20), 124–132.

Doble, M. (2017). Making sense of the updated sepsis definitions. *NursingCenter.* Retrieved from http://www.nursingcenter.com/ncblog/march-2016/making-sense-of-the-updated-sepsis-definitions

Keegan, J., & Wira, C. (2014). Early identification and management of patients with severe sepsis and septic shock in the emergency department. *Emergency Medicine Clinics of North America, 32,* 759–776.

Miller, J. (2014). Surviving sepsis: A review of the latest guidelines. *Nursing, 44*(4), 24–30.

Rhoades, C., Semonin Holleran, R., Carpenter, L., & Grissom, C. (2010). Management of the critical care patient in the emergency department. In P. K. Howard & R. A. Steinmann (Eds.), *Sheehy's emergency nursing: Principles and practice* (6th ed., pp. 211–230). St. Louis, MO: Mosby Elsevier.

---

99. A patient with a history of heroin abuse arrives to the emergency department by ambulance. The patient was found lying on their left side with their head positioned on their forearm for an unknown period of time. The patient is now responsive following an appropriate dose of naloxone (Narcan) and is complaining of severe pain in their left forearm. The extremity is swollen, and skin is taut and cool to touch. The emergency nurse assesses that the patient's left radial pulse is weaker than the right radial pulse, and the patient is unable to rotate the left upper extremity. The emergency nurse anticipates that the patient is exhibiting signs and symptoms of:

A. ecchymosis.
B. upper extremity fracture.
C. rhabdomyolysis.
D. compartment syndrome.

Rationale

A. Ecchymosis is a discoloration of skin caused by blood vessel rupture, which leads to bleeding into the subcutaneous tissue.

B. Fracture occurs from excessive force placed against a bone from an outside source or from a repetitive motion injury. Signs and symptoms of a fracture include pain and swelling over the affected area. Compartment syndrome can occur as a complication of a fracture.

C. Rhabdomyolysis results when significant muscle damage has occurred and myoglobin has been released into the bloodstream. The patient is at risk for renal failure due to myoglobin clogging the renal tubules, leading to acute renal injury. Compartment syndrome may lead to rhabdomyolysis as a result of excessive force or pressure being exercised against the compartment; muscle damage and the release of myoglobin into the bloodstream follow.

D. Increased pressure within the fascial compartment can be caused by an internal hemorrhage or external event (i.e., crush injury). Lying on the limb for an extended period can result in compartment syndrome, and this has been associated with a drug overdose. Classic signs and symptoms of compartment syndrome include pallor, paresthesia, pulselessness, paralysis, pain, and pressure. Additionally, the extremity can be cool to touch.

Category: Maxillofacial, Ocular, Orthopedic, and Wound Emergencies/Orthopedic/Compartment syndrome

Nursing Process: Analysis

Reference

Halpern, J. S. (2013). Musculoskeletal trauma. In B. B. Hammond & P. G. Zimmermann (Eds.), *Sheehy's manual of emergency care* (7th ed., pp. 427–438). St. Louis, MO: Elsevier Mosby.

---

100. A patient is referred for care from an urgent care center to the emergency department for possible costochondritis. On patient assessment, the emergency nurse anticipates this patient will have which of the following findings?

A. The presence of ectopy on electrocardiogram
B. Atelectasis on chest radiograph film
C. Muffled heart sounds
D. Tenderness of the midsternal area

Rationale

A. Ectopy on electrocardiogram is not an assessment finding that is associated with the presence of costochondritis. Costochondritis is an acute, self-limiting inflammation of the costal cartilage of the rib and sternal junctions, not of the cardiac muscle.

B. Atelectasis is the complete or partial collapse of a lung. Palpation over the area of lung collapse will not result in reproducing pain. Costochondritis is an acute, self-limiting inflammation of the costal cartilage of the rib and sternal junctions, not of the lung tissue.

C. Muffled heart sounds are an assessment finding in patients who are experiencing pericardial tamponade and not costochondritis. Costochondritis is an acute, self-limiting inflammation of the costal cartilage of the rib and sternal junctions, not of the cardiac muscle.

D. Costochondritis is an acute, self-limiting inflammation of the costal cartilage of the rib and sternal junctions. Inflammation may result from physical exertion or repetitive movements. Palpation to the area results in a reproducible pain (point tenderness to palpation of chest wall). Factors that worsen or alleviate symptoms are movement and deep inspiration.

Category: Maxillofacial, Ocular, Orthopedic, and Wound Emergencies/Orthopedic/Costochondritis

Nursing Process: Assessment

Reference

Cerepani, M. J., & Ramponi, D. R. (2007). Orthopedic emergencies. In K. S. Hoyt & J. Selfridge-Thomas (Eds.), *Emergency nursing core curriculum* (6th ed., pp. 585–603). St. Louis, MO: Saunders Elsevier.

---

101. A patient arrives to the emergency department after falling out of their wheelchair, injuring their hip. The emergency nurse anticipates that the patient has fractured their hip based on which of the following assessment findings?

A. Absence of pedal pulses
B. Ligamentous instability in the lower leg
C. Misalignment of the extremity
D. Cool extremity

Rationale

A. Absence of pedal pulses is a very late sign of compartment syndrome within the leg. A patient with a hip fracture will have a flexed hip, which is adducted, internally rotated, and shortened on the affected side.

B. Ligamentous instability (which requires disruption of structures), inability to straighten the leg, and peroneal nerve and popliteal artery injury are the most common in injuries of the knee.

C. Clinical findings of a fractured hip include hip flexed, adducted, internally rotated, and shortened. These findings result in a misalignment of the extremity. The patient may also have an associated fracture of femur and the presence of a sciatic nerve injury.

D. An extremity that is cool to touch is a late sign of a decreased perfusion. If perfusion is not restored, permanent dysfunction of the extremity can occur.

Category (Geriatric): Maxillofacial, Ocular, Orthopedic, and Wound Emergencies/Orthopedic/Fractures/dislocations

Nursing Process: Assessment

Reference

Ramponi, D., & Cerepani, M. J. (2007). Orthopedic trauma. In K. S. Hoyt & J. Selfridge-Thomas (Eds.), *Emergency nursing core curriculum* (6th ed., pp. 891–928). St. Louis, MO: Saunders Elsevier.

---

102. A child presents to the emergency department with a suspected "nursemaid's" elbow. The emergency nurse is aware that the correct terminology for this type of injury is which of the following?

A. Radial head subluxation
B. Radial head fracture
C. Olecranon fracture
D. Olecranon dislocation

Rationale

A. A subluxation is a partial or incomplete dislocation. Nursemaid's elbow is defined as the subluxation of the radial head. This injury is considered a pulling injury and occurs when there is traction while the child's arm is in full extension. Children between the ages of 2 and 3 years are the most susceptible to this type of injury.

B. Radial head fracture is not associated with this type of injury. Nursemaid's elbow is a subluxation or partial dislocation injury of the radial head.

C. An olecranon fracture occurs in the bony prominence of the elbow. Nursemaid's elbow is a subluxation injury of the radial head.

D. Olecranon dislocation is a complete dislocation of the elbow. Nursemaid's elbow is a subluxation or partial dislocation of the radial head and is not associated with any fracture or other dislocation.

Category (Pediatric): Maxillofacial, Ocular, Orthopedic, and Wound Emergencies/Orthopedic/Fractures/dislocations

Nursing Process: Assessment

Reference

Ramponi, D., & Cerepani, M. J. (2007). Orthopedic trauma. In K. S. Hoyt & J. Selfridge-Thomas (Eds.), *Emergency nursing core curriculum* (6th ed., pp. 891–928). St. Louis, MO: Saunders Elsevier.

---

103. Before discharging a patient with a lower extremity fracture home with crutches, the emergency nurse is aware that the patient understands the proper use of the crutches when they demonstrate which of the following actions?

A. The patient's elbows remain at a 90-degree angle when using the handgrips.
B. The patient's elbows are slightly bent when using the handgrips.
C. The crutches are placed approximately 3 inches from either side of the patient.
D. The crutches are placed close to the body on either side of the patient.

Rationale

A. If the patient's elbows are at a 90-degree angle, the patient most likely has an incorrect technique when using the crutches. The crutches may be too close to the axilla, or the patient may be leaning forward. The elbow should be only slightly bent when using crutches.

B. The crutches should be about 1.5 inches below the patient's axilla on either side, which allows for a slight bending of the elbow when using the handgrips. The hand grips are used only to absorb the patient's weight.

C. Crutches should be placed at approximately 6 inches from either side of the patient, which allows for good body mechanics and weight distribution.

D. Crutches should be placed at approximately 6 inches from either side of the patient, which allows for good body mechanics and weight distribution

Category: Maxillofacial, Ocular, Orthopedic, and Wound Emergencies/Orthopedic/Fractures/dislocations

Nursing Process: Evaluation

Reference

Ramponi, D., & Cerepani, M. J. (2007). Orthopedic trauma. In K. S. Hoyt & J. Selfridge-Thomas (Eds.), *Emergency nursing core curriculum* (6th ed., pp. 891–928). St. Louis, MO: Saunders Elsevier.

---

104. An elderly male presents to triage complaining of stiff knees every morning, joint pain with movement, and swelling for the past several months. He has not seen his family doctor in over 10 years. The emergency nurse suspects that this patient has the symptoms of:

A. osteoporosis.
B. osteoarthritis.
C. osteomyelitis.
D. osteomalacia.

Rationale

A. Osteoporosis results from inadequate production of bone, excessive removal of bone, or a combination of both, resulting in thin bones. Populations at risk include postmenopausal women, persons who take steroids, and persons who use alcohol.

B. Also known as degenerative joint disease, osteoarthritis is the most common joint disease and results in the degeneration of the articular cartilage in joints. Patients will experience joint stiffness, pain with movement, and occasional swelling of the joint.

C. Osteomyelitis is an inflammatory disorder of bone caused by the presence of an infection. It can lead to necrosis and destruction of the bone, often resulting in amputation.

D. Osteomalacia is characterized by softening of the bone due to poor mineral content, leading to a marked deformity of weight-bearing bones, distortion of the bone structure, and possible pathologic fractures. Osteomalacia, which is caused by inadequate intake of vitamin D, is often referred to as adult rickets.

Category (Geriatric): Maxillofacial, Ocular, Orthopedic, and Wound Emergencies/Orthopedic/Inflammatory conditions

Nursing Process: Analysis

Reference

Cerepani, M. J., & Ramponi, D. (2007). Orthopedic emergencies. In K. S. Hoyt & J. Selfridge-Thomas (Eds.). *Emergency nursing core curriculum* (6th ed., pp. 585–603). St. Louis, MO: Saunders Elsevier.

---

105. A patient arrives to triage with a complaint of joint pain that began the previous day in the small joints of both hands. The joints of the fingers in both hands are swollen, red, and tender to touch. The emergency provider orders a complete blood count and erythrocyte sedimentation rate (ESR). The emergency nurse is aware that the ESR is used as a(n):

A. predictor for the severity of sepsis.
B. definitive diagnosis for the presence of rheumatoid arthritis.
C. indicator of a nonspecific inflammatory process.
D. indicator of tissue damage within the body.

Rationale

A. ESR is not used as a measurement of severity of any disease. There are more appropriate laboratory tests to use when sepsis is suspected, such as a serum lactate level.

B. ESR is not diagnostic of any diseases but may be used to support a diagnosis. If the ESR results are elevated (positive for inflammation, infection, neoplasm, or necrosis), other tests will need to be run to determine if this patient has rheumatoid arthritis.

C. ESR is a nonspecific test that detects inflammation, infection, neoplasms, or necrosis. It can be used if the patient is complaining of vague symptoms or to support a suspected diagnosis; however, it is not diagnostic for a specific disease process or disorder.

D. ESR does not indicate the degree of tissue damage that has occurred within the body. ESR is used as a nonspecific marker to determine whether inflammation, infection, neoplasm, or necrosis is present.

Category: Maxillofacial, Ocular, Orthopedic, and Wound Emergencies/Orthopedic/Inflammatory conditions

Nursing Process: Assessment

Reference

Pagana, K. D., & Pagana, T. J. (2013). *Mosby's manual of diagnostic and laboratory tests* (5th ed.). St. Louis, MO: Mosby.

---

106. A patient presents to the emergency department with lower back pain related to muscle spasms following an acute lumbosacral strain. On providing discharge instructions, the emergency nurse should instruct the patient to do which of the following?

A. Twist gently from side to side to maintain range of motion in the spine.
B. Keep the head elevated slightly and flex the knees when resting in bed.
C. Lying flat, place a small pillow under the upper back to flex the lumbar spine gently.
D. Avoid the use of ice because it will exacerbate the muscle spasms.

Rationale

A. Twisting from side to side will increase tension and pain in the lumbar-sacral area.

B. Resting with the head elevated and knees flexed will reduce the strain on the back and decrease muscle spasms. The knees should be flexed to prevent pressure on the muscles of the lower back and support structures of the spine.

C. A pillow placed under the upper back will cause strain and pain in the lumbar spine. The prone position places more strain on the back and therefore should be avoided.

D. Alternate application of cold and heat should be used to decrease low back pain and muscle spasms.

Category: Maxillofacial, Ocular, Orthopedic, and Wound Emergencies/Orthopedic/Low back pain

Nursing Process: Intervention

Reference

Cerepani, M. J., & Ramponi, D. (2007). Orthopedic emergencies. In K. S. Hoyt & J. Selfridge-Thomas (Eds.), *Emergency nursing core curriculum* (6th ed., pp. 585–603). St. Louis, MO: Saunders Elsevier.

---

107. In caring for a patient who has been diagnosed with an ankle sprain, the patient asks, "What is a grade II ankle sprain?" The most appropriate answer for the emergency nurse to provide is:

A. "A sprain involves injury to the tendon or muscle. There is a partial tear to the tendon or muscle, but the joint is still stable."
B. "A sprain involves injury to the ligaments. With a grade II sprain, there is a partial tear to the ligament, but the ankle joint is still stable."

C. "A sprain involves injury to the ligaments. There is a remarkable tear to the ligament, and the joint is not stable."
D. "A sprain involves injury to the tendon or muscle. The muscle or tendon has ruptured, and the joint is not stable."

Rationale

A. Sprains do not involve injury to the tendon or muscle. A *strain* involves injury to a tendon or muscle and, like a sprain, has three grades. A grade I strain describes stretching of muscle fibers, a grade II strain has partial tearing of the tendon or muscle, and a grade III strain is notable for rupture of the tendon or muscle.

B. A sprain involves injury to the ligaments. There are three grades of sprains. Grade I has minimal damage to the ligament, and the joint is stable. Grade II has partial tearing of the ligament, but the joint is still considered stable. Grade III has remarkable tearing to the ligament, and the joint is not stable.

C. A sprain involves injury to the ligaments. This answer describes a grade III sprain, in which there is remarkable tearing to the ligament, and the joint is not stable. Grade I has minimal damage to the ligament, and the joint is stable. Grade II has partial tearing of the ligament, but the joint is still considered stable.

D. Sprains do not involve injury to the tendon or muscle. A *strain* involves injury to a tendon or muscle and, like a sprain, has three grades. This answer describes a grade III strain, where there is notable rupture of the tendon or muscle. A grade I strain describes stretching of muscle fibers. Grade II has partial tearing of the tendon or muscle.

Category: Maxillofacial, Ocular, Orthopedic, and Wound Emergencies/Orthopedic/Strains/sprains

Nursing Process: Intervention

Reference

Halpren, J. (2013). Musculoskeletal trauma. In B. B. Hammond & P. G. Zimmermann (Eds.), *Sheehy's manual of emergency care* (7th ed., pp. 427–437). St. Louis, MO: Elsevier Mosby.

---

108. An elderly woman is admitted to the emergency department by ambulance after being found lying on the floor at home for the past 6 hours. The patient is alert and states that she tripped and fell. She did not lose consciousness, but she was unable to get up to call for help. The emergency nurse knows that the most common initial finding in the patient with possible rhabdomyolysis is the presence of:

A. pain out of proportion to the injury.
B. a petechial chest rash.
C. tea- or cola-colored urine.
D. shortness of breath at rest.

Rationale

A. Muscle pain, numbness, or changes in sensation is a classic assessment finding with rhabdomyolysis. Pain out of proportion to the injury is indicative of compartment syndrome.

B. Petechial rash found over the chest, axillae, and conjunctiva is an assessment finding of fat emboli syndrome, not rhabdomyolysis.

C. Significant muscle damage and cellular destruction release myoglobin, a muscle protein, into the bloodstream. Because myoglobin is excreted in the kidneys, the risk of acute renal failure is high. Classic assessment findings include dark red or brown urine.

D. Shortness of breath at rest is not an assessment finding of rhabdomyolysis. Shortness of breath at rest may be evident in a patient with multiple injuries.

Category (Geriatric): Maxillofacial, Ocular, Orthopedic, and Wound Emergencies/Orthopedic/Trauma

Nursing Process: Analysis

Reference

Emergency Nurses Association. (2014). Musculoskeletal trauma. In D. Gurney (Ed.), *Trauma Nursing Core Course: Provider manual* (7th ed., pp. 193–204). Des Plaines, IL: Emergency Nurses Association.

---

109. A patient presents to the emergency department complaining of pain around their Achilles tendon after walking several miles earlier in the day. The patient denies any recent injury to the ankle or foot. On reviewing the patient's current medication list, the emergency nurse identifies which of the following medications that places the patient at risk for a tendon rupture?

A. Losartan (Cozaar)
B. Levothyroxine (Synthroid)
C. Levofloxacin (Levaquin)
D. Lisinopril (Zestril)

Rationale

A. Angiotensin receptor blocker medications such as losartan are not associated with tendon rupture.

B. Levothyroxine (Synthroid), a thyroid medication, is not associated with tendon rupture.

C. Fluoroquinolones, such as ciprofloxacin (Cipro) and levofloxacin, are associated with tendon rupture.

D. Angiotensin-converting enzyme inhibitors such as lisinopril are not associated with tendon rupture.

Category: Maxillofacial, Ocular, Orthopedic, and Wound Emergencies/Orthopedic/Trauma

Nursing Process: Analysis

Reference

Halpren, J. (2013). Musculoskeletal trauma. In B. B. Hammond & P. G. Zimmermann (Eds.), *Sheehy's manual of emergency care* (7th ed., pp. 427–438). St. Louis, MO: Elsevier Mosby.

---

110. What should the emergency nurse anticipate in the care of a patient with an avulsed injury to their scalp?

A. Trimming edges of the wound that are gray or dusky in appearance
B. Preparing the wound for local injection of lidocaine with epinephrine before suturing the wound
C. Cleaning and debridement of the devitalized tissue
D. Applying wet-to-dry dressing

Rationale

A. Skin edges of the avulsed segment should be approximated and not trimmed.

B. Lidocaine with epinephrine is contraindicated in the care of avulsed skin because of the vasoconstriction action of epinephrine, which would result in the blood supply to the avulsed fragment being compromised.

C. Cleansing, irrigation, and debridement is an appropriate treatment for avulsed skin.

D. Wet-to-dry dressing is an inappropriate treatment for an avulsed injury.

Category: Maxillofacial, Ocular, Orthopedic, and Wound Emergencies/Wound/Avulsions
Nursing Process: Intervention

Reference

Herr, R. D. (2013). Wound management. In B. B. Hammond & P. G. Zimmermann (Eds.), *Sheehy's manual of emergency care* (7th ed., pp. 147–160). St. Louis, MO: Elsevier.

---

111. An emergency nurse is evaluating a wound that was irrigated with saline via a syringe and attached 18-gauge catheter. The nurse identifies that the wound has been properly irrigated when they observe which of the following?

A. There is the presence of white tissue around the wound without debris.
B. There is no obvious presence of debris.
C. There is no redness surrounding the wound.
D. The wound is no longer actively bleeding.

Rationale

A. A normal wound has signs of inflammation; white tissue may indicate deeper tissue injury.

B. The irrigation solution is meant to remove cellular debris and surface pathogens contained in wound exudates. Contaminated wounds should be irrigated until all visible debris is removed.

C. A syringe with an attached 18-gauge needle typically delivers an output pressure range of 11–31 psi, which may cause wound irritation and redness; however, the removal of bacteria outweighs the tissue trauma.

D. Low-pressure wound irrigation may result in oozing as attached bacteria and debris are removed.

Category: Maxillofacial, Ocular, Orthopedic, and Wound Emergencies/Wound/Foreign bodies
Nursing Process: Evaluation

References

Denke, N. (2010). Wound management. In P. K. Howard & R. A. Steinmann (Eds.), *Sheehy's emergency nursing: Principles and practice* (6th ed., pp. 111–126). St. Louis, MO: Mosby Elsevier.

Gabriel, A. (2015). Wound irrigation. *Medscape*. Retrieved from http://emedicine.medscape.com/article/1895071-overview

112. A dose of LET (lidocaine, epinephrine and tetracaine) gel has been applied to a child in preparation for wound closure. The emergency nurse is aware this preparation has been effective when:

A. redness is observed around wound.
B. 10 minutes have passed.
C. blanching is observed around the wound.
D. 20 minutes have passed and the child is now sleepy.

Rationale

A. LET gel has vasoconstrictive properties and results in a blanching effect of the skin, not redness.

B. LET gel should be applied for at least 15–20 minutes to allow for its properties to take effect and provide adequate anesthesia of the area.

C. LET gel has vasoconstrictive properties that result in a blanching effect of the skin, usually within 20 minutes of application. The absence of blanching indicates that there is incomplete anesthesia of the area.

D. Topical LET gel will not cause the child to become sleepy.

Category: Maxillofacial, Ocular, Orthopedic, and Wound Emergencies/Wound/Lacerations
Nursing Process: Evaluation

Reference

Herr, R. D. (2013). Wound management. In B. B. Hammond & P. G. Zimmermann (Eds.), *Sheehy's manual of emergency care* (7th ed., pp. 147–160). St. Louis, MO: Elsevier Mosby.

---

113. A patient receives sutures to repair a facial laceration. The emergency nurse provides discharge instructions to the patient. The patient acknowledges understanding of their discharge instructions when the patient states the following:

A. "I will return in 3–5 days to have the sutures removed."
B. "I will return in 6–7 days to have the sutures removed."
C. "I will return in 10–14 days to have the sutures removed."
D. "I will return in 7–10 days to have the sutures removed."

Rationale

A. Facial sutures should be removed 3–5 days after they are first placed.

B. Sutures that are placed in the scalp should be removed 6–7 days after they are first placed.

C. Sutures that have been placed over an articulating joint should be removed 10–14 days after they are first placed.

D. Sutures that are not placed on the face, on the scalp, or over an articulating joint should be removed in 7–10 days.

Category: Maxillofacial, Ocular, Orthopedic, and Wound Emergencies/Wound/Lacerations
Nursing Process: Evaluation

Reference

Ramirez, E. G. (2007). Wounds and wound management. In K. S Hoyt & J. Selfridge-Thomas (Eds.), *Emergency nursing core curriculum* (6th ed., pp. 738–759). St. Louis, MO: Saunders Elsevier.

---

114. In caring for a patient who has repeatedly been placed on BiPAP for severe respiratory distress, the emergency nurse observes the presence of a deep open wound across the bridge of the patient's nose under the mask. This wound should be documented as a:

A. stage 1 pressure injury.
B. stage 2 pressure injury.
C. stage 4 pressure injury.
D. unstageable pressure injury.

Rationale

A. The definition of a stage 1 pressure ulcer is inconsistent with the injury described. A stage 1 pressure ulcer is defined as intact skin with nonblanchable redness of a localized area, usually over a bony prominence. Darkly pigmented skin may not have visible blanching; its color may differ from the surrounding area.

B. The definition of a stage 2 pressure ulcer is inconsistent with the injury described. A stage 2 pressure ulcer is defined as partial thickness loss of dermis presenting as a shallow open ulcer with a red pink wound bed, without slough; it may also present as an intact or open/ruptured serum-filled blister.

C. Stage 4 pressure injury is defined as full thickness tissue loss with exposed bone, tendon, or muscle. The bridge of the nose lacks subcutaneous tissue.

D. An unstageable pressure injury is defined as the loss of full thickness skin and tissue, and the extent of the tissue damage cannot be determined because the area is obscured by the presence of eschar or sloughing tissue.

Category: Maxillofacial, Ocular, Orthopedic, and Wound Emergencies/Wound/Pressure ulcers
Nursing Process: Assessment

Reference

National Pressure Ulcer Advisory Panel, European Pressure Ulcer Advisory Panel and Pan Pacific Pressure Injury Alliance. (2014). *Prevention and treatment of pressure ulcers: Quick reference guide* (Emily Haesler, Ed.). Osborne Park, Perth, Australia: Cambridge Media. Retrieved from http://www.npuap.org/wp-content/uploads/2014/08/Updated-10-16-14-Quick-Reference-Guide-DIGITAL-NPUAP-EPUAP-PPPIA-16Oct2014.pdf

---

115. A patient presents to the emergency department with a canine bite to the hand. What is the emergency nurse's priority assessment?

A. The source of the bite
B. Presence of any active bleeding or exudate
C. When the bite occurred
D. Treatment of the bite prior to arrival

Rationale

A. Determining the source of the bite is not the priority assessment.

B. Active bleeding must be controlled. The presence of exudate may indicate a potential wound infection.

C. The timing of the injury is typically important to determine wound closure, but canine bites should not be closed because of the risk of infection.

D. The treatment of the injury is important to determine further wound treatment but is not the priority assessment of the wound.

Category: Maxillofacial, Ocular, Orthopedic, and Wound Emergencies/Wound/Puncture wounds

Nursing Process: Assessment

Reference

Herr, R. D. (2013). Wound management. In B. B. Hammond & P. G. Zimmermann (Eds.), *Sheehy's manual of emergency care* (7th ed., pp. 147–160). St. Louis, MO: Elsevier Mosby.

---

116. A patient presents to the triage nurse with a tooth in their hand. The patient states that they were involved in an altercation approximately 4 hours ago and that the tooth was knocked out at that time. Which of the following is the most appropriate action for the emergency nurse to take?

A. **Determine if the patient has sustained any other injuries and advise that it is likely not possible that the tooth be implanted back into the dental socket.**
B. Inspect and irrigate the dental socket with normal saline sprayed through an 18-gauge bore needle.
C. Place the tooth in milk or Save-a-Tooth solution.
D. Dispose of the tooth.

Rationale

A. Always handle an avulsed tooth by the crown to avoid any damage to the periodontal ligaments. Implantation of the tooth into the socket within 30 minutes of it being removed from the dental socket will increase the likelihood of healing and successful reimplantation. However, after 60 minutes, the dental tissue and ligaments that hold the tooth in the dental socket begin to die, limiting the chance of a successful implantation.

B. Although the irrigation will clean the socket, it will not improve the likelihood of the tooth being successfully implanted into the dental socket.

C. This action will not improve the chances of successful implanting of the tooth but may act to reassure the patient.

D. The emergency provider should exam the patient and discuss potential further options to the patient before final disposition of the tooth.

Category: Maxillofacial, Ocular, Orthopedic, and Wound Emergencies/Maxillofacial/Dental conditions

Nursing Process: Intervention

Reference

Nolan, E. G. (2010). Dental, ear, nose, throat, and facial emergencies. In P. K. Howard & R. A. Steinmann (Eds.), *Sheehy's emergency nursing: Principles and practice* (6th ed., pp. 590–601). St. Louis, MO: Mosby Elsevier.

117. A patient presents to triage with epistaxis (nosebleed). The patient is coughing and spitting blood into a towel. The patient informs the emergency nurse that they are currently taking warfarin (Coumadin). The priority intervention for this patient is to:

A. perform oropharyngeal suction.
B. administer Vitamin K (phytonadione).
C. provide supplemental oxygen.
D. apply direct pressure to the patient's nostrils.

Rationale

A. Coughing and spitting out blood can compromise the airway and is a finding that requires immediate intervention with suctioning to prevent aspiration.

B. It is unknown if the patient has an elevated international normalized ratio (INR) or even if the patient's warfarin level is within therapeutic range. Although the administration of Vitamin K may be needed, it is not the priority intervention.

C. There is no report of breathing difficulty or abnormalities. Maintaining a patent airway is the initial priority, followed by performing the patient's breathing assessment.

D. Applying direct pressure to the patient's nostrils is indicated and should be applied to the bridge of the nose; however, clearing the patient's airway is the priority intervention.

Category: Maxillofacial, Ocular, Orthopedic, and Wound Emergencies/Maxillofacial/Epistaxis

Nursing Process: Intervention

Reference

Smith, D. A. (2007). Dental, ear, nose, and throat emergencies. In K. S. Hoyt & J. Selfridge-Thomas (Eds.), *Emergency nursing core curriculum* (6th ed., pp. 249–289). St. Louis, MO: Saunders Elsevier.

---

118. A patient arrives at the emergency department in full cervical spine precautions following an all-terrain vehicle collision. Initial assessment reveals the presence of rhinorrhea and otorrhea, which tests positive for the presence of glucose. The emergency nurse anticipates that the patient has sustained which type of fracture?

A. Depressed skull fracture
B. Le Fort I fracture
C. Mandibular fracture
D. Cribriform plate fracture

Rationale

A. A depressed skull fracture extends through the skull with pieces of bone depressed toward the brain. Leakage of cerebral spinal fluid (CSF) is found in basilar skull fractures or fractures of the ethmoid bone, which includes the cribriform plate.

B. A Le Fort I fracture is a transverse maxillary fracture characterized by independent movement of the maxilla from the face. Swelling and malocclusion are also common findings. Leakage of CSF is not a common finding with a Le Fort I fracture.

C. The mandible is the lower portion of the jaw bone. A fracture of the mandible is identified by the inability of the patient to open their mouth, also referred to as trismus, and malocclusion of the teeth. Leakage of CSF does not occur with a mandible fracture.

D. Fracture of the cribriform plate, part of ethmoid bone, results in leakage of CSF from the nose and/or ears. CSF will test positive for glucose and produce a halo effect, described as an appearance of rings when the CSF is placed on white paper.

Category: Maxillofacial, Ocular, Orthopedic, and Wound Emergencies/Maxillofacial//Trauma

Nursing Process: Analysis

References

Gisness, C. M. (2010). Maxillofacial trauma. In P. K. Howard, & R. A. Steinmann (Eds.), *Sheehy's emergency nursing: Principles and practice* (6th ed., pp. 355–363). St. Louis, MO: Mosby.

McLaughlin, J. C. (2014). Brain, cranial, and maxillofacial trauma. In D. Gurney (Ed.), *Trauma Nursing Core Course: Provider manual* (7th ed., pp. 105–122). Des Plaines, IL: Emergency Nurses Association.

---

119. A child arrives to the emergency department by emergency medical services, who report that the patient was tackled while playing football and is now complaining of difficulty breathing. Patient assessment reveals swelling and ecchymosis of the neck, subcutaneous emphysema, inspiratory stridor, and a hoarse voice. The emergency nurse anticipates this patient has sustained a:

A. cardiac tamponade.
B. tension pneumothorax.
C. fractured larynx.
D. pulmonary contusion.

Rationale

A. Cardiac tamponade is characterized by hypotension, muffled heart sounds, and distended neck veins, also referred to as Beck's triad. This patient's assessment findings are not specific to the presence of cardiac tamponade.

B. Common symptoms associated with a tension pneumothorax are anxiety, respiratory distress, distended neck veins, and very diminished or absent breath sounds on the affected side. The patient's assessment findings are not consistent with tension pneumothorax.

C. Blunt force trauma to the neck may cause the larynx to fracture. Presenting symptoms such as hoarseness, stridor, and subcutaneous emphysema may progress to the inability of the patient to maintain an adequate airway. This patient's assessment findings are consistent with blunt force neck trauma.

D. Although a pulmonary contusion may result in dyspnea and may require airway intervention, the patient's assessment findings are more consistent with the presence of blunt force neck trauma.

Category (Pediatric): Maxillofacial, Ocular, Orthopedic, and Wound Emergencies/Maxillofacial/Trauma

Nursing Process: Analysis

References

Day, M. W. (2014). Thoracic and neck trauma. In D. Gurney (Ed.), *Trauma Nursing Core Course: Provider manual* (7th ed., pp. 137–150). Des Plaines, IL: Emergency Nurses Association.

Shea, S. S. (2007). Ocular and maxillofacial trauma. In K. S. Hoyt & J. Selfridge-Thomas (Eds.), *Emergency nursing core curriculum* (6th ed., pp. 848–878). St. Louis, MO: Saunders Elsevier.

120. An adult patient weighing 65 kg presents to the emergency department with full thickness burns to the head, chest, and bilateral arms. Using the rule of nines to determine total body surface area burned, how much fluid replacement should the emergency nurse plan to administer based on the Parkland formula?

A. 5850 mL in the first 8 hours and another 5850 mL in the following 16 hours, for a total of 11,700 mL in the first 24 hours

B. 2925 mL in the first 8 hours and another 5850 mL in the following 16 hours, for a total of 8775 mL in the first 24 hours

C. 5850 mL every 8 hours, for a total of 17,550 mL in 24 hours

D. 8775 mL in the first 8 hours and another 5850 mL in the following 16 hours, for a total of 14,625 mL in 24 hours

Rationale

A. The total body surface area (TBSA) burned is 45% (9% right arm, 9% left arm, 18% chest, and 9% head). The formula for replacement of fluids is 2–4 mL × weight in kg × TBSA. 65 × 4 × 45 = 11,700 mL. Half of the fluid should be administered in the first 8 hours, and the other half is administered over the next 16 hours.

B. This is not enough fluid replacement based on TBSA burned and the patient's weight.

C. This is too much fluid replacement based on TBSA burned and the patient's weight.

D. This is too much fluid replacement based on TBSA burned and the patient's weight.

Category: Environment and Toxicology Emergencies, and Communicable Diseases/Environment/Burns
Nursing Process: Intervention

References

Ribbens, K. A., & DeVries, M. (2013). Burns. In B. B. Hammond & P. G. Zimmermann (Eds.), *Sheehy's manual of emergency care* (7th ed., pp. 453–462). St. Louis, MO: Elsevier Mosby.

Wraa, C. (2007). Burn trauma. In K. S. Hoyt & J. Selfridge-Thomas (Eds.), *Emergency nursing core curriculum* (6th ed., pp. 803–819). St. Louis, MO: Saunders Elsevier.

---

121. A 3-year-old is brought to the emergency department after having hydrofluoric acid spilled on their upper legs. In addition to extensive irrigation to decontaminate the area and prevent hypothermia, the nurse needs to monitor:

A. the patient's glucose levels.

B. the pH of the patient's skin where the exposure took place.

C. the need for ongoing pain medication administration.

D. the patient's serum calcium levels.

Rationale

A. Children are at higher risk for developing hypoglycemia; however, monitoring serum glucose levels is not specific to a hydrofluoric acid exposure.

B. Monitoring the patient's skin pH to determine the adequacy of irrigation is important; however, because the chemical involved is hydrofluoric acid, it is also necessary to monitor serum calcium levels.

C. Patient comfort is a concern for all patients and not unique to a hydrofluoric acid exposure.

D. Hydrofluoric acid exposure causes a depletion of serum calcium. The presence of hypocalcemia can result in the patient developing cardiac dysrhythmias.

Category (Pediatric): Environment and Toxicology Emergencies, and Communicable Diseases/ Environment/Burns

Nursing Process: Analysis

Reference

Provins-Churbock, C. (2014). Surface and burn trauma. In D. Gurney (Ed.), *Trauma Nursing Core Course: Provider manual* (7th ed., pp. 205–235). Des Plaines, IL: Emergency Nurses Association.

---

122. A clinical symptom highly characteristic of human scabies is:

A. macular red lesions and vesicular lesions that do not cross the midline.
B. vesicular lesions on the extremities.
C. ring-shaped lesions with central clearing.
D. nocturnal pruritis.

Rationale

A. Macular and vesicular lesions that do not cross the midline are common with herpes zoster. These lesions are not seen in the presence of scabies.

B. Vesicular lesions are not consistent with the presence of scabies.

C. Ring-shaped lesions are a classic sign of tinea corporis. Ring-shaped lesions are not found in the presence of scabies.

D. Intense itching that is worse during the night is a hallmark sign of human scabies. This infestation is highly contagious and is spread through intimate contact or sharing of inanimate objects.

Category: Environment and Toxicology Emergencies, and Communicable Diseases/Environment/ Parasite and fungal infestations

Nursing Process: Assessment

References

Habif, T. P. (2016) Infestations and bites. In *Clinical dermatology* (6th ed., pp. 577–634). Philadelphia, PA: Elsevier.
Peard, A. S. (2007). Communicable and infectious disease emergencies. In K. S. Hoyt & J. Selfridge-Thomas (Eds.), *Emergency nursing core curriculum* (6th ed., pp. 438–482). St. Louis, MO: Saunders Elsevier.

---

123. Which form of radiation exposure is considered to have an expectant or fatal outcome?

A. Central nervous system syndrome
B. Hematopoietic (bone marrow) syndrome
C. Gastrointestinal syndrome
D. Cutaneous radiation injury

Rationale

A. Central nervous system (CNS) syndrome is equated with expectant or fatal outcomes. CNS syndrome includes symptoms such as extreme nervousness, confusion, altered level of consciousness, convulsions, and death. Onset of symptoms occurs within 5–6 hours of exposure, with death occurring within 5 days.

B. Hematopoietic syndrome results in lymphopenia, pancytopenia, sepsis, and hemorrhage but is not associated with a fatal or expectant outcome. Patients can have full recovery within a few weeks and up to 2 years following exposure.

C. Gastrointestinal syndrome is associated with nausea, vomiting, abdominal pain but is not commonly associated with death.

D. Radiation injury to the skin and tissues can occur with doses of radiation as low as 200 rads. This form of radiation exposure produces symptoms of itching, tingling, and edema but does not result in death.

Category: Environment and Toxicology Emergencies, and Communicable Diseases/Environment/Radiation exposure

Nursing Process: Analysis

References

Andress, K. (2010). Nuclear, biologic, and chemical agents of mass destruction. In P. K. Howard & R. A. Steinmann (Eds.), *Sheehy's emergency nursing: Principles and practice* (6th ed., pp. 198–210). St. Louis, MO: Mosby Elsevier.

Assid, P. A. (2014). Disaster management. In D. Gurney (Ed.), *Trauma Nursing Core Course: Provider manual* (7th ed., pp. 311–324). Des Plaines, IL: Emergency Nurses Association.

---

124. Following several hours of observation, a drowning victim is being prepared for discharge home. Which of the following statements by the parent indicates understanding of the discharge instructions?

A. "I will wake my child hourly to make sure they knows where they are."
B. "I will observe my child for any trouble breathing or confusion."
C. "I will provide plenty of liquids that will aid in recovery."
D. "I will have my child lie down with their feet elevated to help promote water drainage from the lungs."

Rationale

A. No evidence is available that shows this is beneficial. Neurological assessments at home would not be indicated unless other neurological-related conditions were present.

B. Asymptomatic patients should be closely observed for approximately 8 hours and admitted if any deterioration occurs. If vital signs, pulse oximetry, and all studies, including a chest radiograph obtained close to the end of the observation period, are normal and no clinical deterioration develops during this period, the patient may be discharged with appropriate follow-up. Clear verbal and written instructions to return to the emergency department immediately for any respiratory or other problems must be given, and the patient must be accompanied by a responsible adult.

C. No evidence is available that shows this is beneficial. Normal hydration would be encouraged, but not overhydration.

D. The Heimlich maneuver, putting arms over head, or postural drainage do not show any benefit in a drowning situation.

Category: Environment and Toxicology Emergencies, and Communicable Diseases/Environment/ Submersion injury

Nursing Process: Evaluation

Reference

Flarity, K. (2007). Environmental emergencies. In K. S. Hoyt & J. Selfridge-Thomas (Eds.), *Emergency nursing core curriculum* (6th ed., pp. 310–348). St. Louis, MO: Saunders Elsevier.

---

125. A 4-year-old is brought to the emergency department after being found locked in a car on a hot day. The patient is agitated and confused, their skin is hot to touch, and their lips are parched. The recommended intervention for this patient is to:

A. prepare to administer a Ringer's lactate solution.
B. immerse the patient in an ice water bath.
C. initiate core temperature monitoring.
D. encourage increased water intake.

Rationale

A. Ringer's lactate solution is not a recommended intervention because the liver may not be able to metabolize lactate.

B. Ice water immersion may cause shivering, which can increase oxygen consumption and can increase body temperature.

C. This patient is experiencing signs and symptoms of heat stroke. Continuous core temperature monitoring is essential during the cooling phase to prevent hypothermia.

D. In the patient experiencing heat stroke, increased water intake is not sufficient in decreasing body temperature. In addition, the agitated and confused child may not be able to tolerate oral hydration.

Category (Pediatric): Environment and Toxicology Emergencies, and Communicable Diseases/ Environment/Temperature-related emergencies

Nursing Process: Intervention

Reference

Flarity, K. (2012). Environmental emergencies. In *Emergency Nursing Pediatric Course: Provider manual* (4th ed., pp. 329–341). Des Plaines, IL: Emergency Nurses Association.

---

126. Which of the following statements made by the child's parent during a heat advisory indicates understanding of discharge instructions to prevent heat injury to their child?

A. "I can briefly leave my child inside my automobile while I run in to the market."
B. "I will provide frequent drink breaks."
C. "I can maintain my child's soccer and sports activity schedule between 11:00 a.m. and 2:00 p.m."
D. "I will keep my child dressed in dark-colored clothing."

Rationale

A. Children should never be left unattended, even briefly, inside a hot automobile. Temperatures rise rapidly, and children's bodies are not able to adequately compensate for the rapid rise in temperature.

B. Taking frequent breaks to drink fluids will help prevent the child from becoming overheated. Also, misting or wetting down with cool water will also help the child to avoid becoming overheated.

C. The sun is at its maximum intensity between 11 a.m. and 2 p.m. Vigorous activity should be scheduled for cooler parts of the day, such as in the early morning or late evening.

D. Light-colored clothing should be worn so that the sun's rays are not easily absorbed by the clothing itself.

Category (Pediatric): Environment and Toxicology Emergencies, and Communicable Diseases/ Environment/Temperature-related emergencies

Nursing Process: Evaluation

Reference

Flarity, K. (2012). Environmental emergencies. In *Emergency Nursing Pediatric Course: Provider manual* (4th ed., pp. 329–341). Des Plaines, IL: Emergency Nurses Association.

---

127. Which of the following patients must receive the series of rabies prophylaxis?

A. The patient who may or may not have been bitten by a guinea pig.
B. The patient with a bite from a pet cat.
C. The patient with a bite from a pet dog.
D. The patient who may or may not have been bitten by a bat.

Rationale

A. Rodent transmission of rabies is unusual. Bites from any animal that can be observed for 2 weeks usually do not require rabies prophylaxis.

B. Bites from any animal that can be observed for 2 weeks usually do not require rabies prophylaxis. Domestic cats have usually been vaccinated against rabies.

C. Bites from any animal that can be observed for 2 weeks usually do not require rabies prophylaxis. Domestic dogs have usually been vaccinated against rabies.

D. Bats are a common carrier of rabies. Prophylaxis is recommended following exposure to a bat.

Category: Environment and Toxicology Emergencies, and Communicable Diseases/Environment/Vector-borne illnesses: Rabies

Nursing Process: Assessment

Reference

Herr, R. D. (2013). Wound management. In B. B. Hammond & P. G. Zimmermann (Eds.), *Sheehy's manual of emergency care* (7th ed., pp. 147–160). St. Louis, MO: Elsevier Mosby.

---

128. The nurse is caring for a patient who complains of muscle weakness on the right side of their face, malaise, headache, and fatigue. The patient has a red bull's-eye-shaped rash on their leg, which presented after removing a tick. The patient's vital signs are: BP 132/76 mm Hg; HR 88 beats/minute; RR 22 breaths/minute; SpO_2 98%; T 37.0°C (98.6°F). Which of the following diagnoses should the nurse suspect?

A. Rocky Mountain spotted fever
B. Lyme disease
C. Cellulitis
D. Tularemia

Rationale

A. Fever, headache, and rash are common signs and symptoms of Rocky Mountain spotted fever. A bull's-eye rash and Bell's palsy would not be expected with this disorder.

B. The patient is presenting with classic signs and symptoms of Lyme disease. Only 25% of patients will develop a bull's-eye rash, that is characteristic of Lyme disease. Bell's palsy is also a common manifestation found in the presence of Lyme disease.

C. Cellulitis generally presents with fever and a red, swollen area on the skin.

D. Tularemia generally presents with a slow-healing ulcer where the tick bite occurred. The systemic signs and symptoms that this patient has would not be characteristic of tularemia.

Category: Environment and Toxicology Emergencies, and Communicable Diseases/Environment/Vector-borne illnesses: Tick-borne illness

Nursing Process: Assessment

References

Centers for Disease Control and Prevention. (2016). *Ticks*. Retrieved from http://www.cdc.gov/ticks/index.html

Sedlak, S. K. (2013). Bite and sting emergencies. In B. B. Hammond & P. G. Zimmermann (Eds.), *Sheehy's manual of emergency care* (7th ed., pp. 232–243). St. Louis, MO: Elsevier Mosby.

---

129. A patient presents to the emergency department after ingesting a full bottle of oxycodone (Oxycontin). Which of the following signs and symptoms is associated with an overdose of oxycodone?

A. Dilated pupils
B. Bradycardia
C. Hypertension
D. Tachypnea

Rationale

A. Patients with opioid overdoses can present with pinpoint pupils, not dilated pupils.

B. Bradycardia can be seen in opioid overdoses, along with hypotension, bradypnea, and a decrease in temperature or hypothermia.

C. Hypotension is an expected sign of opioid overdoses, and hypertension is not an expected sign of opioid overdoses.

D. Slow respirations, or bradypnea, and apnea can occur in the presence of opioid overdoses.

Category: Environment and Toxicology Emergencies, and Communicable Diseases/Toxicology/ Overdose and ingestions

Nursing Process: Assessment

Reference

Badillo, R., Hovseth, K., & Schaffer, S. (2013). Toxicologic emergencies. In B. B. Hammond & P. G. Zimmermann (Eds.), *Sheehy's manual of emergency care* (7th ed., pp. 319–332). St. Louis, MO: Elsevier Mosby.

---

130. An unaccompanied patient suddenly appears in the ambulance entry area of the emergency department. The patient is unresponsive to stimuli. Skin is pale, cool, and dry. The nurse notes bilateral pupil constriction. There are no signs of injury observed. Vital signs are: BP 84/58 mm Hg; HR 52 beats/minute; RR 6 breaths/minute; SpO_2 88%; T 35.4°C (95.7°F). Which of the following is the highest priority intervention for this patient?

A. Open the airway and provide bag-mask device respirations
B. Obtain a serum glucose level to evaluate for hypoglycemia
C. Administer 0.4 to 2 mg of naloxone (Narcan) intravenously
D. Initiate intravenous (IV) access with a large-caliber IV catheter and begin an infusion of normal saline

Rationale

A. The highest priority for this patient is to address the respiratory depression. The patient's vital signs display bradypnea with a decreased oxygen saturation and bradycardia.

B. This is an appropriate intervention for this patient but would not take priority over airway management and resuscitation.

C. It is likely that this patient is experiencing a drug overdose, and naloxone would be an appropriate early intervention. However, resuscitation (with a bag-mask ventilation) takes priority over the administration of naloxone.

D. Inserting an IV line of normal saline is an appropriate intervention, but securing a patent airway and assisting with ventilation is the priority intervention for this patient.

Category: Environment and Toxicology Emergencies, and Communicable Diseases/Toxicology/ Substance abuse

Nursing Process: Intervention

Reference

Stout-Demps, L., & Williams, D. A. (2013). Substance abuse. In B. B. Hammond & P. G. Zimmermann (Eds.), *Sheehy's manual of emergency care* (7th ed., pp. 131–137). St. Louis, MO: Elsevier Mosby.

131. The emergency nurse is preparing to admit a patient to the hospital. After asking the patient a series of alcohol screening questions, the nurse has determined that the patient drinks 6–8 alcoholic drinks every day. How long after the last drink of alcohol would the nurse expect the patient to begin demonstrating early signs and symptoms of acute alcohol withdrawal?

A. 2–3 hours
B. 4–5 hours
C. 6–8 hours
D. 12–72 hours

Rationale

A. Signs and symptoms of alcohol withdrawal do not usually present until 6 hours after the last drink was consumed

B. Signs and symptoms of alcohol withdrawal do not usually present until 6 hours after the last drink was consumed. It is possible that after 6 hours, the patient would begin exhibiting early signs and symptoms of alcohol withdrawal; however, 6–8 hours is the best answer to this question.

C. Early signs and symptoms of alcohol withdrawal often present in the first 6–8 hours after the last drink was consumed.

D. The most serious signs and symptoms of alcohol withdrawal often occur in this time period; however, early signs and symptoms may be present at 6–8 hours following consumption of the last drink.

Category: Environment and Toxicology Emergencies, and Communicable Diseases/Toxicology/ Withdrawal syndrome

Nursing Process: Analysis

Reference

Williamson, D. (2013). Alcohol abuse. In B. B. Hammond & P. G. Zimmermann (Eds.), *Sheehy's manual of emergency care* (7th ed., pp. 137–145). St. Louis, MO: Elsevier Mosby.

---

132. A patient with suspected alcohol intoxication presents to the emergency department. To prevent the onset of Wernicke-Korsakoff syndrome, the nurse should anticipate the administration of which medication to the patient?

A. Thiamine (Vitamin B1)
B. Dextrose 50%
C. Lorazepam (Ativan)
D. Magnesium

Rationale

A. Thiamine 100 mg is given to prevent Wernicke-Korsakoff syndrome, which may manifest as gait ataxia, mental confusion, confabulation, nystagmus, or ophthalmoplegia.

B. Dextrose 50% is given for hypoglycemia and is not indicated for the prevention of Wernicke-Korsakoff syndrome.

C. Lorazepam (Ativan) is given to prevent the onset or progression of signs and symptoms associated with alcohol withdrawal but is not indicated for the prevention of Wernicke-Korsakoff syndrome.

D. Hypomagnesaemia may occur in chronic alcoholism; therefore, magnesium can be given to supplement the patient. Magnesium is also the drug of choice in the presence of the cardiac dysrhythmia torsades de pointes.

Category: Environment and Toxicology Emergencies, and Communicable Diseases/Toxicology/ Withdrawal syndrome

Nursing Process: Intervention

Reference

Williamson, D. M. (2012). Alcohol abuse. In B. B. Hammond & P. G. Zimmermann (Eds.), *Sheehy's manual of emergency care* (7th ed., pp.137–145). St. Louis, MO: Elsevier Mosby.

---

133. You are assessing a patient who has arrived to the emergency department with a 2-day history of watery diarrhea, low-grade fever, loss of appetite, nausea, and abdominal tenderness. On reviewing their medication history, you find the patient just began taking pantoprazole (Protonix) for gastroesophageal reflux disease. What could be the cause of the symptoms the patient is now experiencing?

A. *Escherichia coli*
B. Norovirus
C. ***Clostridium difficile***
D. Salmonella

Rationale

A. Patients with *Escherichia coli (E. coli)* infections experience diarrhea (which may be bloody), vomiting, severe abdominal cramps, and possible low-grade fever (less than 38.5°C). *E. coli* infections are not associated with proton pump inhibitor use.

B. Patients with norovirus have symptoms similar to those for *Clostridium difficile (C. difficile)*; however, it is not associated with the recent administration of proton pump inhibitors.

C. The patient's symptoms recently began after taking pantoprazole (Protonix), a proton pump inhibitor, suggesting *C. difficile* as the cause. *C. difficile* is characterized by symptoms of watery diarrhea, fever, loss of appetite, nausea, abdominal pain/tenderness, and is associated with recent exposure to antibiotics or proton pump inhibitors, gastrointestinal surgery/manipulation, long length of stay in a healthcare setting, advanced age, or the presence of immunosuppression.

D. Patients with salmonella infections also experience diarrhea (which may be bloody), abdominal cramping, fever (almost always present), nausea, vomiting, and headaches. Salmonella infections are not associated with proton pump inhibitor use.

Category: Environment and Toxicology Emergencies, and Communicable Diseases/Communicable Diseases/*C. difficile*

Nursing Process: Analysis

References

Centers for Disease Control and Prevention. (2012). *Frequently asked questions about* clostridium difficile *for healthcare providers*. Retrieved from http://www.cdc.gov/hai/organisms/cdiff/cdiff_faqs_hcp.html

Centers for Disease Control and Prevention. (2013). *General information about norovirus*. Retrieved from http://www.cdc.gov/hai/organisms/norovirus.html

Centers for Disease Control and Prevention. (2015). E. coli (Escherichia coli): *General information*. Retrieved from http://www.cdc.gov/ecoli/general/index.html

Centers for Disease Control and Prevention. (2015). *Salmonella: Technical information*. Retrieved from http://www.cdc.gov/salmonella/general/technical.html

134. You are caring for a 15-year-old female who is being discharged after being diagnosed with infectious mononucleosis. Which of the statements made by the patient shows an understanding of the discharge instructions?

A. "I should remember to always cover my mouth when sneezing or coughing until my doctor says I'm no longer infectious."
B. "I should not shake hands or hug anyone until my doctor says I'm no longer infectious."
C. "I can't kiss my boyfriend for at least the next 2–4 weeks or until my doctor says I'm no longer infectious."
D. "I can go back to school and participate in soccer practice tomorrow."

Rationale

A. It is good infection control practice for patients to cover their mouths when sneezing or coughing. Regarding infectious mononucleosis, direct saliva contact is more likely to cause the infection to spread than contact through airborne transmission.

B. Infectious mononucleosis cannot be spread through simple body contact.

C. Infectious mononucleosis is spread through saliva. Patients with infectious mononucleosis should not kiss or share drinks, food, or personal items like toothbrushes.

D. Patients who are still infectious should not go back to school or engage in other direct contact activities until released by their primary doctor. Patients diagnosed with infectious mononucleosis are at risk for spleen and liver enlargement and should avoid any contact sports until released by doctor.

Category (Pediatric): Environment and Toxicology Emergencies, and Communicable Diseases/Communicable Diseases/Mononucleosis

Nursing Process: Evaluation

Reference

Centers for Disease Control and Prevention. (2016). *Epstein-Barr virus and infectious mononucleosis: About infectious mononucleosis*. Retrieved from http://www.cdc.gov/epstein-barr/about-mono.html

---

135. Several emergency department staff members were involved in the care of a 10-year-old trauma victim, and resuscitation efforts were not successful. Knowing this will have a significant emotional impact on staff members, it is most important that the nurse manager do which of the following?

A. Mandate that all emergency department staff attend a debriefing session within 24 hours of the event
B. Schedule a formal debriefing session within 24–72 hours of the event
C. Meet individually with the involved staff members to discuss their perception of the critical event
D. Arrange for the affected staff to care only for adult patients for the next 2–3 days

Rationale

A. Attendance at and participation in a critical incident stress management debriefing session should be voluntary.

B. Formal debriefing sessions are most effective when organized and convened within 24–72 hours of a critical incident event.

C. An important component of critical incident stress management procedures is the small group structure in which participants can discuss/vent their feelings about the event. Arrangements can be made for the appropriate follow-up for involved providers who require or request individualized counseling sessions.

D. Removing staff from the care of children will not fully address the emotional impact of the event. If not addressed, negative effects of critical events can precipitate behavioral changes in affected individuals, including posttraumatic stress disorder, generalized anxiety, depression, and personality disorders. Left untreated, these conditions may persist indefinitely. Critical incident stress management is intended to halt escalating distress, alleviate the behavioral signs of distress, and restore the individual to an acceptable level of functioning.

Category: Professional Issues/Nurse/Critical Incident Stress Management

Cognitive Level: Application

References

Healey, M. A., & Gurney, D. (2014). Psychological aspects of trauma care. In D. Gurney (Ed.), *Trauma Nursing Core Course: Provider manual* (7th ed., pp. 295–310). Des Plaines, IL: Emergency Nurses Association.

Milici, J. J. (2012). Crisis. In Emergency Nurses Association (Ed.), *Emergency Nursing Pediatric Course: Provider manual* (4th ed., pp. 359–364). Des Plaines, IL: Emergency Nurses Association.

Wuthnow, J., Elwell, S., Quillen, J. M., & Ciancaglione, N. (2016). Implementing an ED critical incident stress management team. *Journal of Emergency Nursing, 42*(6), 474–480.

---

136. The emergency department nurse recognizes that a sentinel event may require the staff directly involved in the event to complete a(n):

A. root cause analysis.
B. incident report.
C. investigation.
D. patient safety report.

Rationale

A. A root cause analysis (RCA) of the event should be prepared to allow both staff members and the organization's management to examine the event for system or process failures. The results of this proactive risk assessment will then be shared with all staff members to prevent similar incidents from occurring in the future.

B. Any sentinel event requires an incident or formal report to be filed with The Joint Commission or your institution's accreditation organization. The highest priority following the event is to complete an RCA so the incident does not reoccur and identified system failures can be corrected.

C. An investigation will only identify how the incident occurred; it does provide a corrective mechanism to prevent similar incidents from happening again in the future. A sentinel event is a threat to patient safety and may have led to permanent harm to, or death of, a patient. An RCA will ensure that a complete comprehensive analysis takes place to prevent a recurrence of a similar event.

D. A patient safety report allows facility personnel involved in a situation to anonymously report a medical event that impacted the safety of patients. The patient safety report may not contain all the needed information to complete a formal RCA.

Category: Professional Issues/System/Performance improvement

Cognitive Level: Application

Reference

The Joint Commission. (2018). Framework for conducting a root cause analysis and action plan. Retrieved from https://www.jointcommission.org/assets/1/18/RCA_framework_10.10.17.docx

---

137. Which of the following is most important to consider when developing evidence-based practice guidelines for the emergency department?

A. Findings from relevant research, combined with practitioner expertise and patient preferences
B. Findings obtained from the results of well-conducted randomized controlled trial research studies alone
C. The availability of published clinical practice guidelines to direct the change in practice
D. The availability of advanced practice nurses or nursing researchers to identify an appropriate clinical research question

Rationale

A. Evidence-based practice consists of the synthesis of the findings from the most relevant research, the experience and expertise of the practitioner, and patient preferences and values.

B. Randomized controlled trial research studies are considered the strongest level of evidence and produce new knowledge. However, the findings, although valid and rigorous, do not always translate into clinical practice. Evidence-based practice is the blending of this new knowledge with practitioner expertise and patient preferences. These blended components guide the decision-making, leading to higher quality care and improved patient outcomes.

C. The ability to apply a published clinical practice guideline to a specific emergency department may not be possible because of institutional differences such as financial resources, physical setting, patient population, or staffing mix.

D. The first step in the development of evidence-based practice guidelines is the support of a culture in which all clinicians, regardless of profession or educational preparation, are encouraged to question their current practices and explore opportunities to improve patient outcomes.

Category: Professional Issues/Nurse/Evidence-based practice

Cognitive Level: Analysis

References

Keough, V. A. Evidence based practice. (2010). In P. K. Howard & R. A. Steinmann (Eds.), *Sheehy's emergency nursing: Principles and practice* (6th ed., pp. 35–45). St. Louis, MO: Mosby.

Melnyk, B. M., & Fineout-Overholt, E. (2011). *Evidence-based practice in nursing & healthcare: A guide to best practices.* Philadelphia, PA: Lippincott, Williams & Wilkins.

---

138. A patient diagnosed with gastroesophageal reflux disease is being discharged and prescribed a proton pump inhibitor. The instructions provided by the emergency nurse should instruct the patient to take the medication at which time?

A. At bedtime
B. 20–30 minutes before a meal
C. At the first indication of stomach pain
D. 2 hours before or after bismuth subsalicylate

Rationale

A. Proton pump inhibitor (PPIs) are activated by an alkaline environment. The stomach environment overnight is typically acid, so the PPI would be ineffective.

B. PPIs are activated by an alkaline stomach environment, so they should be taken 20–30 minutes before a meal.

C. It may take several days of continuous PPI therapy for the patient to obtain relief, and up to 12 weeks of therapy may be needed to reduce the symptoms of gastroesophageal reflux disease.

D. Bismuth subsalicylate is concurrently administered with PPI therapy to eradicate the *H. pylori* bacterium. The two medications can be taken together.

Category: Professional Issues/Patient/Discharge planning

Cognitive Level: Recall

References

Adam, M., Holland, N., & Urban, C. (2017). Drugs for peptic ulcer disease. In *Pharmacology for nurses: A pathophysiologic approach* (5th ed., pp. 676–691). Boston, MA: Pearson.

Russoll, L. W. (2007). Abdominal emergencies. In K. S. Hoyt & J. Selfridge-Thomas (Eds.), *Emergency nursing core curriculum* (6th ed., pp. 159–186). St. Louis, MO: Saunders Elsevier.

---

139. While awaiting the determination of brain death for a patient who has sustained multiple traumatic injuries and is a potential organ donor, the emergency nurse should anticipate which of the following interventions to maintain organ perfusion?

A. Administer intravenous fluids

B. Administer vasoactive agents

C. Administer norepinephrine to avoid hypotension

D. Administer atropine to treat bradydysrhythmias

Rationale

A. Hypotension will occur in most donors secondary to relative hypovolemia exacerbated by reduced systemic vascular resistance. Crystalloid or colloid infusions should be titrated to achieve euvolemia. For refractory hypotension, vasopressin is the drug of choice to maintain adequate pressure and organ perfusion.

B. Brain death may result in cerebral herniation and hypertension, but this is usually self-limiting. If the MAP remains persistently high, vasoactive infusions should be stopped, and short-acting agents should be used (i.e., esmolol, or sodium nitroprusside).

C. Norepinephrine is damaging to the myocardium and is contraindicated when cardiac donation is anticipated.

D. A patient who has lost autoregulation no longer has vagal tone, and anticholinergic drugs such as atropine are ineffective in increasing heart rates. If strong chronotropic agents like isoproterenol are unsuccessful, electrical pacing is indicated to prevent circulatory compromise.

Category: Professional Issues/Patient/End-of-life issues: Organ and tissue donation

Cognitive Level: Application

Reference

Gordon, J. K., & McKinlay, J. (2012). Physiological changes after brain stem death and management of the heart-beating donor. *Continuing Education in Anaesthesia Critical Care and Pain, 12*(5), 225–229.

---

140. A patient who has sustained a self-inflicted gunshot wound is brought to the emergency department. Which of the following interventions describes the appropriate collection and handling of forensic evidence?

A. Projectiles such as bullets or BBs should be secured in a sterile plastic container using a metal instrument.
B. Place the patient's clothing in a plastic bag.
C. Place paper bags over both hands of the patient.
D. Document any personal items that have been returned to the family.

Rationale

A. Projectiles should be wrapped in gauze or gripped with rubber-tipped instruments. Handling projectiles with a bare metal instrument may alter trace evidence or ballistic markings that are used to link the projectile to a weapon.

B. Each piece of the patient's clothing should be placed in a separate paper bag. Placing the clothing in a paper bag rather than a plastic bag will allow air to circulate and prevent moisture from accumulating on the clothing, which can alter the evidence.

C. Placing paper bags over both of the patient's hands will preserve any evidence that is on the hands or under the fingernails.

D. Personal items should not be removed and given to family members or significant others without the approval of law enforcement.

Category: Professional Issues/Patient/Forensic evidence collection

Cognitive Level: Application

References

Baxter, C. S. (2007). Neurologic emergencies. In K. S. Hoyt & J. Selfridge-Thomas (Eds.), *Emergency nursing core curriculum* (6th ed., pp. 510–535). St. Louis, MO: Saunders Elsevier.

Eckes-Roper, J. (2013). Forensics. In B. B. Hammond & P. G. Zimmermann (Eds.), *Sheehy's manual of emergency care* (7th ed., pp. 49–58). St. Louis, MO: Elsevier Mosby.

Sheridan, D., Nash, K. R., & Bresee, H. (2010). Forensic nursing in the emergency department. In P. K. Howard & R. A. Steinmann (Eds.), *Sheehy's emergency nursing: Principles and practice* (6th ed., pp. 174–186). St. Louis, MO: Mosby Elsevier.

---

141. An employee from the hospital's nuclear medicine department arrives at the emergency department stating that they may have been exposed to radioactive material. The patient is pale and diaphoretic and is complaining of a sudden onset of midsternal chest pain that radiates to the jaw. The priority action for the emergency nurse is to:

A. don personal protective equipment.
B. prepare the patient to obtain a 12-lead electrocardiogram.
C. secure intravenous (IV) access and administer atropine 1 mg IV STAT.
D. accompany the patient to the decontamination shower.

Rationale

A. External irradiation exposure does not render a victim radioactive and does not pose a threat to caregivers; therefore, personal protective equipment for the caregiver is not required.

B. The patient presents with symptoms suggestive of a myocardial infarction. The radiation exposure of this patient does not pose a threat to the caregivers. The priority is to medically stabilize the patient, appropriately decontaminate, and then refer for further treatment.

C. Securing IV access is a priority; however, atropine sulfate would not be the initial drug of choice for a patient who is suspected of having a myocardial infarction.

D. An individual who has been exposed to radiation may require decontamination, however, life-saving measures should not be delayed.

Category: Professional Issues/Patient/Patient safety
Cognitive Level: Application

References

Andress, K. (2010). Nuclear, biologic, and chemical agents of mass destruction. In P. K. Howard & R. A. Steinmann (Eds.), *Sheehy's emergency nursing: Principles and practice* (6th ed., pp. 198–210). St. Louis, MO: Mosby Elsevier.
Stopford, B. M., & Colon, W. L. (2007). Weapons of mass destruction. In K. S. Hoyt & J. Selfridge-Thomas (Eds.), *Emergency nursing core curriculum* (6th ed., pp. 970–996). St. Louis, MO: Saunders Elsevier.

---

142. Hand-off communication between providers is most effective when patient information is shared using which type of communication tool?

A. Suitable for use by a care provider with a lower level of knowledge or skill
B. Adaptable to a format for an audiotaped report
C. Standardized
D. Focused solely on the patient and the plan of care

Rationale

A. It is the position of the Emergency Nurses Association that the handoff/transfer of care should only occur between caregivers of equal or higher levels of knowledge, skills, and clinical judgment.

B. The most effective handoff/transfer processes provide an opportunity for the receiving caregiver to ask questions and clarify and confirm information. An audiotaped report would not meet this requirement.

C. The Joint Commission estimates that 80% of serious medical errors occur because of miscommunication during patient handoffs/transfer and requires accredited organizations to use a standardized approach to handoff communications. Chang et al. found that the use of standardized guidelines and processes reduced errors and improved patient outcomes.

D. When possible and appropriate, patients and families should be involved in the information sharing that occurs in handoff communication.

Category: Professional Issues/Patient/Transitions of care: External handoffs

Cognitive Level: Recall

References

Chang, Y. N., Lin, L. H., Chen, W. H., Liao, H. Y., Hu, P. H., Chen, S. F., . . . Peng, Y. C. (2010). Quality control work group focusing on practical guidelines for improving safety of critically ill patient transportation in the emergency department. *Journal of Emergency Nursing, 36*(2), 140–145.

Emergency Nurses Association. (2013). *Position statement: Patient transfers and handoffs*. Des Plaines, IL: Author. Retrieved from https://www.ena.org/docs/default-source/resource-library/practice-resources/position-statements/patienthandofftransfer.pdf?sfvrsn=e2c42cb6_16

---

143. Which of the following is most likely to be related to inadequate communication?

A. **Medication errors**
B. Blood transfusion hypersensitivity reaction
C. Emergency department overcrowding
D. Improper delegation of nursing tasks

Rationale

A. Over 80% of medical errors can be attributed to inadequate communication between caregivers. Medication errors are among the more serious consequences of poor handoff communication.

B. Hypersensitivity reactions occur during a blood transfusion when antibodies in the recipient's blood react with substances in the donor's blood.

C. Emergency department (ED) overcrowding is recognized as a systemwide issue. An ineffective handoff may contribute to a delay in treatment or diagnosis and lead to a prolonged length of ED stay, but it is not the single determining factor in ED overcrowding.

D. Emergency nurses should follow the five rights of delegation when assigning tasks to other nurses or ancillary personnel. These rights include delegating the right task to the right personnel.

Category: Professional Issues/Patient/Transitions of care: Internal handoff

Nursing Process: Analysis

References

Cheung, D., Kelly, J., Beach, C., Berkely, R., Betterman, R., Broida, R., . . .White, M. (2009). Improving hand-offs in the emergency department. *Annals of Emergency Medicine, 55*(2), 171–180. https://doi.org/10.1016/j.annemergmed.2009.07.016

Emergency Nurses Association. (2013). *Position statement: Patient transfers and handoffs*. Des Plaines, IL: Author. Retrieved from https://www.ena.org/docs/default-source/resource-library/practice-resources/position-statements/patienthandofftransfer.pdf?sfvrsn=e2c42cb6_16

144. Which of the following actions would work best to propose a solution to the problem of emergency department (ED) overcrowding?

A. Petition the nursing administration to hire additional transporters to assist with patient flow
B. Serve on a hospital-wide committee to discuss patient flow
C. Participate in a strategic planning session to expand the number of telemetry beds
D. Contribute to the development of ED protocols to divert overflow patients to neighboring hospitals

Rationale

A. Hiring additional ancillary staff will not address the root of the problem, which is an ineffective hospital-wide patient flow system.

B. ED crowding is recognized as a product of ineffective patient flow that results in increased costs and compromised care. There is agreement that it is a hospital-wide and community problem, not an isolated ED issue.

C. Providing additional telemetry beds may ease the holding of cardiac patients in the ED, but the issue affects patients with noncardiac diagnoses as well. Patient boarding in the ED is a hospital-wide patient flow problem, and the solution requires an interdisciplinary team approach.

D. ED crowding is recognized as a hospital and community-wide issue that affects quality of care and access to care. Diverting patients to neighboring hospitals does little to address the root of the problem, which is an ineffective patient flow system.

Category: Professional Issues/Patient/Transitions of care: Patient boarding

Cognitive Level: Application

Reference

Emergency Nurses Association. (2017). *Position statement: Crowding, boarding, and patient throughput*. Des Plaines, IL: Author. Retrieved from https://www.ena.org/docs/default-source/resource-library/practice-resources/position-statements/crowdingboardingandpatientthroughput.pdf?sfvrsn=5fb4e79f_4

---

145. A non–English-speaking patient presents to emergency department triage. To best communicate with the patient, the triage nurse should use which of the following methods?

A. A hospital employee who speaks the patient's native language
B. A member of the patient's family who speaks English
C. A certified translator employed by the hospital
D. A picture-based communication board

Rationale

A. The use of nonprofessional interpreters increases the risk of miscommunication and misunderstanding because the provider may not know if the message has been communicated correctly. Nonprofessional interpreters may have difficulty conveying a message to the patient because of a limitation of knowledge or embarrassment.

B. Family members may have difficulty conveying a message to the patient because of a limitation of knowledge or embarrassment. Children should never be used as interpreters because of their limited ability to understand adult situations.

C. Culturally competent communication has been identified as a patient right and an essential component of the provision of safe and effective health care. Mechanisms to provide effective communication include the use of certified translators either in person or through a video or telephone interpretation service. The use of professional interpreters (in person or via telephone) has been found to increase patient satisfaction, improve adherence and outcomes, and reduce adverse events. Failure to provide such services may be interpreted as an act of discrimination under Title VI of the Civil Rights Act.

D. Picture-based communication tools are an effective means for some aspects of communication, but the use of in-person certified translators or video or telephone interpretation services is preferred as the primary means of communication.

Category: Professional Issues/Patient/Cultural considerations

Cognitive Level: Application

References

Juckett, G., & Unger, K. (2014). Appropriate use of medical interpreters. *American Family Physician, 90*(7), 476–480.

Little, R. (2012, October 4). *New Joint Commission standards for health care interpreting: Myths & truths*. Retrieved from http://blog.cyracom.com/new-joint-commission-standards-healthcare-interpreting

Ruiz-Contreras, A. (2010). Approaching diversity. In P. K. Howard & R. A. Steinmann (Eds.), *Sheehy's emergency nursing: Principles and practice* (6th ed., pp. 27–32). St. Louis, MO: Mosby Elsevier.

---

146. The registered nurse instructs the assistive personnel to reassess the patient's pain level following the administration of pain medications. Is this an appropriate task to delegate to the assistive personnel to perform?

A. Yes
B. No
C. Only if the assistive personnel has been trained in pain scales
D. Only if the assistive personnel feels comfortable doing so

Rationale

A. The registered nurse is accountable for the ongoing monitoring of the outcomes of nursing care. Administering pain medications is part of both nursing care and process. The patient's pain should be reassessed by the nurse. Elements of care may be delegated, but the nursing process itself may not be delegated to assistive personnel.

B. The registered nurse is accountable for the ongoing monitoring of the outcomes of nursing care. Administering pain medications is part of both the nursing care and process. The patient's pain should be reassessed by the registered nurse. Elements of care may be delegated, but the nursing process itself may not be delegated to unlicensed assistive personnel.

C. The registered nurse is accountable for the ongoing monitoring of the outcomes of nursing care. Administering pain medications is part of both nursing care and process. The patient's pain should be reassessed by the nurse. Elements of care may be delegated, but the nursing process itself may not be delegated to assistive personnel. It does not matter if the assistive personnel have been trained in the use of pain scales.

D. The registered nurse is accountable for the ongoing monitoring of the outcomes of nursing care. Administering pain medications is part of both nursing care and process. The patient's pain should be reassessed by the nurse. Elements of care may be delegated, but the nursing process itself may not be delegated to assistive personnel. It does not matter if the assistive personnel feel comfortable in the use of pain scales.

Category: Professional Issues/System/Delegation of tasks to assistive personnel

Cognitive Level: Application

Reference

Bonalumi, N. M., & King, D. (2007). Professionalism and leadership. In K. S. Hoyt & J. Selfridge-Thomas (Eds.), *Emergency nursing core curriculum* (6th ed., pp. 1046–1056). St. Louis, MO: Saunders Elsevier.

---

147. The JumpSTART pediatric triage for mass casualty events uses the same criteria for triage as the adult START triage, with respiratory rate, capillary refill, and mental status; however, JumpSTART triage includes which additional intervention?

A. Rescue breaths
B. Warming
C. Intravenous fluids
D. Glucose

Rationale

A. Emergency management procedures have a few variations in caring for the pediatric population, including the recognition that children have physiological differences compared with an adult patient. The pediatric triage system for mass casualty events is called JumpSTART (Simple Triage and Rapid Treatment) triage. Adult patients typically have circulatory failure before respiratory failure. In the child, respiratory failure tends to affect the child before circulatory failure. For this reason, offering rescue breaths can provide a child with the respiratory support that they need to survive.

B. Remembering to keep the child warm is important because of the availability of less fat stores to maintain body heat in the child. However, remembering to keep the child warm is not included as a component of the JumpSTART triage algorithm.

C. Children have less circulatory volume than adults; therefore, loss of fluids leading to dehydration affects children more quickly than adults. A child will need intravenous fluids to maintain their circulatory volume, however, it is not a part of the JumpSTART triage algorithm.

D. Infants and children have less glucose reserve than adults. The administration of glucose should be considered when treating the child; it is not part of the JumpSTART triage algorithm.

Category: Professional Issues/System/Disaster management

Cognitive Level: Analysis

Reference

Upton, L. A. (2012). Disaster. In *Emergency Nursing Pediatric Course: Provider manual* (4th ed., pp. 365–378). Des Plaines, IL: Emergency Nurses Association.

---

148. A patient presents to the emergency department with chest pain, but the hospital does not accept their medical insurance plan. To be compliant with the Emergency Medical Treatment and Active Labor Act, what must be a component of the medical screening exam for a patient complaining of chest pain?

A. Electrocardiogram
B. Basic laboratory studies, including a troponin level
C. Vital signs
D. Assessment by a physician or physician assistant

Rationale

A. To establish if a life-threatening condition such as a ST elevation myocardial infarction or fatal dysrhythmia is present, an electrocardiogram (ECG) should be a part of the medical screening exam on a patient complaining of chest pain.

B. Although laboratory diagnostic testing would be typical for a chest pain patient, they are not necessary to determine that a life-threatening cardiac condition exists. An ECG is an essential part of determining if the patient's chest pain is related to a cardiac condition and is necessary in any patient with a complaint of chest pain.

C. Vital signs would be a part of the medical screening exam but would not necessarily establish if a life-threatening condition existed.

D. Assessment by physician or physician assistant is necessary for the medical screening exam, but without an ECG, the physician or physician assistant would not be able to determine if a life-threatening cardiac condition existed.

Category: Professional Issues/System/Federal regulations

Cognitive Level: Application

Reference

Jagmin, M. (2007). Legal and regulatory issues. In K. S. Hoyt & J. Selfridge-Thomas (Eds.), *Emergency nursing core curriculum* (6th ed., pp. 1033–1045). St. Louis, MO: Saunders Elsevier.

---

149. An unaccompanied 16-year-old female arrives at triage seeking treatment for a sexually transmitted disease. The patient's request for treatment is:

A. permitted.
B. not permitted.
C. granted only if her parents provide consent.
D. granted only if the patient can provide documentation that she is emancipated.

Rationale

A. Minors are able to consent for treatment in specific areas, such as birth control counseling, sexually transmitted disease treatment, and substance abuse or alcohol rehabilitation, and female patients can seek care for pregnancy-related issues. Because the patient is seeking care for treatment of a sexually transmitted disease, she can consent on her own and receive care in the emergency department (ED) without a parent's consent.

B. Minors are able to consent for treatment in specific areas, such as birth control counseling, sexually transmitted disease treatment, and substance abuse or alcohol rehabilitation, and female patients can seek care for pregnancy-related issues. Because the patient is seeking care for treatment of a sexually transmitted disease, she can consent on her own and receive care in the ED without a parent's consent.

C. The patient can seek treatment alone because minors are able to consent for treatment in specific areas, such as birth control counseling, sexually transmitted disease treatment, and substance abuse or alcohol rehabilitation, and female patients can seek care for pregnancy-related issues. Because the patient is seeking care for treatment of a sexually transmitted disease, she can consent on her own and receive care in the ED without a parent's consent.

D. The patient would not need to be emancipated in this situation because minors are able to consent for treatment in specific areas, such as birth control counseling, sexually transmitted disease treatment, and substance abuse or alcohol rehabilitation, and female patients can seek care for pregnancy-related issues. Because the patient is seeking care for treatment of a sexually transmitted disease, she can consent on her own and receive care in the ED without a parent's consent.

Category (Pediatric): Professional Issues/System/Patient consent for treatment

Cognitive Level: Recall

Reference

Jagmin, M. (2007). Legal and regulatory issues. In K. S. Hoyt & J. Selfridge-Thomas (Eds.), *Emergency nursing core curriculum* (6th ed., pp. 1033–1045). St. Louis, MO: Saunders Elsevier.

---

150. There are five fundamental principles for customer service in the emergency department setting. The acronym for those five principles is AIDET, which stands for Acknowledge, Introduce, Duration, Explanation, and:

A. Trauma.
B. Treatment.
C. Time.
D. Thank You.

Rationale

A. T stands for Thank You. It is important for staff to thank the patient for choosing their emergency department (ED).

B. T stands for Thank You. It is important for staff to thank the patient for choosing their ED.

C. Although it is important to give some time expectations to the patient, that is covered under Duration. The T stands for Thank You. It is important for staff to thank the patient for choosing their ED.

D. Use of the AIDET principles by acknowledging a patient, introducing yourself, giving the patient the amount of time they may expect for what will be done, explaining procedures and diagnostic testing, and thanking the patient for choosing your ED has been proven to improve communication and increase patient satisfaction.

Category: Professional Issues/System/Performance improvement
Cognitive Level: Recall

Reference

Baker, S. (2009). *Excellence in the emergency department: How to get results*. Gulf Breeze, FL: Fire Starter.

SELF-DIAGNOSTIC PROFILE

How to Use the Self-Assessment Worksheet

1. Indicate on your answer sheet whether your answers are correct or incorrect.
2. Note the items you answered incorrectly.
3. Count the total number of items you answered incorrectly in each category.
4. Compare the total number of items you answered incorrectly in each category with the total number of items per category. This information will give you an idea of where you will need to focus your continued study.

Content Category	Questions Answered Incorrectly	Total Number of Questions Answered Incorrectly in Each Category	Total Number of Questions in Each CEN Content Category
Cardiovascular Emergencies			20
Respiratory Emergencies			16
Neurological Emergencies			16
Gastrointestinal, Genitourinary, Gynecology, and Obstetrical Emergencies			21
Psychosocial and Medical Emergencies			25
Maxillofacial, Ocular, Orthopedic, and Wound Emergencies			21
Environment and Toxicology Emergencies, and Communicable Diseases			15
Professional Issues			16

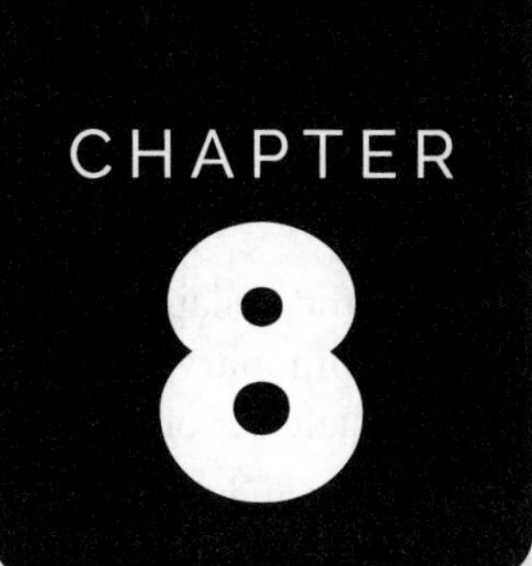

Practice Examination 3
PART 1

1. A patient presents to the emergency department with complaints of chest pain. The 12-lead electrocardiogram (ECG) reveals ST segment elevation in leads I and aVL. The initial blood pressure is 112/69 mm Hg and decreases to a systolic 60 mm Hg following a dose of nitroglycerin 0.4 mg SL. The next most appropriate intervention is to:
   A. complete a fibrinolytic check sheet.
   B. initiate a dopamine drip for blood pressure control.
   C. obtain a right-sided 12-lead ECG.
   D. administer a 0.9% sodium chloride bolus intravenously.

2. A patient presents to the triage nurse complaining of sudden onset of chest pressure that has never been experienced before. The 12-lead electrocardiogram shows ST segment elevation in leads V1–V6. This ST segment pattern is consistent with an occlusion in which coronary artery?
   A. Left anterior descending artery
   B. Circumflex artery
   C. Posterior descending artery
   D. Right coronary artery

3. A 68-year-old female presents to the emergency department with weakness, lightheadedness, and nausea. She has not felt well for the past several hours but had to complete her workday before seeking medical care. She denies the presence of chest pain or shortness of breath. The most appropriate intervention during bedside triage is to:
   A. instruct the patient to chew 325 mg aspirin.
   B. complete the triage process, including obtaining past medical history, current medications, and family history.
   C. obtain vascular access and draw necessary laboratory studies specific to cardiac biomarkers.
   D. perform a 12-lead electrocardiogram.

4. Which symptom points toward a diagnosis of abdominal aortic aneurysm?
   A. Pulsatile mass
   B. Distant heart sounds
   C. Hypertension
   D. Subcutaneous emphysema

5. A patient arrives to emergency department and collapses in front of the triage desk. The patient does not have a pulse and is not breathing. Cardiopulmonary resuscitation is initiated, and the cardiac monitor displays ventricular tachycardia. The immediate action by the emergency nurse is to:
   A. administer amiodarone (Cordarone) 150 mg intravenously.
   B. synchronize cardioversion with 200 joules.
   C. defibrillate using biphasic defibrillator with 120–200 joules.
   D. administer sodium bicarbonate 1 mEq/kg.

6. Which emergency patient would be an ideal candidate for targeted temperature management or induced hypothermia?
   A. A patient with an elevated temperature above 39.4°C (103°F) with a lactic acid level of 6.0 mmol/L
   B. A responsive emergency patient who achieved return of spontaneous circulation (ROSC) following a successful resuscitation by emergency medical services personnel
   C. An unresponsive patient who arrives at the emergency department with ROSC following cardiopulmonary arrest
   D. A patient remaining in ventricular fibrillation following a cardiopulmonary arrest event

7. Which of the following demonstrates that effective cardiopulmonary resuscitation is being delivered to the patient in cardiopulmonary arrest?
   A. Presence of waveform variation on the cardiac monitor
   B. End-tidal CO_2 20 mm Hg
   C. Arterial pH of 6.9
   D. Decreased coronary perfusion pressure

8. Parents arrive to the emergency department with their infant, who has a pulse rate of 30. The infant is limp and not breathing. The immediate action by the emergency nurse would be to:
   A. begin rescue breathing at a rate of 20 breaths per minute.
   B. initiate chest compressions at a rate of 110 per minute.
   C. defibrillate with 100 joules.
   D. administer epinephrine (Adrenalin) 0.01 mg/kg.

9. A patient presents to the emergency department with complaints of a rapid heartbeat, which is identified as an accelerated junctional rhythm. This dysrhythmia is most commonly associated with:
   A. the use of marijuana.
   B. chronic obstructive pulmonary disease.
   C. the use of digoxin.
   D. history of diabetes.

10. A patient presents to the emergency department stating that their heartbeat feels irregular. The emergency nurse assesses an irregular radial pulse. The cardiac monitor displays a cyclic irregular rhythm with an inconsistent PR segment, which becomes progressively longer until dropping a QRS complex. The cyclic pattern repeats each 4 complexes. You determine the cardiac rhythm to be:
    A. second-degree Mobitz I block.
    B. second-degree Mobitz II block.
    C. third-degree heart block.
    D. first-degree heart block.

11. A patient is diagnosed with endocarditis. Which of the following statements indicates that the patient understands a possible cause of this disease?
   A. "I never knew that this type of infection could originate from having the flu."
   B. "I cannot believe I got this disease from a tick bite."
   C. "Endocarditis may have been caused by my recent body piercings."
   D. "Endocarditis is a complication caused by my continued smoking."

12. A patient presents to the emergency department with a left ventricular assistive device (LVAD) in place. Which statement made by the patient demonstrates understanding of the LVAD function?
   A. "You will only be able to hear one number for my blood pressure."
   B. "My LVAD clicks every time it opens and closes."
   C. "I frequently have premature atrial contractions."
   D. "I know my LVAD is working if I do not hear it humming continuously."

13. A female who is 26 weeks pregnant is sent to the emergency department by her OB/GYN physician because of elevated blood pressure. The emergency nurse is aware that gestational hypertension is defined as:
   A. systolic BP above 140 mm Hg or diastolic BP above 90 mm Hg.
   B. systolic BP 10 mm Hg above baseline and elevated pulse rate.
   C. diastolic BP 20 mm Hg above baseline with a corresponding systolic BP 10 mm Hg above baseline.
   D. diastolic BP greater than 90 mm Hg with a systolic BP above 110 mm Hg.

14. The emergency department physician is inserting a 16-guage sheathed needle slowly into the left paraxiphoid area with the needle pointed downward at an approximately 30-degree angle and aimed toward the left shoulder. The trauma nurse understands that this treatment is indicated for which of the following conditions?
   A. Ascites
   B. Pneumothorax
   C. Obstructed airway
   D. Pericardial tamponade

15. A patient arrives at the emergency department complaining of midsternal chest pain that is exacerbated when lying flat and with deep inspiration. Following a 12-lead electrocardiogram, laboratory diagnostic testing, and review of the patient history, the emergency care provider diagnoses the patient with pericarditis. Based on this diagnosis, the nurse anticipates an order to administer which medication to this patient?
   A. Tissue plasminogen activator 0.9 mg/kg intravenously (IV)
   B. Nitroglycerin 0.4 mg sublingual
   C. Furosemide (Lasix) 40 mg IV
   D. Ibuprofen (Motrin) 600 mg PO

16. A patient presents to the emergency department with pain in their left lower leg. The assessment reveals the left lower leg to be pale and cool when compared with the right leg. Femoral pulses are equal, however, the popliteal pulse is significantly diminished on the left leg. The nurse suspects that the patient has which of the following?
    A. Occlusion of the femoral vein
    B. Occlusion of the femoral artery
    C. Occlusion of the popliteal artery
    D. Occlusion of the saphenous vein

17. The nurse suspects a patient of having a pericardial tamponade when the assessment findings reveal:
    A. decreased stroke volume and cardiac output.
    B. distended neck veins and tracheal deviation.
    C. subcutaneous emphysema and air in the mediastinum.
    D. poor cardiovascular response and electrocardiogram abnormalities.

18. Which assessment finding would direct the emergency nurse to suspect that the patient is in compensated shock?
    A. Marked hypotension
    B. Narrowing pulse pressure
    C. Weak, thready pulses
    D. Increased lactic acid level

19. Assessment findings of an unresponsive patient who hit a tree while snow skiing reveal hypotension, bradycardia, and warm, dry skin. The nurse suspects the presence of:
    A. distributive shock.
    B. obstructive shock.
    C. progressive shock.
    D. hypovolemic shock.

20. An infant with a history of cardiomyopathy presents to the emergency department lethargic, pale, and with weak peripheral pulses. After being diagnosed with heart failure, the appropriate medication doses of an inotrope and a diuretic are administered. The emergency nurse can anticipate that the infant will demonstrate which of the following outcomes from the administration of these medications?
    A. Urine output of 0.5 mL/kg per hour
    B. Capillary refill time of 3 seconds
    C. A bounding pulse
    D. Warm extremities

21. A child arrives at the emergency department. While running on the playground, they suddenly experienced severe dyspnea and are unable to run any further. Vital signs: BP: 110/70 mm Hg; HR 120 beats/minute; RR 42 breaths/minute; SpO_2 91% room air; T 37.7°C (99.9°F). The child has audible wheezes with visible chest retractions. The emergency nurse anticipates the child will require:
    A. racemic epinephrine nebulizer treatment.
    B. albuterol nebulizer treatment.
    C. theophylline intravenous infusion.
    D. methylprednisolone (Solu-Medrol).

22. The appropriate dose of albuterol is delivered by nebulizer to an asthmatic child. The emergency nurse would expect which of the following findings following this treatment?
    A. A decreased respiratory rate
    B. An increased peak flow reading
    C. An absence of wheezing
    D. A decrease in heart rate

23. A patient with a history of chronic obstructive pulmonary disease and hypertension arrives at the emergency department in moderate respiratory distress. The patient is alert and oriented. Vital signs: BP 192/110 mm Hg; HR 112 beats/minute; RR 36 breaths/minute; SpO_2 78% room air; T 37.2°C (99.0°F). The initial priority intervention the emergency nurse anticipates for this patient is:
    A. intravenous access.
    B. endotracheal intubation.
    C. biphasic positive airway pressure.
    D. chest radiograph.

24. What is the influenza vaccine recommendation from the Centers for Disease Control and Prevention for 50-year-old patients with stage 1 chronic obstructive pulmonary disease (COPD)?
    A. Patients with COPD should receive an influenza vaccine every year.
    B. Patients with COPD should not receive influenza vaccines because of the high risk of severe side effects.
    C. Patients under the age of 50 are not required to receive the influenza vaccine every year.
    D. Patients who live alone are not required to receive the influenza vaccine each year.

25. The presence of hypoxia in patients with chronic obstructive pulmonary disease is the result of which of the following?
    A. The inability of blood to carry oxygen
    B. Ventilation/perfusion mismatch
    C. The presence of a diminished pulmonary blood flow
    D. The inability of the body's tissues to use the oxygen being delivered to them

26. The most common nosocomial infection that is often fatal in critically ill patients is:
    A. ventilator-associated pneumonia.
    B. urinary tract infection.
    C. central line infection.
    D. pressure ulcer infection.

27. According the guidelines from the Centers for Medicare and Medicaid Services and The Joint Commission, a patient who is diagnosed with pneumonia should receive antibiotics within what time period from the time of arrival at the emergency department?
    A. Within 2 hours
    B. Within 4 hours
    C. Within 6 hours
    D. Within 10 hours

28. The emergency nurse is caring for a patient who was recently intubated. The capnography alarms and indicates a reading of 84 mm Hg. The priority assessment taken by the emergency nurse is to assess for:
   A. equipment failure.
   B. an obstructed or kinked endotracheal tube.
   C. a pneumothorax.
   D. a displaced endotracheal tube.

29. Which patient statement indicates that additional patient education is required for a patient with chronic liver disease and a pleural effusion?
   A. "My shortness of breath was caused by my cirrhosis."
   B. "I can change my diet to avoid shortness of breath."
   C. "I can use my inhaler when I feel short of breath."
   D. "If my shortness of breath gets bad enough, I may need a chest tube thoracostomy."

30. A patient experiences a fall from a horse and arrives via emergency medical services. The patient is complaining of severe right-sided chest pain with respiration. The patient is tachypneic, pulse oximetry is 90% on supplemental oxygen, and endotracheal intubation is immediately performed. Following initiation of mechanical ventilation, a decrease in the patient's blood pressure and a decrease in the oxygen saturation are observed. The emergency nurse identifies that the most likely cause of this sudden change in the patient is related to:
   A. adverse reaction to sedation medication.
   B. dislodged endotracheal tube.
   C. development of a tension pneumothorax.
   D. inadequate mechanical ventilation.

31. A hypoxic patient presents to the emergency department. The patient is immediately stabilized, and arterial blood gases are then drawn. Results are: pH 7.47; pCO_2 33 mm Hg; HCO_3 24 mEq/L. The emergency nurse recognizes these values indicate which of the following abnormalities?
   A. Respiratory acidosis
   B. Respiratory alkalosis
   C. Metabolic acidosis
   D. Metabolic alkalosis

32. When a thromboemboli forms following long periods of immobility, this condition is referred to as:
   A. endothelial injury.
   B. pulmonary vascular pressure.
   C. hypercoagulable state.
   D. venous stasis.

33. The emergency nurse is caring for a patient with pulmonary embolism. An order is expected for which of the following diagnostic tests?
   A. Spiral computed tomography (CT) scan
   B. Chest radiograph
   C. Ventilation/perfusion scan
   D. Chest CT scan without intravenous contrast

34. A patient presents to the emergency department with severe dyspnea. The arterial blood gas results are: pH 7.51; pCO_2 26 mm Hg; HCO_3 24 mEq/L. The emergency nurse interprets these results to indicate the presence of:

A. respiratory alkalosis.
B. metabolic alkalosis.
C. respiratory acidosis.
D. metabolic acidosis.

35. In a patient with acute respiratory distress syndrome, the goal of using a low tidal volume with mechanical ventilation is to:

A. wean the patient from the ventilator.
B. achieve normal blood gas values.
C. prevent volutrauma.
D. prevent ventilator–patient dyssynchrony.

36. A patient who has been stabbed in the right chest arrives to the emergency department via emergency medical services. On assessment, the emergency nurse identifies the presence of a hissing sound with inspiration. The nurse applies a dressing, taped on three sides to the stab wound site. Which of the following indicates to the emergency nurse that this treatment has been effective?

A. Decreased breath sounds
B. Increase in PaO_2 level
C. Increase in respiratory rate
D. Increase in $PaCO_2$ level

37. Which assessment test is the most specific in the diagnosis of multiple sclerosis?

A. Cognitive assessment (processing speed, complex attention, executive function)
B. Respiratory assessment (lung sounds, rate and pattern, cough)
C. Cranial nerve assessment
D. Cardiac assessment

38. A patient presents to the emergency department with complaints of a urinary tract infection. The patient's medical history indicates a diagnosis of multiple sclerosis (MS) within the previous 5 years. Which of the following clinical signs would suggest that the MS treatment the patient has been receiving with interferon has had the desired effect?

A. Urinary incontinence
B. Lower extremity spasticity
C. Resolution of visual disturbances
D. Paresthesia in bilateral feet

39. A patient previously diagnosed with Guillain–Barré syndrome presents to the emergency department with a complaint of progressive weakness and tingling of both upper and lower extremities over the past several weeks. The patient is now complaining of difficulty breathing. Vital signs: BP 130/80 mm Hg; HR 92 beats/minute; RR 28 breaths/minute; SpO_2 90% on room air. Which of the following interventions is most appropriate at this time?

A. Monitor the depth and adequacy of respirations
B. Prepare for an electromyogram
C. Administer immune globulin
D. Prepare for plasmapheresis

40. A patient presents complaining of a headache that feels like someone is squeezing their head in a grip. They say that this type of headache occurs every month. There are no associated signs and symptoms. The emergency nurse is aware that the patient is describing which type of headache?

A. Tension headache
B. Migraine headache
C. Subcortical headache
D. Cluster headache

41. The nurse is discharging a patient following treatment for a migraine headache. The patient discharge medications include sodium valproic acid (Depakote) to be used as a prophylaxis for the treatment of migraine headache. Which of the following statements by the patient indicate the need for further teaching?

A. "The doctor says my liver function tests are normal."
B. "I should avoid medications with aspirin."
C. "My boyfriend and I are not using birth control right now."
D. "If I develop abdominal pain, I will call my doctor."

42. Following a traumatic brain injury, a patient is being treated with mannitol (Osmitrol) for increased intracranial pressure secondary to brain herniation. The emergency nurse is aware that mannitol can result in which of the following abnormalities?

A. Increasing serum creatinine
B. Hyperkalemia
C. Hyponatremia
D. Metabolic alkalosis

43. A patient arrives to the emergency department and is diagnosed with a brain tumor. Interventions are provided to treat the patient's increased intracranial pressure. Which statement made by the family indicates to the emergency nurse that additional education on the patient's condition is required?

A. "Talking quietly and holding hands is helpful."
B. "Lying down to rest is important."
C. "Shaking and stiffness is an emergency."
D. "Speaking may be slow or difficult."

44. A young adult presents to the emergency department complaining of a headache, fever, petechial rash, and neck pain. Which action should the emergency personnel perform before any further contact with this patient?

A. Send a lab specimen to confirm diagnosis
B. Initiate an intravenous access
C. Don personal protective equipment
D. Initiate administration of third-generation cephalosporin and dexamethasone

45. Which patient would be most appropriate to receive levetiracetam (Keppra) for seizure prophylaxis?

A. A patient with an epidural hematoma
B. A patient with a subarachnoid hemorrhage
C. A patient with a subdural hematoma
D. A patient with a cerebral contusion

46. Which of the following children would require 24-hour observation following a tonic–clonic seizure while in the emergency department?

A. A 2-year-old child with a history of seizures who has experienced two seizures that required the administration of rectal diazepam (Valium) to control the seizure activity.
B. A 4-year-old child with no history of a seizure disorder who has had two tonic–clonic seizures that required antiepileptic medications to be administered for control of the seizure activity.
C. A 1-year-old infant who had a tonic–clonic seizure at home, was diagnosed by the emergency provider as having otitis media (middle ear infection), and required acetaminophen (Tylenol) for a fever of 40°C (104°F).
D. An 11-year-old child with a first-time seizure that self-resolved without further treatment.

47. The parent of an 18-month-old arrives to the emergency department stating that the child has had projectile vomiting for the past 24 hours. There is no history of fever or diarrhea. The parent states that their child has a ventriculoperitoneal shunt but no other medical history. The emergency nurse anticipates that the most likely cause of the child vomiting is related to which of the following?

A. Diabetic ketoacidosis
B. Gastroenteritis
C. Shunt malfunction
D. Head injury

48. A patient who sustained a low-velocity fall presents to the emergency department via emergency medical services in full cervical spine precautions. There is an obvious smell of alcohol on their breath. The patient denies any neck pain and can move all extremities. Based on the Nexus criteria, the nurse should:

A. remove the spinal immobilization and allow the patient to sit upright to protect the airway.
B. remove the spine board and keep the patient flat.
C. remove the spinal immobilization and keep the patient flat.
D. await physician exam before removing spinal immobilization

49. A 5-year-old presents with an axial loading injury after diving head first into a shallow pool. The child is unable to move their arms or legs. The radiologic studies of the cervical, thoracic, and lumbar spine are negative for any acute injury. The emergency nurse is aware that the diagnostic study that will provide a clearer diagnosis of the actual injury is:

A. a magnetic resonance imaging study of the cervical spine.
B. a computed tomography scan study.
C. a 3-dimensional ultrasound.
D. repeat radiologic study of the neck.

50. A patient arrives at the emergency department with right-sided hemiparesis and expressive aphasia. The most important information for the emergency nurse to obtain is:

A. history of recent trauma.
B. patient allergies.
C. the last time the patient was seen in their usual state of health.
D. history of recent surgery.

51. An adolescent is being discharged from the emergency department following a mild traumatic brain injury. Which of the following instructions must be included at discharge?
    A. As long as the adolescent did not experience a loss of consciousness, they may return to their usual activities.
    B. The adolescent should rest from activities such as playing video games, texting, watching TV, and doing schoolwork.
    C. As long as the adolescent is headache free, they can resume their normal activities.
    D. The only activity the adolescent should avoid is contact sports; all other activities are permitted.

52. A patient presents to the trauma bay after being kicked in the head during a game of soccer and losing vision a short time later. The provider orders a computed tomography (CT) scan. The emergency nurse anticipates that the CT scan will show an abnormality in what lobe of the brain?
    A. The occipital lobe
    B. The frontal lobe
    C. The temporal lobe
    D. The parietal lobe

53. A patient presents to the emergency department complaining of severe left lower abdominal pain and nausea and vomiting x1. The patient also denies a bowel movement in the past 4 days and has a history of diverticulitis. On exam, the abdomen is firm and rigid with rebound tenderness. Vital signs: BP 94/50 mm Hg; HR 112 beats/minute; RR 28 breaths/minute; T 38.7°C (101.6°F). The patient's symptoms are most consistent with:
    A. appendicitis.
    B. peritonitis.
    C. pancreatitis.
    D. peptic ulcer disease.

54. A patient presents to the triage desk complaining of sharp right upper quadrant abdominal pain that radiates to the right shoulder, along with nausea and vomiting. The emergency nurse suspects this patient may have which clinical condition?
    A. Infectious mononucleosis
    B. Cholecystitis
    C. Pancreatitis
    D. Appendicitis

55. A patient with a history of advanced hepatic disease presents to the emergency department. The patient's family reports that the patient has recently become more confused and now has slurred speech. The patient is diagnosed as having hepatic encephalopathy and is prescribed lactulose. The nurse can expect which of the following outcomes from the administration of this medication?
    A. Decreased clotting time
    B. Decreased liver enzymes
    C. Elevated serum potassium
    D. Decreased serum ammonia level

56. A patient presents to the emergency department complaining of cramping abdominal pain that has localized to the left lower quadrant. The patient's last bowel movement was 24 hours ago, and blood was noted in the stool. The emergency nurse suspects the patient may have:

A. acute pancreatitis.
B. diverticulitis.
C. appendicitis.
D. cholecystitis.

57. A 2-year-old child with a 48-hour history of vomiting and diarrhea is diagnosed with gastroenteritis. The child has been rehydrated in the emergency department and is currently taking fluids by mouth. Initial discharge dietary instructions should direct the child's parents to administer which of the following?

A. Small amounts of a glucose and electrolyte solution
B. Keep the child NPO for the next 24 hours
C. Provide a clear liquid diet of ice pops and apple juice
D. Resume normal eating habits

58. Which of the following statements made by a patient diagnosed with hepatitis A indicates an accurate understanding of their disease?

A. "There must be some mistake, I had the hepatitis vaccine as a baby."
B. "My partner is a recovering intravenous drug abuser. I may have gotten this after we had unprotected sex."
C. "I will be very careful to remember to wash my hands after using the bathroom and when preparing food."
D. "I must be careful from now on so that I don't get this disease again."

59. A patient presents to triage complaining of severe abdominal pain that has worsened over the past 24 hours. The patient has recently started taking infliximab (Remicade). The emergency nurse suspects that the patient's symptoms may be related to which of the following conditions?

A. Diverticulitis
B. Peptic ulcer disease
C. Pancreatitis
D. Crohn's disease

60. Which of the following abnormal laboratory values would the nurse expect to find in a patient diagnosed with acute pancreatitis?

A. Decreased C-reactive protein
B. Elevated serum lipase
C. Elevated serum glucose
D. Decreased serum calcium

61. Following a motor vehicle collision, a patient is brought to the emergency department via emergency medical services. The patient's assessment reveals the presence of lap belt restraint marks on the abdomen and absent bowel sounds, and the patient is complaining of epigastric pain. Based on these assessment findings, the emergency nurse suspects injury to which abdominal structure?

A. Liver
B. Urinary bladder
C. Duodenum
D. Stomach

62. A patient with a history of peptic ulcer disease is treated in the emergency department and discharged with a diagnosis of osteoarthritis. Discharge teaching would include instructions to take which of the following medications to manage the arthritic pain?
   A. Ibuprofen (Motrin)
   B. Acetaminophen (Tylenol)
   C. Omeprazole (Prilosec)
   D. Celecoxib (Celebrex)

63. A patient diagnosed with renal calculi will likely exhibit which signs and symptoms?
   A. Sudden onset of colicky, ipsilateral flank pain radiating to the groin
   B. Urinary frequency and urgency with fever and chills
   C. Unilateral scrotal pain
   D. Sudden onset of severe back pain described as "ripping" or "tearing"

64. The male driver of a vehicle involved in a motor vehicle collision is brought to the emergency department by ambulance. The patient complains of abdominal pain, and on secondary assessment, seatbelt marks are seen across the patient's lower abdomen, and blood is noted at the urinary meatus. Which of the following should the emergency nurse anticipate to be performed next?
   A. Application of a pelvic immobilization device
   B. Insertion of an indwelling urinary catheter
   C. Performance of a retrograde urethrogram
   D. Obtaining a urine specimen for urinalysis

65. A patient being treated for severe nausea and vomiting related to motion sickness is ordered to receive a scopolamine patch. The emergency nurse would verify the order with the emergency care provider when the patient's medical history includes:
   A. irritable bowel disease.
   B. chronic bronchitis.
   C. neurogenic bladder.
   D. glaucoma.

66. The emergency nurse is providing discharge education to a patient who has been diagnosed with pelvic inflammatory disease. Which of the following statements made by the patient leads the nurse to believe further education is needed?
   A. "I don't think I have to tell anyone else about this infection. I'll be fine once I take some pills."
   B. "I should take all of this antibiotic even if I begin feeling better."
   C. "I have an intrauterine device and understand that this may be the cause of my infection."
   D. "This infection is from bacteria that has made its way up to my fallopian tubes and ovaries."

67. A 22-year-old female presents to the emergency department stating that she may have been sexually assaulted the night before. The patient states she was at a nightclub last evening and awoke this morning in an unfamiliar place. She complains of vaginal soreness and bruising of her labia. On examination, the physician determines that forcible intercourse did occur. Which statement made by the patient would likely suggest to the nurse that the assault may have been drug facilitated?
   A. The patient experienced nausea and vomiting on awakening.
   B. The patient states she had one drink and then cannot recall the events of the evening.
   C. The patient states she is missing articles of clothing.
   D. The patient states an individual she did not know bought her a drink.

68. A 38-week-pregnant female presents to the emergency department with a sudden onset of severe abdominal cramping and dark red vaginal bleeding. The patient states the baby is not as active as usual. Vital signs: BP 80/mm Hg by palpation; HR 140 beats/minute; RR 24 breaths/minute. The nurse suspects the patient is experiencing:

A. placental abruption.
B. placenta previa.
C. active labor.
D. amniotic fluid embolism.

69. A patient who is 12 weeks pregnant presents to the emergency department complaining of lower abdominal pain and light vaginal spotting. The patient's risk for having an ectopic pregnancy increases if she relates a history of having which of the following?

A. Maternal age under 25 years
B. An incompetent cervix
C. A previous pregnancy of twins or triplets
D. Pelvic inflammatory disease

70. A 28-year-old female presents to the emergency department via ambulance following her home delivery of a full-term infant. On assessment, the patient's uterus feels boggy and soft. The presence of a boggy and soft uterus places the patient at greatest risk for:

A. postpartum infection.
B. retained products of conception.
C. eclampsia.
D. postpartum hemorrhage.

71. During neonatal resuscitation, which of the following methods will provide the emergency nurse with the most accurate evaluation of the infant's respiratory effectiveness?

A. Pulse oximetry monitoring
B. End-tidal CO_2 measurement
C. Continuous cardiac monitoring
D. Auscultation of the precordium

72. A 36-year-old female who is in the 30th week of her first pregnancy presents with complaints of a headache and swelling of the hands and face. The patient's blood pressure is 150/90 mm Hg. The emergency nurse anticipates administration of which medication?

A. Labetalol (Normodyne)
B. Furosemide (Lasix)
C. Acetaminophen (Tylenol)
D. Magnesium sulfate

73. A 30-week-pregnant female involved in a motor vehicle collision is confirmed to be in labor, and delivery of a preterm infant is anticipated. To stimulate the production of fetal surfactant and reduce the incidence of neonatal respiratory distress, the emergency nurse anticipates administration of which of the following medications to the patient?

A. Oxytocin
B. Magnesium sulfate
C. Terbutaline
D. Betamethasone

74. A young woman states that she has been sexually assaulted. She is ambulatory, alert, and oriented and has no visible injuries. Based on the Emergency Severity Index (ESI) 5-level triage system, the triage nurse assigns the patient an ESI level 1. The triage nurse understands that the rationale for assigning the high acuity level is which of the following?

A. Assessment and evidence collection both constitute a high-risk situation and require time-sensitive interventions.
B. The patient is in custody of the law enforcement officer.
C. The patient should be placed with the general emergency department patient population.
D. The patient will require at least two resources.

75. A school-age child presents to the emergency department with abdominal pain. The nurse notes that this is the third visit this month for a variety of complaints. The patient has followed up with the family physician as directed, but no official diagnosis has been made to account for the child's numerous complaints. The parent reveals the child does not like school and seldom wants to spend time with other children. The emergency nurse suspects the child may have:

A. obsessive compulsive disorder.
B. social anxiety disorder.
C. Tourette syndrome.
D. anorexia nervosa.

76. A patient arrives to triage accompanied by several friends who state the patient has become extremely irritable and impulsive recently and then can be very happy and sociable while acting "normal." The friends report that the irritable and impulsive behavior is not normal for the patient. Which of the following conditions is this patient most likely experiencing?

A. Anxiety
B. Schizophrenia
C. Bipolar disorder
D. Delirium

77. An adolescent patient arrives to triage, accompanied by their parents, after a letter was found in the patient's room revealing a desire to end their life. The letter indicates increased school stressors and a recent injury that could affect their college sport aspirations as reasons for their suicidal thoughts. Which of the following statements by the parents exhibits an understanding of the discharge instructions for the patient?

A. "We will ensure our child sees the therapist tomorrow."
B. "We will make an appointment for our child to see the therapist within 1 week."
C. "We will take time off from work for the next 2 days to monitor our child at all times."
D. "We will take our child out of school until his symptoms of suicidal ideation have resolved."

78. An emergency patient who is agitated, aggressive, and experiencing homicidal ideation is given an injection of haloperidol (Haldol). Within 30 minutes of the injection, the patient is unable to maintain their head in a midline position, resulting in a severe arching of the neck area and pulling of their neck to the left side. The patient's eyes are moving in multiple directions. The patient states that they are unable to sit still and feels like their skin is crawling. The emergency nurse anticipates the administration of benztropine (Cogentin) to treat which of the following symptoms this patient is exhibiting?

A. Hallucination
B. Tonic–clonic seizure
C. Petit mal seizure reaction
D. Torticollis

79. A patient with history of posttraumatic stress disorder and schizophrenia arrives to triage with a case manager. The patient is pacing and screaming repeatedly, "The voices are so loud. Make them stop!" and said they would like to take a gun to "blow your head off right now!" Which Emergency Severity Index (ESI) triage classifications should the emergency nurse assign to this patient?

A. ESI level 2
B. ESI level 1
C. ESI level 5
D. ESI level 3

80. An elderly female is brought to the emergency department by her daughter, who reports that her mother has been unable to sleep for the past 3 days. The daughter states that her mother has been talking to her deceased husband and has been found wandering outside her home. Which of the following is most likely the cause of this change in the patient's behavior?

A. Suicidal ideation
B. Depression
C. Delirium
D. Insomnia

81. A patient with a history of situational depression has asked the nurse about the effects of taking the herb St. John's wort. The patient has heard that it "works better" than the selective serotonin uptake inhibitor (SSRI) that they are currently prescribed. The nurse consults with the pharmacist and tells the patient:

A. "If you combine the herb with the prescription, you should reduce the dose of your SSRI after 2 weeks."
B. "It might be a good idea. The herb will enhance the effectiveness of your prescription."
C. "Yes, you may combine them. Because St. John's Wort is a natural herb, it is safe for you to take."
D. "It is not advised to take this herb with your current prescription without consulting with your provider."

82. A patient is transported to the emergency department from a local restaurant. Emergency medical services reports that the patient was awake and alert on scene and reported rapid-onset difficulty breathing and swelling in their throat and tongue. On arrival, the patient responded only to pain, and their face and tongue appear swollen. BP is 75/40 mm Hg. Their wife states that the patient is allergic to peanuts. What is the first medication the emergency nurse should anticipate administering to the patient?

A. Epinephrine (Adrenalin)
B. Fluid bolus of isotonic crystalloid solution
C. Diphenhydramine (Benadryl)
D. Famotidine (Pepcid)

83. A patient presents to the emergency department with itching, swelling around the lips and tongue, shortness of breath, and anxiety. The patient reports a history of a peanut allergy as a child but has not had a reaction in years, and denies eating any known products that contain peanuts. However, pancakes were eaten earlier in the day just before the symptoms began. What is the most likely cause of the patient's symptoms?

A. The documented peanut allergy
B. Pneumonia
C. Anxiety attack
D. Pulmonary embolism

84. A patient with hemophilia A presents to the emergency department following a mechanical fall resulting in a laceration to the knee that will require suturing. The patient has been applying pressure to the wound, and bleeding is being controlled. The emergency nurse recognizes which of the following to be the highest priority in the care of this patient?

A. Prepare to administer factor VIII
B. Prepare to administer factor IX
C. Prepare to administer desmopressin acetate
D. Prepare to suture the wound on the injured knee

85. A patient presents to the emergency department with complaint of an intermittent headache over the past several days. The patient is currently taking warfarin (Coumadin) for atrial fibrillation. Which international normalized ratio laboratory value would indicate a therapeutic dosage for this medication?

A. 1.2
B. 2.3
C. 5.0
D. 9.6

86. The emergency nurse is aware that the most common form of leukemia diagnosed in children is:

A. acute lymphocytic leukemia.
B. acute myelogenous leukemia.
C. chronic lymphocytic leukemia.
D. chronic myelogenous leukemia.

87. A patient arrives to the emergency department via ambulance with complaints of fatigue and dyspnea. The patient recently completed chemotherapy treatment for acute lymphocytic leukemia. The patient's primary survey is within normal limits. Vital signs: HR 86 beats/minute; RR 18 breaths/minute; SpO_2 94% on room air. Priority interventions for this patient would include which of the following?

A. Preparing the patient for continuous positive airway pressure ventilation
B. Placing the patient in a negative-pressure isolation room
C. Immediate triaging of the patient to the resuscitation room
D. Placing the patient in a private or isolation room

88. A male patient presents to the emergency department with a complaint related to his sickle cell disease. Which of the following complaints should the emergency nurse anticipate?

A. Anasarca
B. Hematemesis
C. Hematochezia
D. Priapism

89. Nursing care of the patient with disseminated intravascular coagulation in the emergency department should include:

A. avoiding suctioning the patient.
B. keeping the patient in a prone position.
C. securing of all invasive lines.
D. administering all medications intramuscularly.

90. A patient has been prescribed spironolactone (Aldactone) for treatment of cirrhosis. The emergency nurse acknowledges that the patient understands the discharge instructions when the patient states:

A. "I should eat more dried fruit, like apricots."
B. "I should eat an extra banana or avocado daily."
C. "I should not eat popcorn or rice cakes."
D. "I should avoid eating bananas and avocados."

91. The priority nursing care goal of a patient with syndrome of inappropriate antidiuretic hormone is directed toward which of the following?

A. Slowly correcting the patient's potassium level
B. Determining the severity of hypernatremia
C. Measuring the specific gravity of the patient's urine
D. Determining the severity of hyponatremia

92. Which of the following conditions caused by excessive amounts of antidiuretic hormone results in a patient developing dilutional hyponatremia?

A. Syndrome of inappropriate antidiuretic hormone
B. Adrenal crisis
C. Diabetes insipidus
D. Cushing's syndrome

93. A patient with a history of Addison's disease presents to the emergency department for treatment of an adrenal crisis. The emergency nurse knows that the following hormone is involved in an adrenal crisis:

A. Antidiuretic hormone
B. Cortisol
C. Follicle-stimulating hormone
D. Thyroid-stimulating hormone

94. Which of the following laboratory studies should the emergency nurse expect in a patient who presents with a diagnosis of diabetic ketoacidosis?

A. Increased pCO_2
B. Elevated creatinine
C. Elevated pH
D. Decreased blood urea nitrogen

95. Which of the following disease processes would *most* likely benefit from prophylactic therapy for deep vein thrombosis?

A. Syndrome of inappropriate antidiuretic hormone
B. Diabetic ketoacidosis
C. Hyperglycemic hyperosmolar syndrome
D. Myxedema coma

96. Several patients complaining of a fever present to triage at the same time. Which of the following patients would be the priority for bed placement?

A. The patient who had surgery 2 weeks ago
B. The patient complaining of a productive cough
C. The patient complaining of a rash
D. The patient who is receiving chemotherapy

97. The emergency nurse should discuss a certain form of health promotion with an immunocompromised patient and each of the patient's frequent visitors. The emergency nurse identifies that the teaching has been effective when the patient states which of the following?

A. "I should limit the number of visitors permitted in the room to only one at a time."
B. "All of my visitors should wash their hands when they enter my room."
C. "I need to remind all my visitors to wear a face mask when they are visiting me."
D. "All my visitors should be screened for infections before entering my room."

98. Which of the following interventions should be initiated for the treatment of a septic patient within 1 hour of presenting to the emergency department?

A. Blood cultures, antibiotics, and 30 mL/kg intravenous fluids for lactate of greater than 2 mmol/L.
B. Blood cultures, vasopressors, and central venous pressure monitoring if the mean arterial pressure is less than 65 mm Hg.
C. Blood cultures, antibiotics, and rapid administration of 30 mL/kg of crystalloids for lactate of greater than or equal to 4 mmol/L.
D. Antibiotics and vasopressors if mean arterial pressure is greater than 65 mm Hg, and lactate level greater than or equal to 4 mmol/L.

99. A patient is transferred from another facility with a fractured tibia/fibula; a splint was applied to the extremity before transfer. The patient is very tearful and is complaining of excessive pain in the injured leg. The emergency nurse is concerned the patient may be experiencing signs and symptoms of compartment syndrome. The most appropriate intervention for the emergency nurse to perform is to:

A. loosen or remove any restrictive devices on the extremity.
B. apply ice packs to the lower portion of the extremity.
C. elevate the extremity immediately above the heart level.
D. apply a tourniquet to the extremity.

100. An unrestrained driver involved in a motor vehicle collision arrives to the emergency department by ambulance. During the secondary assessment, signs and symptoms of a possible fractured femur are observed. The emergency nurse anticipates the patient will have which of the following findings?

A. Excessive hip flexion
B. Shortened length of the injured extremity
C. Hyperextension of the knee in the same extremity as the fractured femur
D. Deformity of the ankle

101. Parents and their child arrive at the emergency department. The child had jumped out of a tree and is complaining of pain in the left ankle and inability to bear weight on the foot. Skin is intact, and the patient has good distal pulses bilaterally (dorsalis pedal and posterior tibial) with no gross deformity, but swelling is present. Initial radiographs are negative for fracture. The emergency nurse suspects the child has a(n):

A. displaced fracture.
B. open fracture.
C. comminuted fracture.
D. Salter–Harris fracture.

102. The emergency nurse is evaluating a patient's understanding of discharge instructions related to gout. The nurse is aware that the patient understands the discharge instructions when the patient states:

A. "I need to limit my water intake because too much fluid can cause a gout flare-up."
B. "My hydrochlorothiazide could have contributed to this flare-up of gout."
C. "I should start the prescription for allopurinol now because it will treat the gout flare-up."
D. "I should eat more seafood to help prevent future gout flare-ups."

103. A patient presents to triage complaining of continuous left knee pain for the past month. The patient denies any history of trauma to the knee. The current pain level is 3/10, and the patient states the pain is more intense on awakening in the morning, but after being up and moving, the pain lessens. The knee will occasionally swell but is currently not swollen. The patient previously trained for marathons and continues to run at least 20 miles each week. Vital signs: BP 108/62 mm Hg; HR 54 beats/minute; RR 14 breaths/minute; SpO_2 97%; T 37°C (98.6°F). The emergency nurse anticipates the patient has:

A. rheumatoid arthritis.
B. osteoarthritis.
C. bursitis.
D. septic arthritis.

104. Following completion of a joint aspiration of the knee by the provider, the emergency nurse should perform which intervention?

A. Apply pressure to the aspiration site for at least 2 minutes
B. Place an ice pack on the aspiration site for 15 minutes
C. Place a heat pack on the aspiration site for 15 minutes
D. Elevate the extremity above the level of the heart

105. A patient presents to the emergency department following their soccer game. The patient states they were running and "rolled" their ankle on an uneven area on the field. Their left ankle is swollen and tender to touch, and the patient experiences increasing pain with weight bearing on the affected foot. On providing discharge instructions for this patient, the emergency nurse acknowledges the need for further instructions when the patient states:

A. "I need to rest my ankle, keep it elevated, ice it, and use an ACE bandage."
B. "It is okay to go back to playing soccer once the swelling is gone."
C. "I should start physical therapy and stretching exercises in about a week."
D. "It is okay for me to take acetaminophen (Tylenol) or ibuprofen (NSAID) for the pain in my ankle."

106. The best way for the emergency nurse to evaluate the effectiveness of teaching a patient with an injured their ankle to crutch walk is to have the patient:

A. teach the skill to a friend in the presence of the emergency nurse.
B. restate the crutch walking instructions.
C. teach back the procedure to the emergency nurse.
D. demonstrate crutch walking.

107. A patient presents to the emergency department with complaints of chest pain and shortness of breath and appears apprehensive and restless. The patient had been discharged the previous day following repair of a fractured femur. Vital signs: BP 132/84 mm Hg; HR 98 beats/minute; RR 22 breaths/minute; T 37.7°C (100°F). The emergency nurse anticipates the most likely explanation for the patient's symptoms is the presence of:

A. hemorrhage.
B. a pulmonary embolism.
C. deep vein thrombosis.
D. myocardial infarction.

108. A baseball player complains of severe pain to the back of their foot above the heel. The patient states they heard a popping noise while running during a recent game. There is tenderness, swelling, and difficulty pointing their toes on examination. The patient's past medical history is significant for traveler's diarrhea over the past month, which has been treated with a fluoroquinolone. The emergency nurse suspects the patient has sustained a(n):

A. ankle dislocation.
B. Achilles tendon rupture.
C. ankle sprain.
D. calcaneal fracture.

109. A patient presents to the emergency department following a motorcycle collision. Multiple abrasions are noted on the patient's left leg, hip, trunk, and arm. While preparing to provide treatment, the emergency nurse explains the goals of wound care to the patient. Which of the following is a goal of wound care?

A. Maintain function
B. Restore thermoregulation
C. Manage pain
D. Obtain homeostasis

110. A patient has undergone an incision and drainage of a large abscess under the axilla. The emergency nurse anticipates which type of further wound treatment for the area?

A. Using a wet-to-dry dressing
B. Suturing of the abscess cavity
C. Using adhesive wound glue to close the abscess cavity
D. Packing with iodinated gauze

111. The emergency nurse is aware that the priority assessment of a patient who has sustained a traumatic laceration with deep tissue injury to the upper arm is to assess which of the following?

A. Capillary refill in the affected extremity
B. Range of motion of the fingers of the affected extremity
C. Distal pulses in the extremity
D. Skin color and temperature

112. In providing discharge instructions to the mother of a toddler who just had a forehead laceration closed with 2-octyl cyanoacrylate (Dermabond), the emergency nurse identifies the mother's proper understanding of the instructions when she states which of the following?

A. "I should wash the wound area daily with soap and water."
B. "I should keep the wound area clean and dry."
C. "It is important for me to keep the wound covered every day."
D. "I must apply antibiotic ointment to the area every day."

113. The emergency nurse is caring for a patient who had been found lying on the floor for 2 days following a fall. The nurse assesses an area of purple discoloration along the patient's greater trochanter, which is boggy and warm to touch. The emergency nurse recognizes this wound to be a(n):

A. area of bruising.
B. stage 1 pressure ulcer.
C. potential deep tissue injury.
D. stage 4 pressure ulcer.

114. A patient presents to emergency triage with a handwritten note indicating that they are experiencing severe throat pain. When attempting to speak, the patient's voice sounds as though they are speaking with a hot potato in their mouth. The emergency nurse immediately recognizes this as a symptom of which of the following?

A. Laryngeal foreign body
B. Epiglottitis
C. Peritonsillar abscess
D. Exudative pharyngitis

115. A patient is brought to the emergency department holding their tooth in their hand, stating the tooth was knocked out while playing soccer. Which of the following interventions is the appropriate method for the emergency nurse to implement to protect the tooth?

A. Hold the avulsed tooth by the crown
B. Wrap the tooth in moist, saline-soaked gauze
C. Place the tooth under the patient's tongue
D. Place the tooth in milk for 2 hours

116. A patient presents to the emergency department complaining of tinnitus and dizziness. Which of the following is the most likely cause of the patient's symptoms that would lead the emergency nurse to suspect this patient has labyrinthitis?

A. Blurred vision
B. Viral illness
C. Unilateral sensorineural hearing loss
D. Episodic vertigo

117. A patient presents to the emergency department with a complaint of severe pain in the left ear. The patient states that they were recently on an airline flight, and during the landing descent, they experienced a sudden onset of sharp pain in the ear that has not decreased. The patient has had no previous difficulty with ear pain when flying. Which of the following assessment findings would indicate the presence of a traumatic ruptured tympanic membrane?

A. Blood in the ear canal, with no accompanying presence of a purulent discharge.
B. Presence of purulent material within the ear canal
C. Redness of the pinna
D. Pain in ear when opening the lower jaw

118. A patient presents to triage, stating that they tripped over a rug, falling directly onto their face. There is noticeable periorbital and facial edema, and ecchymosis is noted around the left eye with the presence of infraorbital hypoesthesia. The patient complains of "seeing double" and is having trouble opening their mouth. There is blood around the nares. The emergency nurse anticipates this patient has sustained which type of facial fracture?

A. Orbital rim fracture
B. Zygomatic fracture
C. Nasal fracture
D. Le Fort II fracture

119. A patient with a history of acute closed-angle glaucoma presents to the emergency department with a complaint of severe unilateral eye pain and blurred vision. What is the priority action for this patient?

A. Immediately notify the emergency provider of the patient's arrival
B. Dilate the eye to determine if the cornea has become edematous
C. Place the patient in a darkened room
D. Treat the patient's accompanying symptoms of nausea and headache

120. Which laboratory test would the emergency nurse anticipate to be ordered on a patient with a potential organophosphate exposure?

A. Platelet count
B. Serum lactate level
C. Urine drug screen
D. Plasma pseudocholinesterase level

121. The most common cardiac rhythm disturbance associated with the presence of an electrical shock injury is:

A. ventricular tachycardia.
B. atrial fibrillation.
C. ventricular fibrillation.
D. premature atrial complexes.

122. A patient presents to the emergency department with an insect bite to the hand. You observe a single puncture wound surrounded by a moderate amount of edema. The patient is complaining of severe cramping in the affected extremity and abdomen. You suspect this puncture wound is the result of a:

A. nonvenomous snake bite
B. brown recluse spider bite.
C. scorpion sting
D. black widow spider bite.

123. You are evaluating a patient complaining of severe abdominal cramping, vomiting, and bloody diarrhea for the last 3 days. The patient has not traveled outside the country in the last 90 days and has had no known ill contacts. The patient's BP is 98/72 mm Hg; HR 124 beats/minute; RR 24 breaths/minute; T 37°C (98.6°F); SpO_2 95%. The priority intervention for this patient is to:

A. initiate intravenous hydration with 0.9% sodium chloride or Ringer's lactate solution.
B. obtain complete blood count, electrolyte panel, and stool for analysis.
C. isolate the patient and institute Ebola precautions.
D. provide oxygen at 2 L/minute via nasal cannula.

124. A young mother presents to the emergency department with her 3-month-old infant, stating the infant has not been taking fluids well for the past several days. The triage nurse notes the infant has a flat fontanelle and normal vital signs and is drooling excessively. Further history includes that the child is breastfed. Assessment of the child's mouth reveals white patches on the mucosa and palate. These findings are most consistent with:

A. strep throat.
B. oral candidiasis.
C. teething syndrome.
D. milk curds.

125. Following a drowning, a patient's arterial blood gas report represents metabolic acidosis as evident by which of the following?

A. pH 7.5; $PaCO_2$ 25 mm Hg; PaO_2 75 mm Hg; HCO_3 24 mEq/L
B. pH 7.4; $PaCO_2$ 40 mm Hg; PaO_2 90 mm Hg; HCO_3 24 mEq/L
C. pH 7.20; $PaCO_2$ 35 mm Hg; PaO_2 75 mm Hg; HCO_3 18 mEq/L
D. pH 7.5; $PaCO_2$ 45 mm Hg; PaO_2 85 mm Hg; HCO_3 28 mEq/L

126. A patient presents to the emergency department with a cold-related tissue injury to their upper right extremity. Which general management principle should be followed in the care of this patient?

A. Use ice or snow and friction to massage the frozen extremity
B. Protect and immobilize the affected extremity after thawing
C. Thaw the affected area even if it is likely the area may become refrozen before definitive care can be obtained
D. Rub the injured tissues in warm circulating water

127. What is the recommended site in adults for the administration of intramuscular human diploid cell vaccine for rabies prophylaxis?

A. Dorsogluteal muscle
B. Deltoid muscle
C. Vastus lateralis muscle
D. Gluteus maximus muscle

128. The emergency nurse is providing discharge instructions for a patient who has been diagnosed with Lyme disease. Which of the following patient responses indicates that the patient understands the discharge instructions being given?

A. "I may continue to experience fatigue for a month or longer."
B. "I will need to take antibiotics twice a day for 7 days."
C. "I should start to feel better after a few days of taking the antibiotics."
D. "I should avoid close contact with other people until I finish my antibiotics."

129. A patient presents to the emergency department with a complaint of increased bleeding of the gums while brushing their teeth. The patient's current medications include warfarin sodium (Coumadin) daily. Which statement by the patient to the emergency nurse demonstrates his understanding of the effects of warfarin?

A. "I have started taking St John's wort and ginseng daily."
B. "I can eat what I want, but avoid high fatty foods."
C. "Ice cream and milk products can cause me to bleed."
D. "I should not drink cranberry juice."

130. A young adult patient arrives to the emergency department accompanied by a friend. According to the friend, the patient was at a party and suddenly became dizzy, confused, and lethargic. The friend is concerned that the patient may have possibly ingested a "date rape" drug. Which of the following medications should the emergency nurse anticipate administering for acute flunitrazepam (Rohypnol) ingestion?

A. Diazepam (Valium)
B. Flumazenil (Romazicon)
C. Naloxone (Narcan)
D. Alprazolam (Xanax)

131. A patient experiencing alcohol withdrawal has been receiving intravenous haloperidol (Haldol) for delirium, delusions, and hallucinations. Which electrocardiogram abnormality would cause the emergency nurse the greatest concern?

A. Peaked T waves
B. QT-interval prolongation
C. Delta waves
D. Osborne waves

132. You are caring for a patient who has arrived by emergency medical services (EMS) from a skilled nursing facility. EMS reports that the patient has a 3-day history of watery diarrhea, low-grade fever, and decreased fluid intake. The patient's medication record reveals the patient is taking levofloxacin (Levaquin) for pneumonia. The patient's vital signs: BP 90/64 mm Hg; HR 112 beats/minute; RR 16 breaths/minute; SpO_2 88% room air; T 38.4°C (101.1°F); Wt 58.1 kg. Which of the following is the priority nursing intervention?

A. Place patient on contact and droplet isolation
B. Administer oxygen
C. Draw blood for cultures and a lactate level
D. Obtain intravenous access

133. A school-age child is brought to the emergency department complaining of fever, headache, muscle aches, loss of appetite, and bilateral swollen salivary glands under both ears. According to the parents the child has not received routine childhood immunizations because of personal beliefs. The emergency nurse determines that these assessment findings are mostly caused by which of the following illnesses?

A. Influenza
B. Mumps
C. Rubella
D. Brucellosis

134. In caring for a patient with diphtheria, which of following findings would alert the emergency nurse that the patient is experiencing a complication from the disease?

A. Abdominal pain
B. ST segment and T wave changes
C. High-grade fever
D. Severe headache

135. Which of the following statements best describes critical incident stress?

A. A combination of complex cognitive, somatic, and behavioral effects caused by psychological trauma
B. A normal response to an abnormal event
C. A unique set of attributes or behaviors that buffer the effects of acute and/or chronic stress
D. A combination of secondary traumatic stress and burnout from exposure to repeated suffering

136. When evaluating research data, which of the following statistical indicators best supports the validity of the data?

A. The relative risk reduction is low.
B. The *p*-value (α) is reported as < 0.05.
C. The confidence interval is 90%.
D. The number needed to treat is high.

137. A young child arrives at the emergency department via emergency medical services after sustaining a near drowning. Cardiopulmonary resuscitation has continued for over 45 minutes, and the child remains in asystole. The child's parents demand to be in the resuscitation room with their child. As the emergency nurse, you should do which of the following?

A. Explain to the parents that their child is critically ill, and staff will provide them with periodic updates on the condition of their child.
B. Ask the social worker or hospital chaplain to be with the parents in the private family waiting room.
C. Designate one person to provide the parents with updates on the condition of their child as indicated.
D. Offer the family presence at the bedside.

138. The family of an elderly patient who has sustained a cardiopulmonary arrest is being approached by the hospital organ procurement agency representative, asking them for consent for organ donation. Which statement, made by a member of the patient's family, indicates an accurate understanding of the organ donation process?

A. "The organs of an elderly person are only suitable for research purposes and not for organ donation."
B. "Our insurance will cover the additional costs related to the organ donation process."
C. "We would not be able to have an open-casket funeral."
D. "Our religion considers organ donation to be a noble gift."

139. The nurse is participating on a committee that is developing guidelines for family presence during an emergency department resuscitation. The committee should define which of the following as a part of the guideline?

A. Who is considered the patient's family
B. The roles and responsibilities of each member of the resuscitation team
C. Situations in which family members should be offered the option of presence
D. Nursing interventions if family members interfere with resuscitation efforts

140. A patient who has been diagnosed with end-stage cardiac disease is receiving palliative care in the emergency department while awaiting placement in the hospice unit. Which of the following interventions is most appropriate for the emergency nurse to implement in the care of this patient?

A. Delegate hygiene care to family members
B. Obtain a 12-lead electrocardiogram
C. Provide oxygen as needed to relieve the patient's dyspnea
D. Restrict visitors to the patient's immediate family

141. Following the death of a patient in the emergency department who may be the victim of crime, the proper collection of forensic evidence includes which of the following actions?

A. Place paper bags over both of the patient's hands
B. Wrap wet clothing in plastic and then place it in a paper bag
C. Return jewelry and religious items to a family member because they are not admissible as evidence
D. Use sterile metal forceps when handling bullets

142. During a cardiac resuscitation, the emergency provider orders amiodarone 600 mg intravenously to be given for ventricular fibrillation. The best action by the emergency nurse is to:

A. ask for clarification of the dose before administering the medication.
B. infuse the ordered dose of amiodarone over 1–2 minutes.
C. mix the amiodarone in 300 mL of 0.9% sodium chloride and infuse over 30 minutes.
D. administer 300 mg of amiodarone as an intravenous bolus and the remaining 300 mg as an infusion drip.

143. Which of the following practices best contributes to patient-reported satisfaction with their emergency department experience?

A. Performing hourly rounding to provide patient information
B. Effective pain management
C. Providing distractions such as television and food
D. Maintaining actual wait times of less than 30 minutes

144. Which of the following definitions best exemplifies the meaning of culture?

A. The patterns of behavior and beliefs shared by persons living in a social group
B. A group of people who share the same attributes, such as social rank or socioeconomic status
C. A group of people who share the same heritage or country of origin
D. An organized or unorganized system of beliefs

145. The registered nurse asks the assistive personnel to reassess vital signs on a patient who had a lumbar puncture performed the previous hour. Is this an appropriate task to delegate to assistive personnel?

A. Yes
B. No
C. Only if the assistive staff member has had specific education on lumbar punctures.
D. Only if the assistive staff member feels comfortable doing so.

146. Following a mass casualty incident, a small child arrives to the emergency department via emergency medical services. The child is not breathing and has no palpable pulse. The child's airway is repositioned, and, following 5 rescue breaths, the child begins breathing on his own. Based on the JumpSTART triage algorithm, which triage category should be assigned to this child?

A. Black (expectant)
B. Yellow (delayed)
C. Red (immediate)
D. Green (minor)

147. It is important to have effective communication among emergency department staff when completing a patient handoff between staff members as well as with other hospital departments. One form of communicating handoff is the SBAR technique. The S in the SBAR communication tool stands for:

A. suggest alternatives.
B. situation.
C. safety.
D. support.

148. A patient delivers a full-term baby in the emergency department of a facility that does not have OB/GYN or women's services available. The ambulance transport crew has arrived to take the mother and baby to an appropriate accepting facility. Based on the Emergency Medical Treatment and Active Labor Act, the emergency nurse identifies this patient cannot be transported unless which of the following has occurred?

A. The mother has not voided urine
B. The nurse completes all necessary documentation
C. The baby is 1 hour old
D. Delivery of the placenta

149. Which type of consent for treatment is recognized when an alert and oriented patient presents for care in the emergency department?

A. Informed consent
B. Implied consent
C. Involuntary consent
D. Express consent

150. Prior to implementing a research study that involves patient outcomes, approval must be obtained from which of the following?

A. The institutional ethics committee
B. The institutional legal consultant
C. The institutional review board
D. The medical staff involved with the patient population

PART 2

1. A patient presents to the emergency department with complaints of chest pain. The 12-lead electrocardiogram (ECG) reveals ST segment elevation in leads I and aVL. The initial blood pressure is 112/69 mm Hg and decreases to a systolic 60 mm Hg following a dose of nitroglycerin 0.4 mg SL. The next most appropriate intervention is to:

   A. complete a fibrinolytic check sheet.
   B. initiate a dopamine drip for blood pressure control.
   C. obtain a right-sided 12-lead ECG.
   D. administer a 0.9% sodium chloride bolus intravenously.

Rationale

A. Although the fibrinolytic check sheet needs to be completed in a timely manner in preparation for the patient to go to interventional radiology, it is not the first priority of care.

B. Blood pressure drop may be a transient response to the nitroglycerin; therefore, a vasopressor is not indicated unless the patient does not respond to fluid bolus resuscitation.

C. The patient's 12-lead ECG reveals an injury pattern that is consistent with a lateral wall myocardial infarction, which is usually not associated with a right ventricular wall myocardial infarction.

D. Patients can be sensitive to vasodilatation effects of nitroglycerin. Initial intervention is the administration of a fluid bolus for the hypotension that occurs secondary to the nitroglycerin.

Category: Cardiovascular Emergencies/Acute coronary syndrome

Nursing Process: Intervention

Reference

American Heart Association. (2016). The ACLS cases: Acute coronary syndrome. In *Advanced cardiovascular life support: Provider manual* (p. 66). Dallas, TX: Author.

---

2. A patient presents to the triage nurse complaining of sudden onset of chest pressure that has never been experienced before. The 12-lead electrocardiogram shows ST segment elevation in leads V1–V6. This ST segment pattern is consistent with an occlusion in which coronary artery?

   A. Left anterior descending artery
   B. Circumflex artery
   C. Posterior descending artery
   D. Right coronary artery

Rationale

A. Occlusion of the LAD will show ST segment elevation in the septal (V1–V2), anterior (V3–V4), and lateral (I, aVL, V5–V6) leads.

B. Circumflex artery occlusion would reflect changes as identified in the anterior and lateral leads (V5, V6, and lead III) of the electrocardiogram (ECG).

C. Posterior descending artery occlusion would reflect changes as identified in an inferior myocardial infarction ECG pattern.

D. RCA occlusion would reflect changes as identified in an inferior wall and right ventricular myocardial infarction ECG pattern.

Category: Cardiovascular Emergencies/Acute coronary syndrome

Nursing Process: Analysis

Reference

Williams, D. A. (2010). Cardiovascular emergencies. In P. K. Howard & R. A. Steinmann (Eds.), *Sheehy's emergency nursing: Principles and practice* (6th ed., pp. 411–444). St. Louis, MO: Mosby Elsevier.

---

3. A 68-year-old female presents to the emergency department with weakness, lightheadedness, and nausea. She has not felt well for the past several hours but had to complete her workday before seeking medical care. She denies the presence of chest pain or shortness of breath. The most appropriate intervention during bedside triage is to:

A. instruct the patient to chew 325 mg aspirin.
B. complete the triage process, including obtaining past medical history, current medications, and family history.
C. obtain vascular access and draw necessary laboratory studies specific to cardiac biomarkers.
D. perform a 12-lead electrocardiogram.

Rationale

A. Having the patient chew aspirin is not the first priority. After obtaining a brief patient history and allergies, the aspirin can be administered.

B. Although this intervention would provide additional pertinent information, it would delay the acquisition of the necessary 12-lead electrocardiogram (ECG).

C. This needs to be completed, but it is not the first priority in the care of this patient.

D. The patient is describing an atypical acute coronary syndrome (ACS) presentation. Women have a unique presentation of signs and symptoms, and their care is at risk of being delayed because of lack of early recognition. The 12-lead ECG should be completed within 10 minutes of arrival at the emergency department.

Category: Cardiovascular Emergencies/Acute coronary syndrome

Nursing Process: Intervention

Reference

Phalen, T., & Aehlert, B. (2012). *The 12-lead ECG in acute coronary syndromes.* Maryland Heights, MO: Elsevier/Mosby.

4. Which symptom points toward a diagnosis of abdominal aortic aneurysm?
   A. **Pulsatile mass**
   B. Distant heart sounds
   C. Hypertension
   D. Subcutaneous emphysema

Rationale

A. Although the presence of a pulsatile mass in the abdomen may not always occur in a patient with an abdominal aortic aneurysm (AAA), when present, the nurse should be highly suspicious of AAA and intervene immediately. Bedside ultrasonography can assist in a rapid diagnosis.

B. Distant heart sounds is an assessment finding in patients with a cardiac tamponade.

C. Hypotension, not hypertension, is an indicator of an abdominal aortic aneurysm.

D. Subcutaneous emphysema is an assessment finding of tension pneumothorax but is not associated with an abdominal aortic aneurysm.

Category: Cardiovascular Emergencies/Aneurysm/dissection
Nursing Process: Assessment

References

Hammond, B. B. (2013). Cardiovascular emergencies. In B. B. Hammond & P. G. Zimmermann (Eds.), *Sheehy's manual of emergency care* (7th ed., pp. 201–211). St. Louis, MO: Elsevier Mosby.

Rubano, E., Mehta, N., Caputo, W., Paladino, L., & Sinert, R. (2013). Systematic review: Emergency department bedside ultrasonography for diagnosing suspected abdominal aortic aneurysm. *Academic Emergency Medicine, 20*, 128–138. https://doi.org/10.1111/acem.12080

---

5. A patient arrives to emergency department and collapses in front of the triage desk. The patient does not have a pulse and is not breathing. Cardiopulmonary resuscitation is initiated, and the cardiac monitor displays ventricular tachycardia. The immediate action by the emergency nurse is to:
   A. administer amiodarone (Cordarone) 150 mg intravenously.
   B. synchronize cardioversion with 200 joules.
   C. **defibrillate using biphasic defibrillator with 120–200 joules.**
   D. administer sodium bicarbonate 1 mEq/kg.

Rationale

A. Amiodarone is used for patients in pulseless ventricular tachycardia at a dose of 300 mg initially. The dose for amiodarone for a patient with ventricular tachycardia with a pulse is 150 mg.

B. Synchronized cardioversion is indicated for unstable patients (with a palatable pulse) in ventricular tachycardia or tachydysrhythmias. Defibrillation is indicated for patients with pulseless ventricular tachycardia.

C. Immediate defibrillation is the recommended treatment for a pulseless ventricular tachycardia, in conjunction with adequate cardiopulmonary resuscitation. Medications are added after the first defibrillation attempt. The defibrillation should be repeated every 2 minutes if a palpable pulse and palatable rhythm do not return. If using a monophasic defibrillator, 360 joules is recommended for defibrillation.

D. Sodium bicarbonate is used for correction of acidosis and may be indicated for a patient in cardiopulmonary arrest, but not in the initial treatment. Administration of sodium bicarbonate should be guided by blood gas analysis.

Category: Cardiovascular Emergencies/Cardiopulmonary arrest

Nursing Process: Intervention

Reference

American Heart Association. (2016). The ACLS cases: Cardiac arrest: Pulseless electrical activity. In *Advanced cardiovascular life support: Provider manual* (pp. 110–119). Dallas, TX: Author.

---

6. Which emergency patient would be an ideal candidate for targeted temperature management or induced hypothermia?

   A. A patient with an elevated temperature above 39.4°C (103°F) with a lactic acid level of 6.0 mmol/L
   B. A responsive emergency patient who achieved return of spontaneous circulation (ROSC) following a successful resuscitation by emergency medical services personnel
   C. An unresponsive patient who arrives at the emergency department with ROSC following cardiopulmonary arrest
   D. A patient remaining in ventricular fibrillation following a cardiopulmonary arrest event

Rationale

A. Targeted temperature management is not used for septic patients to control temperature. Cooling blankets can be used to lower extremely high temperatures but not to a certain target level for an extended period of time. The lactic acid level of 6.0 mmol/L could indicate sepsis.

B. The ideal candidate for targeted temperature management or induced hypothermia is the patient with ROSC following cardiopulmonary arrest who remains unresponsive. According to the American Heart Association 2016 guidelines for postresuscitation care, targeted temperature management should not be routinely initiated in the field using cold intravenous fluids or other invasive methods.

C. The ideal candidate for targeted temperature management or induced hypothermia is the patient with ROSC following cardiopulmonary arrest who remains unresponsive. According to the American Heart Association's 2016 guidelines for postresuscitation care, the described patient should be considered for targeted temperature management immediately on arrival at the emergency department, with optimal reduced temperature reached within 2–3 hours of the cardiopulmonary arrest.

D. The ideal patient for targeted temperature management is a patient returning to spontaneous circulation who remains unresponsive. Ventricular fibrillation does not provide for circulating blood flow; therefore, this patient would not be a candidate for targeted temperature management or induced hypothermia.

Category: Cardiovascular Emergencies/Cardiopulmonary arrest

Nursing Process: Analysis

Reference

American Heart Association. (2016). The ACLS cases: Immediate post cardiac arrest care. In *Advanced cardiovascular life support: Provider manual* (p. 151). Dallas, TX: Author.

7. Which of the following demonstrates that effective cardiopulmonary resuscitation is being delivered to the patient in cardiopulmonary arrest?
   A. Presence of waveform variation on the cardiac monitor
   B. End-tidal CO_2 20 mm Hg
   C. Arterial pH of 6.9
   D. Decreased coronary perfusion pressure

Rationale

A. Movement of the cardiac monitor cable can cause waveform movement on the cardiac monitor during cardiopulmonary resuscitation (CPR). This is not a reliable indicator of adequate CPR performance.

B. End-tidal CO_2 levels greater than 10 mm Hg during CPR efforts demonstrate adequate chest compression depth and good-quality CPR. The higher the end-tidal CO_2 levels during resuscitation, the greater the likelihood of return of spontaneous circulation.

C. An arterial pH of 6.9 demonstrates profound acidosis and would not be an indicator that effective CPR is being performed.

D. An increase in coronary perfusion pressure would be an indicator of good-quality CPR. Coronary perfusion pressures relate to myocardial blood flow and return of spontaneous circulation.

Category: Cardiovascular Emergencies/Cardiopulmonary arrest

Nursing Process: Evaluation

Reference

American Heart Association. (2016). The ACLS cases: Cardiac arrest: VF/pulseless VT. In *Advanced cardiovascular life support: Provider manual* (pp. 102–103). Dallas, TX: Author.

---

8. Parents arrive to the emergency department with their infant, who has a pulse rate of 30. The infant is limp and not breathing. The immediate action by the emergency nurse would be to:
   A. begin rescue breathing at a rate of 20 breaths per minute.
   B. initiate chest compressions at a rate of 110 per minute.
   C. defibrillate with 100 joules.
   D. administer epinephrine (Adrenalin) 0.01 mg/kg.

Rationale

A. Rescue breathing would be indicated for a nonbreathing infant, but chest compressions should also be started immediately due to the presence of a pulse rate less than 60 with poor perfusion.

B. Chest compressions should be started immediately because of the pulse rate less than 60 beats per minute, followed by rescue breathing for a child or infant with a pulse rate of less than 60 with poor perfusion.

C. CPR with compressions and ventilations should be the immediate treatment. Defibrillation should be used in the presence of ventricular tachycardia without a pulse or if ventricular fibrillation rhythm is present. A pulse rate of 30 is described in this infant; therefore, the initiation of chest compressions at 110 per minute is the priority.

D. Epinephrine would be indicated in this scenario, but not before good-quality CPR has been initiated.

Category (Pediatric): Cardiovascular Emergencies/Cardiopulmonary arrest

Nursing Process: Intervention

Reference

American Heart Association. (2015). Pediatric cardiac arrest algorithm. In *2015 handbook of emergency cardiovascular care for healthcare providers* (p. 81). Dallas, TX: Author.

---

9. A patient presents to the emergency department with complaints of a rapid heartbeat, which is identified as an accelerated junctional rhythm. This dysrhythmia is most commonly associated with:

A. the use of marijuana.
B. chronic obstructive pulmonary disease.
C. the use of digoxin.
D. history of diabetes.

Rationale

A. Marijuana use is associated with increases in heart rate that commonly originate in the sinus node, as seen in sinus tachycardia.

B. Chronic obstructive pulmonary disease is not commonly associated with an accelerated junctional rhythm.

C. Digitalis toxicity leads to the development of atrioventricular dysrhythmias, commonly resulting in an accelerated rhythm.

D. Dysrhythmias that are associated with a history of diabetes are frequently related to electrolyte imbalances and usually originate in the sinus node, not the atrioventricular node.

Category: Cardiovascular Emergencies/Dysrhythmias

Nursing Process: Analysis

Reference

Criddle, L. (2007). Cardiovascular emergencies. In K. S. Hoyt & J. Selfridge-Thomas (Eds.), *Emergency nursing core curriculum* (6th ed., pp. 187–248). St. Louis, MO: Saunders Elsevier.

---

10. A patient presents to the emergency department stating that their heartbeat feels irregular. The emergency nurse assesses an irregular radial pulse. The cardiac monitor displays a cyclic irregular rhythm with an inconsistent PR segment, which becomes progressively longer until dropping a QRS complex. The cyclic pattern repeats each 4 complexes. You determine the cardiac rhythm to be:

A. second-degree Mobitz I block.
B. second-degree Mobitz II block.
C. third-degree heart block.
D. first-degree heart block.

Rationale

A. Second-degree Mobitz I block, or Wenckebach rhythm, is described as the progressive lengthening of the PR segment ending in a dropped QRS complex usually occurring after 3–5 beats. One of the P waves fails to be conducted to the ventricles, resulting in a "dropped beat" and then repeating. This is a second-degree Mobitz I block, or Wenckebach rhythm.

B. A second-degree Mobitz II heart block represents a cardiac rhythm where the sinus node impulses occur at regular intervals, but conduction to the ventricles is intermittently absent. The P waves will have a consistent configuration, and the PR interval with the complex that is conducted to the ventricles will remain constant. The P waves that are not conducted below the atria result in failure of the ventricles to contract, and the absence of the QRS complex. Typically, a second-degree Mobitz II block rhythm occurs in conjunction with bradycardia and will require treatment considerations to maintain adequate cardiac output.

C. Third-degree heart block is characterized by the complete absence of conduction between the atria and the ventricles. The sinus node continues to release an impulse, but it is not conducted to the ventricles. As a result, the ventricles release their own impulse to maintain ventricular contraction, resulting in a lower cardiac output. A third-degree heart block rhythm has P waves that occur independent from the QRS complexes. This cardiac rhythm requires immediate lifesaving interventions to improve cardiac output and hemodynamic instability.

D. A first-degree heart block is characterized by a consistent PR interval that is greater than 0.20 seconds.

Category: Cardiovascular Emergencies/Dysrhythmias

Nursing Process: Analysis

Reference

Dubin, D. (2000). Rhythm, part II: Blocks. In *Rapid interpretation of EKG's* (6th ed., pp. 173–202). Tampa, FL: Cover Publishing.

---

11. A patient is diagnosed with endocarditis. Which of the following statements indicates that the patient understands a possible cause of this disease?

A. "I never knew that this type of infection could originate from having the flu."
B. "I cannot believe I got this disease from a tick bite."
C. "Endocarditis may have been caused by my recent body piercings."
D. "Endocarditis is a complication caused by my continued smoking."

Rationale

A. Endocarditis has not been described as occurring as a complication of the flu (influenza).

B. Endocarditis is not considered a tickborne disease. Common tickborne diseases include Rocky Mountain spotted fever and Lyme disease.

C. Infective endocarditis has been shown to occur after recent body piercings or tattooing in addition to recent cardiac surgery, prosthetic valve replacements, and cardiac pacemaker insertions. Poor dental hygiene, intravenous drug abuse, and rheumatic heart disease also have been noted to contribute to endocarditis.

D. Smoking causes significant pulmonary disease and vasoconstriction but is not generally related to endocarditis.

Category: Cardiovascular Emergencies/Endocarditis

Nursing Process: Evaluation

Reference

Criddle, L. (2007). Cardiovascular emergencies. In K. S. Hoyt & J. Selfridge-Thomas (Eds.), *Emergency nursing core curriculum* (6th ed., pp. 187– 248). St. Louis, MO: Saunders Elsevier.

---

12. A patient presents to the emergency department with a left ventricular assistive device (LVAD) in place. Which statement made by the patient demonstrates understanding of the LVAD function?

A. "You will only be able to hear one number for my blood pressure."
B. "My LVAD clicks every time it opens and closes."
C. "I frequently have premature atrial contractions."
D. "I know my LVAD is working if I do not hear it humming continuously."

Rationale

A. LVADs produce a continuous blood flow. A manual BP cuff should be used, with the mean arterial pressure being the first sound heard. The mean arterial pressure generally fluctuates between 70 and 90 mm Hg. Automatic blood pressure devices should not be used with an LVAD patient.

B. A clicking sound is consistent with a mechanical heart valve, not an LVAD. The LVAD typically has a continuous humming sound.

C. Ventricular dysrhythmias are most common in patients with an LVAD, not atrial dysrhythmias.

D. A functioning LVAD will have a continuous humming sound. The provider should listen for the humming as part of the patient assessment.

Category: Cardiovascular Emergencies/Heart failure

Nursing Process: Evaluation

Reference

Cabrera, D., & Decker, W. W. (2012). Management of emergencies related to implanted cardiac devices. In J. G. Adams, E. D. Barton, J. L. Collings, P. M. C. DeBlieux, M. A. Gisondi, & E. S. Nadel (Eds.), *Emergency medicine: Clinical essentials* (2nd ed., pp. 547–557). Philadelphia, PA: Elsevier Saunders.

---

13. A female who is 26 weeks pregnant is sent to the emergency department by her OB/GYN physician because of elevated blood pressure. The emergency nurse is aware that gestational hypertension is defined as:

A. systolic BP above 140 mm Hg or diastolic BP above 90 mm Hg.
B. systolic BP 10 mm Hg above baseline and elevated pulse rate.
C. diastolic BP 20 mm Hg above baseline with a corresponding systolic BP 10 mm Hg above baseline.
D. diastolic BP greater than 90 mm Hg with a systolic BP above 110 mm Hg.

Rationale

A. Gestational hypertension is defined as a systolic BP above 140 mm Hg or diastolic BP above 90 mm Hg.

B. Gestational hypertension is defined as systolic BP above 140 mm Hg or diastolic BP above 90 mm Hg. The patient's pulse rate is not defined in gestational hypertension.

C. Gestational hypertension is defined as systolic BP above 140 mm Hg or diastolic BP above 90 mm Hg. The systolic reading that is 10 mm Hg above baseline and diastolic reading that is 20 mm Hg above baseline are not variations used to define gestational hypertension.

D. Gestational hypertension is defined as systolic BP above 140 mm Hg or diastolic BP above 90 mm Hg. The diastolic value greater than 90 mm Hg and systolic value greater than 110 mm Hg are not correct for the definition for gestational hypertension.

Category: Cardiovascular Emergencies/Hypertension

Nursing Process: Assessment

Reference

Poole, J. H., & Thompson, J. E. (2013). Obstetric emergencies. In B. B. Hammond & P. G. Zimmermann (Eds.), *Sheehy's manual of emergency care* (7th ed., pp. 483–495). St. Louis, MO: Elsevier Mosby.

---

14. The emergency department physician is inserting a 16-guage sheathed needle slowly into the left paraxiphoid area with the needle pointed downward at an approximately 30-degree angle and aimed toward the left shoulder. The trauma nurse understands that this treatment is indicated for which of the following conditions?

A. Ascites
B. Pneumothorax
C. Obstructed airway
D. Pericardial tamponade

Rationale

A. Paracentesis is the procedure used to remove fluid from the abdomen.

B. A needle thoracentesis is the procedure used to decompress the pleural cavity because of a hemothorax or pneumothorax.

C. Needle cricothyroidotomy is the procedure used to establish an emergency airway in a patient in whom intubation and other rescue airway devices have failed.

D. Needle pericardiocentesis is the procedure used to aspirate fluid from around the pericardial space.

Category: Cardiovascular Emergencies/Pericardial tamponade

Nursing Process: Intervention

References

Gurney, D., & Westergard, A. M. (2014). Initial assessment. In D. Gurney (Ed.), *Trauma Nursing Core Course: Provider manual* (7th ed., pp. 39–54). Des Plaines, IL: Emergency Nurses Association.

Mattu, A., & Martinez, J. P. (2013). Pericarditis, pericardial tamponade, and myocarditis. In J. G. Adams, E. D. Barton, J. L. Collings, P. M. C. DeBlieux, M. A. Gisondi, & E. S. Nadel (Eds.), *Emergency medicine: Clinical essentials* (2nd ed., pp. 514–523). Philadelphia, PA: Elsevier Saunders.

---

15. A patient arrives at the emergency department complaining of midsternal chest pain that is exacerbated when lying flat and with deep inspiration. Following a 12-lead electrocardiogram, laboratory diagnostic testing, and review of the patient history, the emergency care provider diagnoses the patient with pericarditis. Based on this diagnosis, the nurse anticipates an order to administer which medication to this patient?

A. Tissue plasminogen activator 0.9 mg/kg intravenously (IV)
B. Nitroglycerin 0.4 mg sublingual
C. Furosemide (Lasix) 40 mg IV
D. Ibuprofen (Motrin) 600 mg PO

Rationale

A. Tissue plasminogen activator (TPA) is used to treat acute ischemic strokes and acute myocardial infarctions. TPA is not recommended in the treatment of pericarditis.

B. Nitroglycerine is used for the treatment of angina; it is not indicated for pericarditis.

C. Furosemide is used to treat heart failure; it is not indicated in the treatment of pericarditis.

D. Anti-inflammatory medications are the recommended treatment for pericarditis.

Category: Cardiovascular Emergencies/Pericarditis

Nursing Process: Intervention

Reference

Hammond, B. B. (2013). Cardiovascular emergencies. In B. B. Hammond & P. G. Zimmermann (Eds.), *Sheehy's manual of emergency care* (7th ed., pp. 201–211). St. Louis, MO: Elsevier Mosby.

---

16. A patient presents to the emergency department with pain in their left lower leg. The assessment reveals the left lower leg to be pale and cool when compared with the right leg. Femoral pulses are equal, however, the popliteal pulse is significantly diminished on the left leg. The nurse suspects that the patient has which of the following?

A. Occlusion of the femoral vein
B. Occlusion of the femoral artery
C. Occlusion of the popliteal artery
D. Occlusion of the saphenous vein

Rationale

A. Venous occlusion generally causes the limb to become engorged and ruddy in appearance, with little change in skin temperature.

B. The femoral artery is the main artery to the lower extremity. If the femoral artery were occluded, the patient would be exhibiting signs and symptoms for the entire leg.

C. Arterial occlusion causes diminished pulses, cooler temperature, and pain as a result of ischemia. The patient has equal femoral pulses, so the occlusion is distal and more likely to be the popliteal artery.

D. Venous occlusion generally causes the limb to be engorged and ruddy, with little change in skin temperature.

Category: Cardiovascular Emergencies/Thromboembolic disease

Nursing Process: Analysis

Reference

Selvin, E., & Erlinger, T. P. (2004, August 10). Prevalence of and risk factors for peripheral arterial disease in the United States: Results from the National Health and Nutrition Examination Survey, 1999–2000. *Circulation, 110*(6), 738–743.

---

17. The nurse suspects a patient of having a pericardial tamponade when the assessment findings reveal:

A. **decreased stroke volume and cardiac output.**
B. distended neck veins and tracheal deviation.
C. subcutaneous emphysema and air in the mediastinum.
D. poor cardiovascular response and electrocardiogram abnormalities.

Rationale

A. Decreased stroke volume and cardiac output are findings associated with pericardial tamponade. These findings are the result of blood collecting in the pericardium, compressing the heart and decreasing the ability of the ventricles to fill.

B. Distended neck veins and tracheal deviation are findings associated with the presence of a tension pneumothorax. As air enters the pleural space resulting in lung collapse, as the pressure continues to increase, the mediastinum shifts to the opposite side resulting in tracheal deviation and distended neck veins as the heart is compressed and no longer able to fill with blood.

C. Subcutaneous emphysema and air in the mediastinum are findings associated with the presence of blunt esophageal injury. Blunt esophageal rupture can be associated with fractures of the first and second rib, and cervical spine fracture.

D. Poor cardiovascular response and electrocardiogram abnormalities are findings of blunt cardiac injury. Blunt cardiac injury can occur following acceleration–deceleration injuries as well as any significant fall.

Category: Cardiovascular Emergencies/Pericardial Tamponade

Nursing Process: Assessment

Reference

Day, M. W. (2014). Thoracic and neck trauma. In D. Gurney (Ed.), *Trauma Nursing Core Course: Provider Manual* (7th ed., pp. 137–150). Des Plaines, IL: Emergency Nurses Association.

---

18. Which assessment finding would direct the emergency nurse to suspect that the patient is in compensated shock?

A. Marked hypotension
B. Narrowing pulse pressure
C. Weak, thready pulses
D. Increased lactic acid level

Rationale

A. Marked hypotension that is unresponsive to vasopressors is a sign of irreversible shock.

B. Narrowing pulse pressure is an assessment finding associated with the presence of compensated shock. A bounding pulse is also an assessment finding that can indicate the presence of compensated shock.

C. Weak, thready pulses are associated with the presence of progressive or decompensated shock.

D. Increased lactic acid level is a symptom of progressive or decompensated shock.

Category: Cardiovascular Emergencies/Shock (cardiogenic and obstructive)

Nursing Process: Assessment

Reference

Pentecost, D. A., & Smith, S. G. (2014). Shock. In D. Gurney (Ed.), *Trauma Nursing Core Course: Provider manual* (7th ed., pp. 73–90). Des Plaines, IL: Emergency Nurses Association.

---

19. Assessment findings of an unresponsive patient who hit a tree while snow skiing reveal hypotension, bradycardia, and warm, dry skin. The nurse suspects the presence of:

A. distributive shock.
B. obstructive shock.
C. progressive shock.
D. hypovolemic shock.

Rationale

A. The patient is at high risk for having sustained a spinal cord injury, resulting in the presence of neurogenic shock, a type of distributive shock. A disruption in the sympathetic regulation of vagal tone leads to venous and arterial vasodilation and loss of vascular resistance, resulting in hypotension, bradycardia, and warm, dry skin.

B. Obstructive shock occurs when there is an obstruction in either the vasculature or the heart, resulting in hypoperfusion of the tissues. The most common cause of obstructive shock is a pulmonary embolus.

C. Progressive shock is decompensated shock. The classic signs of progressive or decompensated shock are increased heart rate, decreased urinary output, decreased blood pressure, and altered mental status.

D. If the patient were exhibiting symptoms of hypovolemic shock, tachycardia and cool, clammy skin would have been present. This patient is exhibiting signs of neurogenic shock, a type of distributive shock with hypotension, bradycardia, and warm, dry skin.

Category: Cardiovascular Emergencies/Shock (cardiogenic and obstructive)

Nursing Process: Assessment

References

Crowley, M. (2014). Spinal cord and vertebral column trauma. In D. Gurney (Ed.), *Trauma Nursing Core Course: Provider manual* (7th ed., pp. 173–182). Des Plaines, IL: Emergency Nurses Association.

Pentecost, D. A. (2014). Shock. In D. Gurney (Ed.), *Trauma Nursing Core Course: Provider manual* (7th ed., pp. 73–90). Des Plaines, IL: Emergency Nurses Association.

---

20. An infant with a history of cardiomyopathy presents to the emergency department lethargic, pale, and with weak peripheral pulses. After being diagnosed with heart failure, the appropriate medication doses of an inotrope and a diuretic are administered. The emergency nurse can anticipate that the infant will demonstrate which of the following outcomes from the administration of these medications?

A. Urine output of 0.5 mL/kg per hour
B. Capillary refill time of 3 seconds
C. A bounding pulse
D. Warm extremities

Rationale

A. Normal urinary output for an infant is 2 mL/kg per hour. A urine output of 0.5 mL/kg per hour would indicate decreased renal and tissue perfusion.

B. A capillary refill time of less than 2 seconds would indicate clinical improvement of increased perfusion and a return to a normal hemodynamic state. A capillary refill time of 3 seconds indicates decreased perfusion.

C. A bounding pulse is a symptom of distributive shock, indicating inappropriate distribution of fluids. The peripheral pulse would be stronger, but not bounding, following administration of the inotrope and diuretic medications.

D. Warm extremities would indicate clinical improvement of increased perfusion and a return to a normal hemodynamic state. The infant's weak peripheral pulses indicate decreased perfusion to the extremities, which results in skin that initially is cool to the touch.

Category (Pediatric): Cardiovascular Emergencies/Shock (cardiogenic and obstructive)

Nursing Process: Evaluation

References

Brandt, C. (2012). Shock. In *Emergency Nursing Pediatric Course: Provider manual* (4th ed., pp. 227–244). Des Plaines, IL: Emergency Nurses Association.

Mecham, N. (2010). Pediatric emergencies. In P. K. Howard & R. A. Steinmann (Eds.), *Sheehy's emergency nursing: Principles and practice* (6th ed., pp. 630–651). St. Louis, MO: Mosby Elsevier.

---

21. A child arrives at the emergency department. While running on the playground, they suddenly experienced severe dyspnea and are unable to run any further. Vital signs: BP: 110/70 mm Hg; HR 120 beats/minute; RR 42 breaths/minute; SpO_2 91% room air; T 37.7°C (99.9°F). The child has audible wheezes with visible chest retractions. The emergency nurse anticipates the child will require:

A. racemic epinephrine nebulizer treatment.
B. albuterol nebulizer treatment.
C. theophylline intravenous infusion.
D. methylprednisolone (Solu-Medrol).

Rationale

A. Racemic epinephrine is not a first-line medication used in asthma control. The most effective evidence-based inhalants for asthma control include beta 2-adrenergic agonists such as albuterol.

B. Asthma is a chronic condition caused by airway inflammation and bronchospasm in response to a stimulus or irritant. The most effective treatment for airway inflammation is the inhaled administration of a beta 2-adrenergic agonist such as albuterol.

C. Theophylline is a bronchodilator administered orally or intravenously. However, the inhalation of bronchodilators is the preferred method of administration for immediate-acting asthma medications.

D. Systemic corticosteroids should be used in individuals who do not respond to short-acting beta 2-agonists; however, they are not a first-line medication used in asthma control.

Category (Pediatric): Respiratory Emergencies/Asthma
Nursing Process: Intervention

References

Brand, P. L., Baraldi, E., Bisgaard, H., Boner, A. L., Castro-Rodriguez, J. A., Custovic, A., . . . Bush, A. (2008). Definition, assessment and treatment of wheezing disorders in preschool children: An evidence-based approach. *European Respiratory Journal, 32*(4), 1096–1099.

Howard, P. K. (2012). Respiratory emergencies. In *Emergency Nursing Pediatric Course* (4th ed., pp. 131–146). Des Plaines, IL: Emergency Nurses Association.

---

22. The appropriate dose of albuterol is delivered by nebulizer to an asthmatic child. The emergency nurse would expect which of the following findings following this treatment?

A. A decreased respiratory rate
B. An increased peak flow reading
C. An absence of wheezing
D. A decrease in heart rate

Rationale

A. A decreased respiratory rate is not necessarily a sign of improvement and may signal impending respiratory failure.

B. When the treatment is effective, the peak flow reading would be expected to increase. A rate of greater than 80% of the child's personal best would be expected.

C. An absence of wheezing may indicate a severe obstruction with very little air exchange.

D. Albuterol would cause the heart rate to increase.

Category (Pediatric): Respiratory Emergencies/Asthma

Nursing Process: Evaluation

Reference

Randolph, R. (2009). Respiratory emergencies. In D. O. Thomas & L. M. Bernardo (Eds.), *Core curriculum for pediatric emergency nursing* (2nd ed., pp. 163–175). Des Plaines, IL: Emergency Nurses Association.

---

23. A patient with a history of chronic obstructive pulmonary disease and hypertension arrives at the emergency department in moderate respiratory distress. The patient is alert and oriented. Vital signs: BP 192/110 mm Hg; HR 112 beats/minute; RR 36 breaths/minute; SpO_2 78% room air; T 37.2°C (99.0°F). The initial priority intervention the emergency nurse anticipates for this patient is:

A. intravenous access.
B. endotracheal intubation.
C. biphasic positive airway pressure.
D. chest radiograph.

Rationale

A. Although an important intervention, intravenous access is not the initial priority. The priority for this patient should be maintaining airway, breathing, and circulation, followed by providing supplemental oxygen such as biphasic positive airway pressure (BiPAP).

B. Patients with chronic obstructive pulmonary disease (COPD) may be difficult to taper (or wean) off from mechanical ventilation. If possible, other airway support measures should be initiated first to improve their oxygenation.

C. BiPAP may help avoid hypoxemia without intubation. The priority for this patient should be maintaining airway, breathing, and circulation, followed by providing supplemental oxygen such as BiPAP. Based on the patient's vital signs and presentation, BiPAP is the best option.

D. A chest radiograph is important to rule out a life-threatening pneumothorax, but this is not the initial priority. COPD is an underlying cause identified in 70% of patients who experience a spontaneous pneumothorax.

Category: Respiratory Emergencies/Chronic obstructive pulmonary disease (COPD)

Nursing Process: Intervention

Reference

Walsh, R. (2013). Respiratory emergencies. In B. B. Hammond & P. G. Zimmermann (Eds.), *Sheehy's manual of emergency care* (7th ed., pp. 185–199). St. Louis, MO: Elsevier Mosby.

24. What is the influenza vaccine recommendation from the Centers for Disease Control and Prevention for 50-year-old patients with stage 1 chronic obstructive pulmonary disease (COPD)?

A. **Patients with COPD should receive an influenza vaccine every year.**
B. Patients with COPD should not receive influenza vaccines because of the high risk of severe side effects.
C. Patients under the age of 50 are not required to receive the influenza vaccine every year.
D. Patients who live alone are not required to receive the influenza vaccine each year.

Rationale

A. The Centers for Disease Control and Prevention (CDC) recommends that any person with a chronic disease be immunized for influenza. Influenza, pneumonia, and other preventable diseases increase the risk of mortality in patients with chronic disease.

B. Severe side effects of the influenza vaccine are rare, and if they occur, they are usually mild and self-limiting. Patients with a chronic disease such as COPD should be immunized for influenza each year.

C. The CDC recommends that people under the age of 50 be immunized against influenza each year.

D. The CDC recommends that everyone 6 months and older receive an annual influenza vaccine, with the only exceptions being for those with life-threatening allergies to the vaccine or any ingredient in the vaccine.

Category: Respiratory Emergencies/Chronic obstructive pulmonary disease (COPD)

Nursing Process: Assessment

Reference

Lung disease including asthma and adult vaccination. (2016). Centers for Disease Control and Prevention. Retrieved from http://www.cdc.gov/vaccines/adults/rec-vac/health-conditions/lung-disease.html

---

25. The presence of hypoxia in patients with chronic obstructive pulmonary disease is the result of which of the following?

A. The inability of blood to carry oxygen
B. **Ventilation/perfusion mismatch**
C. The presence of a diminished pulmonary blood flow
D. The inability of the body's tissues to use the oxygen being delivered to them

Rationale

A. Anemia or high levels of carbon monoxide results in a reduced number of normal cells that can carry oxygen to tissue.

B. In patients with chronic obstructive pulmonary disease, the adequate exchange of oxygen and carbon dioxide is impaired by the presence of damaged alveoli.

C. Decreased blood flow is because of the presence of hypovolemia caused by either trauma or sepsis.

D. Poisonous substances such as cyanide can interfere with the ability of the body's tissues to use oxygen that is being delivered.

Category: Respiratory Emergencies/Chronic obstructive pulmonary disease (COPD)

Nursing Process: Analysis

Reference

West, J. B. (2012). *Respiratory physiology: The essentials* (9th ed.). Baltimore, MD: Lippincott Williams & Wilkins.

---

26. The most common nosocomial infection that is often fatal in critically ill patients is:

A. ventilator-associated pneumonia.
B. urinary tract infection.
C. central line infection.
D. pressure ulcer infection.

Rationale

A. Ventilator-associated pneumonia (VAP) is identified as the most common cause of nosocomial infection deaths. VAP occurs when a patient is intubated and placed on a mechanical ventilator. A patient who is intubated and on mechanical ventilation is commonly sedated; this results in the ability of bacteria to enter the lungs because the patient is unable to clear secretions. As the bacteria colonize the lungs, an infectious process begins within 48–72 hours, resulting in VAP.

B. Although there is a risk of mortality from infection related to the presence of indwelling urinary catheters, this type of infection does not result in as many deaths as VAP.

C. Although there is a risk of mortality from infection related to central line catheters, this type of infection does not result in as many deaths as VAP.

D. Septicemia is unlikely to be caused by an infected pressure ulcer.

Category: Respiratory Emergencies/Infections

Nursing Process: Assessment

References

Stacy, K. M. (2014). Pulmonary therapeutic management. In L. D. Urden, K. M. Stacy, & M. E. Lough (Eds.), *Critical care nursing* (7th ed., pp. 549–586). St. Louis, MO: Elsevier Mosby.

Works, P., & Graunke, S. A. (2010). Respiratory emergencies. In P. K. Howard & R. A. Steinmann (Eds.), *Sheehy's emergency nursing: Principles and practice* (6th ed., pp. 395–310). St. Louis, MO: Mosby.

---

27. According the guidelines from the Centers for Medicare and Medicaid Services and The Joint Commission, a patient who is diagnosed with pneumonia should receive antibiotics within what time period from the time of arrival at the emergency department?

A. Within 2 hours
B. Within 4 hours
C. Within 6 hours
D. Within 10 hours

Rationale

A. According to the Centers for Medicare and Medicaid Services (CMS) and The Joint Commission, the suggested time is within 6 hours from time of arrival at the emergency department (ED). However, administering the antibiotics sooner will act to potentially improve patient outcomes.

B. According to CMS and The Joint Commission, the suggested time is within 6 hours from time of arrival at the ED. However, administering the antibiotics sooner will act to potentially improve patient outcomes.

C. According to guidelines from CMS and The Joint Commission, the suggested time of administration of antibiotics for a patient diagnosed with pneumonia is within 6 hours from time of arrival at the ED.

D. According to CMS and The Joint Commission, the suggested time is within 6 hours, not within 10 hours, from time of arrival at the ED.

Category: Respiratory Emergencies/Infections
Nursing Process: Intervention

Reference

Stacy, K. M. (2014). Pulmonary disorders. In L. D. Urden, K. M. Stacy, & M. E. Lough (Eds.), *Critical care nursing* (7th ed., pp. 514–548). Philadelphia, PA: Wolters Kluwer Health.

---

28. The emergency nurse is caring for a patient who was recently intubated. The capnography alarms and indicates a reading of 84 mm Hg. The priority assessment taken by the emergency nurse is to assess for:
A. equipment failure.
B. an obstructed or kinked endotracheal tube.
C. a pneumothorax.
D. a displaced endotracheal tube.

Rationale

A. Assessing for possible equipment failure is part of the DOPE mnemonic (Displaced, Obstructed, Pneumothorax, Equipment); however, the first intervention is to assess for possible endotracheal tube displacement.

B. Although it is important to assess patency of the endotracheal tube, the primary intervention is to first check for correct placement of the endotracheal tube.

C. Although it is important to assess for the presence of a possible pneumothorax as indicated by the DOPE mnemonic (Displaced, Obstructed, Pneumothorax, Equipment), the first intervention is to assess for possible endotracheal tube displacement.

D. A capnography reading of 84 mm Hg indicates severe hypoventilation with carbon dioxide retention. Assessing for the presence of a displaced endotracheal tube is the primary reevaluation of the placement and effectiveness of an endotracheal tube as indicated by the troubleshooting mnemonic DOPE (Displaced, Obstructed, Pneumothorax, Equipment).

Category: Respiratory Emergencies/Obstruction
Nursing Process: Assessment

Reference

Gurney, D. (2014). Airway and ventilation. In D. Gurney (Ed.), *Trauma Nursing Core Course: Provider manual* (7th ed., pp. 55–72). Des Plaines, IL: Emergency Nurses Association.

---

29. Which patient statement indicates that additional patient education is required for a patient with chronic liver disease and a pleural effusion?

A. "My shortness of breath was caused by my cirrhosis."
B. "I can change my diet to avoid shortness of breath."
C. "I can use my inhaler when I feel short of breath."
D. "If my shortness of breath gets bad enough, I may need a chest tube thoracostomy."

Rationale

A. Chronic liver disease leads to a low amount of albumin found in the blood, known as hypoalbuminemia. Albumin is necessary in maintaining oncotic pressure, which pulls water into the circulatory system. As albumin levels decrease, so does the oncotic pressure, allowing intravascular fluid to move out of capillaries and into the pleural space.

B. Malnutrition may lead to hypoalbuminemia, causing a decreased oncotic pressure, thus allowing fluid to shift into the pleural space. The risk of pleural effusions can be decreased by maintaining good nutrition and adhering to dietary restrictions necessary for management of chronic disease.

C. Pleural effusions are an abnormal collection of fluid in the pleural space. Inhalers work by promoting bronchodilation or reducing inflammation in the airways and would not be beneficial in managing symptoms related to pleural effusions.

D. A chest tube thoracostomy may be required if a pleural effusion is large, causing respiratory distress or accumulating rapidly.

Category: Respiratory Emergencies/Pleural effusion
Nursing Process: Evaluation

Reference

Walsh, R. (2013). Respiratory emergencies. In B. B. Hammond & P. G. Zimmermann (Eds.), *Sheehy's manual of emergency care* (7th ed., pp. 185–199). St. Louis, MO: Elsevier Mosby.

---

30. A patient experiences a fall from a horse and arrives via emergency medical services. The patient is complaining of severe right-sided chest pain with respiration. The patient is tachypneic, pulse oximetry is 90% on supplemental oxygen, and endotracheal intubation is immediately performed. Following initiation of mechanical ventilation, a decrease in the patient's blood pressure and a decrease in the oxygen saturation are observed. The emergency nurse identifies that the most likely cause of this sudden change in the patient is related to:

A. adverse reaction to sedation medication.
B. dislodged endotracheal tube.
C. development of a tension pneumothorax.
D. inadequate mechanical ventilation.

Rationale

A. Sedation medications may cause a decrease in blood pressure but would not have an effect of the oxygen saturation of a mechanically ventilated patient.

B. Dislodgement of an endotracheal tube would result in decreased oxygen saturation because of inadequate ventilation, and a subsequent decrease in cardiac output because of depleting oxygen reserves. In contrast, the building intrathoracic pressure that occurs with a tension pneumothorax results in decreased cardiac output, which will manifest as hypotension and poor tissue perfusion.

C. Because barotrauma is a complication of mechanical ventilation, patients requiring ventilation must be frequently assessed for development of a pneumothorax. The decline in hemodynamics indicates that a life-threatening emergency known as a tension pneumothorax is occurring. Increasing intrathoracic pressure compresses the lungs, heart, and great vessels, resulting in markedly decreased cardiac output, ventilation, and tissue perfusion.

D. Inadequate ventilation would result in decreased oxygen saturation and a subsequent decrease in cardiac output because of depleting oxygen reserves. In contrast, the building intrathoracic pressure that occurs with a tension pneumothorax results in decreased cardiac output, which will manifest as hypotension and poor tissue perfusion.

Category: Respiratory Emergencies/Pneumothorax

Nursing Process: Analysis

References

Everson, F. P. (2013). Chest trauma. In B. B. Hammond & P. G. Zimmermann (Eds.), Sheehy's manual of emergency care (7th ed., pp. 407–417). St. Louis, MO: Elsevier Mosby.

O'Neal, J. V. (2013). Airway management. In B. B. Hammond & P. G. Zimmermann (Eds.), *Sheehy's manual of emergency care* (7th ed., pp. 77–88). St. Louis, MO: Elsevier Mosby.

---

31. A hypoxic patient presents to the emergency department. The patient is immediately stabilized, and arterial blood gases are then drawn. Results are: pH 7.47; pCO_2 33 mm Hg; HCO_3 24 mEq/L. The emergency nurse recognizes these values indicate which of the following abnormalities?

A. Respiratory acidosis
B. Respiratory alkalosis
C. Metabolic acidosis
D. Metabolic alkalosis

Rationale

A. The pH is elevated, indicating alkalosis.

B. The low pCO_2 with an elevated pH is an indication of respiratory alkalosis.

C. The pH is elevated, showing alkalosis, and HCO_3 is normal, indicating that the driving force is the respiratory system, not the metabolic system.

D. The HCO_3 is normal, showing that the driving force of imbalance is related to the respiratory system, not the metabolic system.

Category: Respiratory Emergencies/Pulmonary edema, noncardiac

Nursing Process: Analysis

Reference

Walsh, R. (2013). Respiratory emergencies. In B. B. Hammond & P. G. Zimmermann (Eds.), *Sheehy's manual of emergency care* (7th ed., pp. 185–199). St. Louis, MO: Elsevier Mosby.

---

32. When a thromboemboli forms following long periods of immobility, this condition is referred to as:

A. endothelial injury.
B. pulmonary vascular pressure.
C. hypercoagulable state.
D. venous stasis.

Rationale

A. Endothelial injury is a major risk factor for thromboemboli formation. It is caused by damage to the innermost layer of a vein or artery from trauma, burns, surgery, or infection.

B. Increased pulmonary vascular pressure results in pulmonary edema and does not contribute to thromboemboli formation.

C. Hypercoagulable states are a major risk factor for thromboemboli formation. Contributing factors include postpartum period, contraceptive use, malignancy, major surgery, and disease processes.

D. Venous stasis is a major risk factor for thromboemboli formation. Heart failure, limb immobilization, prolonged lying or sitting, obesity, pregnancy, and venous insufficiency can result in venous stasis.

Category: Respiratory Emergencies/Pulmonary embolus

Nursing Process: Assessment

Reference

Walsh, R. (2013). Respiratory emergencies. In B. B. Hammond & P. G. Zimmermann (Eds.), *Sheehy's manual of emergency care* (7th ed., pp. 185–199). St. Louis, MO: Elsevier Mosby.

---

33. The emergency nurse is caring for a patient with pulmonary embolism. An order is expected for which of the following diagnostic tests?

A. Spiral computed tomography (CT) scan
B. Chest radiograph
C. Ventilation/perfusion scan
D. Chest CT scan without intravenous contrast

Rationale

A. A CT scan is the recommended study for evaluating the perfusion of blood through the lungs to identify the presence of a pulmonary embolism. Using intravenous (IV) contrast, CT angiography has the sensitivity and specificity comparable to that of contrast pulmonary angiography.

B. A chest radiograph (CXR) may be used for preliminary findings; however, it does not provide the detail needed for diagnosis of a pulmonary embolism. On rare occasions, the CXR may show a dilation of the pulmonary vessels proximal to an embolism, along with collapse of distal vessels referred to as Westermark's sign.

C. Although performing a ventilation/perfusion scan is an option for patients with allergies to IV contrast or when a multidetector CT angiography is not available, it is not the recommended study for diagnosis of a pulmonary embolism.

D. Without timed contrast to evaluate blood flow through the lungs, a chest CT scan may be unable to detect the presence of a pulmonary embolism.

Category: Respiratory Emergencies/Pulmonary embolus
Nursing Process: Intervention

Reference

Walsh, R. (2013). Respiratory emergencies. In B. B. Hammond & P. G. Zimmermann (Eds.), *Sheehy's manual of emergency care* (7th ed., pp. 185–199). St. Louis, MO: Elsevier Mosby.

---

34. A patient presents to the emergency department with severe dyspnea. The arterial blood gas results are: pH 7.51; pCO_2 26 mm Hg; HCO_3 24 mEq/L. The emergency nurse interprets these results to indicate the presence of:

A. respiratory alkalosis.
B. metabolic alkalosis.
C. respiratory acidosis.
D. metabolic acidosis.

Rationale

A. The pH is high, indicating alkalosis; the pCO_2 is low, indicating that the cause is not metabolic but the result of the patient's respiratory status.

B. The pH is high, indicating alkalosis; the pCO_2 is low, indicating that the cause is respiratory; and the HCO_3 remains within normal limits of 22 mEq/L–26 mEq/L. For the arterial blood gas result to indicate metabolic alkalosis, the HCO_3 would need to be greater than 26 mEq/L.

C. The pH is high, indicating alkalosis. The pCO_2 is low, indicating that the cause is respiratory; the pCO_2 is low, indicating that the patient is retaining CO_2, and the cause is respiratory because the result is less than 35; and the HCO_3 is within normal limits of 22 mEq/L–26 mEq/L, indicating the cause of the patient's abnormal values is not metabolic.

D. The pH is high, indicating alkalosis. The pCO_2 is low, indicating that the cause is respiratory. For acidosis to occur, the pH would need to be below 7.35. The pCO_2 is low, indicating that the patient is retaining CO_2, and the cause is respiratory. The HCO_3 remains stable, indicating that the blood is being adequately buffered by HCO_3 from the kidneys.

Category: Respiratory Emergencies/Pulmonary embolus
Nursing Process: Analysis

Reference

Walsh, R. (2013). Respiratory emergencies. In B. B. Hammond & P. G. Zimmermann (Eds.), *Sheehy's manual of emergency care* (7th ed., pp. 185–199). St. Louis, MO: Elsevier Mosby.

35. In a patient with acute respiratory distress syndrome, the goal of using a low tidal volume with mechanical ventilation is to:

A. wean the patient from the ventilator.
B. achieve normal blood gas values.
C. prevent volutrauma.
D. prevent ventilator–patient dyssynchrony.

Rationale

A. Weaning the patient from the ventilator is not the goal of low tidal ventilation; the goal of low tidal ventilation is to prevent further lung injury so that the patient can be removed from the ventilator earlier than anticipated.

B. The goal of treatment in caring for a patient with acute respiratory distress syndrome (ARDS) is to provide the best oxygenation possible without further injury to lung tissue. A patient with ARDS will not have normal blood gas values.

C. High tidal volumes can lead to ventilator-associated lung injury caused by overstretching of the lung tissue.

D. Ventilator–patient dyssynchrony is caused by spontaneous breathing during mechanical ventilation and can lead to lack of control of the tidal volumes being delivered.

Category: Respiratory Emergencies/Respiratory distress syndrome
Nursing Process: Analysis

Reference

Guo, R., & Fan, E. (2014). Beyond low tidal volumes: Ventilating the patient with acute respiratory distress syndrome. In L. B. Ware, J. A. Bastarache, & C. S. Calfee (Eds.), *Acute respiratory distress syndrome* (pp. 729–741). Philadelphia, PA: Elsevier.

---

36. A patient who has been stabbed in the right chest arrives to the emergency department via emergency medical services. On assessment, the emergency nurse identifies the presence of a hissing sound with inspiration. The nurse applies a dressing, taped on three sides to the stab wound site. Which of the following indicates to the emergency nurse that this treatment has been effective?

A. Decreased breath sounds
B. Increase in PaO_2 level
C. Increase in respiratory rate
D. Increase in $PaCO_2$ level

Rationale

A. In the presence of a pneumothorax that has the potential to become a tension pneumothorax, an increase in the presence of breath sounds indicates a positive patient response to the intervention. A decrease in breath sounds is an indication of continued deterioration of the patient's condition.

B. An improvement in the patient's PaO_2 level is an indication that the patient's oxygenation and gas exchange have improved.

C. The patient should experience a respiratory rate decrease in response to the intervention.

D. Continued retention of $PaCO_2$ indicates that the patient is experiencing hypercapnia and continued respiratory difficulty with inadequate gas exchange.

Category: Respiratory Emergencies/Trauma

Nursing Process: Evaluation

References

Day, M. W. (2014). Thoractic and neck trauma. In D. Gurney (Ed.), *Trauma Nursing Core Course: Provider manual* (7th ed., pp. 137–150). Des Plaines, IL: Emergency Nurses Association.

Denke, N. (2010). Thoracic trauma. In P. K. Howard & R. A. Steinmann (Eds.), *Sheehy's emergency nursing: Principles and practice* (6th ed., pp. 285–300). St. Louis, MO: Mosby Elsevier.

---

37. Which assessment test is the most specific in the diagnosis of multiple sclerosis?

A. Cognitive assessment (processing speed, complex attention, executive function)

B. Respiratory assessment (lung sounds, rate and pattern, cough)

C. Cranial nerve assessment

D. Cardiac assessment

Rationale

A. Patients with multiple sclerosis (MS) will experience cognitive difficulty approximately 40–60% of time in the early stages of the disease course before the development of other symptoms. A balance assessment is also useful in the diagnosis of MS.

B. This is a component of the emergency nurse's standard patient assessment and does not assist in the diagnosis of MS.

C. This assessment is helpful in cranial nerve disorders such as Bell's palsy but is not beneficial in the diagnosis of MS.

D. This should be part of the emergency department nurse's standard assessment but does not assist in the diagnosis of MS.

Category: Neurological Emergencies/Chronic neurological disorders

Nursing Process: Assessment

References

Faguy, K. (2016). Multiple sclerosis: An update. *Radiologic Technology, 87*(5), 529–553.

Niccolai, C., Portaccio, E., Goretti, B., Hakiki, B., Giannini, M., Pastò, L., . . . Viterbo, R. G. (2015). A comparison of the brief international cognitive assessment for multiple sclerosis and the brief repeatable battery in multiple sclerosis patients. *BMC Neurology, 15*, 1–5. https://doi.org/10.1186/s12883-015-0460-8

---

38. A patient presents to the emergency department with complaints of a urinary tract infection. The patient's medical history indicates a diagnosis of multiple sclerosis (MS) within the previous 5 years. Which of the following clinical signs would suggest that the MS treatment the patient has been receiving with interferon has had the desired effect?

A. Urinary incontinence

B. Lower extremity spasticity

C. Resolution of visual disturbances

D. Paresthesia in bilateral feet

Rationale

A. The most common symptoms of MS include sensory disturbances of the extremities, spasticity, weakness of the legs, bowel and bladder dysfunction, ataxia, and paresthesia. The presence of urinary incontinence would indicate that treatment with interferon has not had the desired effect.

B. The most common symptoms of MS include sensory disturbances of the extremities, spasticity, weakness of the legs, bowel and bladder dysfunction, ataxia, and paresthesia. The presence of lower extremity spasticity would indicate that the patient's treatment with interferon has not had the desired effect.

C. Initial signs and symptoms for MS include blurred vision, diplopia, red-green color distortion, and possible blindness in one eye. Frequently, complete remission of the patient's initial symptoms occurs with interferon treatment.

D. The most common symptoms of MS include sensory disturbances of the extremities, spasticity, weakness of the legs, bowel and bladder dysfunction, ataxia, and paresthesia. The presence of bilateral paresthesia in the patient's feet would indicate that treatment with interferon has not had the desired effect.

Category: Neurological Emergencies/Chronic neurological disorders

Nursing Process: Evaluation

Reference

Dunphy, L., Winland-Brown, J., Porter, B., & Thomas, D. (2015). *Primary care: The art and science of advanced practice nursing* (4th ed.). Philadelphia, PA: F. A. Davis.

---

39. A patient previously diagnosed with Guillain–Barré syndrome presents to the emergency department with a complaint of progressive weakness and tingling of both upper and lower extremities over the past several weeks. The patient is now complaining of difficulty breathing. Vital signs: BP 130/80 mm Hg; HR 92 beats/minute; RR 28 breaths/minute; SpO_2 90% on room air. Which of the following interventions is most appropriate at this time?

A. Monitor the depth and adequacy of respirations
B. Prepare for an electromyogram
C. Administer immune globulin
D. Prepare for plasmapheresis

Rationale

A. There is potential for hypoventilation because of the patient's respiratory muscle weakness, so careful monitoring of the patient's respiratory pattern is important. Mechanical ventilation may be required until the patient's respiratory muscle weakness spontaneously resolves, which is generally weeks after its onset.

B. Electromyograms are used to identify peripheral nerve demyelination to establish a diagnosis; however, it is not an emergent diagnostic study. In addition, performing a diagnostic study will not treat the patient's current symptoms of increasing muscle weakness.

C. Intravenous immune globulin is frequently given to Guillain–Barré syndrome patients, but this will not immediately treat the patient's symptoms of hypoventilation.

D. Plasmapheresis may be prescribed, but this will not immediately treat the patient's symptoms of hypoventilation.

Category: Neurological Emergencies/Guillain–Barré syndrome

Nursing Process: Intervention

References

Guillain–Barré syndrome (GBS). (n.d.). GBS/CIDP Foundation International. Retrieved from https://www.gbs-cidp.org/gbs

Walsh, R. (2013). Neurologic emergencies. In B. B. Hammond & P. G. Zimmerman (Eds.), *Sheehy's manual of emergency care* (7th ed., pp. 265–274). St. Louis, MO: Elsevier Mosby.

---

40. A patient presents complaining of a headache that feels like someone is squeezing their head in a grip. They say that this type of headache occurs every month. There are no associated signs and symptoms. The emergency nurse is aware that the patient is describing which type of headache?

A. **Tension headache**
B. Migraine headache
C. Subcortical headache
D. Cluster headache

Rationale

A. A tension headache is associated with a report of tightening- or squeezing-type pain. It is frequently described as being a dull nonpulsating pain that begins in the occipital area and moves bilaterally to the frontal region.

B. A migraine headache is most often unilateral, has a pulsating quality, and rarely occurs without other associated symptoms such as nausea or photophobia.

C. Subcortical means below the cortex of the brain and is not a type of headache.

D. A cluster headache causes a severe sharp burning sensation. The associated pain is excruciating and results in tearing and nasal congestion with redness of the eye, diaphoresis, and pallor.

Category: Neurological Emergencies/Headache

Nursing Process: Assessment

References

Baxter, C. S. Neurologic emergencies (2007). In K. S. Hoyt & J. Selfridge-Thomas (Eds.), *Emergency nursing core curriculum* (6th ed., pp. 510–535). St. Louis, MO: Saunders Elsevier.

Brown, A., & King, D. (2010). Neurologic emergencies. In P. K. Howard & R. Steinmann (Eds.), *Sheehy's emergency nursing: Principles and practice* (6th ed., pp. 457–466). St. Louis, MO: Mosby Elsevier.

41. The nurse is discharging a patient following treatment for a migraine headache. The patient discharge medications include sodium valproic acid (Depakote) to be used as a prophylaxis for the treatment of migraine headache. Which of the following statements by the patient indicate the need for further teaching?

A. "The doctor says my liver function tests are normal."
B. "I should avoid medications with aspirin."
C. "My boyfriend and I are not using birth control right now."
D. "If I develop abdominal pain, I will call my doctor."

Rationale

A. Before valproic acid is prescribed, the provider screens the patient and checks liver function tests.

B. Aspirin increases the concentration of valproic acid.

C. Valproic acid is considered one of the most teratogenic drugs. It can result in neural tube, cardiac, and facial defects; therefore, birth control measures are indicated when taking this medication.

D. Patients who are taking valproic acid are at risk of developing abdominal pain secondary to the presence of pancreatitis.

Category: Neurological Emergencies/Headache

Nursing Process: Evaluation

Reference

Collins-Yoder, A., & Lowell, J. (2017). Valproic acid: Special considerations and targeted monitoring. *Journal of Neuroscience Nursing, 49*(1), 59–60.

---

42. Following a traumatic brain injury, a patient is being treated with mannitol (Osmitrol) for increased intracranial pressure secondary to brain herniation. The emergency nurse is aware that mannitol can result in which of the following abnormalities?

A. Increasing serum creatinine
B. Hyperkalemia
C. Hyponatremia
D. Metabolic alkalosis

Rationale

A. Mannitol can cause acute renal failure, resulting in an increase of serum creatinine if intravascular volume is not replaced. The most common acid–base balance imbalance is metabolic acidosis. It can also exacerbate heart failure and asthma symptoms because of pulmonary congestion that results from an initial episode of fluid retention.

B. The most common electrolyte abnormalities include hypernatremia and hypokalemia. The most common acid–base balance imbalance is metabolic acidosis.

C. The most common electrolyte abnormalities include hypernatremia and hypokalemia. The most common acid–base balance imbalance is metabolic acidosis. In addition, mannitol can cause acute renal failure if intravascular volume is not replaced, as well as exacerbate heart failure and asthma symptoms because of pulmonary congestion that results from an initial episode of fluid retention.

D. Mannitol is a potent diuretic with numerous side effects that cause electrolyte and acid–base imbalances and other abnormalities. The most common acid–base imbalance is metabolic acidosis. The most common electrolyte abnormalities include hypernatremia and hypokalemia. In addition, mannitol can cause acute renal failure if intravascular volume is not replaced, as well as exacerbate heart failure and asthma symptoms because of pulmonary congestion that results from an initial episode of fluid retention.

Category: Neurological Emergencies/Increased intracranial pressure (ICP)

Nursing Process: Analysis

Reference

Shawkat, H., Westwood, M. M., & Mortimer, A. (2012). Mannitol: A review of its clinical uses. *Continuing Education in Anesthesia, Critical Care, & Pain, 12*(2), 82–85.

---

43. A patient arrives to the emergency department and is diagnosed with a brain tumor. Interventions are provided to treat the patient's increased intracranial pressure. Which statement made by the family indicates to the emergency nurse that additional education on the patient's condition is required?

A. "Talking quietly and holding hands is helpful."
B. "Lying down to rest is important."
C. "Shaking and stiffness is an emergency."
D. "Speaking may be slow or difficult."

Rationale

A. Intracranial pressure may increase because of noxious stimuli such as suctioning, rectal temperatures, pain, or agitation. Reassurance and closeness of family provides a soothing, calming presence.

B. Maintaining a 30-degree or higher elevation of the head promotes drainage of cerebrospinal fluid and/or blood, resulting in decreasing intracranial pressure. The family requires education on proper positioning, which also includes keeping the head and neck aligned to further promote drainage.

C. Seizures are a complication of increased intracranial pressure and may indicate declining neurological status. Families participate in care by learning to recognize situations that require intervention.

D. Varying centers of the brain may be affected by increased pressure or tumor location. Families should be aware that personality, behavior, or speech may be different.

Category: Neurological Emergencies/Increased intracranial pressure (ICP)

Nursing Process: Evaluation

Reference

March, K. S., & Hickey, J. V. (2014). Intracranial hypertension: Theory and management of increased intracranial pressure. In J. V. Hickey, *The clinical practice of neurological and neurosurgical nursing* (7th ed.) [Kindle version]. Philadelphia, PA: Lippincott Williams & Wilkins.

44. A young adult presents to the emergency department complaining of a headache, fever, petechial rash, and neck pain. Which action should the emergency personnel perform before any further contact with this patient?

A. Send a lab specimen to confirm diagnosis
B. Initiate an intravenous access
C. Don personal protective equipment
D. Initiate administration of third-generation cephalosporin and dexamethasone

Rationale

A. Lab confirmation of the diagnosis is low on the list of priorities for this patient. The patient will require a lumbar puncture to confirm the diagnosis of meningococcemia. Meningitis can be fatal up to 56% of the time and has a high morbidity.

B. An intravenous access is priority; however, protection of the team is the first priority before proceeding with further patient care.

C. This patient has a high degree of suspicion for meningococcemia, which is most commonly spread by respiratory droplet. The first priority is for the team to don personal protective equipment. To minimize the risk of exposure, the patient should be placed in respiratory isolation as indicated.

D. These are the drugs of choice for treatment of meningococcemia, but the first priority is protection of the team with PPE.

Category: Neurological Emergencies/Meningitis

Nursing Process: Intervention

References

Richard, G. C., & Lepe, M. (2013). Meningitis in children: Diagnosis and treatment for the emergency clinician. *Clinical Pediatric Emergency Medicine, 14*(2),146–156. http://dx.doi.org/10.1016/j.cpem.2013.04.008

Viale, P., Scudeller, L., Pea, F., Tedeschi, S., Lewis, R., Bartoletti, M., . . . Giannella, M. (2015). Implementation of a meningitis care bundle in the emergency room reduces mortality associated with acute bacterial meningitis. *Annals of Pharmacotherapy, 49*(9), 978–985. https://doi.org/10.1177/1060028015586012

---

45. Which patient would be most appropriate to receive levetiracetam (Keppra) for seizure prophylaxis?

A. A patient with an epidural hematoma
B. A patient with a subarachnoid hemorrhage
C. A patient with a subdural hematoma
D. A patient with a cerebral contusion

Rationale

A. Levetiracetam is indicated for seizure prophylaxis in patients with traumatic brain injury and diagnosed with a subdural hematoma. There has been no benefit shown in seizure prophylaxis for patients diagnosed with an epidural hematoma.

B. There has been no benefit shown in seizure prophylaxis for patients diagnosed with a subarachnoid hemorrhage. Levetiracetam is indicated for seizure prophylaxis in patients with traumatic brain injury and those diagnosed with a subdural hematoma. The duration of treatment is 7 days.

C. Levetiracetam (Keppra) is indicated for seizure prophylaxis in patients with traumatic brain injury and those diagnosed with a subdural hematoma. The duration of treatment is 7 days. There has been no benefit shown in seizure prophylaxis for patients diagnosed with other forms of traumatic brain injury.

D. Levetiracetam is indicated for seizure prophylaxis in patients with traumatic brain injury and diagnosed with a subdural hematoma. There has been no benefit shown in seizure prophylaxis for patients diagnosed with a cerebral contusion.

Category: Neurological Emergencies/Seizure disorders

Nursing Process: Analysis

Reference

Patanwala, A. E. (2016). Low-dose levetiracetam for seizure prophylaxis after traumatic brain injury. *Brain Injury, 30*(2), 156–158. https://doi.org/10.3109/02699052.215.1089596

---

46. Which of the following children would require 24-hour observation following a tonic–clonic seizure while in the emergency department?

A. A 2-year-old child with a history of seizures who has experienced two seizures that required the administration of rectal diazepam (Valium) to control the seizure activity.

B. A 4-year-old child with no history of a seizure disorder who has had two tonic–clonic seizures that required antiepileptic medications to be administered for control of the seizure activity.

C. A 1-year-old infant who had a tonic–clonic seizure at home, was diagnosed by the emergency provider as having otitis media (middle ear infection), and required acetaminophen (Tylenol) for a fever of 40°C (104°F).

D. An 11-year-old child with a first-time seizure that self-resolved without further treatment.

Rationale

A. Provided that parents are comfortable managing this patient (evidenced by the administration of diazepam), this child can be safely managed as an outpatient. Parents who demonstrate a familiarity with managing their child's seizure activity, as evidenced by the administration of rectal diazepam, can safely manage the child as an outpatient; therefore, the child should not require hospitalization.

B. Any child with no history of seizures who requires antiepileptic medications for control of seizure activity while at the emergency department requires close observation.

C. A child who has experienced a febrile seizure will not normally require hospitalization unless the child required the administration of antiepileptic medications to be administered for the presence of status epilepticus.

D. It is considered standard of care to discharge patients who have experienced a first-time seizure and whose results of the diagnostic studies are all within normal limits.

Category (Pediatric): Neurological Emergencies/Seizure disorders

Nursing Process: Analysis

References

Chen, C., Yang, W., Wu, K., & Wu, H. (2012). Clinical assessment of children with first-attack seizures admitted to the ED. *American Journal of Emergency Medicine, 30*(7), 1080–1088. http://dx.doi.org/10.1016/j.ajem.2011.07.008

Friese, G., & Collopy, K. (2010). Febrile seizures. *EMS Magazine, 39*(5), 52–57.

Yamamoto, L., Olaes, E., & Lopez, A. (2004). Challenges in seizure management: Neurologic versus cardiac emergencies. *Topics in Emergency Medicine, 26*(3), 212–224.

---

47. The parent of an 18-month-old arrives to the emergency department stating that the child has had projectile vomiting for the past 24 hours. There is no history of fever or diarrhea. The parent states that their child has a ventriculoperitoneal shunt but no other medical history. The emergency nurse anticipates that the most likely cause of the child vomiting is related to which of the following?

A. Diabetic ketoacidosis
B. Gastroenteritis
C. Shunt malfunction
D. Head injury

Rationale

A. There is no history of diabetes, so the presence of diabetic ketoacidosis is very unlikely.

B. Although gastroenteritis causes vomiting, it can also result in diarrhea, which this child does not have. The history of a ventriculoperitoneal (VP) shunt contributes to the likelihood that the patient's projectile vomiting is related to increased intracranial pressure secondary to the shunt being clotted or dislodged.

C. VP shunts from brain to peritoneum can become occluded or displaced, requiring replacement as a child grows. The malfunctioning shunt results in hydrocephalus and the signs and symptoms of increased intracranial pressure, such as an altered level of consciousness, tense fontanelles (in children under 18 months), and projectile vomiting.

D. There is no history of a recent traumatic brain injury or assessment findings to indicate this is the cause of the patient's vomiting.

Category: Neurological Emergencies/Shunt dysfunctions

Nursing Process: Assessment

References

Cohen, J. S., Jamal, N., Dawes, C., Chamberlain, J. M., & Atabaki, S. M. (2014). Cranial computed tomography utilization for suspected ventriculoperitoneal shunt malfunction in a pediatric emergency department. *Journal of Emergency Medicine, 46*(4), 449–455. https://doi.org/10.1016/j.jemermed.2013.08.137

Mater, A., Shroff, M., Al-Farsi, S., Drake, J., & Goldman, R. D. (2008). Test characteristics of neuroimaging in the emergency department evaluation of children for cerebrospinal fluid shunt malfunction. *CJEM: Canadian Journal of Emergency Medicine, 10*(2), 131–135.

48. A patient who sustained a low-velocity fall presents to the emergency department via emergency medical services in full cervical spine precautions. There is an obvious smell of alcohol on their breath. The patient denies any neck pain and can move all extremities. Based on the Nexus criteria, the nurse should:

A. remove the spinal immobilization and allow the patient to sit upright to protect the airway.
B. remove the spine board and keep the patient flat.
C. remove the spinal immobilization and keep the patient flat.
D. await physician exam before removing spinal immobilization.

Rationale

A. This patient is potentially intoxicated, so these criteria may not be used to evaluate for the presence of a cervical spine injury.

B. This patient is potentially intoxicated, so these criteria may not be used to evaluate for the presence of a cervical spine injury.

C. This patient is potentially intoxicated, so these criteria may not be used to evaluate for the presence of a cervical spine injury.

D. The NEXUS criteria state that a patient with suspected cervical spine injury can be cleared providing the following are present: (1) No posterior midline cervical spine tenderness is present; (2) no evidence of intoxication is present; (3) the patient has a normal level of alertness; and (4) no focal neurologic deficit is present. This patient is potentially intoxicated, so these criteria may not be used to evaluate for the presence of a cervical spine injury.

Category: Neurological Emergencies/Spinal cord injuries

Nursing Process: Intervention

References

Crowley, M. (2014). Spinal cord and vertebral column trauma. In D. Gurney (Ed.), *Trauma Nursing Core Course: Provider manual* (7th ed., pp. 173–192). Des Plaines, IL: Emergency Nurses Association.

Davenport, M. (2016). Cervical spine fracture workup. *Medscape*. Retrieved from http://emedicine.medscape.com/article/824380-workup

---

49. A 5-year-old presents with an axial loading injury after diving head first into a shallow pool. The child is unable to move their arms or legs. The radiologic studies of the cervical, thoracic, and lumbar spine are negative for any acute injury. The emergency nurse is aware that the diagnostic study that will provide a clearer diagnosis of the actual injury is:

A. a magnetic resonance imaging study of the cervical spine.
B. a computed tomography scan study.
C. a 3-dimensional ultrasound.
D. repeat radiologic study of the neck.

Rationale

A. Magnetic resonance imaging (MRI) studies are the gold standard to determine extent and presence of spinal cord imaging. Early imaging in patients with a suspected spinal cord injury can decrease a patient's length of stay.

B. A computed tomography scan is useful for diagnosis of a bone injury such as a fracture, but it does not identify soft tissue injury. An MRI study differentiates between bone injuries and soft tissue injuries.

C. A 3-dimensional ultrasound study is not helpful in initial diagnosis and management of a spinal cord injury.

D. These studies may be useful after the initial recovery period but will not aid in the diagnosis of a soft tissue injury.

Category: Neurological Emergencies/Spinal cord injuries

Nursing Process: Analysis

Reference

Easter, J. S., Barkin, R., Rosen, C. L., & Ban, K. (2011). Cervical spine injuries in children, Part II: Management and special considerations. *Journal of Emergency Medicine*, *41*(3), 252–256. https://doi.org/10.1016/j.jemermed.2010.03.018

---

50. A patient arrives at the emergency department with right-sided hemiparesis and expressive aphasia. The most important information for the emergency nurse to obtain is:

A. history of recent trauma.
B. patient allergies.
C. the last time the patient was seen in their usual state of health.
D. history of recent surgery.

Rationale

A. Although recent trauma may be considered an exclusion to the administration of tissue plasminogen activator (TPA), it must first be determined if the patient is within the treatment window of 3 to 4.5 hours for certain eligible patients to receive this drug.

B. Although allergies are important, the ability to administer TPA safely requires knowing the last time the patient was seen in usual state of health.

C. The last time seen in usual state of health will help to determine if this patient is a candidate to receive TPA. The patient is considered within the treatment window if "last seen well" is 3 to 4.5 hours in eligible patients.

D. Although recent surgery may be considered an exclusion to TPA, first we must determine if the patient is within the treatment window of 3 to 4.5 hours for certain eligible patients to receive this drug.

Category: Neurological Emergencies/Stroke (ischemic or hemorrhagic)

Nursing Process: Assessment

References

Hemphill, J. C., Greenberg, S. M., Anderson, C. S., Becker, K., Bendok, B. R., Cushman, M., . . . Wood, D.; American Heart Association Stroke Council, Council on Cardiovascular and Stroke Nursing, and Council on Clinical Cardiology. (2015). Guidelines for the management of spontaneous intracerebral hemorrhage: A guideline for healthcare professionals from the American Heart Association/American Stroke Association. *Stroke, 46*(7), 2032–2060. https://doi.org/10.1161/STR.0000000000000069

Powers, W. J., Derdeyn, C. P., Biller, J., Coffey, C. S., Hoh, B. L., Jauch, E. C., . . .Yavagal, D. R.; American Stroke Association Stroke Council. (2015). 2015 AHA/ASA focused update of the 2013 guidelines for the early management of patients with acute ischemic stroke regarding endovascular treatment: A guideline for healthcare professionals from the American Heart Association/American Stroke Association. *Stroke, 46*(10):3020–3035. https://doi.org/10.1161/STR.0000000000000074

---

51. An adolescent is being discharged from the emergency department following a mild traumatic brain injury. Which of the following instructions must be included at discharge?

A. As long as the adolescent did not experience a loss of consciousness, they may return to their usual activities.

B. The adolescent should rest from activities such as playing video games, texting, watching TV, and doing schoolwork.

C. As long as the adolescent is headache free, they can resume their normal activities.

D. The only activity the adolescent should avoid is contact sports; all other activities are permitted.

Rationale

A. Only 10% of patients with an mTBI experience a loss of consciousness; however, the patient still has a brain injury that occurred without a loss of consciousness.

B. A mild traumatic brain injury (mTBI) is a functional brain injury and requires both physical and cognitive rest.

C. Concussions may take 7–10 days or longer to resolve.

D. An mTBI is a brain injury, and both physical and cognitive rest are important to support recovery.

Category (Pediatric): Neurological Emergencies/Trauma

Nursing Process: Intervention

Reference

Cartwright, C. (2014). Pediatric athletic concussion. *Journal of Neuroscience Nursing, 46*(6), 313.

52. A patient presents to the trauma bay after being kicked in the head during a game of soccer and losing vision a short time later. The provider orders a computed tomography (CT) scan. The emergency nurse anticipates that the CT scan will show an abnormality in what lobe of the brain?

A. The occipital lobe

B. The frontal lobe

C. The temporal lobe

D. The parietal lobe

Rationale

A. The occipital lobe is responsible for vision and balance.

B. The frontal lobe is responsible for personality and motor function but not vision.

C. The temporal lobe is responsible for hearing but not vision.

D. The parietal lobe is responsible for sensory integration but not vision.

Category: Neurological Emergencies/Trauma

Nursing Process: Analysis

Reference

Rea, P. (2015). *Essential anatomy and function of the brain.* Philadelphia, PA: Elsevier.

53. A patient presents to the emergency department complaining of severe left lower abdominal pain and nausea and vomiting x1. The patient also denies a bowel movement in the past 4 days and has a history of diverticulitis. On exam, the abdomen is firm and rigid with rebound tenderness. Vital signs: BP 94/50 mm Hg; HR 112 beats/minute; RR 28 breaths/minute; T 38.7°C (101.6°F). The patient's symptoms are most consistent with:

A. appendicitis.
B. peritonitis.
C. pancreatitis.
D. peptic ulcer disease.

Rationale

A. Presentation of appendicitis would include a mild fever, periumbilical pain shifting to the right lower quadrant, nausea, and anorexia.

B. Peritonitis can occur when abdominal organs perforate and release their contents into the peritoneal cavity. Given the patient's history of diverticulitis, the clinical symptoms, and vital signs, the presentation of hypovolemic shock is most likely because of the massive shift of fluid into the peritoneum from bowel perforation, secondary to diverticulitis.

C. Pain with pancreatitis is generally located in the left upper abdomen or epigastrium and may radiate through to the back. The cause of pancreatitis is usually excessive ethanol ingestion or blockage of the common bile duct secondary to the presence of gallstones.

D. Peptic ulcer is generally the result of a disruption of the protective mucosal barriers and increased acid secretion. Symptoms include episodic gnawing or burning pain accompanied by a feeling of fullness or bloating. Pain may be relieved or exacerbated by food.

Category: Gastrointestinal, Genitourinary, Gynecology, and Obstetrical Emergencies/ Gastrointestinal/Acute abdomen

Nursing Process: Analysis

Reference

Wolf, L., & Zimmermann, P. G. (2013). Abdominal pain and emergencies. In B. B. Hammond & P. G. Zimmermann (Eds.), *Sheehy's manual of emergency care* (7th ed., pp. 291–301). St. Louis, MO: Elsevier Mosby.

54. A patient presents to the triage desk complaining of sharp right upper quadrant abdominal pain that radiates to the right shoulder, along with nausea and vomiting. The emergency nurse suspects this patient may have which clinical condition?

A. Infectious mononucleosis
B. Cholecystitis
C. Pancreatitis
D. Appendicitis

Rationale

A. Infectious mononucleosis is an acute viral illness. Symptoms include a sore throat and cervical lymphadenopathy. Abdominal tenderness resulting from splenomegaly or hepatomegaly may be present, but nausea and vomiting are not experienced.

B. Right upper quadrant pain that radiates to the right shoulder or scapula and is accompanied by nausea and vomiting is the characteristic presentation of cholecystitis.

C. The discomfort associated with pancreatitis is more likely to be described as dull, steady, and localized in the left upper abdomen or epigastrium.

D. The typical presentation of a patient with appendicitis includes periumbilical pain that localizes in the right lower quadrant and is associated with mild fever, anorexia, and nausea. The pain associated with appendicitis does not radiate to the right shoulder or scapula.

Category: Gastrointestinal, Genitourinary, Gynecology, and Obstetrical Emergencies/ Gastrointestinal/Cholecystitis

Nursing Process: Assessment

Reference

Wolf, L., & Zimmerman, P. G. (2013). Abdominal pain and emergencies. In B. B. Hammond & P. G. Zimmermann (Eds.), *Sheehy's manual of emergency care* (7th ed., pp. 291–301). St. Louis, MO: Elsevier Mosby.

---

55. A patient with a history of advanced hepatic disease presents to the emergency department. The patient's family reports that the patient has recently become more confused and now has slurred speech. The patient is diagnosed as having hepatic encephalopathy and is prescribed lactulose. The nurse can expect which of the following outcomes from the administration of this medication?

A. Decreased clotting time
B. Decreased liver enzymes
C. Elevated serum potassium
D. Decreased serum ammonia level

Rationale

A. The laxative effect of lactulose only removes ammonia produced in the intestines and does not affect the clotting functions of the liver. Therefore, the production of clotting factors by the liver would not be affected by the lactulose treatment.

B. Lactulose only removes ammonia from the intestines. It does not lessen the degree of hepatic disease.

C. Lactulose does not affect the serum potassium level; in fact, an excessive diarrhea effect of lactulose may cause the patient's serum potassium levels to decrease, resulting in hypokalemia.

D. Dietary proteins and intestinal bacteria produce ammonia. The cognitive changes associated with hepatic encephalopathy are because of the inability of the liver to convert this ammonia to urea so it can be eliminated from the body. In excessive quantity, ammonia is a central nervous system toxin. Lactulose reduces the ammonia produced in the intestines, and the laxative effect assists in eliminating the ammonia from the body, thereby reducing the serum ammonia level.

Category: Gastrointestinal, Genitourinary, Gynecology, and Obstetrical Emergencies/ Gastrointestinal/Cirrhosis

Nursing Process: Evaluation

References

Lilly, L. L., Collins, S. R., & Snyder, J. S. (2014). *Pharmacology and the nursing process* (7th ed.). St. Louis, MO: Elsevier.

Wolf, L., & Zimmermann, P. G. (2013). Abdominal pain and emergencies. In B. B. Hammond & P. G. Zimmermann (Eds.), *Sheehy's manual of emergency care* (7th ed., pp. 291–301). St. Louis, MO: Elsevier Mosby.

56. A patient presents to the emergency department complaining of cramping abdominal pain that has localized to the left lower quadrant. The patient's last bowel movement was 24 hours ago, and blood was noted in the stool. The emergency nurse suspects the patient may have:

A. acute pancreatitis.
B. diverticulitis.
C. appendicitis.
D. cholecystitis.

Rationale

A. Acute pancreatitis can be caused by an obstruction from gallstones, injury, or infection. The pain associated with pancreatitis is described as a sharp, boring-type pain that is localized in the epigastric area, with radiation to the chest and back.

B. Diverticulitis is an inflammation of the diverticuli of the colon, which can become obstructed with food or fecal matter. The pain associated with diverticulitis is typically described as cramping and is localized to the left lower abdominal quadrant. The patient may also experience constipation, fever, chills, nausea, and vomiting.

C. The pain associated with appendicitis usually begins in the periumbilical area and is diffuse in nature. Later, the pain localizes in the right lower abdominal quadrant.

D. Cholecystitis is an inflammation of the gallbladder. The pain is sharp and constant and occurs in the right upper quadrant, with radiation to the right shoulder or scapula. Symptoms frequently occur after ingesting a meal high in fat content.

Category: Gastrointestinal, Genitourinary, Gynecology, and Obstetrical Emergencies/ Gastrointestinal/Diverticulitis

Nursing Process: Assessment

Reference

Wolf, L., & Zimmermann, P. G. (2013). Abdominal pain and emergencies. In B. B. Hammond & P. G. Zimmermann (Eds.), *Sheehy's manual of emergency care* (7th ed., pp. 291–301). St. Louis, MO: Elsevier Mosby.

---

57. A 2-year-old child with a 48-hour history of vomiting and diarrhea is diagnosed with gastroenteritis. The child has been rehydrated in the emergency department and is currently taking fluids by mouth. Initial discharge dietary instructions should direct the child's parents to administer which of the following?

A. Small amounts of a glucose and electrolyte solution
B. Keep the child NPO for the next 24 hours
C. Provide a clear liquid diet of ice pops and apple juice
D. Resume normal eating habits

Rationale

A. This solution will help to replace needed electrolytes and minimize additional stomach irritation.

B. Patients who have been rehydrated and are able to take fluids by mouth are generally discharged with instructions to maintain a clear liquid diet.

C. This patient should be discharged with instructions for a clear liquid diet. Ice pops would be appropriate, but apple juice is hyperosmolar and would worsen the diarrhea.

D. The early resumption of a regular diet may cause additional stomach stimulation and can worsen symptoms of vomiting and diarrhea.

Category (Pediatric): Gastrointestinal Gastrointestinal, Genitourinary, Gynecology, and Obstetrical Emergencies/Gastrointestinal/Gastroenteritis

Nursing Process: Intervention

Reference

Mecham, N. L. (2010). Pediatric emergencies. In P. K. Howard & R. A. Steinmann (Eds.), *Sheehy's emergency nursing: Principles and practice* (6th ed., pp. 630–651). St. Louis, MO: Mosby Elsevier.

---

58. Which of the following statements made by a patient diagnosed with hepatitis A indicates an accurate understanding of their disease?

A. "There must be some mistake, I had the hepatitis vaccine as a baby."
B. "My partner is a recovering intravenous drug abuser. I may have gotten this after we had unprotected sex."
C. "I will be very careful to remember to wash my hands after using the bathroom and when preparing food."
D. "I must be careful from now on so that I don't get this disease again."

Rationale

A. The hepatitis B vaccine is administered to the pediatric population. The hepatitis A vaccine is recommended for anyone who plans to travel to, or reside for a long period of time in, an area where the population is at risk for hepatitis infection or after exposure to the hepatitis A virus.

B. Intravenous drug abusers are more likely to be infected with hepatitis B and can transmit that infection through unprotected sexual contact. Hepatitis A is acquired through the fecal–oral route, most often through ingestion of contaminated food or water.

C. Hepatitis A is spread by the fecal–oral route. Enteric precautions, such as handwashing after using the bathroom, are recommended for the first 2 weeks of the illness and for 1 week after the onset of jaundice.

D. Hepatitis A antibodies (IgG anti-HAV) appear early in the course of the disease and provide the patient with life-long protection against the disease. There is no chronic form of hepatitis A. The patient will have no immunity to other forms of hepatitis, such as hepatitis B or hepatitis C.

Category: Gastrointestinal, Genitourinary, Gynecology, and Obstetrical Emergencies/Gastrointestinal/Hepatitis

Nursing Process: Evaluation

References

Lai, M., & Chopra, S. (2013). Patient information: Hepatitis A (beyond the basics). *UpToDate.* Retrieved from http://www.uptodate.com/contents/hepatitis-a-beyond-the-basics

Short, W. R., Kemper, M., & Jackson, J. (2013). Infectious diseases. In B. B. Hammond & P. G. Zimmermann (Eds.), *Sheehy's manual of emergency care* (7th ed., pp. 233–243). St. Louis, MO: Elsevier Mosby.

59. A patient presents to triage complaining of severe abdominal pain that has worsened over the past 24 hours. The patient has recently started taking infliximab (Remicade). The emergency nurse suspects that the patient's symptoms may be related to which of the following conditions?

A. Diverticulitis
B. Peptic ulcer disease
C. Pancreatitis
D. Crohn's disease

Rationale

A. Treatment of diverticulitis includes rehydration and possibly antibiotics; a monoclonal antibody such as infliximab is not appropriate therapy for diverticulitis.

B. Treatment of peptic ulcer disease is likely to include the use of histamine (H2) blockers or proton pump inhibitors. Infliximab is not indicated as a treatment for peptic ulcer disease.

C. Treatment of pancreatitis includes intravenous fluids, pain management, antiemetics, and antibiotics. Infliximab is not the appropriate medication for pancreatitis.

D. Infliximab is a monoclonal antibody agent that is used for multiple inflammatory diseases. This drug is prescribed in the management of Crohn's disease.

Category: Gastrointestinal, Genitourinary, Gynecology, and Obstetrical Emergencies/Gastrointestinal/Inflammatory bowel disease

Nursing Process: Analysis

References

Lilley, L. L., Collins, S. R., & Snyder, J. S. (2014). *Pharmacology and the nursing process* (7th ed.). St. Louis, MO: Elsevier.

Wolf, L., & Zimmermann, P. G. (2013). Abdominal pain and emergencies. In B. B. Hammond & P. G. Zimmermann (Eds.), *Sheehy's manual of emergency care* (7th ed., pp. 291–301). St. Louis, MO: Elsevier Mosby.

---

60. Which of the following abnormal laboratory values would the nurse expect to find in a patient diagnosed with acute pancreatitis?

A. Decreased C-reactive protein
B. Elevated serum lipase
C. Elevated serum glucose
D. Decreased serum calcium

Rationale

A. An elevated C-reactive protein, an inflammatory marker, is a late indicator of pancreatic disease and usually is indicative of pancreatic necrosis.

B. Elevations in both serum amylase and serum lipase are highly suggestive of pancreatitis. The serum amylase will return to baseline quickly, whereas the serum lipase level will remain elevated for several days following the onset of symptoms, making it the more specific and sensitive indicator of acute pancreatitis.

C. Insulin secretion may be altered when the pancreas is inflamed, causing the patient to be hyperglycemic, but this is not a diagnostic indicator.

D. Hypocalcemia can occur as a complication of acute pancreatitis, but it is not a diagnostic indicator of the presence of acute pancreatitis.

Category: Gastrointestinal, Genitourinary, Gynecology, and Obstetrical Emergencies/ Gastrointestinal/Pancreatitis

Nursing Process: Assessment

References

Carroll, J. K., Herrick, B., Gipson, T., & Lee, S. P. (2007). Acute pancreatitis: Diagnosis, prognosis, and treatment. *American Family Physician, 75*(10), 1513–1520.

Herrington, A. (2010). Gastrointestinal emergencies. In P. K. Howard & R. A. Steinmann (Eds.), *Sheehy's emergency nursing: Principles and practice* (6th ed., pp. 467–477). St. Louis, MO: Mosby Elsevier.

Russoll, L. W. (2007). Abdominal emergencies. In K. S. Hoyt & J. Selfridge-Thomas (Eds.), *Emergency nursing core curriculum* (6th ed., pp. 159–186). St. Louis, MO: Saunders Elsevier.

---

61. Following a motor vehicle collision, a patient is brought to the emergency department via emergency medical services. The patient's assessment reveals the presence of lap belt restraint marks on the abdomen and absent bowel sounds, and the patient is complaining of epigastric pain. Based on these assessment findings, the emergency nurse suspects injury to which abdominal structure?

A. Liver
B. Urinary bladder
C. Duodenum
D. Stomach

Rationale

A. Liver injuries are more likely to occur as a result of a direct blow to the right upper quadrant. Injury to the liver will produce right upper quadrant pain, abdominal spasm, and rigidity. Based on the mechanism of injury in this patient, an intestinal injury is more likely.

B. Bladder injuries as a result of blunt trauma are unlikely unless the bladder was distended at the time of injury. Symptoms would include hematuria, the inability to void, abdominal distention, suprapubic pain, and tenderness and ecchymosis over the bladder and thighs.

C. Because both the small and large intestines are susceptible to injury with blunt abdominal trauma, the nurse should have a high index of suspicion for intestinal injury when lap belt restraint marks are noted across the abdomen. Signs and symptoms of intestinal injury include vague generalized abdominal or epigastric pain with abdominal rigidity, spasm, or guarding. Bowel sounds are usually hypoactive or absent.

D. The stomach is not usually injured with blunt trauma because it is easily displaced; it is more often injured with penetrating trauma. Signs and symptoms would include left upper quadrant pain and tenderness, free air under the diaphragm on radiograph, and aspiration of blood drainage through a nasogastric tube.

Category: Gastrointestinal, Genitourinary, Gynecology, and Obstetrical Emergencies/ Gastrointestinal/Trauma

Nursing Process: Analysis

References

Bacidore, V. (2010). Abdominal and genitourinary trauma. In P. K. Howard & R. A. Steinmann (Eds.), *Sheehy's emergency nursing: Principles and practice* (6th ed., pp. 301–312). St. Louis, MO: Mosby Elsevier.

Harris, C. (2013). Abdominal trauma. In B. B. Hammond & P. G. Zimmermann (Eds.), *Sheehy's manual of emergency care* (7th ed., pp. 419–426). St. Louis, MO: Elsevier Mosby.

---

62. A patient with a history of peptic ulcer disease is treated in the emergency department and discharged with a diagnosis of osteoarthritis. Discharge teaching would include instructions to take which of the following medications to manage the arthritic pain?

A. Ibuprofen (Motrin)
B. Acetaminophen (Tylenol)
C. Omeprazole (Prilosec)
D. Celecoxib (Celebrex)

Rationale

A. Patients with a history of peptic ulcer disease should be advised to avoid the use of nonsteroidal anti-inflammatory medications.

B. Acetaminophen is the initial treatment of choice for osteoarthritis. It does not cause gastrointestinal bleeding or contribute to gastric ulcer formation.

C. Omeprazole is a proton pump inhibitor, which is effective in the management of peptic ulcer disease but will not alleviate the discomfort associated with osteoarthritis.

D. COX-2 inhibitors such as celecoxib may provide effective pain relief for patients with osteoarthritis but are contraindicated for patients with a history of peptic ulcer disease because of an increased risk for serious gastrointestinal bleeding.

Category: Gastrointestinal, Genitourinary, Gynecology, and Obstetrical Emergencies/ Gastrointestinal/Ulcers

Nursing Process: Intervention

Reference

Adams, M., Holland, N., & Urban, C. (2017). Drugs for peptic ulcer disease. In *Pharmacology for nurses: A pathophysiologic approach* (5th ed., pp. 676–691). Boston, MA: Pearson.

---

63. A patient diagnosed with renal calculi will likely exhibit which signs and symptoms?

A. Sudden onset of colicky, ipsilateral flank pain radiating to the groin
B. Urinary frequency and urgency with fever and chills
C. Unilateral scrotal pain
D. Sudden onset of severe back pain described as "ripping" or "tearing"

Rationale

A. The pain associated with renal colic typically begins in the flank area of the lower back and radiates to the groin.

B. Patients with renal colic may have a low-grade fever. Fever and chills are more suggestive of an infectious process such as pyelonephritis.

C. The discomfort associated with renal calculi originates in the flank area and may radiate to the groin and scrotum. Pain that originates in the scrotum is more likely to be associated with the etiologies of conditions such as acute epididymitis or testicular torsion.

D. Symptoms associated with a dissecting aortic aneurysm, such as a sudden onset of a pain described as "ripping" or "tearing," can mimic those of renal colic but are associated with greater hemodynamic instability and loss of distal pulses.

Category: Gastrointestinal, Genitourinary, Gynecology, and Obstetrical Emergencies/Genitourinary/Renal calculi

Nursing Process: Assessment

References

Hammond, B. B. (2013). Cardiovascular emergencies. In B. B. Hammond & P. G. Zimmermann (Eds.), *Sheehy's manual of emergency care* (7th ed., pp. 201–211). St. Louis, MO: Elsevier Mosby.

Quallich, S. (2013). Genitourinary emergencies. In B. B. Hammond & P. G. Zimmermann (Eds.), *Sheehy's manual of emergency care* (7th ed., pp. 353–360). St. Louis, MO: Elsevier Mosby.

---

64. The male driver of a vehicle involved in a motor vehicle collision is brought to the emergency department by ambulance. The patient complains of abdominal pain, and on secondary assessment, seatbelt marks are seen across the patient's lower abdomen, and blood is noted at the urinary meatus. Which of the following should the emergency nurse anticipate to be performed next?

A. Application of a pelvic immobilization device
B. Insertion of an indwelling urinary catheter
C. Performance of a retrograde urethrogram
D. Obtaining a urine specimen for urinalysis

Rationale

A. Urethral disruption can be associated with a pelvic fracture but can also be linked to other injuries, so application of a pelvic immobilization device would not be initially indicated for this patient.

B. In trauma patients, the presence of blood at the urinary meatus may indicate urethral disruption, and a urinary catheter should not be attempted until a retrograde urethrogram is performed.

C. The presence of urethral injuries is more common in males than in females. Blood at the urinary meatus may be an indication of urethral injury, and a retrograde urethrogram should be performed to rule out urethral injury.

D. A urine specimen will eventually be collected from this trauma patient, but the retrograde urethrogram to determine a partial or total urethral disruption is the priority intervention.

Category: Gastrointestinal, Genitourinary, Gynecology, and Obstetrical Emergencies/Genitourinary/Trauma

Nursing Process: Intervention

References

Armenakas, N. A. (2018). Urethral trauma. *Merck Manual Online*. Retrieved from http://www.merckmanuals.com/professional/injuries-poisoning/genitourinary-tract-trauma/urethral-trauma

Campbell, M. R. (2007). Abdominal and urologic trauma. In K. S. Hoyt & J. Selfridge-Thomas (Eds.), *Emergency nursing core curriculum* (6th ed., pp. 800–801). St. Louis, MO: Saunders Elsevier.

65. A patient being treated for severe nausea and vomiting related to motion sickness is ordered to receive a scopolamine patch. The emergency nurse would verify the order with the emergency care provider when the patient's medical history includes:

A. irritable bowel disease.
B. chronic bronchitis.
C. neurogenic bladder.
D. glaucoma.

Rationale

A. Cholinergic blocking (anticholinergic) drugs decrease gastrointestinal motility and are commonly used in the management of irritable bowel disease.

B. Cholinergic blocking (anticholinergic) drugs are indicated in the treatment of chronic bronchitis because they reduce bronchial secretions and promote bronchodilation.

C. Cholinergic blocking (anticholinergic) drugs decrease spasms of the detrusor muscles of the bladder and tighten the internal bladder sphincter, reducing episodes of incontinence.

D. Cholinergic blocking (anticholinergic) drugs, such as scopolamine, must be used with caution in the patient with glaucoma. Cholinergic blocking action keeps the sphincter muscles of the iris from constricting. This causes the pupil to dilate and increases the patient's intraocular pressure, which could result in blindness.

Category: Gastrointestinal, Genitourinary, Gynecology, and Obstetrical Emergencies/Genitourinary/Urinary retention

Nursing Process: Intervention

References

4 drugs linked to urinary incontinence. (2016). *WebMD*. Retrieved from http://www.webmd.com/urinary-incontinence-oab/4-medications-that-cause-or-worsen-incontinence?page=2

Lilley, L. L., Collins, S. R., & Snyder, J. S. (2017). In *Pharmacology and the nursing process* (8th ed., pp. 331–339). St. Louis, MO: Elsevier.

The National Institute of Diabetes and Digestive and Kidney Diseases Health Information Center. (2014). *Urinary retention*. Retrieved from https://www.niddk.nih.gov/health-information/health-topics/urologic-disease/urinary-retention/Pages/facts.aspx

---

66. The emergency nurse is providing discharge education to a patient who has been diagnosed with pelvic inflammatory disease. Which of the following statements made by the patient leads the nurse to believe further education is needed?

A. "I don't think I have to tell anyone else about this infection. I'll be fine once I take some pills."
B. "I should take all of this antibiotic even if I begin feeling better."
C. "I have an intrauterine device and understand that this may be the cause of my infection."
D. "This infection is from bacteria that has made its way up to my fallopian tubes and ovaries."

Rationale

A. The treatment of pelvic inflammatory disease (PID). requires treatment of all current and recent sexual partners.

B. Antibiotics are the recommended treatment for PID. It is important that the patient complete the entire course of antibiotic medication because a patient with PID may continue to be infected yet remain asymptomatic.

C. The presence of an intrauterine device, a recent abortion, and having multiple sexual partners are all possible risk factors for developing PID.

D. PID is an infection of the upper genital tract and can develop from bacteria that migrate upward from the lower genital tract.

Category: Gastrointestinal, Genitourinary, Gynecology, and Obstetrical Emergencies/ Gynecology/Infection

Nursing Process: Evaluation

Reference

Kelly, L. (2013). Gynecological emergencies. In B. B. Hammond & P. G. Zimmermann (Eds.), *Sheehy's manual of emergency care* (7th ed., pp. 497–503). St. Louis, MO: Elsevier Mosby.

---

67. A 22-year-old female presents to the emergency department stating that she may have been sexually assaulted the night before. The patient states she was at a nightclub last evening and awoke this morning in an unfamiliar place. She complains of vaginal soreness and bruising of her labia. On examination, the physician determines that forcible intercourse did occur. Which statement made by the patient would likely suggest to the nurse that the assault may have been drug facilitated?

A. The patient experienced nausea and vomiting on awakening.
B. The patient states she had one drink and then cannot recall the events of the evening.
C. The patient states she is missing articles of clothing.
D. The patient states an individual she did not know bought her a drink.

Rationale

A. Nausea and vomiting may be a reaction to alcohol intake and does not independently suggest ingestion of GHB or Ecstasy.

B. A patient who has been given a drug such as GHB or Ecstasy will typically progress quickly to a high level of intoxication, with impaired motor skills and drowsiness. The patient will quickly lose consciousness with little to no recall of the events.

C. Victims of a drug-facilitated sexual assault may find that their clothes are torn or they are wearing their clothes improperly, such as inside-out or backward.

D. Date rape drugs are usually dissolved in beverages and the taste is not detectable, so women are cautioned to not accept a drink from a stranger unless they watch the drink being poured/prepared. Consuming the drink along with experiencing the amnesic effects associated with the drugs would lead the nurse to strongly suspect drug ingestion.

Category: Gastrointestinal, Genitourinary, Gynecology, and Obstetrical Emergencies/Gynecology/ Sexual assault/battery

Nursing Process: Evaluation

References

Erneohazy, W., & Shlamovitz, G. (2015, November 10). Sexual assault. *Medscape*. Retrieved from http://emedicine.medscape.com/article/806120-overview

Ruiz-Contreras, A. (2010). Sexual assault. In P. K. Howard & R. A. Steinmann (Eds.), *Sheehy's emergency nursing: Principles and practice* (6th ed., pp. 698–703). St. Louis, MO: Mosby Elsevier.

U.S. Department of Health and Human Services: Office on Women's Health. (2012). *Date rape drugs*. Retrieved from https://www.womenshealth.gov/publications/our-publications/fact-sheet/date-rape-drugs.html

68. A 38-week-pregnant female presents to the emergency department with a sudden onset of severe abdominal cramping and dark red vaginal bleeding. The patient states the baby is not as active as usual. Vital signs: BP 80/mm Hg by palpation; HR 140 beats/minute; RR 24 breaths/minute. The nurse suspects the patient is experiencing:

A. placental abruption.
B. placenta previa.
C. active labor.
D. amniotic fluid embolism.

Rationale

A. Placental abruption (abruptio placenta) is the premature separation of the placenta from its implantation site. Clinical presentation typically includes a sudden onset of abdominal pain and frank, dark red vaginal bleeding. Depending on the extent of separation, fetal and maternal death can occur as a result of hemorrhage and hypovolemic shock. Placental abruption should be suspected in any pregnant female in the third trimester who presents with abdominal pain and vaginal bleeding.

B. Placenta previa refers to a placenta implanted over, or in close proximity to, the internal cervical os. The most characteristic clinical finding is painless, bright red bleeding.

C. During labor, the patient presents with contractions that may be mild to severe in nature. There is an increase in bloody show. The patient's vital signs are normal, not hypotensive.

D. Amniotic fluid embolism is a catastrophic event in which amniotic fluid leaks into the mother's circulation during labor or delivery, causing sudden respiratory distress and cardiopulmonary arrest. An amniotic fluid embolus can occur as a result of a placental abruption, but this patient's symptoms of hypotension and tachycardia are consistent with hypovolemia as a result of bleeding.

Category: Gastrointestinal, Genitourinary, Gynecology, and Obstetrical Emergencies/Obstetrical/Abruptio placenta

Nursing Process: Analysis

References

Benrubi, G. (2010). *Obstetric and gynecologic emergencies* (4th ed.). Philadelphia, PA: Lippincott Williams & Wilkins.

Jordan, K. S. (2007). Obstetric and gynecologic emergencies. In K. S. Hoyt & J. Selfridge-Thomas (Eds), *Emergency nursing core curriculum* (6th ed., pp. 536–570). St. Louis, MO: Saunders Elsevier.

Mason, D. (2010). Obstetric emergencies. In P. K. Howard & R. A. Steinmann (Eds.), *Sheehy's emergency nursing: Principles and practice* (6th ed., pp. 619–629). St. Louis, MO: Mosby Elsevier.

Poole, J. H., & Thompson, J. E. (2013). Obstetric emergencies. In B. B. Hammond & P. G. Zimmermann (Eds.), *Sheehy's manual of emergency care* (7th ed., pp. 483–495). St. Louis, MO: Elsevier Mosby.

69. A patient who is 12 weeks pregnant presents to the emergency department complaining of lower abdominal pain and light vaginal spotting. The patient's risk for having an ectopic pregnancy increases if she relates a history of having which of the following?

A. Maternal age under 25 years
B. An incompetent cervix
C. A previous pregnancy of twins or triplets
D. Pelvic inflammatory disease

Rationale

A. The incidence of an ectopic pregnancy is greater when the mother's age is 35 years of age or older.

B. An incompetent cervix will increase the mother's risk for a spontaneous abortion but does not increase the risk for an ectopic pregnancy.

C. A history of a multiple gestational pregnancy does not increase the mother's risk for a subsequent ectopic pregnancy.

D. A history of prior inflammation of the fallopian tubes significantly raises the mother's risk for having an ectopic pregnancy.

Category: Gastrointestinal, Genitourinary, Gynecology, and Obstetrical Emergencies/Obstetrical/Ectopic pregnancy

Nursing Process: Assessment

References

Mason, D. L. (2010). Obstetric emergencies. In P. K. Howard & R. A. Steinmann (Eds.), *Sheehy's emergency nursing: Principles and practice* (6th ed., pp. 619–629). St. Louis, MO: Mosby Elsevier.

Poole, J. H., & Thompson, J. E. (2013). Obstetric emergencies. In B. B. Hammond & P. G. Zimmermann (Eds.), *Sheehy's manual of emergency care* (7th ed., pp. 483–495). St. Louis, MO: Elsevier Mosby.

---

70. A 28-year-old female presents to the emergency department via ambulance following her home delivery of a full-term infant. On assessment, the patient's uterus feels boggy and soft. The presence of a boggy and soft uterus places the patient at greatest risk for:

A. postpartum infection.
B. retained products of conception.
C. eclampsia.
D. postpartum hemorrhage.

Rationale

A. The symptoms associated with a postpartum infection are generally evident between 1 and 3 days following delivery; they include abdominal tenderness and a low-grade fever, and may include a malodorous vaginal discharge.

B. After a home birth, it is important to ensure that the patient has fully delivered the placenta. However, presentation for retained products of conception includes severe abdominal pain, abnormal bleeding, and fever.

C. Eclampsia in the postpartum patient is characterized by seizure activity.

D. A soft, boggy uterus is the assessment finding for uterine atony. Uterine atony is the most common cause of a significant postpartum hemorrhage. The nurse should perform manual massage of the uterus to help expel retained clots and restore uterine tone.

Category: Gastrointestinal, Genitourinary, Gynecology, and Obstetrical Emergencies/Obstetrical/Hemorrhage

Nursing Process: Analysis

References

Moldenhauer, J. S. (2016). Postpartum care. *Merck Manual.* Retrieved from http://www.merckmanuals.com/professional/gynecology-and-obstetrics/postpartum-care-and-associated-disorders/postpartum-care

Poole, J. H., & Thompson, J. E. (2013). Obstetric emergencies. In B. B. Hammond & P. G. Zimmermann (Eds.), *Sheehy's manual of emergency care* (7th ed., pp. 483–495). St. Louis, MO: Elsevier Mosby.

Smith, J. R. (2017, July 21). Postpartum hemorrhage. *Medscape*. Retrieved from http://emedicine.medscape.com/article/275038-overview#a10

---

71. During neonatal resuscitation, which of the following methods will provide the emergency nurse with the most accurate evaluation of the infant's respiratory effectiveness?

A. Pulse oximetry monitoring
B. End-tidal CO_2 measurement
C. Continuous cardiac monitoring
D. Auscultation of the precordium

Rationale

A. Changes in the heart rate of a newborn have been found to be the most sensitive indicator of the infant's respiratory effectiveness. Measurement of the heart rate by pulse oximetry has not been found to be an accurate means to evaluate heart rate. Pulse oximetry often underestimates the infant's heart rate, which could potentially lead to unnecessary interventions.

B. End-tidal CO_2 monitoring and measurement is the most reliable method for evaluating endotracheal tube placement and also reflects alveolar gas exchange, but the heart rate more accurately assesses respiratory effectiveness.

C. An increase in the newborn's heart rate is considered the most sensitive indicator of improvement in respiratory effectiveness. When compared to rate determination by either auscultation or pulse oximetry measurement, the 3-lead electrocardiogram provided data with greater accuracy within a shorter period of time.

D. In previous treatment guidelines, auscultation of the precordium was recommended as the preferred method to evaluate heart rate. However, this method was determined to be unreliable and inaccurate because providers tended to underestimate the infant's pulse rate, potentially leading to unnecessary interventions. In its 2015 Neonatal Resuscitation Guidelines, the American Heart Association recommends cardiac monitoring as the best method to evaluate changes in the infant's heart rate.

Category (Pediatric): Gastrointestinal, Genitourinary, Gynecology, and Obstetrical Emergencies/ Obstetrical/Neonatal resuscitation

Nursing Process: Analysis

Reference

Wyckoff, M. H., Aziz, K., Escobedo, M. B., Kapadia, V. S., Kattwinkel, J., Perlman, J. M., . . . Zaichkin, J. G. (2015). Part 13: Neonatal resuscitation: 2015 American Heart Association guidelines update for cardiopulmonary resuscitation and emergency cardiovascular care. *Circulation, 132*(18), S543–S560. https://doi.org/10.1161/CIR.0000000000000267

72. A 36-year-old female who is in the 30th week of her first pregnancy presents with complaints of a headache and swelling of the hands and face. The patient's blood pressure is 150/90 mm Hg. The emergency nurse anticipates administration of which medication?

A. Labetalol (Normodyne)
B. Furosemide (Lasix)
C. Acetaminophen (Tylenol)
D. Magnesium sulfate

Rationale

A. BP of 140/90 mm Hg is considered hypertension, however, lowering the diastolic BP to less than 90–100 mm Hg may result in placental hypoperfusion and lead to fetal distress.

B. This patient is exhibiting signs and symptoms of preeclampsia. The edema associated with preeclampsia is a result of vasospasm causing intravascular fluid to leak into the surrounding tissues. Intravascular volume is therefore low. The administration of furosemide would cause further dehydration and potentially elevate the mother's risk for seizures.

C. This patient is exhibiting signs and symptoms of preeclampsia. Preeclampsia is frequently associated with elevated liver enzymes. Administration of acetaminophen, a drug known to cause hepatotoxicity, therefore would be contraindicated for this patient.

D. This patient is exhibiting signs and symptoms of preeclampsia. Magnesium sulfate is given to decrease the seizure threshold in a patient who has preeclampsia.

Category: Gastrointestinal, Genitourinary, Gynecology, and Obstetrical Emergencies/Obstetrical/Preeclampsia, eclampsia, HELLP syndrome

Nursing Process: Intervention

References

Jordan, K. S. (2007). Obstetric and gynecologic emergences. In K. S. Hoyt & J. Selfridge-Thomas (Eds.), *Emergency nursing core curriculum* (6th ed., pp. 536–570). St. Louis, MO: Saunders Elsevier.

Mason, D. L. (2010). Obstetric emergencies. In P. K. Howard & R. A. Steinmann (Eds.), *Sheehy's emergency nursing: Principles and practice* (6th ed., pp. 619–629). St. Louis, MO: Mosby Elsevier.

---

73. A 30-week-pregnant female involved in a motor vehicle collision is confirmed to be in labor, and delivery of a preterm infant is anticipated. To stimulate the production of fetal surfactant and reduce the incidence of neonatal respiratory distress, the emergency nurse anticipates administration of which of the following medications to the patient?

A. Oxytocin
B. Magnesium sulfate
C. Terbutaline
D. Betamethasone

Rationale

A. Oxytocin is indicated to stimulate labor contractions and would be contraindicated in this case.

B. When administered to a patient in preterm labor, magnesium sulfate may help reduce the risk of neurological injury that is associated with early birth. Magnesium sulfate is not indicated in the treatment of neonatal respiratory distress.

C. Terbutaline is a tocolytic medication that will delay preterm delivery from 2 to 7 days. It does not directly affect fetal lung development but will allow time for a full course of antenatal corticosteroids to be administered.

D. The American College of Obstetricians and Gynecologists advocates the use of steroids to hasten neonatal lung maturity for women between 24 and 34 weeks' gestation who are at risk for delivery.

Category (Pediatric): Gastrointestinal, Genitourinary, Gynecology, and Obstetrical Emergencies/ Obstetrical/Preterm labor

Nursing Process: Intervention

References

American College of Obstetricians and Gynecologists. (2017). *Preterm (premature) labor and delivery: Frequently asked questions*. Retrieved from http://www.acog.org/Patients/FAQs/Preterm-Premature-Labor-and-Birth

Hunter, L. A. (2013). Preterm labor. In D. J. Angelini & D. LaFonteanine (Eds.), *Obstetric triage and emergency care protocols* (pp. 119–127). New York, NY: Springer.

---

74. A young woman states that she has been sexually assaulted. She is ambulatory, alert, and oriented and has no visible injuries. Based on the Emergency Severity Index (ESI) 5-level triage system, the triage nurse assigns the patient an ESI level 1. The triage nurse understands that the rationale for assigning the high acuity level is which of the following?

A. **Assessment and evidence collection both constitute a high-risk situation and require time-sensitive interventions.**
B. The patient is in custody of the law enforcement officer.
C. The patient should be placed with the general emergency department patient population.
D. The patient will require at least two resources.

Rationale

A. Identification of life-threatening injuries is a priority. Additionally, collection of evidence may be done before full patient assessment or treatment of nonlife-threatening injuries.

B. This is not a criterion for assigning the triage level of acuity. Although she is with the police to ensure that the forensic chain of evidence is followed, the patient may not be under arrest or in police custody.

C. Placing the patient in a safe, private environment is a priority, yet there is no reason that the patient should not be exposed to other patients in the emergency department.

D. Resource utilization alone is not the main reason the patient receives a high acuity level. Assessment and evidence collection are time-sensitive, high-priority interventions, indicating that this patient should be assigned an ESI level 1.

Category: Psychosocial and Medical Emergencies/Psychosocial/Abuse and neglect

Nursing Process: Analysis

References

Gilboy, N., Tanabe, P., Travers, D., & Rosenau, A. M. (2011). *Emergency Severity Index (ESI): A triage tool for emergency department care, Version 4 implementation handbook 2012 edition. Agency for Healthcare Research and Quality Publication No. 12-0014*. Rockville, MD: U.S. Department of Health and Human Services. Retrieved from https://www.ahrq.gov/sites/default/files/wysiwyg/professionals/systems/hospital/esi/esihandbk.pdf

Weintraub, B. (2013). Sexual assault. In B. B. Hammond & P. G. Zimmermann (Eds.), *Sheehy's manual of emergency care* (7th ed., pp. 537–546). St. Louis, MO: Elsevier Mosby.

---

75. A school-age child presents to the emergency department with abdominal pain. The nurse notes that this is the third visit this month for a variety of complaints. The patient has followed up with the family physician as directed, but no official diagnosis has been made to account for the child's numerous complaints. The parent reveals the child does not like school and seldom wants to spend time with other children. The emergency nurse suspects the child may have:

A. obsessive compulsive disorder.
B. social anxiety disorder.
C. Tourette syndrome.
D. anorexia nervosa.

Rationale

A. Obsessive compulsive disorder is a disorder in which children form an obsession that becomes associated with a compulsive behavior presenting as rituals needed to reduce the anxiety caused by the obsession.

B. Social anxiety disorder (SAD) is the typical "shy child," but the disorder affects the child's ability to function, possibly leading them to avoid other children and refuse to go to school. Further, children with SAD may present frequently to the emergency department with various complaints without organic cause. The more nonspecific the symptomology a child manifests, the more likely that anxiety plays a role in the presentation.

C. Tourette syndrome is associated with uncontrollable verbal and nonverbal tics.

D. Although eating disorders often appear comorbidly with anxiety disorders, neither the patient nor parent reported symptoms are consistent with anorexia nervosa, such as vomiting or excessive diarrhea.

Category: Psychosocial and Medical Emergencies/Psychosocial/Anxiety/panic

Nursing Process: Analysis

References

Lewis. G. C. (2016). Eating disorders. In J. E. Tintinalli, J. Stapczynski, O. Ma, D. M. Yealy, & G. D. Meckler, & D. M. Cline (Eds.), *Tintinalli's emergency medicine: A comprehensive study guide* (8th ed.). Retrieved from http://access emergencymedicine.mhmedical.com/Content.aspx?bookid=1658&Sectionid=109448456

Wagers, B., Hariharan, S., Wagers, B., & Hariharan, S. (2014). Psychiatric emergencies. In C. K. Stone, R. L. Humphries, D. Drigalla, & M. Stephan (Eds.), *CURRENT Diagnosis & Treatment: Pediatric Emergency Medicine.* Retrieved from http://accessemergencymedicine.mhmedical.com/content.aspx?bookid=1175&Sectionid=65115102

---

76. A patient arrives to triage accompanied by several friends who state the patient has become extremely irritable and impulsive recently and then can be very happy and sociable while acting "normal." The friends report that the irritable and impulsive behavior is not normal for the patient. Which of the following conditions is this patient most likely experiencing?

A. Anxiety
B. Schizophrenia
C. Bipolar disorder
D. Delirium

Rationale

A. Anxiety is often related to a perceived threat to self. The patient experiences the feeling of nervousness or increased apprehension, and in severe cases of anxiety, the patient may have shortness of breath or chest pain.

B. Schizophrenia is a chronic psychotic disorder that manifests with hallucinations, delusions, flattened affect, and impaired social skills. The typical age of onset is adolescence or young adulthood.

C. This patient is exhibiting classic signs of bipolar disorder. Bipolar disorder manifests with alternating bouts of depression and mania. Mania can include hyperactivity, exaggerated actions, including risky behaviors, and sometimes paranoia.

D. Delirium is characterized by a rapid change in mental status, including memory loss, and may include hallucinations and nightmares.

Category: Psychosocial and Medical Emergencies/Psychosocial/Bipolar disorder

Nursing Process: Analysis

References

Gagnon, L. (2007). Psychiatric/psychosocial emergencies. In K. S. Hoyt & J. Selfridge-Thomas (Eds.), *Emergency nursing core curriculum* (6th ed., pp. 659–684). St. Louis, MO: Saunders Elsevier.

Gagnon, L. (2010). Behavioral health emergencies. In P. K. Howard & R. A. Steinmann (Eds.), *Sheehy's emergency nursing: Principles and practice* (6th ed., pp. 677–688). St. Louis, MO: Mosby Elsevier.

---

77. An adolescent patient arrives to triage, accompanied by their parents, after a letter was found in the patient's room revealing a desire to end their life. The letter indicates increased school stressors and a recent injury that could affect their college sport aspirations as reasons for their suicidal thoughts. Which of the following statements by the parents exhibits an understanding of the discharge instructions for the patient?

A. "We will ensure our child sees the therapist tomorrow."
B. "We will make an appointment for our child to see the therapist within 1 week."
C. "We will take time off from work for the next 2 days to monitor our child at all times."
D. "We will take our child out of school until his symptoms of suicidal ideation have resolved."

Rationale

A. If the adolescent has an effective support system that can ensure patient observation with appropriate follow-up within 24 hours, this is a good plan of action for the acutely depressed or possibly suicidal patient. Acknowledgment that the family will ensure the patient's safety is also a sign of acceptance of the follow-up plan of care. Adolescents with a clear plan of possible suicide often require admission to an inpatient facility.

B. The best plan of action is to ensure the patient has a confirmed appointment for adequate follow-up with a mental health provider as soon as possible. An adolescent who has written a potential suicide note is considered high risk and should be seen as soon as possible or admitted to an inpatient facility.

C. Although staying with the child to ensure his safety is important, the child should have an appointment with a mental health provider within the next 24–48 hours.

D. Taking the child out of school until the symptoms of suicidal ideation resolve does not ensure the proper prescribed follow-up and may delay the patient in receiving an adequate mental health evaluation and care.

Category (Pediatric): Psychosocial and Medical Emergencies/Psychosocial/Depression
Nursing Process: Evaluation

References

Gagnon, L. (2010). Behavioral health emergencies. In P. K. Howard & R. A. Steinmann (Eds.), *Sheehy's emergency nursing: Principles and practice* (6th ed., pp. 677–688). St. Louis, MO: Mosby Elsevier.
Manton, A. (2013). Mental health emergencies. In B. B. Hammond & P. G. Zimmermann (Eds.), *Sheehy's manual of emergency care* (7th ed., pp. 505–520). St. Louis, MO: Elsevier Mosby.

---

78. An emergency patient who is agitated, aggressive, and experiencing homicidal ideation is given an injection of haloperidol (Haldol). Within 30 minutes of the injection, the patient is unable to maintain their head in a midline position, resulting in a severe arching of the neck area and pulling of their neck to the left side. The patient's eyes are moving in multiple directions. The patient states that they are unable to sit still and feels like their skin is crawling. The emergency nurse anticipates the administration of benztropine (Cogentin) to treat which of the following symptoms this patient is exhibiting?

A. Hallucination
B. Tonic–clonic seizure
C. Petit mal seizure reaction
D. Torticollis

Rationale

A. Benztropine is used to treat dystonic reaction; it will not be effective for treating or eliminating the patient's hallucinations.

B. Benztropine is used to treat dystonic reaction related to the administration of haloperidol. Benztropine will not be effective in eliminating the patient's tonic–clonic seizure.

C. Benztropine may cause some drowsiness but would not be indicated in the activity associated with a petit mal seizure disorder.

D. Torticollis is a particular spasm of the neck muscles that causes the twisting of the neck that the patient cannot control. Opisthotonos is a hyperextension of the neck muscles caused by muscular spasm that places the patient in a hyperextended state that he cannot control. These behaviors are considered a dystonic reaction.

Category: Psychosocial and Medical Emergencies/Psychosocial/Homicidal ideation
Nursing Process: Evaluation

Reference

Manton, A. (2013). Mental health emergencies. In B. B. Hammond & P. G. Zimmermann (Eds.), *Sheehy's manual of emergency care* (7th ed., pp. 505–520). St. Louis, MO: Elsevier Mosby.

---

79. A patient with history of posttraumatic stress disorder and schizophrenia arrives to triage with a case manager. The patient is pacing and screaming repeatedly, "The voices are so loud. Make them stop!" and said they would like to take a gun to "blow your head off right now!" Which Emergency Severity Index (ESI) triage classifications should the emergency nurse assign to this patient?

A. ESI level 2
B. ESI level 1
C. ESI level 5
D. ESI level 3

Rationale

A. A patient who is actively aggressive, has homicidal thoughts, and does not have control of normal thought processes would fall into the category of high-risk situation, which places him into the ESI level 2 category. The patient's heart rate and respiratory pattern are most likely elevated, and they will require multiple resources for care, again placing this patient into ESI level 2.

B. ESI level 1 is designated for patients who require immediate lifesaving interventions. The patient has a patent airway and is not demonstrating unstable vital signs or signs of uncontrolled hemorrhage. Although suicidal and homicidal thoughts can be an emergent situation, the patient in this scenario is out of control and needs to be cared for immediately for both their safety and the safety of others. They are demonstrating the criteria for ESI level 2.

C. ESI level 5 is designated for patients who require no resources for care; their condition is considered minor in nature, and care could be delayed if necessary. Any patient who has active suicidal or homicidal thoughts and actions would not be designated an ESI level 5.

D. Patients who might fall into the ESI level 3 triage category may have suicidal or homicidal thoughts, but they are calm and cooperative and seeking help for their current mental health.

Category: Psychosocial and Medical Emergencies/Psychosocial/Homicidal ideation
Nursing Process: Analysis

References

Gilboy, N. (2010). Triage. In P. K. Howard & R. A. Steinmann (Eds.), *Sheehy's emergency nursing: Principles and practice* (6th ed., pp. 59–72). St. Louis, MO: Mosby Elsevier.
Manton, A. (2013). Mental health emergencies. In B. B. Hammond & P. G. Zimmermann (Eds.), *Sheehy's manual of emergency care* (7th ed., pp. 505–520). St. Louis, MO: Elsevier Mosby.

80. An elderly female is brought to the emergency department by her daughter, who reports that her mother has been unable to sleep for the past 3 days. The daughter states that her mother has been talking to her deceased husband and has been found wandering outside her home. Which of the following is most likely the cause of this change in the patient's behavior?

A. Suicidal ideation
B. Depression
C. Delirium
D. Insomnia

Rationale

A. Suicidal ideation would involve the patient voicing the desire to injure herself. The patient may have a plan as well as access to things that could harm her, including a weapon.

B. Depression is manifested by several symptoms, including a low mood, lack of interest in activities, anxiety, and sleep disturbances. It has a slow onset of symptoms.

C. Delirium is an acutely disturbed, potentially reversible neuropsychiatric emergency that involves changes in attention, awareness, and cognition. The symptoms may occur acutely or develop over a number of days. Causes of delirium include illnesses such as a urinary tract infection or pneumonia, metabolic disturbances such as hyponatremia, and medications, especially in patients who take multiple medications.

D. Insomnia is a sleep disorder that involves problems with falling and staying asleep. The patient may manifest some abnormal behaviors and problems with cognition, especially if she has not been able to sleep for long periods of time. It would be important to evaluate if the patient has a history of insomnia, but it generally does not cause acute behavioral changes by itself.

Category (Geriatric): Psychosocial and Medical Emergencies/Psychosocial/Psychosis

Nursing Process: Assessment

References

Deal, N., & Matorin, A. (2015). Stabilization and management of the acutely agitated or psychotic patient. *Emergency Medicine Clinics of North America, 33*, 739–752.

Seeganna, C., & Antai-Otong, D. (2016). Managing the care of the older patient with delirium and dementia. *Nursing Clinics of North America, 51*, 261–273.

Wheat, S., & Taleri, M. (2016). Psychiatric emergencies. *Primary Care: Clinics in Office Practice, 43*(2), 341–354.

---

81. A patient with a history of situational depression has asked the nurse about the effects of taking the herb St. John's wort. The patient has heard that it "works better" than the selective serotonin uptake inhibitor (SSRI) that they are currently prescribed. The nurse consults with the pharmacist and tells the patient:

A. "If you combine the herb with the prescription, you should reduce the dose of your SSRI after 2 weeks."

B. "It might be a good idea. The herb will enhance the effectiveness of your prescription."

C. "Yes, you may combine them. Because St. John's Wort is a natural herb, it is safe for you to take."

D. "It is not advised to take this herb with your current prescription without consulting with your provider."

Rationale

A. Patients should always be educated to discuss use of herbs and supplements with their provider. Reduction in the prescribed medication dose should be given by the prescribing physician.

B. Although it may potentiate the effects of the SSRI, the combination of St. John's Wort and the SSRI might have serious side effects.

C. This is a common but inaccurate belief. Many natural supplements interact with prescribed medications, resulting in untoward effects.

D. St. John's Wort, although often recommended to treat mild depression, can interact with SSRIs. Providers should be aware of any prescribed or over-the-counter herbs or supplements the patient may be taking.

Category: Psychosocial and Medical Emergencies/Psychosocial/Situational crisis

Nursing Process: Intervention

Reference

Sweet, V. (2007). Complementary/alternative therapies. In K. S. Hoyt & J. Selfridge-Thomas (Eds.), *Emergency nursing core curriculum* (6th ed., pp. 69–77). St. Louis, MO: Saunders Elsevier.

---

82. A patient is transported to the emergency department from a local restaurant. Emergency medical services reports that the patient was awake and alert on scene and reported rapid-onset difficulty breathing and swelling in their throat and tongue. On arrival, the patient responded only to pain, and their face and tongue appear swollen. BP is 75/40 mm Hg. Their wife states that the patient is allergic to peanuts. What is the first medication the emergency nurse should anticipate administering to the patient?

    A. **Epinephrine (Adrenalin)**
    B. Fluid bolus of isotonic crystalloid solution
    C. Diphenhydramine (Benadryl)
    D. Famotidine (Pepcid)

Rationale

A. Epinephrine is the first-line treatment for hemodynamically unstable anaphylaxis. Epinephrine will result in vasoconstriction and bronchodilation. Failure to promptly administer epinephrine is associated with mortality, hypoxic encephalopathy, and biphasic anaphylaxis.

B. The patient will require a fluid bolus to fill the intravascular space, however, the administration of epinephrine is the first-line treatment for anaphylactic shock.

C. An antihistamine is used to treat allergic reactions, however, it is not the immediate medication of choice in a patient who is demonstrating signs of anaphylactic shock.

D. An H2 receptor antagonist is used to treat allergic reactions, however, the administration of epinephrine is the first-line treatment in patients with anaphylactic shock.

Category: Psychosocial and Medical Emergencies/Medical/Allergic reactions and anaphylaxis

Nursing Process: Intervention

Reference

Yunker, N. S., & Wagner, B. J. (2014). A pharmacologic review of anaphylaxis. *Plastic Surgical Nursing, 34*(4), 183–189. http://dx.doi.org.webproxy.ouhsc.edu/10.1097/PSN.00

---

83. A patient presents to the emergency department with itching, swelling around the lips and tongue, shortness of breath, and anxiety. The patient reports a history of a peanut allergy as a child but has not had a reaction in years, and denies eating any known products that contain peanuts. However, pancakes were eaten earlier in the day just before the symptoms began. What is the most likely cause of the patient's symptoms?

    A. **The documented peanut allergy**
    B. Pneumonia
    C. Anxiety attack
    D. Pulmonary embolism

Rationale

A. Although unexpected, pancakes and other baked goods sometimes contain peanut oil or peanut products. The patient should be advised to carry an epinephrine auto-injector (EpiPen) in case of future reactions. Approximately 20% of children with peanut allergies eventually outgrow their allergy.

B. The patient has a history of a peanut allergy and the symptoms began suddenly after eating. Despite experiencing shortness of breath, pneumonia is unlikely to be the cause of the patient's symptoms.

C. Despite experiencing shortness of breath and anxiety, the patient does not appear to be experiencing an anxiety attack. The patient needs emergent treatment for anaphylaxis, secondary to the documented peanut allergy.

D. Although the symptoms of shortness of breath and anxiety can be caused by a pulmonary embolism, this patient's presentation, history, and onset of symptoms are more consistent with anaphylaxis, secondary to the documented peanut allergy.

Category: Psychosocial and Medical Emergencies/Medical/Allergic reactions and anaphylaxis
Nursing Process: Assessment

Reference

Food Allergy Research & Education. (2016). *Peanut allergy*. Retrieved from https://www.foodallergy.org/allergens/peanut-allergy

---

84. A patient with hemophilia A presents to the emergency department following a mechanical fall resulting in a laceration to the knee that will require suturing. The patient has been applying pressure to the wound, and bleeding is being controlled. The emergency nurse recognizes which of the following to be the highest priority in the care of this patient?

A. Prepare to administer factor VIII
B. Prepare to administer factor IX
C. Prepare to administer desmopressin acetate
D. Prepare to suture the wound on the injured knee

Rationale

A. The highest priority of care for this patient is the replacement of factor VIII, the deficient factor in the patient with hemophilia A (classic hemophilia).

B. Factor IX is the deficient factor in patients with hemophilia B (Christmas disease).

C. Desmopressin acetate (DDAVP) may be helpful in the presence of a mild bleeding episode; however, the administration of DDAVP is not the highest priority. DDAVP will stimulate the release of factor VIII and von Willebrand factor and is not a replacement for factor VIII. The patient should have factor VIII administered directly, not DDAVP, which will stimulate the release of factor VIII.

D. The patient will require sutures to further control bleeding, but the highest priority is to administer the deficient factor VIII. Continued pressure should be applied to any uncontrolled bleeding sites before suturing of the wound.

Category: Psychosocial and Medical Emergencies/Medical/Blood dyscrasias: Hemophilia
Nursing Process: Intervention

References

Carringer, C. J., & Hammond, B. B. (2013). Hematologic and immunologic emergencies. In B. B. Hammond & P. G. Zimmermann (Eds.), *Sheehy's manual of emergency care* (7th ed., pp. 245–254). St. Louis, MO: Elsevier Mosby.

Golder, D. (2012). Childhood illness. In *Emergency Nursing Pediatric Course: Provider manual* (4th ed., pp. 147–170). Des Plaines, IL: Emergency Nurses Association.

Smith, D. A. (2010). Hematologic and oncologic emergencies. In P. K. Howard & R. A. Steinmann (Eds.), *Sheehy's emergency nursing: Principles and practice* (6th ed., pp. 554–563). St. Louis, MO: Mosby Elsevier.

---

85. A patient presents to the emergency department with complaint of an intermittent headache over the past several days. The patient is currently taking warfarin (Coumadin) for atrial fibrillation. Which international normalized ratio laboratory value would indicate a therapeutic dosage for this medication?

A. 1.2
B. 2.3
C. 5.0
D. 9.6

Rationale

A. A level of 1.2 is subtherapeutic and would not provide an adequate level of anticoagulation for the patient.

B. The recommended international normalized ratio range is usually 2–3 for most patients. Levels below this are subtherapeutic and not effective for anticoagulation. Levels greater than the therapeutic range can cause the patient to experience bleeding episodes.

C. A level of 5.0 is above the therapeutic range and could result in the patient experiencing bleeding.

D. A level of 9.6 is well above the therapeutic range and can be life threatening. This value would require immediate intervention to reverse the effects of the warfarin.

Category: Psychosocial and Medical Emergencies/Medical/Blood dyscrasias: Other coagulopathies
Nursing Process: Assessment

Reference

Wolters Kluwer. (2017). Warfarin sodium. In *Nursing 2017 drug handbook* (pp. 1512–1515). Philadelphia, PA: Author.

---

86. The emergency nurse is aware that the most common form of leukemia diagnosed in children is:

A. acute lymphocytic leukemia.
B. acute myelogenous leukemia.
C. chronic lymphocytic leukemia.
D. chronic myelogenous leukemia.

Rationale

A. Acute lymphocytic leukemia (ALL) is the most common type of leukemia diagnosed in children.

B. Acute myelogenous leukemia is not frequently diagnosed in pediatrics; ALL is the most common form of leukemia in children.

C. Chronic lymphocytic leukemia (CLL) is the most common leukemia diagnosed in adults, however, CLL is very rare in the pediatric population.

D. The presence of chronic myelogenous leukemia is very rare in children; ALL is the most common form of leukemia diagnosed in the pediatric population.

Category (Pediatric): Psychosocial and Medical Emergencies/Medical/Blood dyscrasias: Leukemia
Nursing Process: Assessment

References

McQueen, A., & Place, A. E. (2016). Oncologic emergencies. In K. N. Shaw & R. G. Bachur (Eds.), *Fleisher and Ludwig's textbook of pediatric emergency medicine* (7th ed., pp. 934–968). Philadelphia, PA: Wolters Kluwer.

Mueller, L. (2015). Leukemia. In J. J. Schaider, A. Z. Barkin, R. M. Barkin, P. Shayne, . . . P. Rosen (Eds.), *Rosen and Barkin's 5-minute emergency medicine consult* (5th ed., pp. 652–653). Philadelphia, PA: Wolters Kluwer.

---

87. A patient arrives to the emergency department via ambulance with complaints of fatigue and dyspnea. The patient recently completed chemotherapy treatment for acute lymphocytic leukemia. The patient's primary survey is within normal limits. Vital signs: HR 86 beats/minute; RR 18 breaths/minute; SpO_2 94% on room air. Priority interventions for this patient would include which of the following?

A. Preparing the patient for continuous positive airway pressure ventilation
B. Placing the patient in a negative-pressure isolation room
C. Immediate triaging of the patient to the resuscitation room
D. Placing the patient in a private or isolation room

Rationale

A. This patient is not in acute respiratory distress and does not require this level of airway support.

B. A negative pressure room circulates air from outside the room into the room. This creates the possibility of introducing infectious organisms into the room. Negative pressure is used to keep infectious organisms from entering the general air circulation. This patient does not require a negative pressure room environment.

C. The patient is stable and is not in need of emergent resuscitative interventions.

D. Immature white blood cells in leukemic patients result in increased vulnerability to infection. The patient must be isolated from other potentially infectious emergency department patients.

Category: Psychosocial and Medical Emergencies/Medical/Blood dyscrasias: Leukemia
Nursing Process: Intervention

References

Braun, C. A., & Anderson, C. M. (2011). *Pathophysiology: A clinical approach* (2nd ed.) [Kindle version]. Philadelphia, PA: Wolters Kluwer/Lippincott Williams & Wilkins.

Smith, D. (2010). Hematologic and oncologic emergencies. In P. K. Howard & R. A. Steinmann (Eds.), *Sheehy's emergency nursing: Principles and practice* (6th ed., pp. 554–563). St. Louis, MO: Mosby Elsevier.

88. A male patient presents to the emergency department with a complaint related to his sickle cell disease. Which of the following complaints should the emergency nurse anticipate?

A. Anasarca
B. Hematemesis
C. Hematochezia
D. Priapism

Rationale

A. Anasarca (generalized edema) is not a common complaint associated with sickle cell. It is common in patients with a history of heart failure or kidney failure.

B. Hematemesis (vomiting bright red blood) is common in upper gastrointestinal bleeding.

C. Hematochezia (bright red blood in the stool) is not a common complaint associated with sickle cell. It is a common finding in lower gastrointestinal bleeding.

D. Priapism is a painful erection and a genitourinary emergency. It is a common complication for male patients with sickle cell disease to experience priapism. It will occur when the red blood cells become misshapen, sickle, and become lodged in the microvasculature, leading to entrapment of blood in the penis.

Category: Psychosocial and Medical Emergencies/Medical/Blood dyscrasias: Sickle cell crisis

Nursing Process: Analysis

Reference

Smith, D. A. (2010). Hematologic and oncologic emergencies. In P. K. Howard & R. A. Steinmann (Eds.), *Sheehy's emergency nursing: Principles and practice* (6th ed., pp. 554–563). St. Louis, MO: Mosby Elsevier.

---

89. Nursing care of the patient with disseminated intravascular coagulation in the emergency department should include:

A. avoiding suctioning the patient.
B. keeping the patient in a prone position.
C. securing of all invasive lines.
D. administering all medications intramuscularly.

Rationale

A. The patient's airway must be kept patent. However, suctioning should be done only as necessary to minimize the risk of oral bleeding.

B. The patient should be turned and positioned for comfort to prevent skin injury and/or skin breakdown and minimize the risk of bleeding. Additional personnel should be used to move and position the patient as gently as possible.

C. Securing invasive lines minimizes the risk of bleeding as a result of unintentional or intentional dislodgement of the line.

D. Medications should primarily be administered intravenously to avoid the risk of bleeding.

Category: Psychosocial and Medical Emergencies/Medical/Disseminated intravascular coagulation (DIC)

Nursing Process: Intervention

References

Holleran, R., & Lambie, D. (2014). Caring for patients with blood disorders. In K. Osborn, C. Wraa, A. Watson, & R. Holleran (Eds.), *Medical surgical nursing: Preparation for practice* (2nd ed., pp. 1716–1764). Boston, MA: Pearson.

Parker, R. (2013). Coagulopathies in the PICU: DIC and liver disease. *Critical Care Clinics, 29*, 319–333.

---

90. A patient has been prescribed spironolactone (Aldactone) for treatment of cirrhosis. The emergency nurse acknowledges that the patient understands the discharge instructions when the patient states:

A. "I should eat more dried fruit, like apricots."
B. "I should eat an extra banana or avocado daily."
C. "I should not eat popcorn or rice cakes."
D. "I should avoid eating bananas and avocados."

Rationale

A. Dried apricots are high in dietary potassium and therefore should be avoided by patients taking spironolactone.

B. Bananas and avocados are potassium rich and should be avoided with potassium-sparing diuretics.

C. Popcorn and rice cakes do not contain potassium and therefore will not alter the patient's serum potassium levels.

D. Spironolactone is a potassium-sparing diuretic. Patients should receive education to avoid foods that are high in potassium. Both bananas and avocados provide high levels of nutritional potassium.

Category: Psychosocial and Medical Emergencies/Medical/Electrolyte/fluid imbalance

Nursing Process: Evaluation

Reference

Karch, A. M. (2013). Diuretic agents. In *Focus on nursing pharmacology* (7th ed., pp. 882–898). Philadelphia, PA: Lippincott Williams & Wilkins.

---

91. The priority nursing care goal of a patient with syndrome of inappropriate antidiuretic hormone is directed toward which of the following?

A. Slowly correcting the patient's potassium level
B. Determining the severity of hypernatremia
C. Measuring the specific gravity of the patient's urine
D. Determining the severity of hyponatremia

Rationale

A. The patient's serum potassium level is often normal and may not need to be corrected. The sodium level is the most important electrolyte to treat and often must be aggressively corrected or the patient may die.

B. The patient with syndrome of inappropriate antidiuretic hormone (SIADH) will not have an elevated serum sodium level; instead, the patient will have a sodium level often as low as 125 mEq/L.

C. The specific gravity of the patient's urine will be elevated because of the presence of severe hyponatremia. This, however, is not the highest priority of care for the nurse.

D. The patient with SIADH will present with a severe dilutional hyponatremia (low serum sodium levels). Often this level will be less than 125 mEq/L. Symptomatic patients may require 3–5% hypertonic saline to be administered intravenously to correct the severe hyponatremia. Normal serum sodium level is 135 mEq/L–145 mEq/L.

Category: Psychosocial and Medical Emergencies/Medical/Endocrine conditions

Nursing Process: Intervention

References

Marett, B. E. (2013). Metabolic emergencies. In B. B. Hammond & P. G. Zimmermann (Eds.), *Sheehy's manual of emergency care* (7th ed., pp. 303–318). St. Louis, MO: Elsevier Mosby.

Morey, C. M. (2010). Endocrine emergencies. In P. K. Howard & R. A. Steinmann (Eds.), *Sheehy's emergency nursing: Principles and practice* (6th ed., pp. 499–512). St. Louis, MO: Mosby Elsevier.

---

92. Which of the following conditions caused by excessive amounts of antidiuretic hormone results in a patient developing dilutional hyponatremia?

A. Syndrome of inappropriate antidiuretic hormone
B. Adrenal crisis
C. Diabetes insipidus
D. Cushing's syndrome

Rationale

A. The patient will present with dilutional hyponatremia and water intoxication, which can result in seizures. The patient will also complain of headache, fatigue, and weight gain without the presence of edema. Treatment depends on the severity of the patient's hyponatremia. Fluid restriction should be initiated. Severe hyponatremia is treated with hypertonic saline and the administration of furosemide (Lasix).

B. Adrenal crisis, also known as acute adrenal insufficiency, is a life-threatening condition caused by a decrease in cortisol and aldosterone levels. This result is sodium and water loss from both the kidneys and gastrointestinal track, causing the patient to become hypotensive and hypovolemic. As the body loses sodium, there is an increase in potassium leading to hyperkalemia and the development of fatal dysrhythmias. Treatment includes fluid replacement, correction of hyperkalemia, and hydrocortisone administration.

C. Diabetes insipidus (DI) is a life-threatening condition caused by the presence of insufficient antidiuretic hormone (ADH) being produced by the hypothalamus or not being released by the posterior pituitary gland. DI results in the patient to excrete large amounts of diluted urine and complain of associated fatigue and weight loss. Treatment for DI is both fluid replacement and ADH replacement with medications such as desmopressin acetate.

D. Cushing's syndrome is the result of a prolonged exposure to glucocorticoids (either endogenous or exogenous), causing the patient to develop a cushingoid appearance. There is an increased amount of adipose tissue to the face, upper back, and base of the neck.

Category: Psychosocial and Medical Emergencies/Medical/Endocrine conditions
Nursing Process: Assessment

References

Marett, B. (2013). Metabolic emergencies. In B. B. Hammond & P. G. Zimmermann (Eds.), *Sheehy's manual of emergency care* (7th ed., pp. 303–318). St. Louis, MO: Elsevier Mosby.
Morey, C. (2010). Endocrine emergencies. In P. K. Howard & R. A. Steinmann (Eds.), *Sheehy's emergency nursing: Principles and practice* (6th ed., pp. 499–512). St. Louis, MO: Mosby Elsevier.
Wall, S. M. (2007). Endocrine emergencies. In K. S. Hoyt & J. Selfridge-Thomas (Eds.), *Emergency nursing core curriculum* (6th ed., pp. 290–309). St. Louis, MO: Saunders Elsevier.

---

93. A patient with a history of Addison's disease presents to the emergency department for treatment of an adrenal crisis. The emergency nurse knows that the following hormone is involved in an adrenal crisis:

A. Antidiuretic hormone
B. Cortisol
C. Follicle-stimulating hormone
D. Thyroid-stimulating hormone

Rationale

A. Antidiuretic hormone is produced in the pituitary gland and is not involved in an adrenal crisis.

B. Adrenal crisis is an endocrine emergency caused by a lack of glucocorticoids (cortisol) and mineralocorticoids (aldosterone).

C. Follicle-stimulating hormone is a female reproductive hormone produced in the pituitary gland and is not involved in an adrenal crisis.

D. Thyroid-stimulating hormone is produced in the pituitary gland and is not involved in an adrenal crisis.

Category: Psychosocial and Medical Emergencies/Medical/Endocrine conditions: Adrenal
Nursing Process: Assessment

Reference

Sommers, M. S., & Fannin, E. (2015). *Diseases and disorders: A nursing therapeutics manual* (5th ed.). Philadelphia, PA: F. A. Davis.

---

94. Which of the following laboratory studies should the emergency nurse expect in a patient who presents with a diagnosis of diabetic ketoacidosis?

A. Increased pCO_2
B. Elevated creatinine
C. Elevated pH
D. Decreased blood urea nitrogen

Rationale

A. Decreased pCO_2 occurs as a compensatory effect of acidosis. Kussmaul respirations, defined as a deep, rapid respiratory pattern, result in the decreased pCO_2.

B. An elevated creatinine and BUN level should be expected in a patient who is experiencing an episode of diabetic ketoacidosis (DKA) because of dehydration. The dehydration occurs because of the osmotic diuresis from the increased osmolality that accompanies the DKA disease process.

C. The pH level is expected to be deceased, consistent with the presence of metabolic acidosis. An elevated pH level indicates the presence of an alkalosis, not acidosis.

D. The blood urea nitrogen level would be expected to be increased because of the dehydrated state of the patient in diabetic ketoacidosis. This dehydration is caused by an osmotic dehydration because of the increase in the blood glucose level in the serum.

Category: Psychosocial and Medical Emergencies/Medical/Endocrine conditions: Glucose-related conditions

Nursing Process: Analysis

References

Marett, B. (2013). Metabolic emergencies. In B. B. Hammond & P. G. Zimmermann (Eds.), *Sheehy's manual of emergency care* (7th ed., pp. 303–318). St. Louis, MO: Elsevier Mosby.

Morey, C. (2010). Endocrine emergencies. In P. K. Howard & R. A. Steinmann (Eds.), *Sheehy's emergency nursing: Principles and practice* (6th ed., pp. 499–512). St. Louis, MO: Mosby Elsevier.

---

95. Which of the following disease processes would *most* likely benefit from prophylactic therapy for deep vein thrombosis

A. Syndrome of inappropriate antidiuretic hormone
B. Diabetic ketoacidosis
C. Hyperglycemic hyperosmolar syndrome
D. Myxedema coma

Rationale

A. Syndrome of inappropriate antidiuretic hormone does not create dehydration; rather, it increases the amount of water held inside the body and causes a dilutional hyponatremia and a decreased serum osmolality. In this situation, fluids would be restricted.

B. This malady rarely causes thrombotic events to occur. Individuals are usually younger, and though dehydration is part of the diabetic ketoacidosis process, it is not as pronounced as in hyperglycemic hyperosmolar syndrome (HHS).

C. HHS creates extreme dehydration for the patient as well as a hyperosmolar state. The patients are also often bedfast or sedentary either for their age or because of the critical nature of their illness. Therefore, prophylaxis for deep vein thrombosis that can lead to other thrombotic events is necessary.

D. Myxedema coma is a complication of hypothyroidism. This does not cause dehydration in the individual experiencing this progression of hypothyroidism.

Category: Psychosocial and Medical Emergencies/Medical/Endocrine conditions: Glucose-related conditions

Nursing Process: Intervention

References

Marett, B. (2013). Metabolic emergencies. In B. B. Hammond & P. G. Zimmermann (Eds.), *Sheehy's manual of emergency care* (7th ed., pp. 303–318). St. Louis, MO: Elsevier Mosby.

Morey, C. (2010). Endocrine emergencies. In P. K. Howard & R. A. Steinmann (Eds.), *Sheehy's emergency nursing: Principles and practice* (6th ed., pp. 499–512). St. Louis, MO: Mosby Elsevier.

---

96. Several patients complaining of a fever present to triage at the same time. Which of the following patients would be the priority for bed placement?

A. The patient who had surgery 2 weeks ago
B. The patient complaining of a productive cough
C. The patient complaining of a rash
D. The patient who is receiving chemotherapy

Rationale

A. A postop patient is at increased risk of infection, but usually within a few days of the surgery. The febrile patient who underwent surgery 2 weeks earlier requires evaluation, but it does not need to be performed immediately.

B. The complaint of a fever and productive cough warrants assessment, however, the cancer patient who has been receiving chemotherapy and is at risk for neutropenia has the highest priority for care.

C. Though the presence of a rash and fever is concerning, it is common for some viral illnesses to cause a rash. The cancer patient who has been receiving chemotherapy and is at risk for neutropenia has the highest priority for care.

D. Cancer patients, especially those receiving chemotherapy, who present with a fever should be given priority given the concern for neutropenia, their suppressed immune system, and the risk for rapid onset of sepsis.

Category: Psychosocial and Medical Emergencies/Medical/Fever
Nursing Process: Analysis

References

Schillo, G. M., & Williams, J. (2015). The cancer patient in the emergency department. In A. B. Wolfson (Ed.), *Harwood-Nuss' clinical practice of emergency medicine* (6th ed., pp. 984–990). Philadelphia, PA: Wolters Kluwer.

Sterling, S. A., & Jones, A. E. (2015). Fever. In A. B. Wolfson (Ed.), *Harwood-Nuss' clinical practice of emergency medicine* (6th ed., pp. 74–79). Philadelphia, PA: Wolters Kluwer.

---

97. The emergency nurse should discuss a certain form of health promotion with an immunocompromised patient and each of the patient's frequent visitors. The emergency nurse identifies that the teaching has been effective when the patient states which of the following?

A. "I should limit the number of visitors permitted in the room to only one at a time."
B. "All of my visitors should wash their hands when they enter my room."
C. "I need to remind all my visitors to wear a face mask when they are visiting me."
D. "All my visitors should be screened for infections before entering my room."

Rationale

A. There is no minimum number of visitors attributed to a decrease in transmission of infection. As long as the patient is feeling well and desires visitors, there is no need for a strict limit to the number of visitors permitted in the patient's room at one time unless otherwise directed by the health facility policy.

B. All visitors should perform hand hygiene before entering a patient room and immediately after leaving the room. Hand hygiene is a well-established means of reducing the microbial burden on hands and preventing pathogen transmission. In the healthcare setting, hand hygiene can prevent the spread of microorganisms between patients and visitors.

C. This is not necessary unless the patient has been placed in isolation for airborne precautions or the visitor feels they are may be ill.

D. Screening all visitors for infection may not be feasible. Proper hand hygiene is proved to be one of the most effective infection control measures.

Category: Psychosocial and Medical Emergencies/Medical/Immunocompromise

Nursing Process: Evaluation

Reference

Munoz-Price, L. S., Banach, D. B., Bearman, G., Gould, J. M., Leekha, S., Morgan, D. J., . . . Wiemken, T. L. (2015). Isolation precautions for visitors. *Infection Control & Hospital Epidemiology, 36*(7), 747–758. http://dx.doi.org/10.1017/ice.2015.67

---

98. Which of the following interventions should be initiated for the treatment of a septic patient within 1 hour of presenting to the emergency department?

A. Blood cultures, antibiotics, and 30 mL/kg intravenous fluids for lactate of greater than 2 mmol/L.

B. Blood cultures, vasopressors, and central venous pressure monitoring if the mean arterial pressure is less than 65 mm Hg.

C. Blood cultures, antibiotics, and rapid administration of 30 mL/kg of crystalloids for lactate of greater than or equal to 4 mmol/L.

D. Antibiotics and vasopressors if mean arterial pressure is greater than 65 mm Hg, and lactate level greater than or equal to 4 mmol/L.

Rationale

A. Begin rapid administration of crystalloids for hypotension or lactate level greater than or equal to 4 mmol/L.

B. Central venous pressure monitoring may be initiated but is not included in the 1-hour sepsis bundle.

C. These are all included in the 1-hour sepsis bundle.

D. Vasopressors are indicated if the patient is hypotensive during or after fluid resuscitation to maintain a mean arterial pressure of greater than or equal to 65 mm Hg.

Category: Psychosocial and Medical Emergencies/Medical/Sepsis and septic shock

Nursing Process: Intervention

Reference

Levy, M. M., & Rhodes, A. (2018). The surviving sepsis campaign bundle: 2018 update. *Critical Care Medicine, 46*(6), 997–1000. https://doi.org10.1097/CCM.0000000000003119

---

99. A patient is transferred from another facility with a fractured tibia/fibula; a splint was applied to the extremity before transfer. The patient is very tearful and is complaining of excessive pain in the injured leg. The emergency nurse is concerned the patient may be experiencing signs and symptoms of compartment syndrome. The most appropriate intervention for the emergency nurse to perform is to:

A. loosen or remove any restrictive devices on the extremity.
B. apply ice packs to the lower portion of the extremity.
C. elevate the extremity immediately above the heart level.
D. apply a tourniquet to the extremity.

Rationale

A. Remove restrictive items, such as circumferential tape or elastic wraps, and ice bags in patients who are demonstrating possible signs and symptoms of compartment syndrome. Signs and symptoms of compartment syndrome are pain that is disproportional to the injury; pressure or tightness over the injury site; pale and cool skin; lack of or diminished pulses distal to the injury site; numbness/tingling (paresthesia) in the affected extremity; and paralysis.

B. The application of ice is contraindicated because this promotes further vasoconstriction in the presence of compartment syndrome.

C. Maintain the extremity in a neutral position and elevate the limb only to the level of the heart to promote circulation. Further elevation above the level of the heart inhibits arterial perfusion to the affected tissue.

D. A tourniquet may be used to control bleeding for amputations. For compartment syndrome, a fasciotomy may be indicated to decompress the compartment in order to prevent muscle and/or neurovascular damage and loss of limb.

Category: Maxillofacial, Ocular, Orthopedic, and Wound Emergencies/Orthopedic/Compartment syndrome

Nursing Process: Intervention

Reference

Halpern, J. S. (2013). Musculoskeletal trauma. In B. B. Hammond & P. G. Zimmermann (Eds.), *Sheehy's manual of emergency care* (7th ed., pp. 427–438). St. Louis, MO: Elsevier Mosby.

100. An unrestrained driver involved in a motor vehicle collision arrives to the emergency department by ambulance. During the secondary assessment, signs and symptoms of a possible fractured femur are observed. The emergency nurse anticipates the patient will have which of the following findings?

A. Excessive hip flexion
B. Shortened length of the injured extremity
C. Hyperextension of the knee in the same extremity as the fractured femur
D. Deformity of the ankle

Rationale

A. Assessment findings of femur fractures include pain and the inability to bear weight; shortening of the affected leg; internal or external rotation; edema of the thigh; deformity of the thigh; and evidence of hypovolemic shock (this may or may not be present). Excessive hip flexion indicates a possible hip injury in conjunction with the femur fracture.

B. Assessment findings of femur fractures include pain and the inability to bear weight; shortening of the affected leg; internal or external rotation; edema of the thigh; deformity of the thigh; and evidence of hypovolemic shock (this may or may not be present).

C. Assessment findings of femur fractures include pain and the inability to bear weight; shortening of the affected leg; internal or external rotation; edema of the thigh; deformity of the thigh; and evidence of hypovolemic shock (this may or may not be present). Hyperextension of the knee on the affected side would indicate a secondary injury in the knee joint, not a fractured femur.

D. Assessment findings of femur fractures include pain and the inability to bear weight; shortening of the affected leg; internal or external rotation; edema of the thigh; deformity of the thigh; and evidence of hypovolemic shock (this may or may not be present). Deformity of the ankle would indicate an injury in the ankle, not a fractured femur.

Category: Maxillofacial, Ocular, Orthopedic, and Wound Emergencies/Orthopedic/Fractures/dislocations

Nursing Process: Assessment

Reference

Bratcher, C. M. (2014). Musculoskeletal trauma. In D. Gurney (Ed.), *Trauma Nursing Core Course: Provider manual* (7th ed., pp. 193–203). Des Plaines, IL: Emergency Nurses Association.

---

101. Parents and their child arrive at the emergency department. The child had jumped out of a tree and is complaining of pain in the left ankle and inability to bear weight on the foot. Skin is intact, and the patient has good distal pulses bilaterally (dorsalis pedal and posterior tibial) with no gross deformity, but swelling is present. Initial radiographs are negative for fracture. The emergency nurse suspects the child has a(n):

A. displaced fracture.
B. open fracture.
C. comminuted fracture.
D. Salter–Harris fracture.

Rationale

A. Although swelling is observed, there is no bone displacement evident on radiographs.

B. Open fractures are graded 1–3 according to degree of soft tissue injury. The skin is intact on this patient, so the fracture is considered "closed."

C. Comminuted fractures result in splintering of bone with the presence of obvious fragments. Radiographs show no obvious fracture pattern or bone fragments in this patient.

D. The classification of Salter–Harris fractures (type I–type V) involves the disruption of the epiphysis (growth plate). These fractures have implications for treatment, prognosis, and healing. A type V Salter–Harris fracture generally involves an axial load, and initial radiographs may be negative but can result in a poor functional outcome. Diagnosis is often made retrospectively after premature closure of the epiphysis.

Category (Pediatric): Maxillofacial, Ocular, Orthopedic, and Wound Emergencies/Orthopedic/Fractures/dislocations

Nursing Process: Analysis

References

Cerepani, M. J. (2010). Orthopedic and neurovascular trauma. In P. K. Howard & R. A. Steinmann (Eds.), *Sheehy's emergency nursing: Principles and practice* (6th ed., pp. 313–339). St. Louis, MO: Mosby Elsevier.

Crowley, M. (2014). Spinal cord and vertebral column trauma. In D. Gurney (Ed.), *Trauma Nursing Core Course: Provider manual* (7th ed., pp. 173–192). Des Plaines, IL: Emergency Nurses Association.

Denske, N. (2012). Trauma. In *Emergency Nursing Pediatric Course: Provider manual* (4th ed., pp. 261–294). Des Plaines, IL: Emergency Nurses Association.

Moore, W. H. (2017). Salter-Harris fracture imaging. Retrieved from https://emedicine.medscape.com/article/412956-overview

---

102. The emergency nurse is evaluating a patient's understanding of discharge instructions related to gout. The nurse is aware that the patient understands the discharge instructions when the patient states:

A. "I need to limit my water intake because too much fluid can cause a gout flare-up."
B. "My hydrochlorothiazide could have contributed to this flare-up of gout."
C. "I should start the prescription for allopurinol now because it will treat the gout flare-up."
D. "I should eat more seafood to help prevent future gout flare-ups."

Rationale

A. Staying hydrated will help decrease the incidence of the patient experiencing a gout flare-up. Not staying well hydrated will increase the incidence of gout flare-up.

B. Thiazide diuretics can contribute to gout flare-ups because they cause loss of fluid in the body. This causes the remaining body fluids to become more concentrated, which increases the likelihood that urate crystals will then deposit in joint spaces.

C. Allopurinol is a preventive medication that is indicated in the treatment of gout. It can actually increase the severity of the gout flare-up if it is started immediately after the flare-up occurs. The patient should wait until the gout flare-up has subsided completely to start allopurinol.

D. Patients should eat foods low in purine; therefore, patients with gout should avoid organ meats, red meats, and seafood. In addition, patients need to limit their intake of alcohol and drink plenty of water to reduce the occurrence of flare-ups.

Category: Maxillofacial, Ocular, Orthopedic, and Wound Emergencies/Orthopedic/Inflammatory conditions

Nursing Process: Evaluation

Reference

Lazier, S. E., & Roberts, A. (2007). Medical emergencies. In K. S. Hoyt & J. Selfridge-Thomas (Eds.), *Emergency nursing core curriculum* (6th ed., pp. 483–509). St. Louis, MO: Saunders Elsevier.

---

103. A patient presents to triage complaining of continuous left knee pain for the past month. The patient denies any history of trauma to the knee. The current pain level is 3/10, and the patient states the pain is more intense on awakening in the morning, but after being up and moving, the pain lessens. The knee will occasionally swell but is currently not swollen. The patient previously trained for marathons and continues to run at least 20 miles each week. Vital signs: BP 108/62 mm Hg; HR 54 beats/minute; RR 14 breaths/minute; SpO_2 97%; T 37°C (98.6°F). The emergency nurse anticipates the patient has:

A. rheumatoid arthritis.
B. osteoarthritis.
C. bursitis.
D. septic arthritis.

Rationale

A. Rheumatoid arthritis is an autoimmune disorder associated with inflammation around the synovial joints. Rheumatoid arthritis often affects the little joints of the fingers and usually affects the joints bilaterally. The disorder should be managed by a rheumatologist because it will require long-term management to prevent permanent disability.

B. Osteoarthritis is associated with pain in one or more joints. The pain is not always bilateral but can be. Swelling may or may not be present and is marked by stiffness when not active but improvement in stiffness when active. Osteoarthritis can be associated with sports such as running, which can cause a lot of wear and tear on weight-bearing joints such as knees and hips.

C. Bursitis is an inflammation of a bursa. It usually occurs over bony prominences such as the elbow but can also occur in the knees or hips. It can be caused by trauma, repetitive use (such as always resting elbows on a hard surface), or infection in the bursa.

D. Septic arthritis occurs when a joint becomes infected with bacteria. It is commonly seen in the presence of trauma to the joint space or surrounding area, such as a puncture wound where bacteria are able to enter into the joint space. The joint will be red, swollen, and warm to touch, and it will be painful for the patient to move.

Category: Maxillofacial, Ocular, Orthopedic, and Wound Emergencies/Orthopedic/Inflammatory conditions

Nursing Process: Analysis

Reference

Cerepani, M. J., & Ramponi, D. R. (2007). Orthopedic emergencies. In K. S. Hoyt & J. Selfridge-Thomas (Eds.), *Emergency nursing core curriculum* (6th ed., pp. 585–603). St. Louis, MO: Saunders Elsevier.

---

104. Following completion of a joint aspiration of the knee by the provider, the emergency nurse should perform which intervention?

A. Apply pressure to the aspiration site for at least 2 minutes
B. Place an ice pack on the aspiration site for 15 minutes

C. Place a heat pack on the aspiration site for 15 minutes
D. Elevate the extremity above the level of the heart

Rationale

A. Applying direct pressure for 2 minutes is the first thing that should be performed following the procedure to stop further bleeding at the site. Other interventions, like applying ice or a pressure dressing, can be delayed until the bleeding has stopped.

B. Application of an ice pack is an appropriate intervention after the dressing has been applied, but applying pressure to the aspiration site is the priority intervention.

C. Placing heat on an aspiration site following the procedure is not recommended because this can increase blood flow to the area and increase the risk of bleeding.

D. This is a recommended intervention and is thought to reduce swelling, but applying direct pressure to the site for 2 minutes, followed by the application of a pressure dressing, is the priority intervention.

Category: Maxillofacial, Ocular, Orthopedic, and Wound Emergencies/Orthopedic/Joint effusion
Nursing Process: Intervention

Reference

Halpern, J. S. (2013). Musculoskeletal trauma. In B. B. Hammond & P. G. Zimmermann (Eds.), *Sheehy's manual of emergency care* (7th ed., pp. 427–438). St. Louis, MO: Elsevier Mosby.

---

105. A patient presents to the emergency department following their soccer game. The patient states they were running and "rolled" their ankle on an uneven area on the field. Their left ankle is swollen and tender to touch, and the patient experiences increasing pain with weight bearing on the affected foot. On providing discharge instructions for this patient, the emergency nurse acknowledges the need for further instructions when the patient states:

A. "I need to rest my ankle, keep it elevated, ice it, and use an ACE bandage."
B. "It is okay to go back to playing soccer once the swelling is gone."
C. "I should start physical therapy and stretching exercises in about a week."
D. "It is okay for me to take acetaminophen (Tylenol) or ibuprofen (NSAID) for the pain in my ankle."

Rationale

A. This statement shows understanding of correct discharge instructions. RICE (Rest, Ice, Compress, Elevate) principles are used to decrease swelling/inflammation and decrease pain.

B. This injury is consistent with an ankle sprain. There are different grades of ankle sprains, and although the swelling may go down, the ankle may still be unstable. It will be important for the patient to have the ankle reevaluated with their primary care provider once the swelling is gone to determine ankle stability and the need for possible further treatment, especially if the patient continues is having difficulty weight bearing.

C. This statement shows understanding of correct discharge instructions for ankle sprains. Physical therapy or a sports provider can recommend stretching and strengthening exercises that will increase the strength and stability of the joint.

D. This statement shows understanding of correct discharge instructions for ankle sprains. Anti-inflammatories like ibuprofen and pain medications like acetaminophen may help decrease inflammation and decrease pain.

Category (Pediatric): Maxillofacial, Ocular, Orthopedic, and Wound Emergencies/Orthopedic/Strains/sprains

Nursing Process: Evaluation

Reference

Rouzier, P. (2010). *The sports medicine patient advisor* (3rd ed.). Amherst, MA: SportsMedPress.

---

106. The best way for the emergency nurse to evaluate the effectiveness of teaching a patient with an injured their ankle to crutch walk is to have the patient:

A. teach the skill to a friend in the presence of the emergency nurse.
B. restate the crutch walking instructions.
C. teach back the procedure to the emergency nurse.
D. demonstrate crutch walking.

Rationale

A. Teach-back has been proved as an effective technique for cognitive learning, however, demonstration of the skill is superior in psychomotor situations.

B. Verbalization of the steps may indicate a cognitive understanding; however, it does not indicate the ability to perform the procedure.

C. Teach-back has been proved as an effective technique for cognitive learning, however, demonstration of the skill is superior in psychomotor situations.

D. The return demonstration of the proper techniques offers the best ability to evaluate learning.

Category: Maxillofacial, Ocular, Orthopedic, and Wound Emergencies/Orthopedic/Strains/sprains

Nursing Process: Evaluation

References

Cerepani, M. J. (2010). Orthopedic and neurovascular trauma. In P. K. Howard & R. A. Steinmann (Eds.), *Sheehy's emergency nursing: Principles and practice* (6th ed., pp. 313–339). St. Louis, MO: Mosby Elsevier.

EuroMed Info. (n.d.). *Evaluating teaching and learning*. Retrieved from http://www.euromedinfo.eu/evaluating-teaching-and-learning.html/

---

107. A patient presents to the emergency department with complaints of chest pain and shortness of breath and appears apprehensive and restless. The patient had been discharged the previous day following repair of a fractured femur. Vital signs: BP 132/84 mm Hg; HR 98 beats/minute; RR 22 breaths/minute; T 37.7°C (100°F). The emergency nurse anticipates the most likely explanation for the patient's symptoms is the presence of:

A. hemorrhage.
B. a pulmonary embolism.
C. deep vein thrombosis.
D. myocardial infarction.

Rationale

A. The patient's vital signs do not indicate any signs or symptoms of excessive bleeding.

B. Patients who have sustained recent trauma with long bone injuries that require surgery and immobility are at a high risk for the development of a pulmonary embolism. Patients with a pulmonary embolism often appear anxious and restless.

C. Impaired gas exchange is more likely to present with pulmonary embolism rather than deep vein thrombosis. This patient is restless and anxious and has a respiratory rate of 22, all of which indicate the potential for impaired gas exchange. The patient does not indicate any calf tenderness, redness, or swelling.

D. The patient's history of trauma with long bone fracture and recent surgery is more likely the cause of the pulmonary embolism. More information and diagnostic studies are needed to rule out the presence of a myocardial infarction.

Category: Maxillofacial, Ocular, Orthopedic, and Wound Emergencies/Orthopedic/Trauma

Nursing Process: Analysis

Reference

Selfridge-Thomas, J., & Hoyt, K. S. (2007). Respiratory emergencies. In K. S. Hoyt & J. Selfridge-Thomas (Eds.), *Emergency nursing core curriculum* (6th ed., pp. 685–720). St. Louis, MO: Saunders Elsevier.

---

108. A baseball player complains of severe pain to the back of their foot above the heel. The patient states they heard a popping noise while running during a recent game. There is tenderness, swelling, and difficulty pointing their toes on examination. The patient's past medical history is significant for traveler's diarrhea over the past month, which has been treated with a fluoroquinolone. The emergency nurse suspects the patient has sustained a(n):

A. ankle dislocation.
B. Achilles tendon rupture.
C. ankle sprain.
D. calcaneal fracture.

Rationale

A. Symptoms of dislocation include joint deformity and swelling over the affected area. Ambulation would be unlikely with an ankle dislocation.

B. Symptoms of Achilles tendon rupture include pain along the back of the foot and above the heel, especially when stretching the ankle or standing on toes; tenderness; swelling; stiffness; a popping noise during injury; and difficulty flexing the foot or pointing the toes. The administration of fluoroquinolones is a known risk factor for tendinitis and tendon rupture.

C. Sprain symptoms include swelling and pain over the lateral and/or medial malleolus.

D. Symptoms include pain in the heel, but the mechanism of running is unlikely to cause a fracture calcaneus.

Category: Maxillofacial, Ocular, Orthopedic, and Wound Emergencies/Orthopedic/Trauma

Nursing Process: Assessment

Reference

Lewis, T., & Cook, J. (2014). Fluoroquinolones and tendinopathy: A guide for athletes and sports clinicians and a systematic review of the literature. *Journal of Athletic Training, 49*(3), 422–427.

---

109. A patient presents to the emergency department following a motorcycle collision. Multiple abrasions are noted on the patient's left leg, hip, trunk, and arm. While preparing to provide treatment, the emergency nurse explains the goals of wound care to the patient. Which of the following is a goal of wound care?

A. Maintain function
B. Restore thermoregulation
C. Manage pain
D. Obtain homeostasis

Rationale

A. Maintaining or preserving function is a goal or desired outcome of wound care and management of the trauma patient. Additional goals are prevention of complications such as infection, and promotion of wound healing.

B. Thermoregulation, an essential integumentary function, is restored through the process of wound healing but is not a goal of wound healing.

C. Pain management is an overall goal of managing the trauma patient. Interventions to manage pain are beneficial before performing wound care.

D. A phase of wound healing, homeostasis occurs with the formation of a clot through platelet aggregation, the clotting cascade, and vasoconstriction. Interventions to control bleeding, such as direct pressure or tourniquets, are used to obtain and maintain homeostasis, which is a goal of treating surface trauma.

Category: Maxillofacial, Ocular, Orthopedic, and Wound Emergencies/Wound/Abrasions

Nursing Process: Evaluation

Reference

Churbock, C. P. Surface and burn trauma. (2014). In D. Gurney (Ed.), *Trauma Nursing Core Course: Provider manual* (7th ed., pp. 205–224). Des Plaines, IL: Emergency Nurses Association.

---

110. A patient has undergone an incision and drainage of a large abscess under the axilla. The emergency nurse anticipates which type of further wound treatment for the area?

A. Using a wet-to-dry dressing
B. Suturing of the abscess cavity
C. Using adhesive wound glue to close the abscess cavity
D. Packing with iodinated gauze

Rationale

A. Application of a wet-to-dry dressing would not be appropriate for this type of wound.

B. Abscesses are typically not sutured to allow for continued drainage from the abscess cavity.

C. Adhesive wound glue is not indicated for the closure of an abscess cavity following incision and drainage.

D. Following incision and drainage, an abscess is packed with iodinated gauze to prevent the premature closure of the skin and to facilitate further drainage from the area.

Category: Maxillofacial, Ocular, Orthopedic, and Wound Emergencies/Wound/Infections

Nursing Process: Intervention

Reference

Herr, R. D. (2013). Wound management. In B. B. Hammond & P. G. Zimmermann (Eds.), *Sheehy's manual of emergency care* (7th ed., pp. 147–160). St. Louis, MO: Elsevier Mosby.

---

111. The emergency nurse is aware that the priority assessment of a patient who has sustained a traumatic laceration with deep tissue injury to the upper arm is to assess which of the following?

A. Capillary refill in the affected extremity
B. Range of motion of the fingers of the affected extremity
C. Distal pulses in the extremity
D. Skin color and temperature

Rationale

A. Decreased capillary refill can indicate impaired perfusion to the extremity but is not as reliable an indicator of tissue perfusion as the presence of a radial pulse and ulnar pulse.

B. Limited range of motion in the affected extremity may indicate that a tendon has been compromised by the injury, but it is not the priority assessment.

C. Lack of a distal pulse may indicate vascular compromise to the arm and requires an immediate intervention because perfusion to the extremity has been compromised.

D. Altered skin color and temperature can indicate decreased perfusion to the arm but is not as reliable an indicator as the presence of a radial pulse and ulnar pulse.

Category: Maxillofacial, Ocular, Orthopedic, and Wound Emergencies/Wound/Lacerations

Nursing Process: Assessment

Reference

Herr, R. D. (2013). Wound management. In B. B. Hammond & P. G. Zimmermann (Eds.), *Sheehy's manual of emergency care* (7th ed., pp. 147–160). St. Louis, MO: Elsevier Mosby.

---

112. In providing discharge instructions to the mother of a toddler who just had a forehead laceration closed with 2-octyl cyanoacrylate (Dermabond), the emergency nurse identifies the mother's proper understanding of the instructions when she states which of the following?

A. "I should wash the wound area daily with soap and water."
B. "I should keep the wound area clean and dry."
C. "It is important for me to keep the wound covered every day."
D. "I must apply antibiotic ointment to the area every day."

Rationale

A. Wounds closed with surgical glue, 2-octyl cyanoacrylate (Dermabond) should be kept clean and dry; if wetness develops during bathing, the area should be pat dry gently.

B. Wounds closed with surgical glue, 2-octyl cyanoacrylate (Dermabond), should be kept clean and dry.

C. The wound should be kept open to the air and observed for signs of possible infection.

D. Application of an ointment will weaken the integrity of the 2-octyl cyanoacrylate (Dermabond) and should be avoided.

Category: Maxillofacial, Ocular, Orthopedic, and Wound Emergencies/Wound/Lacerations

Nursing Process: Evaluation

Reference

Ethicon. (1997). *Dermabond.* Retrieved from https://www.accessdata.fda.gov/cdrh_docs/pdf/P960052c.pdf

---

113. The emergency nurse is caring for a patient who had been found lying on the floor for 2 days following a fall. The nurse assesses an area of purple discoloration along the patient's greater trochanter, which is boggy and warm to touch. The emergency nurse recognizes this wound to be a(n):

A. area of bruising.
B. stage 1 pressure ulcer.
C. potential deep tissue injury.
D. stage 4 pressure ulcer.

Rationale

A. Bruise is the extravasation of blood in the tissues as a result of blunt force impact to the body. The wound sustained by this patient is described as a purple or maroon localized area of discolored intact skin or blood-filled blister that is a result of damage to underlying soft tissue from pressure and/or shear.

B. A stage 1 pressure ulcer is described as intact skin with nonblanchable redness of a localized area, usually over a bony prominence. The wound sustained by this patient is described as a purple or maroon localized area of discolored intact skin or blood-filled blister that is a result of damage to underlying soft tissue from pressure and/or shear.

C. A deep tissue injury is described as a purple or maroon localized area of discolored intact skin or blood-filled blister that is a result of damage to underlying soft tissue from pressure and/or shear. This injury results from intense and/or prolonged pressure and shear forces at the bone–muscle interface, which is consistent with the patient's history of lying on the floor for 2 days.

D. A stage 4 pressure ulcer is described as full thickness tissue loss with exposed bone, tendon, or muscle. The wound sustained by this patient is described as a purple or maroon localized area of discolored intact skin or blood-filled blister that is a result of damage to underlying soft tissue from pressure and/or shear.

Category: Maxillofacial, Ocular, Orthopedic, and Wound Emergencies/Wound/Pressure ulcers

Nursing Process: Assessment

References

National Pressure Ulcer Advisory Panel. (n.d.). *Deep tissue injury* [White paper]. Retrieved from http://www.npuap.org/wp-content/uploads/2012/01/DTI-White-Paper.pdf

National Pressure Ulcer Advisory Panel. (n.d.). *NPUAP pressure injury stages.* Retrieved from http://www.npuap.org/resources/educational-and-clinical-resources/npuap-pressure-injury-stages/

---

114. A patient presents to emergency triage with a handwritten note indicating that they are experiencing severe throat pain. When attempting to speak, the patient's voice sounds as though they are speaking with a hot potato in their mouth. The emergency nurse immediately recognizes this as a symptom of which of the following?

A. Laryngeal foreign body
B. Epiglottitis
C. Peritonsillar abscess
D. Exudative pharyngitis

Rationale

A. Laryngeal foreign body typically occurs in children under the age of 6 years. The most common foreign bodies include peanuts, hot dogs, grapes, and other small objects that can obstruct the main stem bronchi or distal trachea, leading to airway obstruction.

B. Epiglottitis occurs most commonly in children under the age of 7 years. Hallmark signs of epiglottitis are sudden onset with fever and severe sore throat; speech is muffled and drooling is present because of the increased difficulty swallowing.

C. Peritonsillar abscess results from an infection affecting the tonsils and surrounding tissue. Patients experience a severe sore throat and have difficulty speaking and swallowing. The tonsils may become so enlarged that the uvula can be displaced, and the patient is unable to swallow.

D. Microorganisms that result in pharyngitis can also affect the tonsils. Patients will experience enlarged tonsils, sore throat, difficulty swallowing, and cervical lymphadenopathy.

Category: Maxillofacial, Ocular, Orthopedic, and Wound Emergencies/Maxillofacial/Abscess

Nursing Process: Assessment

Reference

Smith, D. A. (2007). Dental, ear, nose, and throat emergencies. In K. S. Hoyt & J. Selfridge-Thomas (Eds.), *Emergency nursing core curriculum* (6th ed., pp. 249–289). St. Louis, MO: Saunders Elsevier.

---

115. A patient is brought to the emergency department holding their tooth in their hand, stating the tooth was knocked out while playing soccer. Which of the following interventions is the appropriate method for the emergency nurse to implement to protect the tooth?

A. Hold the avulsed tooth by the crown
B. Wrap the tooth in moist, saline-soaked gauze
C. Place the tooth under the patient's tongue
D. Place the tooth in milk for 2 hours

Rationale

A. Handling the tooth by the crown protects any periodontal ligament fragments that may still be attached to the tooth. These fragments will aid in healing when the tooth is reimplanted.

B. Wrapping the tooth may damage the periodontal ligament fragments and endanger the success of reimplantation. Moist saline gauze may be applied to the avulsion site to relieve pain or control bleeding.

C. Although placing the tooth under the tongue or between the cheek and gum will preserve the tooth, this places the patient at risk for aspiration.

D. It is appropriate to transport an avulsed tooth in milk; however, successful reimplantation is best accomplished within 30 minutes after the tooth has been avulsed.

Category (Pediatric): Maxillofacial, Ocular, Orthopedic, and Wound Emergencies/Maxillofacial/Dental conditions

Nursing Process: Intervention

References

Olson, C. (2003). Dental, ear, nose, and throat emergencies. In L. Newberry (Ed.), *Sheehy's emergency nursing: Principles and practice* (5th ed., pp. 691–706). St. Louis, MO: Mosby.

Smith, D. A. (2007). Dental, ear, nose, and throat emergencies. In K. S. Hoyt & J. Selfridge-Thomas (Eds.), *Emergency nursing core curriculum* (6th ed., pp. 249–289). St. Louis, MO: Saunders Elsevier.

---

116. A patient presents to the emergency department complaining of tinnitus and dizziness. Which of the following is the most likely cause of the patient's symptoms that would lead the emergency nurse to suspect this patient has labyrinthitis?

A. Blurred vision
B. Viral illness
C. Unilateral sensorineural hearing loss
D. Episodic vertigo

Rationale

A. Visual disturbance is frequently associated with Meniere's disease, not labyrinthitis.

B. Labyrinthitis is an inflammatory response of the inner ear and can result from a recent viral or bacterial infection. The inflammation affects the cochlea, resulting in tinnitus and dizziness.

C. Unilateral sensorineural hearing loss is a hallmark symptom of Meniere's disease, along with episodic vertigo and tinnitus. Labyrinthitis may result in decreased hearing.

D. Episodic vertigo is a hallmark symptom of Meniere's disease, along with unilateral hearing loss and tinnitus.

Category: Maxillofacial, Ocular, Orthopedic, and Wound Emergencies/Maxillofacial/Acute vestibular dysfunction

Nursing Process: Analysis

Reference

Smith, D. A. (2007). Dental, ear, nose, and throat emergencies. In K. S. Hoyt & J. Selfridge-Thomas (Eds.), *Emergency nursing core curriculum* (6th ed., pp. 249–289). St. Louis, MO: Saunders Elsevier.

117. A patient presents to the emergency department with a complaint of severe pain in the left ear. The patient states that they were recently on an airline flight, and during the landing descent, they experienced a sudden onset of sharp pain in the ear that has not decreased. The patient has had no previous difficulty with ear pain when flying. Which of the following assessment findings would indicate the presence of a traumatic ruptured tympanic membrane?

A. Blood in the ear canal, with no accompanying presence of a purulent discharge.
B. Presence of purulent material within the ear canal
C. Redness of the pinna
D. Pain in ear when opening the lower jaw

Rationale

A. In the presence of a traumatic ruptured tympanic membrane, normal ear canal landmarks are lost and cannot be visualized; blood will be visualized within the ear canal.

B. Otitis media shows a white or bulging tympanic membrane. If the tympanic membrane ruptures because of increased pressure from the presence of purulent material in the middle ear, visualization of purulent material will be visualized in the ear canal.

C. Redness of the pinna is associated with otitis externa, also referred to as "swimmer's ear," and is the result of water that accumulates within the ear canal. The patient will experience intense pain when the tragus of the ear is pulled or moved. The ear canal is narrowed because of the presence of purulent material that is lining the canal.

D. The temporomandibular joint (TMJ) lies just under the ear canal. Pain that is localized to the TMJ is the result of arthritis or unusual stress that is placed on the TMJ. The pain can occur from crunching hard food such as ice cubes or carrots or be the result of a direct blow to the mandible on the affected side.

Category: Maxillofacial, Ocular, Orthopedic, and Wound Emergencies/Maxillofacial/Ruptured tympanic membrane

Nursing Process: Assessment

References

Nolan, E. G. (2010). Dental, ear, nose, throat, and facial emergencies. In P. K. Howard & R. A. Steinmann (Eds.), *Sheehy's emergency nursing: Principles and practice* (6th ed., pp. 590–601). St. Louis, MO: Mosby Elsevier.

Solheim, J. (2013). Facial, ocular, ENT, and dental trauma. In B. B. Hammond & P. G. Zimmermann (Eds.), *Sheehy's manual of emergency care* (7th ed., pp. 439–452). St. Louis, MO: Elsevier Mosby.

118. A patient presents to triage, stating that they tripped over a rug, falling directly onto their face. There is noticeable periorbital and facial edema, and ecchymosis is noted around the left eye with the presence of infraorbital hypoesthesia. The patient complains of "seeing double" and is having trouble opening their mouth. There is blood around the nares. The emergency nurse anticipates this patient has sustained which type of facial fracture?

A. Orbital rim fracture
B. Zygomatic fracture
C. Nasal fracture
D. Le Fort II fracture

Rationale

A. Orbital rim fracture is associated with visible or palpable deformity around the orbit, ocular entrapment, diplopia, enophthalmos, infraorbital paresthesia, and subconjunctival hemorrhage.

B. Symptoms of a zygomatic fracture are trismus, infraorbital hypoesthesia, diplopia, epistaxis, symmetrical abnormality, and the presence of facial edema and ecchymosis. The mechanism of injury for this patient was a direct blow to the face, which is indicative in the presence of a zygomatic fracture.

C. Nasal fracture can involve nasal deformity, crepitus, ecchymosis, and edema, as well as anterior or posterior epistaxis.

D. Le Fort II fracture extends above the nose in a pyramidal manner. The nose and upper palate are separated from the rest of the face. If the upper teeth are manipulated, the nose and upper palate will remain mobile, while the orbits remain fixed. The patient will complain of midfacial pain and flattened nares. The patient may also exhibit subconjunctival hemorrhage.

Category: Maxillofacial, Ocular, Orthopedic, and Wound Emergencies/Maxillofacial/Trauma

Nursing Process: Analysis

Reference

Solheim, J. (2013). Facial, ocular, ENT, and dental trauma. (2013). In B. B. Hammond & P. G. Zimmermann (Eds.), *Sheehy's manual of emergency care* (7th ed., pp. 439–452). St. Louis, MO: Elsevier Mosby.

---

119. A patient with a history of acute closed-angle glaucoma presents to the emergency department with a complaint of severe unilateral eye pain and blurred vision. What is the priority action for this patient?

A. Immediately notify the emergency provider of the patient's arrival
B. Dilate the eye to determine if the cornea has become edematous
C. Place the patient in a darkened room
D. Treat the patient's accompanying symptoms of nausea and headache

Rationale

A. The emergency department provider can complete tonometry and, if elevated pressures are present, provide prompt definitive treatment to preserve vision. The patient will most likely also require an examination by an ophthalmologist.

B. It is very important that the examiner not dilate the eye because dilatation may further exacerbate the increased intraocular pressure.

C. A darkened room may cause pupillary dilation and exacerbate the presence of increased intraocular pressure.

D. The presence of nausea and a headache can be treated with the appropriate medication; however, these symptoms usually resolve without treatment once the increased intraocular pressures have been decreased.

Category: Maxillofacial, Ocular, Orthopedic, and Wound Emergencies/Ocular/Glaucoma

Nursing Process: Intervention

Reference

Goolsby, M. (2015). The eye. In M. Goolsby & L. Grubbs (Eds.), *Advanced assessment* (3rd ed., pp. 96–122). Philadelphia, PA: F. A. Davis.

---

120. Which laboratory test would the emergency nurse anticipate to be ordered on a patient with a potential organophosphate exposure?

A. Platelet count
B. Serum lactate level
C. Urine drug screen
D. Plasma pseudocholinesterase level

Rationale

A. Blood platelets are not altered by exposure to organophosphates, so a platelet count is not indicated.

B. Serum lactate levels are not indicated to confirm organophosphate exposure; serum lactate level is indicated in the presence of suspected sepsis.

C. Urine drug screen will not confirm a patient's exposure to organophosphates.

D. Organophosphate poisoning may be confirmed by measuring the patient's plasma pseudocholinesterase level.

Category: Environment and Toxicology Emergencies, and Communicable Diseases/Environment/Chemical exposure

Nursing Process: Analysis

Reference

Sturt, P. (2010). Toxicological emergencies. In P. K. Howard & R. A. Steinmann (Eds.), *Sheehy's emergency nursing: Principles and practice* (6th ed., pp. 564–577). St. Louis, MO: Mosby Elsevier.

---

121. The most common cardiac rhythm disturbance associated with the presence of an electrical shock injury is:

A. ventricular tachycardia.
B. atrial fibrillation.
C. ventricular fibrillation.
D. premature atrial complexes.

Rationale

A. Causes of ventricular tachycardia may be because of myocardial infarction, digitalis toxicity, or hypokalemia, but it is not the result of an electric shock injury.

B. Atrial fibrillation may be caused by heart failure, hypertension, and atrial enlargement. The presence of atrial fibrillation is not associated with an electrical shock injury. Patients may develop atrial fibrillation because of excitation of atrial tissue, which may lead to a tachydysrhythmia.

C. Alternating current that travels through the body can lead to ventricular fibrillation, requiring immediate defibrillation and resuscitation. All patients who have experienced significant electrical shock should have cardiac monitoring as soon as possible following the injury. The presence of any cardiac dysrhythmias should be evaluated for immediate intervention.

D. Premature atrial complexes can be because of caffeine, nicotine, cocaine, alcohol, or anxiety; they are not the result of an electrical shock injury.

Category: Environment and Toxicology Emergencies, and Communicable Diseases/Environment/ Electrical injuries

Nursing Process: Assessment

References

Criddle, L. (2007). Cardiovascular emergencies. In K. S. Hoyt & J. Selfridge-Thomas (Eds.), *Emergency nursing core curriculum* (6th ed., pp. 187–248). St. Louis, MO: Saunders Elsevier.

Wraa, C. (2010). Burns. In P. K. Howard & R. A. Steinmann (Eds.), *Sheehy's emergency nursing: Principles and practice* (6th ed., pp. 340–354). St. Louis, MO: Mosby Elsevier.

---

122. A patient presents to the emergency department with an insect bite to the hand. You observe a single puncture wound surrounded by a moderate amount of edema. The patient is complaining of severe cramping in the affected extremity and abdomen. You suspect this puncture wound is the result of a:

A. nonvenomous snake bite
B. brown recluse spider bite.
C. scorpion sting
D. black widow spider bite.

Rationale

A. Nonvenomous snakes have rows of teeth and demonstrate scratch marks rather than a single puncture wound. Although edema may be present, muscle cramps are not present.

B. A brown recluse spider bite is defined as necrotoxic, resulting in tissue destruction. Initially the bite will appear red and swollen, followed by a burning sensation at the site. The typical bite mark has a bluish discoloration with tissue toxicity occurring over several hours.

C. The stings of most scorpions are considered harmless to humans and require no specific care or treatment. The sting causes immediate painful tingling at the site with local erythema and heightened sensitivity in the area.

D. A black widow spider bite is considered neurotoxic, causing initial stinging at the bite site followed by muscle cramps in the affected extremity and the larger muscles in the abdomen. Moderate edema is typically evident, along with a halo around the single bite mark. The patient may also experience hypertension and diaphoresis.

Category: Environment and Toxicology Emergencies, and Communicable Diseases/Environment/ Envenomation emergencies

Nursing Process: Analysis

Reference

Sedlak, K. (2013). Bite and sting emergencies. In B. B. Hammond & P. G. Zimmermann (Eds.), *Sheehy's manual of emergency care* (7th ed., pp. 345–352). St. Louis, MO: Elsevier Mosby.

123. You are evaluating a patient complaining of severe abdominal cramping, vomiting, and bloody diarrhea for the last 3 days. The patient has not traveled outside the country in the last 90 days and has had no known ill contacts. The patient's BP is 98/72 mm Hg; HR 124 beats/minute; RR 24 breaths/minute; T 37°C (98.6°F); SpO_2 95%. The priority intervention for this patient is to:

A. initiate intravenous hydration with 0.9% sodium chloride or Ringer's lactate solution.
B. obtain complete blood count, electrolyte panel, and stool for analysis.
C. isolate the patient and institute Ebola precautions.
D. provide oxygen at 2 L/minute via nasal cannula.

Rationale

A. Inflammatory diarrhea is caused by agents such as rotavirus, Norwalk virus, *S. Dysenteriae*, Salmonella, *E. coli*, and *Campylobacter jejuni*. They invade the intestinal mucosa and secrete toxins that destroy the intestinal mucosal epithelial cells and result in bloody diarrhea, lower abdominal cramping, and fever. Patients vomiting and unable to tolerate oral rehydration should have an intravenous established for administration of crystalloid fluid and medication.

B. The laboratory testing would be ordered for this patient but is not considered a priority intervention.

C. When obtaining the history, mention is made that the patient has not been out of the country, nor were there any sick contacts. Isolating the patient and initiating Ebola precautions would not be indicated for this patient.

D. The patient's respiratory rate is within normal parameters, and oxygen saturation level is 95%, so supplemental oxygen would not be indicated.

Category: Environment and Toxicology Emergencies, and Communicable Diseases/Environment/Food poisoning

Nursing Process: Intervention

Reference

Russoll, L. W. (2007). Abdominal emergencies. In K. S. Hoyt & J. Selfridge-Thomas (Eds.), *Emergency nursing core curriculum* (6th ed., pp. 159–186). St. Louis, MO: Saunders Elsevier.

---

124. A young mother presents to the emergency department with her 3-month-old infant, stating the infant has not been taking fluids well for the past several days. The triage nurse notes the infant has a flat fontanelle and normal vital signs and is drooling excessively. Further history includes that the child is breastfed. Assessment of the child's mouth reveals white patches on the mucosa and palate. These findings are most consistent with:

A. strep throat.
B. oral candidiasis.
C. teething syndrome.
D. milk curds.

Rationale

A. Strep throat is caused by streptococcal bacteria (group A strep). Symptoms include inflammation and swelling in the back of the throat, and white patches may be noted in the oropharynx; however, white patches do not appear on the tongue.

B. Oral candidiasis, or thrush, is a yeast infection that is common in young infants who are breastfed/nursing. Symptoms include the presence of white patches on the mucous membrane and palate of the mouth.

C. Drooling is often present with teething, but white patches are not noted on the mucous membranes of the mouth. At 3 months of age, the infant is too young to be teething; first teeth do not erupt until at least 6–12 months of age.

D. Milk curds can be regurgitated but usually are noted on the tongue, not the oral mucosa.

Category (Pediatric): Environment and Toxicology Emergencies, and Communicable Diseases/Environment/Parasite and fungal infestations

Nursing Process: Analysis

References

Cadwell, S. (2003). Dermatologic conditions. In D. O. Thomas & L. M. Bernardo (Eds.), *Core curriculum for pediatric emergency nursing* (2nd ed., pp. 265–272). Des Plaines, IL: Emergency Nurses Association.

Pammi, M. (2016). Treatment of candida infection in neonates. *UpToDate*. Retrieved from https://www.uptodate.com/contents/treatment-of-candida-infection-in-neonates

---

125. Following a drowning, a patient's arterial blood gas report represents metabolic acidosis as evident by which of the following?

A. pH 7.5; $PaCO_2$ 25 mm Hg; PaO_2 75 mm Hg; HCO_3 24 mEq/L
B. pH 7.4; $PaCO_2$ 40 mm Hg; PaO_2 90 mm Hg; HCO_3 24 mEq/L
C. pH 7.20; $PaCO_2$ 35 mm Hg; PaO_2 75 mm Hg; HCO_3 18 mEq/L
D. pH 7.5; $PaCO_2$ 45 mm Hg; PaO_2 85 mm Hg; HCO_3 28 mEq/L

Rationale

A. These blood gas values represent respiratory alkalosis, which consists of a pH greater than 7.45 and $PaCO_2$ less than 35 with a normal PaO_2. The pH is above 7.45, indicating alkalosis. The PaO_2 is low (less than 80 mm Hg), and the $PaCO_2$ is less than 35.

B. This blood gas demonstrates represents normal values.

C. Metabolic acidosis consists of low pH, normal $PaCO_2$, and low HCO_3. This blood gas result demonstrates metabolic acidosis, with a pH less than 7.35. The normal $PaCO_2$ is 35–45 mm Hg, and the HCO_3 is low at 18, with a normal value being 22–28 mEq/L.

D. Metabolic alkalosis is demonstrated with these blood gas values. Metabolic alkalosis consists of a pH greater than 7.45 and a HCO_3 greater than 26. The pH is alkalotic with an increased HCO_3 level, indicating alkalosis.

Category: Environment and Toxicology Emergencies, and Communicable Diseases/Environment/Submersion injury

Nursing Process: Assessment

Reference

Selfridge-Thomas, J., & Hoyt, K. S. (2007). Respiratory emergencies. In K. S. Hoyt & J. Selfridge-Thomas (Eds.), *Emergency nursing core curriculum* (6th ed., pp. 685–720) St. Louis, MO: Saunders Elsevier.

126. A patient presents to the emergency department with a cold-related tissue injury to their upper right extremity. Which general management principle should be followed in the care of this patient?

A. Use ice or snow and friction to massage the frozen extremity
B. Protect and immobilize the affected extremity after thawing
C. Thaw the affected area even if it is likely the area may become refrozen before definitive care can be obtained
D. Rub the injured tissues in warm circulating water

Rationale

A. This intervention is now considered outmoded and promotes further tissue destruction, resulting in damage to capillaries and the small vasculature within the extremity.

B. The cold-related tissue injured extremity should be immobilized with a splint and bulky sterile dressings after the thawing process. This intervention will help prevent further trauma to the extremity. Deep cold-related tissue injury or frostbite produces local vascular and tissue changes, resulting in cellular injury and death.

C. Repeated freeze-thaw cycles lead to the development of additional tissue destruction and tissue necrosis.

D. Rubbing the injured tissue can lead to tissue destruction and additional trauma to the extremity.

Category: Environment and Toxicology Emergencies, and Communicable Diseases/Environment/Temperature-related emergencies

Nursing Process: Intervention

Reference

Sedlak, K. (2013). Environmental emergencies. In B. B. Hammond & P. G. Zimmermann (Eds.), *Sheehy's manual of emergency care* (7th ed., pp. 333–343). St. Louis, MO: Elsevier Mosby.

---

127. What is the recommended site in adults for the administration of intramuscular human diploid cell vaccine for rabies prophylaxis?

A. Dorsogluteal muscle
B. Deltoid muscle
C. Vastus lateralis muscle
D. Gluteus maximus muscle

Rationale

A. Human diploid cell vaccine (HDCV) should never be administered in the gluteal area because it results in lower neutralizing antibody titers.

B. The deltoid muscle area is the only acceptable site of vaccination for adults and older children. For young children, the recommended site of HDCV administration is the anterolateral aspect of the thigh.

C. The deltoid muscle area is the only acceptable site of vaccination for adults and older children. For young children, the recommended site of HDCV administration is the anterolateral aspect of the thigh.

D. HDCV should never be administered in the gluteal area because it results in lower neutralizing antibody titers.

Category: Environment and Toxicology Emergencies, and Communicable Diseases/Environment/ Vector-borne illnesses: Rabies

Nursing Process: Intervention

References

Denke, N. (2010). Wound management. In P. K. Howard & R. A. Steinmann (Eds.), *Sheehy's emergency nursing: Principles and practice* (6th ed., pp. 111–126). St. Louis, MO: Mosby Elsevier.

Flarity, K. (2007). Environmental emergencies In K. S. Hoyt & J. Selfridge-Thomas (Eds.), *Emergency nursing core curriculum* (6th ed., pp. 328–330). St. Louis, MO: Saunders Elsevier.

Rupprecht, C. E., Briggs, D., Brown, C. M., Franka, R., Katz, S. L., Kerr, H. D., . . . Cieslak, P. R. (2010). Use of a reduced (4-dose) vaccine schedule for postexposure prophylaxis to prevent human rabies: Recommendations of the Advisory Committee on Immunization Practices. *Morbidity and Mortality Weekly Report (MMWR), 59*(RR-2). Retrieved from http://www.cdc.gov/mmwr/preview/mmwrhtml/rr5902a1.htm

---

128. The emergency nurse is providing discharge instructions for a patient who has been diagnosed with Lyme disease. Which of the following patient responses indicates that the patient understands the discharge instructions being given?

A. "I may continue to experience fatigue for a month or longer."

B. "I will need to take antibiotics twice a day for 7 days."

C. "I should start to feel better after a few days of taking the antibiotics."

D. "I should avoid close contact with other people until I finish my antibiotics."

Rationale

A. It is common for patients with Lyme disease to experience fatigue for the 2–4 weeks of treatment and even longer. Some patients will experience fatigue for months following treatment.

B. Antibiotics are required for 21 days.

C. It is common for people with Lyme disease to experience lingering signs and symptoms after they have completed a full course of antibiotics.

D. There is no evidence that Lyme disease can be spread by direct person-to-person contact.

Category: Environment and Toxicology Emergencies, and Communicable Diseases/Environment/ Vector-borne illnesses: Tick-borne illness

Nursing Process: Evaluation

References

Centers for Disease Control and Prevention. (2016). *Ticks.* Retrieved from http://www.cdc.gov/ticks/index.html

Sedlak, S. K. (2013). Bite and sting emergencies. In B. B. Hammond & P. G. Zimmermann (Eds.), *Sheehy's manual of emergency care* (7th ed., pp. 345–352). St. Louis, MO: Elsevier Mosby.

---

129. A patient presents to the emergency department with a complaint of increased bleeding of the gums while brushing their teeth. The patient's current medications include warfarin sodium (Coumadin) daily. Which statement by the patient to the emergency nurse demonstrates his understanding of the effects of warfarin?

A. "I have started taking St. John's wort and ginseng daily."

B. "I can eat what I want, but avoid high fatty foods."

C. "Ice cream and milk products can cause me to bleed."
D. "I should not drink cranberry juice."

Rationale

A. Some herbal remedies and treatments may have an adverse effect on warfarin sodium. St. John's wort and ginseng may reduce the action of warfarin sodium.

B. Foods high in fat do not have an effect on coagulation. Patients on anticoagulation therapy such as warfarin sodium need to avoid certain foods, including green leafy vegetables and brussels sprouts. These foods are high in Vitamin K and may impair anticoagulation when combined with warfarin sodium.

C. Dairy products do not cause an interaction with warfarin sodium. Individuals with lactose intolerance should avoid these products.

D. Cranberry juice may increase the risk of severe bleeding. Patients who take anticoagulants should also avoid foods high in Vitamin K, such as green leafy vegetables and broccoli. Excessive alcohol may also impair the effects of anticoagulation.

Category: Environment and Toxicology Emergencies, and Communicable Diseases/Toxicology/Drug interactions

Nursing Process: Evaluation

References

Rotblatt, M., & Ziment, I. (2002). *Evidence based herbal medicine*. Philadelphia, PA: Haney & Belfus.
Wolters Kluwer. (2017). Warfarin sodium. *Nursing 2017 drug handbook* (pp. 1512–1515). Philadelphia: Author.

---

130. A young adult patient arrives to the emergency department accompanied by a friend. According to the friend, the patient was at a party and suddenly became dizzy, confused, and lethargic. The friend is concerned that the patient may have possibly ingested a "date rape" drug. Which of the following medications should the emergency nurse anticipate administering for acute flunitrazepam (Rohypnol) ingestion?

A. Diazepam (Valium)
B. Flumazenil (Romazicon)
C. Naloxone (Narcan)
D. Alprazolam (Xanax)

Rationale

A. Diazepam is a benzodiazepine, like flunitrazepam, so it would not be an appropriate choice to treat this patient.

B. Flunitrazepam is a benzodiazepine. Flumazenil is the correct medication choice because it is used for benzodiazepine reversal. Flumazenil acts to antagonize the actions of benzodiazepines on the central nervous system.

C. Naloxone is used for opiate reversal and would not be indicated for the reversal of a benzodiazepine.

D. Alprazolam is a benzodiazepine, like flunitrazepam, so it would not be an appropriate choice to treat this patient.

Category: Environment and Toxicology Emergencies, and Communicable Diseases/Toxicology/Substance abuse

Nursing Process: Analysis

Reference

Stout-Demps, L., & Williams, D. A. (2013). Substance abuse. In B. B. Hammond & P. G. Zimmermann (Eds.), *Sheehy's manual of emergency care* (7th ed., pp. 131–136). St. Louis, MO: Elsevier Mosby.

---

131. A patient experiencing alcohol withdrawal has been receiving intravenous haloperidol (Haldol) for delirium, delusions, and hallucinations. Which electrocardiogram abnormality would cause the emergency nurse the greatest concern?

A. Peaked T waves
B. QT-interval prolongation
C. Delta waves
D. Osborne waves

Rationale

A. Peaked T waves occur in hyperkalemia but are not associated with the administration of haloperidol.

B. QT-interval prolongation in the cardiac cycle may occur, which may predispose the patient to ventricular dysrhythmias. Continuous electrocardiogram monitoring should be maintained with intravenous haloperidol use.

C. Delta waves are present in Wolff–Parkinson–White syndrome but are not associated with the administration of haloperidol.

D. Osborne waves occur in the presence of hypothermia but are not associated with the administration of haloperidol.

Category: Environment and Toxicology Emergencies, and Communicable Diseases/Toxicology/Withdrawal syndrome

Nursing Process: Evaluation

Reference

Sturt, P. (2010). Toxicologic emergencies. In B. B. Hammond & P. G. Zimmermann (Eds.), *Sheehy's manual of emergency care* (6th ed., pp. 564–577). St. Louis, MO: Elsevier Mosby.

---

132. You are caring for a patient who has arrived by emergency medical services (EMS) from a skilled nursing facility. EMS reports that the patient has a 3-day history of watery diarrhea, low-grade fever, and decreased fluid intake. The patient's medication record reveals the patient is taking levofloxacin (Levaquin) for pneumonia. The patient's vital signs: BP 90/64 mm Hg; HR 112 beats/minute; RR 16 breaths/minute; SpO_2 88% room air; T 38.4°C (101.1°F); Wt 58.1 kg. Which of the following is the priority nursing intervention?

A. Place patient on contact and droplet isolation
B. Administer oxygen
C. Draw blood for cultures and a lactate level
D. Obtain intravenous access

Rationale

A. This is the priority intervention to protect the staff and other patients from infection.

B. Oxygen administration is likely to be needed depending on the patient's normal baseline oximetry level, but protection of the staff and other patients takes priority.

C. Blood for cultures and a lactate level are indicated, but protection of the staff and other patients takes priority.

D. Intravenous access is indicated, but protection of the staff and other patients takes priority.

Category: Environment and Toxicology Emergencies, and Communicable Diseases/Communicable Diseases/*C. difficile*

Nursing Process: Intervention

Reference

Centers for Disease Control and Prevention. (2012). *Frequently asked questions about* clostridium difficile *for healthcare providers*. Retrieved from http://www.cdc.gov/HAI/organisms/cdiff/Cdiff_faqs_HCP.html

---

133. A school-age child is brought to the emergency department complaining of fever, headache, muscle aches, loss of appetite, and bilateral swollen salivary glands under both ears. According to the parents the child has not received routine childhood immunizations because of personal beliefs. The emergency nurse determines that these assessment findings are mostly caused by which of the following illnesses?

A. Influenza
B. Mumps
C. Rubella
D. Brucellosis

Rationale

A. Fever, headache, muscle aches, and loss of appetite are all common signs and symptoms of influenza; however, swollen salivary glands is not a sign of influenza. Given the immunization status of this patient, the diagnosis of mumps is more probable.

B. The signs and symptoms exhibited in this case are classic findings in a child with mumps. In particular, the swollen salivary glands should alert the emergency nurse that this child may have mumps.

C. This child is at risk for rubella because of the immunization status and would likely experience many of these signs and symptoms. The first sign of rubella is generally a red rash that starts on the face and spreads.

D. Brucellosis is an infection caused by eating or drinking unpasteurized dairy products. Signs and symptoms include malaise, fever, lack of appetite, headache, and muscle pain, but not swollen salivary glands.

Category (Pediatric): Environment and Toxicology Emergencies, and Communicable Diseases/Communicable Diseases/Childhood diseases

Nursing Process: Assessment

Reference

Centers for Disease Control and Prevention. (2016). *Diseases and conditions.* Retrieved from http://www.cdc.gov/DiseasesConditions/index.html

---

134. In caring for a patient with diphtheria, which of following findings would alert the emergency nurse that the patient is experiencing a complication from the disease?

A. Abdominal pain
B. ST segment and T wave changes
C. High-grade fever
D. Severe headache

Rationale

A. The presence of abdominal pain can be seen in many illnesses, but it is not a finding in patients with diphtheria.

B. In patients who have been diagnosed with diphtheria, changes in electrocardiogram indicate the presence of myocarditis and other possible cardiac involvement.

C. A high-grade fever can be found in many different infectious processes, but it is not a finding in patients with diphtheria. Patients with diphtheria will present with a low-grade fever.

D. A severe headache can be experienced by many patients, but it is not an assessment finding in patients with diphtheria.

Category: Environment and Toxicology Emergencies, and Communicable Diseases/Communicable Diseases/Childhood diseases

Nursing Process: Assessment

References

Peard, A. S. (2007). Communicable and infectious disease emergencies. In K. S. Hoyt & J. Selfridge-Thomas (Eds.), *Emergency nursing core curriculum* (6th ed., pp. 438–482). St. Louis, MO: Saunders Elsevier.

Short, W. R., Kemper, M., & Jackson, J. (2013). Infectious diseases. In B. B. Hammond & P. G. Zimmermann (Eds.), *Sheehy's manual of emergency care* (7th ed., pp. 233–244). St. Louis, MO: Elsevier Mosby.

---

135. Which of the following statements best describes critical incident stress?

A. A combination of complex cognitive, somatic, and behavioral effects caused by psychological trauma

B. A normal response to an abnormal event

C. A unique set of attributes or behaviors that buffer the effects of acute and/or chronic stress

D. A combination of secondary traumatic stress and burnout from exposure to repeated suffering

Rationale

A. This is the definition of posttraumatic stress disorder (PTSD). People suffering from this relate intrusive thoughts, nightmares, and flashbacks. Ultimately, if not treated, PTSD will lead to social, occupational, and interpersonal dysfunction.

B. Critical incident stress creates a struggle for those affected to regain control of their lives and a sense of normalcy. Critical Incident Stress Debriefing (CISD) is a valuable tool to assist with the psychological symptoms that are generally associated with exposure to these events.

C. This is the definition of resilience. Possession of these traits provides coping mechanisms in the face of stress and thus allows for a positive work experience.

D. This is a definition of compassion fatigue. Possession of these traits negatively impacts job satisfaction, productivity, and performance.

Category: Professional Issues/Nurse/Critical Incident Stress Management

Cognitive Level: Application

References

Davis, J. A. (2013). Critical Incident Stress Debriefing from a traumatic event. *Psychology Today*. Retrieved from https://www.psychologytoday.com/blog/crimes-and-misdemeanors/201302/critical-incident-stress-debriefing-traumatic-event

Healy, M. N., & Gurney, D. (2014). Psychosocial aspects of trauma care. In *Trauma Nursing Core Course* (7th ed., pp. 295–310). Des Plaines, IL: Emergency Nurses Association.

---

136. When evaluating research data, which of the following statistical indicators best supports the validity of the data?

A. The relative risk reduction is low.
B. The *p*-value (α) is reported as < 0.05.
C. The confidence interval is 90%.
D. The number needed to treat is high.

Rationale

A. The relative risk reduction is the mathematical difference in the outcomes of the experimental and control group. This statistic can be misleading because a small difference in numbers, when calculated into percentages, may appear larger and more significant.

B. The *p*-value indicates the probability that the findings are due simply to chance. A *p*-value of < 0.5 is generally accepted as being statistically significant and suggests that the findings are not because of chance alone.

C. This is a poor result in that there is a 10% chance that the findings are wrong. Most researchers consider a confidence interval between 95% and 99% to be acceptable.

D. The number needed to treat (NNT) indicates how many patients would need to be treated with a new therapy in order to achieve an outcome that is better than the current therapy. The ideal NNT = 1. An NNT < 10 is considered acceptable by most researchers.

Category: Professional Issues/Nurse/Research

Cognitive Level: Analysis

Reference

Keough, V. A. (2010). Evidence-based practice. (2010). In P. K. Howard & R. A. Steinmann (Eds.), *Sheehy's emergency nursing: Principles and practice* (6th ed., pp. 35–44). St. Louis, MO: Mosby Elsevier.

137. A young child arrives at the emergency department via emergency medical services after sustaining a near drowning. Cardiopulmonary resuscitation has continued for over 45 minutes, and the child remains in asystole. The child's parents demand to be in the resuscitation room with their child. As the emergency nurse, you should do which of the following?

A. Explain to the parents that their child is critically ill, and staff will provide them with periodic updates on the condition of their child.
B. Ask the social worker or hospital chaplain to be with the parents in the private family waiting room.
C. Designate one person to provide the parents with updates on the condition of their child as indicated.
D. Offer the family presence at the bedside.

Rationale

A. This may anger the parents further if staff do not permit them to see or be with their child during the actual resuscitation.

B. The social worker or chaplain should be notified to assist the family of a critically ill patient. The chaplain or social worker should be open and honest, and ensure that the family members are aware of what they will see, allowing them to then decide if they wish to be at the bedside. If the family requests to be at the bedside, staff should attempt to honor the wishes of the family.

C. Designation of one person as the patient advocate is important, but assisting the family to be at the bedside will often help them during the grieving process, as they talk to their child as treatment continues.

D. The Emergency Nurses Association has long advocated for family members to have the option to be at their loved one's bedside. Emergency nurses have an obligation to provide the opportunity for the family to be in the treatment room. One designated healthcare team member should be assigned to be with the family members, explain in nonmedical terminology what is taking place, and provide the rationale as to why.

Category: Professional Issues/Patient/End-of-life issues

Cognitive Level: Application

References

Hammond, B. (2013). Cardiopulmonary arrest. in B. B. Hammond & P. G. Zimmerman *Sheehy's manual of emergency care* (7th ed., pp. 89–96). St. Louis, MO: Elsevier Mosby.

Kingsnorth-Hinrichs, J. (2010). Family presence during resuscitation. In P. K. Howard & R. A. Steinmann (Eds.), *Sheehy's emergency nursing: Principles and practice* (6th ed., pp. 148–154). St. Louis, MO: Mosby Elsevier.

---

138. The family of an elderly patient who has sustained a cardiopulmonary arrest is being approached by the hospital organ procurement agency representative, asking them for consent for organ donation. Which statement, made by a member of the patient's family, indicates an accurate understanding of the organ donation process?

A. "The organs of an elderly person are only suitable for research purposes and not for organ donation."
B. "Our insurance will cover the additional costs related to the organ donation process."
C. "We would not be able to have an open-casket funeral."
D. "Our religion considers organ donation to be a noble gift."

Rationale

A. There is no age limit that defines organ donation. The suitability of the organs for transplant is determined by the transplant team at the time of the donor's death.

B. All costs associated with the organ donation process are assumed by the organ recipient. No costs are billed to the donor or donor family.

C. Organ and tissue donation does not alter the appearance of the body. An open-casket funeral is still possible.

D. Most major religions have published documents in support of organ donation.

Category: Professional Issues/Patient/End-of-life issues: Organ and tissue donation

Cognitive Level: Application

Reference

U.S. Department of Health and Human Services. (2016). *How organ donation works*. Retrieved from https://organdonor.gov/about/process.html

---

139. The nurse is participating on a committee that is developing guidelines for family presence during an emergency department resuscitation. The committee should define which of the following as a part of the guideline?

A. Who is considered the patient's family
B. The roles and responsibilities of each member of the resuscitation team
C. Situations in which family members should be offered the option of presence
D. Nursing interventions if family members interfere with resuscitation efforts

Rationale

A. The committee will need to determine whether a family member is defined as one who is a blood relative or someone who plays a significant role in the patient's life.

B. The roles and responsibilities of the physicians, nurses, and ancillary care personnel should not be affected by family presence in the resuscitation area.

C. All families should be offered the option of presence during a family member's resuscitation.

D. Current studies have found little to no evidence that the presence of family members negatively affects resuscitation efforts or time to treatments.

Category: Professional Issues/Patient/End-of-life issues: Family presence

Cognitive Level: Application

References

Chan, G. K. (2007). Palliative and end-of-life care in the emergency department. In K. S. Hoyt & J. Selfridge-Thomas (Eds.), *Emergency nursing core curriculum* (6th ed., pp. 164–173). St. Louis, MO: Saunders Elsevier.

Kingsnorth-Hinrichs, J. (2010). Family presence during resuscitation. In P. K. Howard & R. A. Steinmann (Eds.), *Sheehy's emergency nursing: Principles and practice* (6th ed., pp. 148–154). St. Louis, MO: Mosby Elsevier.

140. A patient who has been diagnosed with end-stage cardiac disease is receiving palliative care in the emergency department while awaiting placement in the hospice unit. Which of the following interventions is most appropriate for the emergency nurse to implement in the care of this patient?

A. Delegate hygiene care to family members
B. Obtain a 12-lead electrocardiogram
C. Provide oxygen as needed to relieve the patient's dyspnea
D. Restrict visitors to the patient's immediate family

Rationale

A. In palliative care, the patient's family should be encouraged and supported to participate in the care of the patient, but it cannot be assumed that the family is willing or able to assume to the responsibility of any part of the patient's care.

B. For the patient receiving palliative care, diagnostic testing should be cautiously considered. If the results obtained from the testing will not change the course of treatment or management, the diagnostic test may not be appropriate.

C. Palliative care is symptom management. Providing oxygen, pain medications, or medications to relieve coughs or excessive fluids are appropriate interventions that ease symptoms but do not attempt to treat the underlying disease process.

D. The emergency nurse should provide a private and quiet space within the emergency department in which care can be provided and where the patient, the patient's family, and significant others can be together.

Category: Professional Issues/Patient/End-of-life issues: Withholding, withdrawing, and palliative care

Cognitive Level: Application

References

Chan, G. K. (2007). Palliative and end-of-life care in the emergency department. In K. S. Hoyt & J. Selfridge-Thomas (Eds.), *Emergency nursing core curriculum* (6th ed., pp. 164–173). St. Louis, MO: Saunders Elsevier.

Granero-Molina, J., Diaz-Cortez, M., Hernandez-Padilla, J. M., Garcia-Caro, M. P., & Fernandez-Sola, C. (2016). Loss of dignity in end-of-life care in the emergency department: A phenomenological study with health professionals. *Journal of Emergency Nursing, 42*(3), 233–239.

---

141. Following the death of a patient in the emergency department who may be the victim of crime, the proper collection of forensic evidence includes which of the following actions?

A. Place paper bags over both of the patient's hands
B. Wrap wet clothing in plastic and then place it in a paper bag
C. Return jewelry and religious items to a family member because they are not admissible as evidence
D. Use sterile metal forceps when handling bullets

Rationale

A. Placing paper bags over the patient's hands will act to preserve any evidence that may be on the hands or under the fingernails.

B. Each article of clothing should be placed in its own separate paper bag to avoid possible cross-contamination. Wet articles should either be allowed to dry or placed while still wet into paper bags. Moisture collection on items wrapped in plastic could potentially alter the evidence.

C. All items associated with the patient are considered evidence and should not be returned to the family or a significant other without the express permission of law enforcement.

D. Metal forceps may alter forensic markings on the outside of bullets. If necessary, place a plastic shield over the teeth of the forceps before touching the bullet.

Category: Professional Issues/Patient/Forensic evidence collection

Cognitive Level: Application

References

Eckes-Roper, J. (2013). Forensics. In B. B. Hammond & P. G. Zimmermann (Eds.), *Sheehy's manual of emergency care* (7th ed., pp. 49–58). St. Louis, MO: Elsevier Mosby.

Ferrell, J. J. (2007). Forensic aspects of emergency nursing. In K. S. Hoyt & J. Selfridge-Thomas (Eds.), *Emergency nursing core curriculum* (6th ed., pp. 1025–1032). St. Louis, MO: Saunders Elsevier.

---

142. During a cardiac resuscitation, the emergency provider orders amiodarone 600 mg intravenously to be given for ventricular fibrillation. The best action by the emergency nurse is to:

A. ask for clarification of the dose before administering the medication.
B. infuse the ordered dose of amiodarone over 1–2 minutes.
C. mix the amiodarone in 300 mL of 0.9% sodium chloride and infuse over 30 minutes.
D. administer 300 mg of amiodarone as an intravenous bolus and the remaining 300 mg as an infusion drip.

Rationale

A. The nurse should recognize that the dose ordered is not the recommended dose and should ask for clarification and be prepared to state the correct recommended dose: amiodarone is 300 mg intravenous (IV) push initially, followed by 150 mg IV push. Safety measures should include closed-loop communication, readback protocols, and double-checking medication calculations before medication administration.

B. The dose ordered is not the recommended dose. Clarification must be obtained to prevent a medication error.

C. The dose ordered is not the recommended dose for amiodarone. In the presence of ventricular fibrillation, amiodarone is initially administered as an IV bolus.

D. This is not the ACLS protocol for amiodarone in ventricular fibrillation. All members of the healthcare team must take responsibility to prevent medication errors by speaking up and asking for clarification. Patient safety and medication error prevention is a national initiative.

Category: Professional Issues/Patient/Patient safety

Cognitive Level: Analysis

References

Fazio, J. (2010). Emergency nursing practice. In P. K. Howard & R. A. Steinmann (Eds.), *Sheehy's emergency nursing: Principles and practice* (6th ed., pp. 8–15). St. Louis, MO: Mosby Elsevier.

Hohenhaus, S. M. (2013). Patient safety in the emergency department. In B. B. Hammond & P. G. Zimmermann (Eds.), *Sheehy's manual of emergency care* (7th ed., pp. 37–41). St. Louis, MO: Elsevier Mosby.

---

143. Which of the following practices best contributes to patient-reported satisfaction with their emergency department experience?

A. Performing hourly rounding to provide patient information
B. Effective pain management
C. Providing distractions such as television and food
D. Maintaining actual wait times of less than 30 minutes

Rationale

A. Providing patient information is an important component leading to patient satisfaction; however, information should be provided as it is available or pertinent, not just hourly.

B. Research has shown a correlation between emergency department (ED) pain management and satisfaction with the ED experience. This is especially true of parental satisfaction when the patient is a child.

C. Data collected indicate that the although patients may appreciate distractions such as television and food, they do not contribute significantly to overall patient satisfaction.

D. *Perceived,* not *actual*, wait times are an important component of patient satisfaction with the ED experience.

Category: Professional Issues/Patient/Patient satisfaction

Cognitive Level: Recall

References

American College of Emergency Physicians. (2011). *Clinical and practice management: Patient satisfaction*. Retrieved from https://www.acep.org/patientsatisfaction/

Emergency Nurses Association. (2014). *Patient experience/satisfaction with the emergency department experience.* Des Plaines, IL: Author.

Welch, S. J. (2010). Twenty years of patient satisfaction research applied to the emergency department: A qualitative review. *American Journal of Medical Quality, 25*(1), 64–72. Retrieved from http://journals.sagepub.com/doi/abs/10.1177/1062860609352536

---

144. Which of the following definitions best exemplifies the meaning of culture?

A. The patterns of behavior and beliefs shared by persons living in a social group
B. A group of people who share the same attributes, such as social rank or socioeconomic status
C. A group of people who share the same heritage or country of origin
D. An organized or unorganized system of beliefs

Rationale

A. Culture is defined as the patterns of behavior and beliefs shared by persons living in a social group.

B. A group of people who share the same attributes, such as social rank or socioeconomic status, is the definition of class.

C. The beliefs, values, and practices shared by a group of people based on heritage or the country of origin of one's ancestors is the definition of ethnicity.

D. An organized or unorganized system of beliefs is the definition of religion.

Category: Professional Issues/Patient/Cultural considerations

Cognitive Level: Recall

Reference

Ruiz-Contreras, A. (2010). Approaching diversity. (2010). In P. K. Howard & R. A. Steinmann (Eds.), *Sheehy's emergency nursing: Principles and practice* (6th ed., pp. 27–32). St. Louis, MO: Mosby Elsevier.

---

145. The registered nurse asks the assistive personnel to reassess vital signs on a patient who had a lumbar puncture performed the previous hour. Is this an appropriate task to delegate to assistive personnel?

A. Yes
B. No
C. Only if the assistive staff member has had specific education on lumbar punctures.
D. Only if the assistive staff member feels comfortable doing so.

Rationale

A. The registered nurse is accountable for the ongoing monitoring of the outcomes of nursing care. Elements of care may be delegated, but the nursing process itself may not be delegated. Reassessing vital signs postprocedure would be an appropriate element of care to delegate to the assistive personnel.

B. The registered nurse is accountable for the ongoing monitoring of the outcomes of nursing care. Elements of care may be delegated, but the nursing process itself may not be delegated. Reassessing vital signs postprocedure would be an appropriate element of care to delegate to the assistive personnel.

C. The registered nurse is accountable for the ongoing monitoring of the outcomes of nursing care. Elements of care may be delegated, but the nursing process itself may not be delegated. Reassessing vital signs postprocedure would be an appropriate element of care to delegate to the assistive personnel. Specific education on lumbar punctures would not be necessary to reassess vital signs.

D. The registered nurse is accountable for the ongoing monitoring of the outcomes of nursing care. Elements of care may be delegated, but the nursing process itself may not be delegated. Reassessing vital signs postprocedure would be an appropriate element of care to delegate to the assistive personnel. If the assistive staff member does not feel comfortable doing a delegated task, the registered nurse must be informed.

Category: Professional Issues/System/Delegation of tasks to assistive personnel

Cognitive Level: Application

Reference

Bonalumi, N. M., & King, D. (2007). Professionalism and leadership. In K. S. Hoyt & J. Selfridge-Thomas (Eds.), *Emergency nursing core curriculum* (6th ed., pp. 1046–1056). St. Louis, MO: Saunders Elsevier.

146. Following a mass casualty incident, a small child arrives to the emergency department via emergency medical services. The child is not breathing and has no palpable pulse. The child's airway is repositioned, and, following 5 rescue breaths, the child begins breathing on his own. Based on the JumpSTART triage algorithm, which triage category should be assigned to this child?

A. Black (expectant)
B. Yellow (delayed)
C. Red (immediate)
D. Green (minor)

Rationale

A. The black (expectant) category is designated for patients who are not expected to survive and for whom palliative care and/or pain medication be given. The child who regains their ability to breathe after 5 rescue breaths and has a palpable pulse is to be placed in the red (immediate) JumpSTART triage category.

B. The yellow (delayed) category is indicated for patients whose transport can be delayed and who have either serious or potentially life-threatening injuries but are not expected to deteriorate within the next several hours. The child who regains their ability to breathe after 5 rescue breaths and has a palpable pulse is to be placed in the red (immediate) JumpSTART triage category.

C. If a child regains breathing and has a palpable pulse following rescue breaths, they are assigned the red JumpSTART (immediate) category.

D. The green (minor) category is for children who are able to walk when initially triaged. This patient had no spontaneous respirations or palpable pulse on initial assessment and would therefore be assigned a red (immediate) triage category.

Category (Pediatric): Professional Issues/System/Disaster management

Cognitive Level: Analysis

Reference

Upton, L. A. (2012). Disaster. In *Emergency Nursing Pediatric Course: Provider manual* (4th ed., pp. 365–382). Des Plaines, IL: Emergency Nurses Association.

---

147. It is important to have effective communication among emergency department staff when completing a patient handoff between staff members as well as with other hospital departments. One form of communicating handoff is the SBAR technique. The S in the SBAR communication tool stands for:

A. suggest alternatives.
B. situation.
C. safety.
D. support.

Rationale

A. Suggesting alternatives is used in the DESC tool for communication, which is used in conflict management. In using SBAR, the S stands for describing the situation, which includes the chief complaint and reasons the patient has come to the emergency department (ED), or why the patient is being admitted to the hospital.

B. Describing the situation includes the chief complaint and reasons the patient has come to the ED, or why the patient is being admitted to the hospital.

C. Safety is used in the CUS tool for communication when a team member recognizes an unsafe situation and "stops the line." The CUS tool stands for concern, uncomfortable, and safety. In using SBAR, the S stands for describing the situation, which includes the chief complaint and reasons the patient has come to the ED, or why the patient is being admitted to the hospital.

D. The S in the SBAR communication tool represents situation. Describing the situation includes the chief complaint and reasons the patient has come to the ED, or why the patient is being admitted to the hospital.

Category: Professional Issues/System/Performance improvement

Cognitive Level: Recall

Reference

Hohenhaus, S. B., & Nierstedt, P. (2014). Teamwork and trauma care. In D. Gurney (Ed.), *Trauma Nursing Core Course: Provider manual* (7th ed., pp. 5–8). Des Plaines, IL: Emergency Nurses Association.

---

148. A patient delivers a full-term baby in the emergency department of a facility that does not have OB/GYN or women's services available. The ambulance transport crew has arrived to take the mother and baby to an appropriate accepting facility. Based on the Emergency Medical Treatment and Active Labor Act, the emergency nurse identifies this patient cannot be transported unless which of the following has occurred?

A. The mother has not voided urine
B. The nurse completes all necessary documentation
C. The baby is 1 hour old
D. Delivery of the placenta

Rationale

A. The lack of voided urine by the mother following delivery would not be an indication for withholding transport if a patient is stable for transfer.

B. Nursing documentation is not affected by Emergency Medical Treatment and Active Labor Act (EMTALA). The nurse can finish any additional charting that was not complete after the patient is transported to another facility.

C. The age of the newborn infant is not affected by EMTALA. The patient and baby can leave after the delivery of the placenta and the mother and baby are both deemed to be in stable condition.

D. According to EMTALA, women who are in active labor are not considered stabilized until after the delivery of the placenta.

Category: Professional Issues/System/Federal regulations

Cognitive Level: Application

Reference

Jagim, M. (2007). Legal and regulatory issues. In K. S. Hoyt & J. Selfridge-Thomas (Eds.), *Emergency nursing core curriculum* (6th ed., pp. 1033–1045). St. Louis, MO: Saunders Elsevier.

---

149. Which type of consent for treatment is recognized when an alert and oriented patient presents for care in the emergency department?

A. Informed consent
B. Implied consent
C. Involuntary consent
D. Express consent

Rationale

A. Before a procedure, a physician describes the procedure to be performed, alternatives to the procedure, risks and benefits of the procedure, and the patient's understanding of the procedure, alternatives, risks, and benefits.

B. Implied consent for treatment occurs when an individual is in either a life-threatening or limb-threatening situation and unable to provide express consent. Implied consent for treatment is a legal consent and occurs even while all attempts are being made to contact the patient's family members and obtain consent for treatment from them.

C. Involuntary consent is used when an incompetent individual refuses to consent to needed medical treatment. It is often used to ensure a that mentally incompetent individual receives necessary medical treatment.

D. Express consent is the voluntary consent of an individual seeking medical treatment and is predicated on one's mental competency.

Category: Professional Issues/System/Patient consent for treatment

Cognitive Level: Recall

Reference

Jagim, M. (2007). Legal and regulatory issues. In K. S. Hoyt & J. Selfridge-Thomas (Eds.), *Emergency nursing core curriculum* (6th ed., pp. 1033–1045). St. Louis, MO: Saunders Elsevier.

---

150. Prior to implementing a research study that involves patient outcomes, approval must be obtained from which of the following?

A. The institutional ethics committee
B. The institutional legal consultant
C. The institutional review board
D. The medical staff involved with the patient population

Rationale

A. The institutional review board is charged with overseeing that the study complies with all ethical standards.

B. The institutional review board is charged with overseeing that the study complies with all federal regulations regarding the use of human subjects.

C. All research studies that involve human subjects must be reviewed and approved by an institutional review board prior to the start of the study.

D. It is important that members of the medical staff are aware of any nursing research that is being conducted, and their cooperation may be beneficial. However, their approval is not required for nursing research to be conducted.

Category: Professional Issues/Nurse/Research

Cognitive Level: Recall

References

Barnason, S. (2010). Research. In P. K. Howard & R. A. Steinmann (Eds.), *Sheehy's emergency nursing: Principles and practice* (6th ed., pp. 46–55). St. Louis, MO: Mosby Elsevier

Carlon, S. (2008). Legal and regulatory considerations. In J. Houser (Ed.), *Nursing research* (pp. 75–99). Sudbury, MA: Jones and Bartlett.

SELF-DIAGNOSTIC PROFILE

How to Use the Self-Assessment Worksheet

1. Indicate on your answer sheet whether your answers are correct or incorrect.
2. Note the items you answered incorrectly.
3. Count the total number of items you answered incorrectly in each category.
4. Compare the total number of items you answered incorrectly in each category with the total number of items per category. This information will give you an idea of where you will need to focus your continued study.

Content Category	Questions Answered Incorrectly	Total Number of Questions Answered Incorrectly in Each Category	Total Number of Questions in Each CEN Content Category
Cardiovascular Emergencies			20
Respiratory Emergencies			16
Neurological Emergencies			16
Gastrointestinal, Genitourinary, Gynecology, and Obstetrical Emergencies			21
Psychosocial and Medical Emergencies			25
Maxillofacial, Ocular, Orthopedic, and Wound Emergencies			21
Environment and Toxicology Emergencies, and Communicable Diseases			15
Professional Issues			16

Practice Examination 4

PART 1

1. A patient presents who had experienced chest pain but is now pain free. Electrocardiograms have been repeated twice, and troponin levels repeated at 4-hour intervals are within normal limits. The patient has no significant risk factors for heart disease. The nurse anticipates:

A. admission to the ICU to rule out myocardial infarction.
B. admission to cardiac catheterization lab for evaluation of coronary anatomy.
C. that the patient will be discharged to home, with instructions for close follow-up with their primary care provider because the risk of an adverse coronary event is low.
D. admission to the telemetry unit to rule out myocardial infarction.

2. A patient who became unconscious during ascent while scuba diving arrives via emergency medical services. The patient is unconscious and hypotensive. What is the most appropriate position in which to place this patient during their examination by the physician?

A. Left lateral decubitus, head down
B. Right lateral decubitus, head down
C. Left lateral decubitus, head up
D. Supine

3. In which patient would the nurse question an order for morphine sulfate?

A. A patient with aortic dissection
B. A patient with a ST elevation myocardial infarction
C. A patient with unstable angina
D. A patient with non-ST elevation myocardial infarction

4. Following the administration of 2 L of intravenous (IV) crystalloids, the emergency nurse begins to administer IV dobutamine (Dobutrex) to a patient who has been diagnosed with a right ventricular infarction. The emergency nurse identifies that this medication has been effective when the patient demonstrates which of the following?

A. Bradycardia
B. Increase in blood pressure
C. Presence of distended neck veins
D. Onset of atrial fibrillation

5. The nurse has instituted applied oxygen and is to reduce the patient's heart rate and blood pressure. Which of the following findings would be expected after applying oxygen, initiating two large-caliber intravenous (IV) lines, and administering IV beta-blockers?
   A. Difference of > 20 mm Hg blood pressure when comparing in both arms
   B. Chest pain radiating to the left shoulder
   C. Orthopnea and jugular venous distention
   D. Petechial lesions on the patient's palms or soles

6. A 3-month-old infant weighing 11 pounds (5 kg) arrives at the emergency department in full cardiopulmonary arrest. The monitor shows ventricular fibrillation. Good-quality cardiopulmonary resuscitation is being performed, and the infant has been defibrillated once. Which medication should be administered next?
   A. Epinephrine 0.05 mg intravenously/intraosseously (IV/IO)
   B. Atropine 0.1 mg IV/IO
   C. Amiodarone (Cordarone) 25 mg IV/IO
   D. Sodium bicarbonate 5 mEq IV

7. A patient in cardiopulmonary arrest remains in ventricular fibrillation despite having been defibrillated 6 times, receiving good quality cardiopulmonary resuscitation, and the administration of epinephrine (Adrenalin) and amiodarone (Cordarone). Arterial blood gases reveal a pH of 7.02, PO_2 96 mm Hg, and pCO_2 40 mm Hg. What medication order should the emergency nurse anticipate next for this patient?
   A. Adenosine (Adenocard) 6 mg
   B. Calcium chloride 1 g
   C. Vasopressin (Pitressin) 40 units
   D. Sodium bicarbonate 1 mEq/kg

8. A patient presents via emergency medical services in cardiopulmonary arrest. Chest compressions and bag-mask ventilation are being performed. The cardiac monitor shows ventricular tachycardia. While the defibrillator is charging for defibrillation, the nurse should ensure that:
   A. no one is touching the patient.
   B. high-quality cardiopulmonary resuscitation is continued.
   C. oxygen delivery via nasal cannula continues at 6 L/minute.
   D. the defibrillator pads have been placed on the patient.

9. A teenaged patient presents to triage stating that they have the sensation that their heart is jumping out of their chest for the past several hours. The patient denies routine drug use and states that they have been studying for end-of-the-semester final exams for the past 3 days and took a pill to help him study. You palpate a radial pulse that is 170 beats/minute and regular. Which of the following dysrhythmias would be suspected?
   A. Supraventricular tachycardia
   B. Ventricular tachycardia
   C. Atrial fibrillation
   D. Sinus rhythm with premature atrial complexes

10. The emergency nurse is participating in the treatment of a patient in cardiopulmonary arrest. Cardiopulmonary resuscitation is ongoing, an advanced airway is present, and vascular access has been obtained. The monitor shows an organized rhythm, but no palpable pulse is detected. In addition to evaluating the "Hs and Ts" as causes of pulseless electrical activity (PEA), the nurse anticipates the use of what device or procedure to better evaluate for potentially reversible causes of PEA?
    A. Electrocardiogram
    B. Point of care ultrasound
    C. Bedside chest radiograph
    D. Glucometer

11. Echocardiography determines that a patient has infective endocarditis with bacterial or fungal growth isolated to the tricuspid valve. In addition to a heart murmur, what other pertinent signs or symptoms would the emergency department nurse include in the assessment related to this finding?
    A. Blood-tinged frothy sputum
    B. Jugular vein distension
    C. Sharp, piercing chest pain that decreases when leaning forward
    D. Severe chest pain radiating to the back, 20 mm Hg difference in blood pressure between arms

12. A dyspnic patient presents to the emergency department. Physical assessment reveals an S3 heart sound and auscultated bilateral crackles, in addition to an ultrasound finding of bilateral "B-lines" when scanning the anterior lung fields. The nurse suspects:
    A. right-sided heart failure.
    B. left-sided heart failure.
    C. pneumonia.
    D. pulmonary embolism.

13. Nitroprusside is ordered for a patient with a hypertensive emergency. This medication works to reduce blood pressure by:
    A. decreasing heart rate and causing vasodilation.
    B. inhibiting the influx of calcium ions.
    C. relaxing vascular smooth muscle to reduce afterload and preload.
    D. dilating arterioles.

14. Emergency medical services arrives with an elderly patient, the victim of a single-vehicle collision with a tree. The patient was not wearing a seat or shoulder restraint, was not ejected from the vehicle, and the airbag did not deploy. The patient has equal breath sounds and symmetrical chest rise and fall. The patient appears anxious and is complaining of sternal pain to palpation, although no crepitus is present. Vital signs: BP 128/74 mm Hg with the presence of a pulsus paradoxus of 15 mm Hg; HR 86 beats/minute; RR 28 breaths/minute. The emergency nurse anticipates that this patient will require the following intervention:
    A. Needle thoracentesis
    B. Pericardiocentesis
    C. Administration of a 1000 mL warm 0.9% sodium chloride bolus
    D. Endotracheal intubation

15. The definition of afterload is:
   A. the amount of force needed by the ventricle walls during systole.
   B. the amount of force needed by the atria during systole.
   C. the volume of blood found within the venous system.
   D. the volume of blood found within the arterial system.

16. A patient presents to the emergency department 2 weeks postoperative following a coronary artery bypass graft via an open sternotomy. The patient has a temperature of 37.8°C (100°F). The sternal wound is intact with no redness or drainage present. The patient describes a sudden onset of midsternal chest pain, increasing with inspiration. The emergency nurse auscultates a leathery grating sound with S1S2. The patient describes relief from the pain when leaning forward. The patient is describing symptoms associated with:
   A. acute aortic dissection.
   B. coronary artery occlusion.
   C. wound infection.
   D. pericarditis.

17. A patient has been diagnosed with Raynaud's disease. Which of the following statements made by the patient would reflect an understanding of this disease?
   A. "I developed this disease because I am female and live in a cold climate."
   B. "I am fearful that I may require a liver transplant if the disease does not improve."
   C. "If I take an antibiotic for a while, the disease should go away."
   D. "I noticed the onset of the symptoms when I started coughing, usually at night."

18. During the implementation of the massive transfusion protocol, the emergency nurse should observe for which of the following?
   A. Hypercalcemia
   B. Hyperkalemia
   C. Acidosis
   D. Hypercoagulopathy

19. An obese patient presents to the emergency department complaining of leg pain. The patient relates no history of trauma. The lower leg appears swollen, slightly reddened, and painful to touch. When asked to dorsiflex the foot, the patient complains of increasing pain in the calf area of the leg. Based on this assessment, the emergency nurse would suspect which of the following?
   A. Acute arthritis
   B. Deep vein thrombosis
   C. Chronic arterial occlusion
   D. Raynaud's syndrome

20. Damage control resuscitation (DCR) is a principle of treating hemorrhage that focuses on prevention rather than intervention. Which of the following outcomes would demonstrate successful DCR?
   A. Rapid infusion of isotonic crystalloid
   B. Calcium chloride replacement
   C. Hemostatic resuscitation
   D. Autotransfusion

21. A patient who has been treated for an asthmatic attack is being discharged from the emergency department. The emergency nurse identifies that the patient requires additional instruction when they state:
   A. "I will use my rescue inhaler if I become short of breath suddenly."
   B. "I will avoid aggravating allergens."
   C. "I will stop my corticosteroid therapy as soon as I feel better."
   D. "In conjunction with my medications, I will use relaxation techniques and controlled breathing exercises when I begin to feel short of breath."

22. Chronic obstructive pulmonary disease is diagnosed by:
   A. arterial blood gas.
   B. chest radiograph.
   C. forced expiratory volume in 1 second per forced vital capacity by spirometry.
   D. 6-minute walk test.

23. A well-known patient with chronic obstructive pulmonary disease arrives to the emergency department with a history of increasing respiratory difficulty over the past several days. On assessment, the patient has diminished breath sounds bilaterally and is extremely anxious. The emergency provider orders an albuterol and atrovent nebulized treatment for this patient. The nurse anticipates which of the following responses to this intervention?
   A. Increased respiratory rate
   B. Auscultation of bilateral wheezing
   C. Decreased heart rate
   D. Increase in $PaCO_2$ level

24. A patient with an endotracheal tube in place is at increased risk for the development of ventilator-associated pneumonia when which of the following occurs?
   A. The endotracheal tube acts to impair the lungs' normal defense mechanism.
   B. A silver-coated endotracheal tube is used for intubation.
   C. The patient's subglottic secretions are removed frequently.
   D. No leaks are present in the cuff of the endotracheal tube.

25. A person with acute bronchitis is most likely to have the presence of:
   A. infiltrates on their chest radiograph.
   B. a dry cough initially that develops into a productive cough.
   C. wheezing on physical exam.
   D. course crackles on physical exam.

26. A patient with a gastrostomy tube is diagnosed with aspiration pneumonia. Which of the following interventions would the emergency nurse perform last?
   A. Identifying the time of the patient's last tube feeding
   B. Suctioning the patient's oropharyngeal area
   C. Initiating mechanical ventilation if indicated
   D. Administering oxygen

27. A patient arrives at the emergency department via emergency medical services. The patient has sustained burns to the face, neck, and chest from a fire. The patient is alert and has a productive cough of carbonaceous sputum. The priority intervention for the emergency nurse to perform is to:

    A. prepare for intubation.
    B. obtain a full set of vital signs.
    C. place the patient on continuous pulse oximetry.
    D. remove all clothing and jewelry.

28. A young patient presents to the emergency department with difficulty swallowing, drooling, inspiratory stridor, and an elevated temperature of 39.2°C (102.6°F). The physician suspects the patient may have acute epiglottitis. What is the priority intervention that the emergency nurse should anticipate for this patient?

    A. Administer high-flow humidified oxygen
    B. Establish intravenous access
    C. Prepare for endotracheal intubation
    D. Attempt to visualize the oropharynx using a tongue blade

29. A patient arrives at the emergency department complaining of mild pleuritic chest pain and a productive cough. The nurse notes the presence of a pleural friction rub. What plan of care would be most appropriate for this patient?

    A. Prepare for hospital admission
    B. Provide comfort measures
    C. Obtain blood cultures and administer antibiotics
    D. Identify underlying disease process

30. Which of the following is the leading risk factor for the development of a spontaneous pneumothorax?

    A. Cigarette smoking
    B. Barotrauma
    C. Rupture of bleb
    D. Chronic obstructive pulmonary disease

31. An unresponsive patient arrives via emergency medical services following a motor vehicle collision. Patient assessment reveals absent breath sounds and bruising on the left side of the chest, a deviated trachea, and the appearance of sudden cyanosis. The emergency nurse suspects the patient has developed a:

    A. tension pneumothorax.
    B. rupture of the diaphragm.
    C. flail chest.
    D. right mainstem bronchial intubation.

32. The emergency nurse is caring for the victim of a motor vehicle collision. The patient has experienced a large pneumothorax on the right side, and a chest tube has been inserted. The emergency nurse anticipates this treatment has been effective when the patient has which of the following responses?

    A. Sucking sound heard with respiration
    B. Increase in heart rate
    C. Absence of fluctuation in water seal chamber
    D. Decreasing respiratory rate

33. A patient presents to triage with chest wall pain and worsening cough after cliff-diving 90 feet into the water below. The patient complains of pink, frothy sputum when coughing. Based on the patient's history, the emergency nurse is concerned this patient may have which of the following?

A. Pulmonary embolism
B. Pulmonary edema
C. Asthma
D. Pleural effusion

34. A patient presents with increased shortness of breath. Vital signs: BP 128/72 mm Hg; HR 115 beats/minute; RR 20 breaths/minute; SpO_2 88% room air; T 37.1°C (98.9°F). The patient reports recently having been a passenger on a transcontinental airline flight. The emergency nurse would use which of the following anatomical areas to initiate an intravenous line prior to a computerized tomography scan?

A. Exterior jugular vein
B. Cephalic vein
C. Dorsal metacarpal veins
D. Median cubital vein

35. A patient arrives complaining of dyspnea and mild right-sided chest pain that began last evening and now increases with exertion. The patient states that 3 days ago, they sustained an injury to their right lower leg. The patient has a previous history of deep vein thrombosis that occurred 15 years ago. The emergency nurse is aware that the laboratory test that is most specific for the presence of a pulmonary embolus is:

A. complete blood count.
B. D-dimer.
C. complete metabolic panel.
D. B-type natriuretic peptide.

36. Extracorporeal membrane oxygenation may be used in the treatment of a patient with severe acute respiratory distress syndrome in order to:

A. circumvent the damaging effects of mechanical ventilation.
B. maintain the patient's oxygen levels while allowing the lungs to rest.
C. provide hemodynamic support.
D. prevent respiratory failure.

37. An elderly male with dementia is brought to the emergency department by his family, who state, "We just can't handle him at home anymore." The patient frequently attempts to get out of bed, and the emergency nurse is afraid the patient will fall. Which intervention is most appropriate to prevent falls in this patient?

A. Place the patient in a vest restraint
B. Provide the patient with the call light
C. Have family remain with the patient
D. Place the patient in a geriatric chair near the nurse's station

38. A young mother presents to triage with her 6-week-old infant. The mother states the infant has a had a fever and "acts funny." While drawing blood, the emergency nurse observes the infant to rapidly move her right leg in a bicycling fashion. The emergency nurse is concerned that this behavior indicates which of the following?

A. Intracerebral bleeding
B. A temper tantrum
C. Seizure
D. Electrolyte imbalance

39. A patient who is 26 weeks pregnant arrives at the emergency department exhibiting left-sided weakness and slurred speech that began 20 minutes before arrival. The computed tomography scan comes back negative for cerebral hemorrhage. Which intervention should the emergency team prepare for next?
   A. Induction of labor
   B. Administration of fibrinolytics
   C. Emergency cesarean section
   D. Transfer to a labor and delivery unit

40. An elderly patient arrives at the emergency department via emergency medical services from an assisted living facility with a history of a "brain shunt" and contractures. Recent history indicates that the patient is "less interactive than usual," has been "sleepy," and has had no bowel movement for 3 days. The computed tomography scan exam reveals evidence of hydrocephalus, and the abdominal radiograph shows a large amount of feces, causing the ventriculoperitoneal shunt to kink. The emergency nurse anticipates which intervention for this patient?
   A. An enema to clear feces from the bowel
   B. Immediate transfer of the patient to an ICU
   C. Preparing the patient for surgery to replace the shunt
   D. Performing a digital rectal exam

41. A patient presents to triage complaining that they have experienced increasing difficulty walking. The patient has an uneven gait and feels "unsteady" when standing. Speech is clear, and vital signs are stable. Which assessment criteria would the emergency nurse use to evaluate the patient for the presence of cerebellar dysfunction?
   A. Extraocular eye movements
   B. Appropriate decision making
   C. Finger-to-nose coordination
   D. Visual acuity assessment

42. The emergency nurse is preparing to discharge a patient who has been treated for a migraine headache. The patient asks how similar headaches in the future can be prevented. The most appropriate response by the emergency nurse would be:
   A. "Maintaining a headache diary to identify what triggers your headache is often helpful in preventing similar episodes in the future."
   B. "Reducing stress levels will reduce the incidence of migraine headaches."
   C. "Avoid foods that contain tyramine, such as aged cheeses, pickled food, and red wine."
   D. "Herbal products such as butterbur or feverfew are helpful."

43. The emergency nurse understands that the purpose of the Glasgow Coma Scale is to:
   A. allow the provider to predict outcomes for the trauma patient.
   B. assess the level of consciousness in all patients.
   C. identify interventions to improve outcomes for unconscious patients.
   D. assess the level of consciousness in head-injured patients.

44. The emergency nurse is preparing to discharge a child who has been diagnosed with epilepsy. Which information is essential for the child's parents and caregivers to understand regarding this diagnosis?
   A. The types of surgery available for patients with epilepsy
   B. Completion of a cardiopulmonary resuscitation course
   C. How to find an epilepsy support group
   D. Basic first aid for epilepsy

45. The emergency nurse is caring for a patient with increased intracranial pressure following a traumatic head injury. Which of the following vital signs should the nurse immediately report to the physician?

A. Heart rate 94 beats/minute
B. Temperature of 38.5°C (101.3°F)
C. Capnography of 30 mm Hg
D. Mean arterial pressure 70 mm Hg

46. The emergency nurse is preparing to administer intranasal midazolam to a patient in status epilepticus. The nurse is aware of which of the following regarding intranasal administration of midazolam?

A. Onset of the drug action may be delayed.
B. Onset of action is similar to the doses administered intramuscularly.
C. The drug rapidly crosses the blood–brain barrier.
D. The dose is given in one nostril.

47. A patient presents to the emergency department with a headache, and the diagnosis of subarachnoid hemorrhage is confirmed. When reviewing the patient's presenting chief complaint, the emergency nurse would expect to find:

A. a report of a recent traumatic injury to the head.
B. a sudden, brief loss of consciousness followed by a period of lucidity.
C. an insidious onset of headache with progressive worsening.
D. a report of the worst headache of the patient's life.

48. A patient presents to the emergency department following an all-terrain vehicle collision. During the neurological assessment, the emergency nurse notes motor paralysis and a loss of pain and temperature sensation below the level of T2. However, proprioception, touch, and vibratory sense are preserved. What is the most likely spinal cord injury associated with this clinical presentation?

A. Anterior cord syndrome
B. Brown-Sequard syndrome
C. Posterior cord syndrome
D. Central cord syndrome

49. Which of the following assessment findings would represent increased intracranial pressure according to the Cushing reflex?

A. Narrowing pulse pressure
B. Hypotension
C. Tachycardia
D. Cheyne–Stokes respirations

50. A patient presents to the emergency department complaining of a headache for the past 10 hours after being tackled and kicked in the head during a football game the previous day. A concussion is suspected without the presence of any neurological deficits. While continuing to evaluate the patient, which of the following would indicate to the emergency nurse the need for a computed tomography scan of the head?

A. Presence of cervical spine pain
B. Continued report of a headache
C. A Glasgow Coma Scale score of 12
D. Intermittent amnesia of the event

51. A patient presents to the emergency department via emergency medical services with a cervical collar in place following an altercation in the nearby pub. The patient reports being struck in the head, torso, and pelvic region numerous times with a bar stool. On assessment, the emergency nurse observes an obvious deformity of the left upper extremity, tenderness to the chest on palpation, and multiple abrasions and contusions to the face and head. The patient is able to move all extremities but has no recollection of the event and is oriented to person only. The presence of right otorrhea is also observed. Vital signs: BP 110/60 mm Hg; HR 106 beats/minute; RR 20 breaths/minute; SpO_2 98% on 4 L nasal cannula. The most appropriate intervention to be performed for this patient is which of the following?
    A. Removal of the cervical collar
    B. Computed tomography scan of the neck
    C. Application of a long spine board
    D. Obtain blood alcohol level

52. A patient presents to the emergency department with a history of a prior cerebrovascular infarction. The family reports that the patient was functioning independently before suddenly becoming confused, screaming, and throwing things at home. The nurse recognizes these symptoms are an indication of which of the following?
    A. Delirium
    B. Dementia
    C. Lacunar stroke
    D. Hyperoxia

53. A patient presents to the emergency department with complaints of bright red blood with clots in their stool for the past 2 weeks. The patient is in no apparent distress and has normal vital signs, and laboratory values are within normal limits. The emergency nurse suspects the source of the bleeding is:
    A. ulcerative colitis.
    B. esophageal varices.
    C. hemorrhoids.
    D. Mallory–Weiss syndrome

54. A patient with recent history of gastric bypass surgery presents to the emergency department with a 3-day history of right upper quadrant pain that radiates to the right shoulder. The emergency nurse suspects these symptoms are associated with:
    A. pyelonephritis.
    B. pancreatitis.
    C. appendicitis.
    D. cholecystitis.

55. A patient with a history of cirrhosis presents to the emergency department stating that they are "spitting up bright red blood." The patient's abdomen is severely distended, with numerous bruises in various stages of healing. The emergency nurse suspects the source of the patient's bleeding is most likely which of the following?
    A. Tuberculosis
    B. Intraoral abscess
    C. Esophageal varices
    D. Peptic ulcer disease

56. A patient with a diagnosis of esophagitis secondary to gastroesophageal reflux disease is treated in the emergency department and prepared for discharge. Which statement, made by the patient, indicates a correct understanding of the discharge instructions?

A. "I should take only small sips of water with any of my pills."
B. "I should lie on my left side after I eat to aid in my digestion."
C. "I should eat several small meals a day instead of three large meals."
D. "I should follow a gluten-free diet."

57. A patient presents to the emergency department with complaints of a burning, gnawing type pain in the left upper quadrant, and epigastrium that is associated with nausea and vomiting. The patient is diagnosed with acute gastritis. Based on the patient's symptoms, the nurse would expect which diagnostic test to yield abnormal results?

A. Serum creatinine
B. Liver enzymes
C. Serum electrolytes
D. Serum lipase

58. A patient presents to the emergency department complaining of fatigue, joint pain, and anorexia for the past 3 months. On assessment, the patient has an elevated temperature, yellowed sclera, and tenderness in the right upper quadrant. The patient admits to intravenous drug use. The emergency nurse would anticipate a positive result to which diagnostic test?

A. Hepatitis B antigen
B. Hepatitis A antigen
C. Human immunodeficiency virus immunoassay
D. Enzyme-linked immunosorbent assay test

59. An elderly male presents to triage complaining of intense pain in his lower abdomen. The patient states it started as a mild ache but has become more severe over the past week. The emergency nurse palpates the area and feels a mass in the mid-abdominal area. The emergency nurse suspects which of the following conditions?

A. Abdominal aortic aneurysm
B. Hernia
C. Appendicitis
D. Small bowel obstruction

60. A patient presents to the emergency department complaining of the feeling that something is caught in their throat. It began after the patient swallowed a piece of meat. After assessing that the patient's airway is not compromised, the nurse would anticipate the intravenous administration of what medication?

A. Omeprazole (Prilosec)
B. Glucagon
C. Metoclopramide (Reglan)
D. Nitroglycerin

61. The most common cause of acute pancreatitis is:

A. alcohol abuse.
B. abdominal trauma.
C. endoscopic retrograde cholangiopancreatography.
D. diabetes mellitus.

62. A patient presents to the emergency department complaining of recurrent "stomach" pain that occurs before meals and is relieved by eating. The patient has no significant medical history and takes 200 mg ibuprofen daily for chronic shoulder pain. Based on this information, the nurse suspects the patient's symptoms are most likely the result of:

A. gastroesophageal reflux disease.
B. gastric ulcer.
C. duodenal ulcer.
D. Mallory–Weiss syndrome.

63. A patient is being discharged home with a diagnosis of renal calculi. Which of the following statements by the patient indicates the need for further education regarding the discharged instructions?

A. "I may still see some blood in my urine until the stone passes."
B. "Once the pain is relieved, I should strain my urine and check the filter for stones."
C. "I will need to increase my intake of fluids, especially water."
D. "If I should experience any pain tonight, I should return to the emergency department immediately."

64. Which of the following conditions is caused by a sexually transmitted infection?

A. Priapism
B. Epididymitis
C. Prostatitis
D. Testicular torsion

65. The emergency nurse anticipates that the treatment for a patient with the diagnosis of vaginitis would most likely include the administration of:

A. antimicrobial medications.
B. probiotic medications.
C. antiviral medications.
D. immune-response modifier medications.

66. A woman with a history of ovarian cysts presents to the emergency department complaining of severe lower abdominal pain. Which of the following diagnostic testing would best confirm the presence of an ovarian cyst?

A. Serum beta HCG
B. Pelvic examination
C. Pelvic ultrasound
D. Clean-catch urine specimen

67. A patient with sudden onset of severe testicular pain is diagnosed with testicular torsion. The next appropriate intervention for the emergency nurse to perform is to:

A. elevate the scrotum.
B. insert an indwelling urinary catheter.
C. administer an antibiotic.
D. prepare the patient for emergency surgery.

68. If left untreated, a male who experiences a penile fracture resulting from the rupture of the tunica albuginea may develop which complication?

A. Erectile difficulties
B. Impaired urinary function
C. Penile ischemia
D. Infertility

69. A patient with bacterial vaginosis is prescribed clindamycin vaginal cream. It is important to include which information in the patient's discharge instructions for the use of this antibiotic?

A. Clindamycin cream should be applied immediately on arising in the morning.
B. Clindamycin cream may weaken a condom.
C. Clindamycin is the only medication needed to treat this infection.
D. Continue to use the medication until your symptoms are no longer present.

70. A 40-year-old female in the first trimester of her pregnancy presents to the emergency department complaining of severe left-sided abdominal tenderness with vaginal bleeding. The patient is lethargic, pale, hypotensive, and tachycardic. The emergency nurse recognizes the priority intervention for this patient is to:

A. prepare the patient for a transvaginal ultrasound.
B. prepare for the administration of a methotrexate injection.
C. prepare the patient for surgery.
D. obtain a serum beta human chorionic gonadotropin level.

71. The recommended method of performing chest compressions on a neonate is:

A. cardiac compression using two thumbs with the fingers encircling the chest and supporting the back.
B. cardiac compressions with two fingers and the opposite hand supporting the back.
C. compressions with the heel of one hand depressing the sternum not more than 4 cm (1.5 in).
D. five back blows followed by five chest thrust compressions.

72. Following the delivery of a full-term neonate in the emergency department, the emergency nurse administers a dose of intravenous pitocin to the mother. The nurse can expect which of the following outcomes from the administration of this medication?

A. Facilitated delivery of the placenta
B. Reduction of postpartum bleeding
C. Stimulated breast milk production
D. Prevention of Rh incompatibility between the mother and the fetus

73. A 36-week-pregnant female presents to the emergency department with a sudden onset of painless, bright red vaginal bleeding. Placenta previa is suspected. The emergency nurse should prepare this patient for which procedure?

A. Manual pelvic examination
B. Assessment of fetal heart tones
C. Immediate cesarean delivery
D. Pelvic ultrasound.

74. The triage nurse suspects a patient may be the victim of intimate partner violence. The primary survey is within normal limits, and there is no visible acute injury. Which of the following is a priority intervention for this patient?

A. Ask hospital security personnel to sit with the patient during the triage interview
B. Provide a private area for the assessment interview
C. Allow the patient to remain dressed in their own clothing during the provider examination
D. Document the name of the suspected offender in the patient record

75. The nurse considers which statement regarding pediatric posttraumatic stress disorder (PTSD) to be *false*?

A. Children under the age of 3 do not exhibit signs of pediatric PTSD.
B. School-aged children typically do not have "flashbacks" of the traumatic event.
C. How a parent responds to an infant's needs after a traumatic event has an effect on the child.
D. Teenagers may be expected to be hypervigilant and exhibit impulsive behaviors.

76. The acting out of the emotions of fear or anger is a definition of which of the following?

A. Anxiety
B. Paranoia
C. Violence
D. Panic

77. A patient presents to the emergency department hyperventilating. On further assessment, the emergency nurse determines that the patient is having a panic attack and encourages the patient to use slow, regular breathing. Which of the following interventions would next be most effective in assisting this patient?

A. Teach the patient the correct way to deal with anxiety
B. Assure the patient that things are going to be OK
C. Listen to the patient with empathy and concern
D. Tell the patient that the emergency team is in control, and everything will be fine.

78. A teenaged patient presents to the emergency department reporting recent suicidal thoughts. The patient has never experienced these thoughts in the past. The patient's only history is anxiety, which began several months ago for which the family physician recently prescribed some medication. The emergency nurse is aware that which of the following medications can lead to possible suicidal ideation and actions?

A. Benzodiazepine
B. Beta-blocker
C. Selective serotonin reuptake inhibitor
D. Tricyclic antidepressant

79. A female adolescent presents to triage accompanied by her father. The patient has a deep linear abrasion with yellow drainage surrounded by a reddened area on her forearm. The emergency nurse observes numerous linear abrasions and scars in various stages of healing on both arms. The patient denies suicidal thoughts or attempts. The patient's father states he recently obtained custody of the patient after her mother was arrested, and his daughter has been diagnosed with depression. He asks the nurse why his daughter is cutting herself. What is the best explanation for the emergency nurse to provide for this behavior?

A. "When people cut themselves, they are seeking attention."
B. "Patients who report feeling numb from their depression induce physical pain, which allows them to 'feel something.'"
C. "Your daughter attempted suicide by cutting herself."
D. "Your daughter is seeking pain medication."

80. A patient arrives to the emergency department via emergency medical services after being found "passed out in a park." The patient is now awake, smells of alcohol, appears to be intoxicated, and states, "Go away and leave me alone." The patient's spouse reports that the patient has been suffering from depression since their son died a few years ago but believed he had recently been improving. The patient had cleaned out the garage and given items away to friends, and the previous evening, he had spoken of making a will and "getting things in order." This morning, a large amount of alcohol and sleeping pills were found in the home with a letter telling the family "goodbye." Once medically cleared, the emergency nurse anticipates the next step in the patient's treatments will be:

A. to discharge the patient home once he is less intoxicated.
B. to admit the patient to a psychiatric facility.
C. to provide the patient and family with resources for help with alcoholism.
D. to contact adult protective services because the patient was found intoxicated in a park.

81. A patient has just been treated for an allergic reaction to a bee sting. On discharge, the patient is given a prescription for an epinephrine auto injector (EpiPen). What education should the emergency nurse provide to the patient regarding their condition and the use of the EpiPen?

A. If symptoms resolve after use of the EpiPen, the patient does not need to seek further care in the emergency department (ED).
B. The patient must administer the EpiPen at the onset of symptoms following a bee sting and then proceed to the nearest ED immediately after use.
C. The EpiPen should be stored in a safe place at home so the patient always knows where it is located.
D. Because the patient has had one severe anaphylactic reaction, they will likely not experience another similar episode.

82. A patient with a history of bipolar disorder presents to the emergency department complaining of increased thirst, excessive urination, a headache, and vision changes. The emergency nurse identifies that which of the following medications is the most likely cause of the patient's symptoms?

A. Ziprasidone (Geodon)
B. Haloperidol (Haldol)
C. Lithium
D. Carbamazepine (Tegretol)

83. What is the most common physical complaint exhibited by children being evaluated in the emergency department that is symptomatic of both depression and mood disorders?

A. Increased fatigue
B. Recent change in the child's weight
C. Changes in sleep
D. Frequent unexplained "stomach pains"

84. A schizophrenic patient who has been hearing voices telling them to kill their children is presently in a manic state after receiving haloperidol (Haldol) in the emergency department for their aggressive behavior. The emergency nurse should be prepared to administer which of the following medications if the patient should develop side effects related to haloperidol?

A. Lorazepam (Ativan)
B. Diphenhydramine (Benadryl)
C. Promethazine (Phenergan)
D. Ziprasidone (Geodon)

85. Which of the following medications would be administered to manage a patient's severe agitation in the emergency department?
   A. Ketamine
   B. Haloperidol (Haldol)
   C. Lorazepam (Ativan)
   D. Fentanyl (Duragesic)

86. Hemorrhagic signs that indicate the presence of disseminated intravascular coagulation include:
   A. purpura.
   B. gangrene of the fingers.
   C. bowel infarction.
   D. renal failure.

87. The emergency nurse is caring for a patient who states they are receiving chemotherapy for breast cancer. The patient lives alone and has a pet. Which type of pet would be most concerning as a possible source of infection for this patient?
   A. Fish
   B. Cat
   C. Dog
   D. Ant farm

88. Which of the following diagnostic interventions would have the highest priority to be performed in a patient with hemophilia who presents to the emergency department with altered mental status following a fall?
   A. Cervical spine radiograph
   B. Serum coagulation studies
   C. Computed tomography scan of the head
   D. Blood gas

89. Which of the following skin conditions is most closely associated with leukemia?
   A. Petechiae
   B. Skin bronzing
   C. Jaundice
   D. Erythematous rash

90. A patient presents to triage with a history of increasing fatigue and extreme pallor. The patient is suspected of having undiagnosed leukemia. Which of the following interventions should the emergency nurse prepare for?
   A. Lumbar puncture
   B. Initiation of the first dose of chemotherapy
   C. Administration of nonsteroidal anti-inflammatory drugs
   D. Bone marrow aspiration

91. A major trauma victim has received multiple transfusions of blood products. Which of the following electrolytes has the highest priority for the emergency nurse to monitor?
   A. Serum calcium
   B. Serum glucose
   C. Serum sodium
   D. Serum phosphate

92. A patient presents to the emergency department and states they are experiencing a sickle cell episode. The nurse knows that a pathophysiologic change occurs in a sickle cell episode when:

A. leukocytes assume a sickled shape and clump together in the micro vasculature.
B. platelets assume a sickled shape and clump together in the micro vasculature.
C. red blood cells assume a sickled shape and clump together in the micro vasculature.
D. neutrophils assume a sickled shape and clump together in the microvasculature.

93. Which medication does the emergency nurse anticipate to be administered to a patient who is being treated for an adrenal crisis because of the lack of aldosterone?

A. Spironolactone (Aldactone)
B. Metoprolol (Lopressor)
C. Dexamethasone (Decadron)
D. Nicardipine (Cardene)

94. The emergency nurse is caring for a patient with diabetic ketoacidosis. Which of the following values would *best* indicate that this patient is improving?

A. Respiratory rate of 16 breaths/minute
B. Pulse rate of 108 beats/minute
C. Blood pressure 138/72
D. Pulse oximetry 98%

95. Which of the following statements made by the patient reveals to the emergency nurse an understanding of the discharge instructions regarding how to avoid further episodes of hypoglycemia?

A. "As long as I check my glucose daily, I will not have further hypoglycemic reactions."
B. "I will keep a couple of pieces of candy with me at all times."
C. "I will eat small, frequent meals throughout the day and monitor my blood glucose before meals and at bedtime."
D. "I will keep my glucose oral gel with me at work, at school, and when I play sports."

96. A patient with elevated T3 and T4 levels has a temperature of 40.1°C (104.3°F). Which medication should be avoided to control this patient's fever?

A. Ibuprofen (Motrin)
B. Acetaminophen (Tylenol)
C. Naproxen (Naprosyn)
D. Aspirin (acetylsalicylic acid)

97. Which of the following assessment findings should the emergency nurse be most concerned about in a patient who presents with a fever of unknown origin?

A. Altered mental status
B. Tachycardia
C. Nasal congestion
D. Rash

98. A patient presents to the emergency department complaining of swollen lymph nodes, generalized aches and pains, and a headache. The patient has recently been receiving chemotherapy for breast cancer. The patient states they live alone, and their only companion is their pet cat. In providing education to the patient, the emergency nurse acknowledges the patient's understanding of the cause of the infection when they makes the following statement:

A. "I should have had someone clean my fish tank for me, instead of doing it myself."
B. "I should have had someone clean the cat litter box for me."
C. "I'll have to have someone help me by walking my dog."
D. "I'll have to get rid of the ant farm that I maintain for work."

99. A patient has unintentionally amputated the distal end of their middle finger. The emergency department nurse is aware that the proper care of the amputated part is to perform which of the following?

A. Rinse the amputated part in normal saline, wrap in saline moistened gauze, secure it in a plastic bag, and then place it on a bed of ice.
B. Place the amputated part directly in ice water.
C. Immediately rinse the amputated part with distilled water to remove dirt and debris, place it back onto the injury site, and secure it with a sterile gauze dressing.
D. Place the amputated part in a sterile dressing and then place it into a cold milk solution.

100. An elderly male presents to the emergency department complaining of a swollen left knee that is reddened and warm to touch. Bursitis of the knee is diagnosed, and the emergency provider performs a knee aspiration in order to:

A. administer prophylactic antibiotics directly into the joint space.
B. obtain a gram stain and culture of the synovial fluid.
C. remove the knee cyst.
D. prevent further infection.

101. A patient has sustained a forearm fracture. Following the application of a short-arm cast, the emergency nurse will assess sensation and motion of the patient's fingers. Numbness and tingling at the tips of the index and middle fingers may indicate compromise of which nerve?

A. Radial nerve
B. Peroneal nerve
C. Median nerve
D. Ulnar nerve

102. Which of the following assessment findings would lead the emergency nurse to suspect that a patient with a fracture of the left femur may be developing a fat embolus?

A. Acute dyspnea
B. Numbness and tingling of the left leg
C. Clusterlike headaches
D. Muscle spasms of the left leg

103. The emergency nurse is caring for a patient who presented with increasing arm pain following a long-arm splint application 2 days ago for an olecranon fracture. Assessment of the affected extremity reveals +1 radial pulse, a pale hand, and inability to wiggle or move the fingers. The patient is requesting pain medication. The emergency nurse identifies that the priority intervention for this patient is to:

A. apply ice to the extremity.
B. administer pain medication to the patient.
C. remove or loosen the long-arm splint.
D. elevate the extremity.

104. A patient presents to the emergency department following blunt trauma to the right upper leg and is diagnosed with a contusion. On receiving discharge instructions, the emergency nurse identifies the patient's understanding when they state:

A. "I will apply heat and ice to my leg and keep a loose gauze dressing over the injured area."
B. "I will apply heat to my leg, have my leg dangle, and leave the wound open to air."
C. "I will apply ice to the bruise on my leg, make sure the ace wrap is secure around my leg, and keep my leg elevated."
D. "I will let the leg dangle, and I will apply loose gauze directly over the injured area."

105. A patient presents to the emergency department after falling and sustaining multiple contusions to their trunk, right upper extremity, and right lower extremity. On reviewing the patient's list of current prescribed medications, the emergency nurse identifies that the patient is at risk for complications from their multiple contusions related to which of the following?

A. Hydroxychloroquine (Plaquenil)
B. Clopidogrel (Plavix)
C. Ciprofloxacin (Cipro)
D. Acetaminophen (Tylenol)

106. A patient presents to triage with a complaint of chest pain. The patient has a recent history of upper respiratory infection and a prescription for an antitussive medication that is taken as indicated. Vital signs: BP 150/88 mm Hg; HR 92 beats/minute; RR 20 breaths/minute; SpO_2 95%; T 38.1°C (100.6°F). The chest pain increases with deep inspiration, and the area around the patient's sternum is tender to palpation. An electrocardiogram shows regular sinus rhythm; a chest radiograph and serum troponins are normal. What is the most likely cause of this patient's chest pain?

A. Pleurisy
B. Myocardial infarction
C. Costochondritis
D. Pulmonary embolism

107. Numerous patients arrive to the emergency department with multiple lacerations over their entire bodies following a suspected pipe bomb that was detonated into a crowd. The emergency nurse anticipates that these injuries are the result of which category of blast injury?

A. Primary
B. Secondary
C. Tertiary
D. Quaternary

108. Which of the following findings would the emergency nurse expect to assess in a patient who had received procedural sedation before the reduction of a right radius and ulna fracture?

A. The patient is unarousable.
B. There is purposeful response following repeated painful stimulation.
C. There is a purposeful response to verbal/tactile stimulus.
D. The patient is awake, tracking the team.

109. An elderly patient presents to the emergency department after being found on the floor for an unknown period of time. The patient is awake and responsive. Head trauma has been ruled out, and the patient has been diagnosed with rhabdomyolysis. The patient has received a total of five liters of intravenous crystalloid solution. The emergency nurse identifies that the treatment has been effective when:

A. the urine output is 80 mL/hour.
B. the patient's urine appears clear.
C. the blood urea nitrogen approaches 35 mg/dL.
D. the serum creatinine approaches 3.0 mg/dL.

110. An elderly male patient is complaining of severe back pain that began 2 days ago and has increasingly gotten worse. The patient has no prior history of a similar episode. Unable to walk unassisted because of a loss of sensation in the groin area, the patient presents to the exam room in a wheelchair. The patient does not recall any heavy lifting, pushing, or pulling. When performing the patient assessment, the emergency nurse would be most concerned regarding the presence of:

A. positive left straight leg raise.
B. patellar and Achilles reflex +3 bilaterally.
C. a distended bladder on abdominal exam.
D. monofilament test 3/10 bilaterally.

111. A patient presents to the emergency department complaining of pain in their nondominant hand after being bitten by their cat 3 days previously. On assessment of the hand, it is noted to be red, swollen, and warm to touch. The nurse suspects the patient may have:

A. pasteurellosis.
B. rabies.
C. wound botulism.
D. gas gangrene.

112. The emergency nurse is conducting discharge teaching for a patient with a forehead laceration that has been closed with adhesive wound glue. The patient acknowledges understanding of discharge instructions when stating the following:

A. "I need to avoid showering for 24 hours."
B. "It is important for me to apply a thin layer of antibiotic ointment to the laceration every day after showering."
C. "I will be sure to wear sunscreen over the area."
D. "I must return to the emergency department for removal of adhesive glue in 3 days."

113. A patient presents to the emergency department with a human bite to the hand. The patient states they were the victim of an assault. What is the emergency nurse's priority in the care of this patient?

A. Assess the wound for the presence of exudate
B. Determine the source of the bite
C. Ask the patient when the bite occurred
D. Treatment of the bite before arrival

114. A patient arrives to the emergency department from an extended care facility. The emergency nurse is assessing the sacrum of the patient and notes an area of nonblanching erythema. What intervention would be most appropriate to protect the patient's skin from further pressure injury?

A. Place the patient in the Trendelenburg position
B. Insert an indwelling urinary catheter
C. Place the patient in a left lateral recumbent position
D. Calculate a Braden score

115. The patient presents to triage with a complaint of a persistent toothache for over 1 week. The patient has been traveling and has been unable to see a dentist. On assessment, the emergency nurse observes that the affected tooth is loose, with marked edema and inflammation in the surrounding gum. The emergency nurse anticipates that the patient will require which of the following from the emergency provider?

A. Acetaminophen (Tylenol) for the pain control
B. Tooth extraction
C. Antibiotic
D. Referral to a dentist

116. A patient presents to the emergency department complaining of severe, stabbing pain in the right side of the cheek and jaw after shoveling snow. The patient reports prior episodes of severe pain while eating. The nurse suspects a disorder of which cranial nerve?

A. Cranial nerve V
B. Cranial nerve VII
C. Cranial nerve IX
D. Cranial nerve XII

117. The presence of labyrinthitis is associated with which of the following signs and symptoms?

A. Periauricular cellulitis
B. Pain with movement of the tragus
C. Headache
D. History of recent infective process

118. An elderly patient presents to triage stating, "I can't see out of my right eye." The patient states the vision began to change when it appeared that a shade was lowering over the eye, and vision began to deteriorate. The patient denies pain in the right eye and has a history of diabetes and hypertension. The right pupil is dilated. The immediate intervention of the emergency nurse is to:

A. advise the patient that the loss of their vision is painless and a benign event, and assign the patient an Emergency Severity Index category 3.
B. perform a 12-lead electrocardiogram immediately.
C. contact the emergency provider and initiate an emergent consult with an ophthalmologist immediately.
D. perform a Snellen visual acuity assessment.

119. A patient presents to the emergency department for treatment of a laceration to their eyelid. What is the priority assessment for the emergency nurse to perform?

A. Assessment of cranial nerve II and cranial nerve III.
B. Assessment of cranial nerve I and cranial nerve II
C. Assessment of cranial nerve V and cranial nerve VII
D. Assessment of cranial nerve III and cranial nerve VII.

120. An adult patient presents to the emergency department with thermal burns to the face, chest, bilateral arms, and groin. Primary assessment reveals that the patient is alert, agitated, and having difficulty speaking. The patient has blisters around their mouth, and decreased breath sounds are noted auscultation. Vital signs: BP 180/120 mm Hg; HR 140 beats/minute; RR 36 breaths/minute; T 35.8°C (96.4°F); SpO_2 85% on 6 L/minute via mask; pain 10/10. The priority intervention for this patient is to:

A. administer pain medication.
B. establish intravenous access.
C. maintain a patent airway.
D. adhere to universal precautions to prevent infection.

121. A patient with suspected *Escherichia coli* food poisoning is at risk for developing which potentially life-threatening complication?
   A. Central nervous system syndrome
   B. Disseminated intravascular coagulation
   C. Toxoplasmosis
   D. Hemolytic uremic syndrome

122. The hospital is notified that two victims of radiation exposure are en route from the nearby nuclear power plant. What is the priority of care for these patients on arrival to the hospital?
   A. Notifying law enforcement
   B. Decontamination
   C. Medical stabilization
   D. Consulting the hospital radiation safety officer

123. A patient is brought into the emergency department via ambulance after participating in 8 hours of intense outdoor physical training. The patient is combative and confused. Vital signs: BP 80/48 mm Hg; HR 166 beats/minute; RR 30 breaths/minute and shallow; T 41°C (105.8°F) core temperature; SpO_2 90% on room air. The priority nursing intervention for this patient is to:
   A. administer supplemental oxygen by the most appropriate method for the patient's level of consciousness.
   B. administer 1–2 L of 0.9% sodium chloride over the first 4 hours.
   C. apply cooling blankets and continuously monitor the patient's core temperature.
   D. place the patient on the cardiac monitor and observe for signs of high-output cardiac failure.

124. After providing discharge instructions to the mother of a child diagnosed with head lice, the nurse acknowledges the mother understands the instructions when she states:
   A. "I will apply the pyrethrins 0.33%/piperonyl butoxide 4% (RID®) shampoo to dry hair."
   B. "I will take my child to the barber to have his head shaved, which will remove the lice."
   C. "I will shampoo my child's hair in hot soapy water to kill the lice."
   D. "I will apply bleach to my child's head to kill the lice."

125. A patient presents to the emergency department requesting post exposure rabies prophylaxis after being bitten by a fox. The patient has open wounds on the right buttock and right forearm. The patient reports having previously not received rabies vaccines. The site that would be the most appropriate for the nurse to administer the rabies vaccine is:
   A. any large muscle used for intramuscular injections.
   B. left deltoid.
   C. right buttock.
   D. right deltoid.

126. A patient presents to triage complaining of fever, muscle pain, headache, and a small, flat, pink rash on the palms, wrists, forearms, soles, and ankles. The patient reports that the symptoms began a few days after returning home from a camping trip. The triage nurse suspects that the patient has which of the following disorders?
   A. Rocky Mountain spotted fever
   B. Lyme disease
   C. Tularemia
   D. Colorado tick fever

127. A toddler is brought to triage with general malaise, fever, and a pruritic rash on the face and trunk that has progressed from macules to vesicles over the past several days. The nurse should plan to implement which of the following precautions?

A. Droplet precautions
B. Standard precautions
C. Contact precautions
D. Airborne precautions

128. A firefighter presents to the emergency department with seizures, hypotension, and hypoxia after fighting a house fire. Which substance may the firefighter have been exposed to that is causing these symptoms?

A. Iron
B. Pesticides
C. Petroleum distillates
D. Cyanide

129. Treatment is initiated for a patient who presents to the emergency department with signs and symptoms of an acute digoxin (Lanoxin) overdose. Which of the following changes in the patient's status would indicate to the nurse that the treatment is having its intended effect?

A. Hypoglycemia
B. Bradycardia
C. Potassium level within normal limits (3.5–5.0 mEq/L)
D. Signs and symptoms of hypovolemia

130. A patient with a history of alcohol abuse is being admitted to the hospital for pneumonia. Which early sign of alcohol withdrawal should the emergency nurse observe for in this patient?

A. Hallucinations
B. Tremulousness
C. Delirium
D. Low-grade fever

131. A patient presents to the emergency department suspected of ingesting an overdose of acetaminophen. The emergency nurse should anticipate to administer which medication as the appropriate antidote for acetaminophen overdose?

A. N-acetylcysteine (Mucomyst)
B. Flumazenil (Romazicon)
C. Octreotide (Sandostatin)
D. Diphenhydramine (Benadryl)

132. A patient is discharged from the emergency department with a prescription for doxycycline monohydrate (Doxycycline). Which statement made by the patient to the emergency nurse demonstrates an understanding of the side effects of this medication?

A. "I must stay out of the sun while taking this medicine."
B. "I must take calcium carbonate (Maalox) with my medication to avoid diarrhea."
C. "This medication is safe while I am breastfeeding."
D. "This medication may discolor my teeth."

133. A 16-year-old patient presents to the emergency department after being tackled early in a football game. The patient is complaining of left shoulder pain. History reveals the patient just returned to school following an extended absence related to infectious mononucleosis. The patient's vital signs: BP 96/48 mm Hg; HR 104/beats minute; RR 22 breaths/minute; SpO_2 97%; T 37.2°C (99.0°F); Wt 86.3 kg. What is the most likely cause of the patient's vital signs?

A. Hypovolemia related to splenic injury
B. Recurrence of the infectious mononucleosis
C. Dehydration related to physical activity
D. The patient's vital signs are within normal limits and intervention isn't necessary

134. The patient reports a history of having been diagnosed with tuberculosis. Which of the following would indicate that the patient is no longer infectious?

A. Patient has been compliant taking the prescribed medications for 1 week.
B. Patient had two consecutive negative sputum cultures for acid-fast bacillus.
C. Patient reports less coughing at night, and temperature is 37.7°C (99.9°F).
D. Patient's earlier tuberculin skin test induration diameter is less than 10 mm.

135. The development of secondary traumatic stress (STS) can occur as the result of caring for those who are exposed to suffering or traumatic events. Symptoms of STS include which of the following signs and symptoms?

A. Emotional exhaustion
B. The repeated reliving of disturbing events
C. Difficulty making decisions
D. Presence of reduced empathy toward patients or their families

136. A patient with terminal cancer arrives at the emergency department in septic shock. The patient refuses to have any life-sustaining interventions initiated. The emergency nurse states they cannot morally care for this patient because it is against their beliefs. What document supports transferring the care of this patient to another nurse?

A. Emergency Nurses position statement: Patient handoff/transfer
B. The patient's bill of rights
C. The Patient Self-Determination Act
D. American Nurses Association code of ethics

137. Along with identifying the best available research and their clinical expertise, emergency nurses incorporate which other component to make evidence-based practice decisions in the clinical area?

A. Education level of nursing staff
B. Administrative support
C. Traditional practices
D. Patient preferences

138. The emergency nurse is aware that a patient with which of the following preexisting medical conditions is not eligible to donate organs or tissues for transplantation?

A. Diabetes mellitus
B. History of cancer
C. Human immunodeficiency virus
D. Coronary artery disease

139. A patient with end-stage lung cancer is brought to the emergency department with progressive dyspnea. The patient is diagnosed with a pleural effusion secondary to the lung malignancy. Which of the following interventions is appropriate and consistent with the patient's palliative care management at home?

A. Administer intravenous antibiotics
B. Perform chest physiotherapy
C. Prepare the patient for a paracentesis
D. Prepare the patient for a thoracentesis

140. The victim of multiple gunshot wounds arrives to the emergency department via emergency medical services. The emergency nurse is aware that a key principle of preserving clothing evidence of the victim of a violent crime is to perform which of the following actions?

A. Place each piece of clothing in an individual paper bag; label, seal with tape, and include appropriate patient identification.
B. Place the clothing in a plastic bag because of saturation of blood on the clothing.
C. Cut the clothing off immediately to expose the patient as quickly as possible; because it is a trauma patient, you may cut through bullet holes, tears, rips, or holes.
D. Place all the clothing in a large paper bag; label, seal with tape, and include appropriate patient identification

141. Which agent administered intravenously before procedural sedation has the shortest duration of action?

A. Ketalar (Ketamine)
B. Midazolam (Versed)
C. Propofol (Diprivan)
D. Fentanyl (Sublimaze)

142. Research has demonstrated that patients who report satisfaction with the care they received in an emergency department (ED) are more likely to perform which of the following actions?

A. Frequently access the ED
B. Use the ED as a source for primary care
C. Require hospital admission
D. Adhere to their treatment plan

143. Studies have shown that patients report increased satisfaction with the care they received during their emergency department (ED) visit when they are provided with which of the following?

A. The ability to fill the prescription provided at discharge in the hospital pharmacy
B. Distraction devices such as televisions or laptop computers
C. Frequent interactions with the ED registered nurse
D. Additional blankets and pillows

144. When using a certified translator to communicate with a non-English-speaking patient, the emergency nurse should direct questions to which participant in the conversation?

A. The patient
B. The certified translator
C. The patient's oldest male family member
D. The patient's designated family spokesperson

145. The Five Rights of Delegation are: right task, right circumstances, right person, right direction and communication, and which of the following?
   A. Right equipment and supplies
   B. Right documentation
   C. Right supervision and evaluation
   D. Right assessment and reassessment

146. A nurse leaves a patient's chart open on a portable work station. A patient's family member is observed looking at the open chart on the work station. This action by the nurse is considered a violation of the:
   A. patient's bill of rights.
   B. Emergency Medical Treatment and Active Labor Act.
   C. Health Insurance Portability and Accountability Act.
   D. Patient Self-Determination Act.

147. A terminally ill patient is admitted to the emergency department (ED). The patient informs the and nurse that they have a living will (advance directive) with a Do Not Resuscitate (DNR) order. The emergency nurse would:
   A. make the patient a full code because nothing will likely happen while in the ED.
   B. document in the chart that the patient is a DNR and ask the patient for a copy of their living will and DNR to place in their medical record.
   C. ask the patient's family members what lifesaving interventions they would like performed in the event of a cardiopulmonary arrest.
   D. take no action, because the advance directive and the DNR only apply once the patient is admitted to the hospital.

148. The emergency department provider directs the nurse who is caring for a patient to suture the patient's forearm laceration. The nurse should do which of the following on receiving this order?
   A. Do not perform the procedure
   B. Perform the procedure
   C. Perform the procedure with a physician assistant present
   D. Delegate the task to assistive personnel

149. A child is transported to the emergency department following a mass casualty incident. The child is unable to ambulate, has spontaneous respirations of 32 breaths/minute, has a palpable pulse, and is alert. Which JumpSTART triage category should be assigned to this child?
   A. Yellow (delayed)
   B. Red (immediate)
   C. Black (expectant)
   D. Green (minor)

150. A pediatric traumatic cardiopulmonary arrest is in progress when the charge nurse comes to assist the primary emergency department nurse with the resuscitation. At first glance, the patient looks similar to the son the charge nurse recently loss due to a terminal illness. The charge nurse is unable to stay focused on the necessary resuscitation tasks for this patient. Upon debriefing, the code team discusses the charge nurse's challenges. The best response to encourage resiliency is which of the following?

A. "This experience should help you get you back to the bedside. You are a "super nurse." You can take care of anyone that rolls through those doors."

B. "This is a tough place to work. Management didn't give you enough time off to grieve, staff members don't take initiative to help, and you are tired and overworked. Have you considered looking to work somewhere else that will support you in a better way?"

C. "Don't forget, we are a team and you are part of our team. Some of us want to pray with you at the end of the shift and join you when you go to visit your son's grave site."

D. "We need more situation awareness from this team. If one us is not able to step up, we need to speak up and get someone else in who can do the job. We cannot risk patient safety."

PART 2

1. A patient presents who had experienced chest pain but is now pain free. Electrocardiograms have been repeated twice, and troponin levels repeated at 4-hour intervals are within normal limits. The patient has no significant risk factors for heart disease. The nurse anticipates:
   A. admission to the ICU to rule out myocardial infarction.
   B. admission to cardiac catheterization lab for evaluation of coronary anatomy.
   C. that the patient will be discharged to home, with instructions for close follow-up with their primary care provider because the risk of an adverse coronary event is low.
   D. admission to the telemetry unit to rule out myocardial infarction.

Rationale

A. Patients who do not exhibit concerning symptoms for acute coronary syndrome and who have no risk factors for coronary artery disease do not benefit from ICU admission.

B. Patients without ongoing concerning symptoms and having no diagnostic testing concerning for acute coronary syndrome do not need urgent cardiac catheterization.

C. In adult patients with chest pain who demonstrate two negative findings for serial biomarkers, nonconcerning vital signs, and nonischemic electrocardiographic findings, short-term clinically relevant adverse cardiac events are rare and commonly iatrogenic, suggesting that routine inpatient admission may not be a beneficial strategy for this group.

D. Patients who are not exhibiting ongoing symptoms of myocardial ischemia and who have no significant risk factors for heart disease do not benefit from hospital admission.

Category: Cardiovascular Emergencies/Acute coronary syndrome

Nursing Process: Analysis

Reference

Weinstock, M., Weingart, S., Orth, F., VanFossen, D., Kaide, C., Anderson, J., & Newman, D. H. (2015). Risk for clinically relevant adverse cardiac events in patients with chest pain at hospital admission. *JAMA Internal Medicine, 175*(7), 1207–1212. Retrieved from http://archinte.jamanetwork.com

---

2. A patient who became unconscious during ascent while scuba diving arrives via emergency medical services. The patient is unconscious and hypotensive. What is the most appropriate position in which to place this patient during their examination by the physician?
   A. Left lateral decubitus, head down
   B. Right lateral decubitus, head down
   C. Left lateral decubitus, head up
   D. Supine

Rationale

A. Positioning the patient in a left lateral decubitus, head down position prevents air from traveling through the right side of the heart into the pulmonary arteries, leading to a possible right ventricular outflow obstruction.

B. Placing the patient on their right side would potentiate the obstruction of the pulmonary arteries by the presence of an air embolism.

C. Placing the patient with their head up would act to increase the passage of air through the vasculature increasing the possibility of an air embolism. Placing the patient head down limits the passage of air through the right side of the heart.

D. Placing the patient in a supine position will not limit the possibility of an air embolism entering the right side of the heart and leading to a possible right ventricular outflow obstruction. The best position is for the patient to be placed in a left lateral decubitus position with head down.

Category: Cardiovascular Emergencies/Shock (cardiogenic and obstructive)

Nursing Process: Intervention

References

Moon, R. E. (2003). Air or gas embolism. In J. J. Feldmeier (Ed.), *Hyperbaric oxygen therapy: Committee report* (pp. 5–10). Kensington, MD: Undersea and Hyperbaric Medical Society.

Schellar, N. A., & Sterk, W. (2012). Venous gas embolism after an open-water air dive and identical repetitive dive. *Undersea and Hyperbaric Medicine, 39*(1), 577–587.

---

3. In which patient would the nurse question an order for morphine sulfate?
   A. A patient with aortic dissection
   B. A patient with a ST elevation myocardial infarction
   C. A patient with unstable angina
   D. A patient with non-ST elevation myocardial infarction

Rationale

A. Morphine sulfate is a reasonable order for a patient with aortic dissection.

B. Morphine sulfate is a reasonable order for a patient with ST segment elevation myocardial infarction.

C. Morphine sulfate is a reasonable order for a patient with unstable angina.

D. An increase in mortality has been associated with the use of morphine sulfate in patients with non-ST segment elevation myocardial infarction (NSTEMI). Investigators from the CRUSADE registry looked at over 50,000 patients with NSTEMI and found that those patients receiving morphine had a 48% greater risk of death.

Category: Cardiovascular Emergencies/Acute coronary syndrome

Nursing Process: Analysis

References

American Heart Association. (2016). The ACLS cases: Acute coronary syndrome. In *Advanced cardiovascular life support: Provider manual* (pp. 59–72). Dallas, TX: Author.

Meine, T. J., Roe, M. T., Chen, A. Y., Patel, M. R., Washam, J. B., Ohman, E. M., . . . Peterson, E. D.; CRUSADE Investigators. (2005). Association of intravenous morphine use and outcomes in acute coronary syndromes: Results from the CRUSADE Quality Improvement Initiative. *American Heart Journal, 149*(6), 1043–1049. https://doi.org/10.1016/j.ahj.2005.02.010

4. Following the administration of 2 L of intravenous (IV) crystalloids, the emergency nurse begins to administer IV dobutamine (Dobutrex) to a patient who has been diagnosed with a right ventricular infarction. The emergency nurse identifies that this medication has been effective when the patient demonstrates which of the following?

   A. Bradycardia
   B. Increase in blood pressure
   C. Presence of distended neck veins
   D. Onset of atrial fibrillation

Rationale

A. The presence of bradycardia in a patient who has experienced a right ventricular infarction (RVI) is an indication of impaired cardiac function and contractility.

B. Patients who experience an RVI are preload dependent and require additional fluids to increase their blood pressure. If the patient's blood pressure does not respond to the additional fluid administration, the administration of dobutamine is indicated to increase the patient's cardiac output, thereby increasing the blood pressure.

C. The presence of distended neck veins indicates an increase in central venous pressure, thereby indicating right ventricular failure and impaired ventricular contraction and emptying. Dobutamine is indicated in the presence of decreased contractility to enhance cardiac output and increase the patient's heart rate, in addition to increasing the patient's blood pressure.

D. New-onset atrial fibrillation following a RVI indicates the presence of atrial infarction and/or atrial dilation, and, therefore, impaired atrial contraction and ventricular filling.

Category: Cardiovascular Emergencies/Acute coronary syndrome

Nursing Process: Evaluation

References

Criddle, L. (2007). Cardiovascular emergencies. In K. S. Hoyt & J. Selfridge-Thomas (Eds.), *Emergency nursing core curriculum* (6th ed., pp. 187–248). St. Louis, MO: Saunders Elsevier.

Hammond, B. B. (2013). Cardiovascular emergencies. In B. B. Hammond & P. G. Zimmermann (Eds.), *Sheehy's manual of emergency care* (7th ed., pp. 201–211). St. Louis, MO: Elsevier Mosby.

---

5. The nurse has instituted applied oxygen and is to reduce the patient's heart rate and blood pressure. Which of the following findings would be expected after applying oxygen, initiating two large-caliber intravenous (IV) lines, and administering IV beta-blockers?

   A. Difference of > 20 mm Hg blood pressure when comparing in both arms
   B. Chest pain radiating to the left shoulder
   C. Orthopnea and jugular venous distention
   D. Petechial lesions on the patient's palms or soles

Rationale

A. Difference of > 20 mm Hg blood pressure in both arms is suggestive of aortic dissection. Treatment for aortic dissection includes the insertion of two large-caliber IV lines, application of oxygen, and administration of beta-blockers to reduce the patient's heart rate and blood pressure.

B. Chest pain radiating to the left shoulder is a symptom of pericarditis. The treatment for pericarditis is IV access with administration of anti-inflammatory agents and a possible pericardiocentesis.

C. Orthopnea and jugular venous distention are symptoms of congestive heart failure (CHF). The treatment for CHF includes the administration of sedatives, diuretics, morphine sulfate, and vasodilators.

D. Petechial lesions of the palms or soles (Janeway lesions) are indicative of infective endocarditis. Treatment for infective endocarditis consists of administering antipyretics and antibiotics.

Category: Cardiovascular Emergencies/Aneurysm/dissection

Nursing Process: Evaluation

Reference

Criddle, L. (2007). Cardiovascular emergencies. In K. S. Hoyt & J. Selfridge-Thomas (Eds.), *Emergency nursing core curriculum* (6th ed., pp. 187–248). St. Louis, MO: Saunders Elsevier.

---

6. A 3-month-old infant weighing 11 pounds (5 kg) arrives at the emergency department in full cardiopulmonary arrest. The monitor shows ventricular fibrillation. Good-quality cardiopulmonary resuscitation is being performed, and the infant has been defibrillated once. Which medication should be administered next?

A. Epinephrine 0.05 mg intravenously/intraosseously (IV/IO)
B. Atropine 0.1 mg IV/IO
C. Amiodarone (Cordarone) 25 mg IV/IO
D. Sodium bicarbonate 5 mEq IV

Rationale

A. Epinephrine is the first-line drug for an infant in cardiopulmonary arrest because of ventricular fibrillation. The correct dose is 0.01 mg/kg. The correct IV/IO dose for this infant would be 0.01 mg × 5 kg, or 0.05 mg.

B. Atropine is not indicated in the treatment of ventricular fibrillation.

C. Amiodarone is not considered the first drug for ventricular fibrillation; it would be administered after epinephrine. The dose of amiodarone is 5 mg/kg, or 25 mg.

D. Although sodium bicarbonate may be indicated during cardiopulmonary arrest for correction of acidosis, it is not considered a first-line treatment. The correct dose for sodium bicarbonate is 1 mEq/kg, or 5 mEq IV.

Category (Pediatric): Cardiovascular Emergencies/Cardiopulmonary arrest

Nursing Process: Intervention

Reference

American Heart Association. (2016). *Pediatric advanced life support: Provider manual.* Dallas, TX: Author.

---

7. A patient in cardiopulmonary arrest remains in ventricular fibrillation despite having been defibrillated 6 times, receiving good quality cardiopulmonary resuscitation, and the administration of epinephrine (Adrenalin) and amiodarone (Cordarone). Arterial blood gases reveal a pH of 7.02, PO_2 96 mm Hg, and pCO_2 40 mm Hg. What medication order should the emergency nurse anticipate next for this patient?

A. Adenosine (Adenocard) 6 mg
B. Calcium chloride 1 g
C. Vasopressin (Pitressin) 40 units
D. Sodium bicarbonate 1 mEq/kg

Rationale

A. Adenosine is an antidysrhythmic used to slow conduction at the AV node. Ventricular fibrillation is a dysrhythmia of the ventricles. Adenosine is typically used for supraventricular tachycardia.

B. Calcium chloride would be indicated for hypocalcemia or other electrolyte abnormalities such as hyperkalemia, hypermagnesemia, or hyperphosphatemia.

C. Vasopressin is currently not recommended for administration for ventricular fibrillation according to the 2016 guidelines of the American Heart Association.

D. Sodium bicarbonate is indicated for documented acidosis during cardiopulmonary arrest. Arterial gases indicate a pH of 7.0, or acidosis. Sodium bicarbonate will act as an alkalinizer to raise the pH to a value closer to a normal range of 7.35–7.45. This arterial blood gas does not reflect a respiratory cause for the acidosis in the presence of a normal pCO_2 value. The latest recommendation from the American Heart Association is to administer sodium bicarbonate at 1 mEq/kg.

Category: Cardiovascular Emergencies/Cardiopulmonary arrest

Nursing Process: Intervention

References

American Heart Association. (2016). The ACLS cases: Cardiac arrest: VF/pulseless VT. In *Advanced cardiac life support: Provider manual* (pp. 92–109). Dallas, TX: Author.

Wolters Kluwer. (2016). *Nursing 2016 drug handbook* (pp. 88, 256, 1309). Philadelphia, PA: Author.

---

8. A patient presents via emergency medical services in cardiopulmonary arrest. Chest compressions and bag-mask ventilation are being performed. The cardiac monitor shows ventricular tachycardia. While the defibrillator is charging for defibrillation, the nurse should ensure that:

A. no one is touching the patient.
B. high-quality cardiopulmonary resuscitation is continued.
C. oxygen delivery via nasal cannula continues at 6 L/minute.
D. the defibrillator pads have been placed on the patient.

Rationale

A. High-quality cardiopulmonary resuscitation (CPR) should continue up to the moment just before the actual defibrillation. It is important that no one is touching the patient when the actual defibrillation occurs because the current can travel through a rescuer and possibly induce a lethal dysrhythmia.

B. The 2016 American Heart Association guidelines include the continuation of high-quality CPR with optimal oxygen delivery to the patient while the defibrillator is charging. This results in a reduction of the time between stopping compression and defibrillation, thereby increasing the success of the defibrillation.

C. Because of the risk of sparking or ignition during defibrillation, all oxygen administration should be discontinued.

D. Defibrillation pads (no touch pads) should be placed on the patient's chest during the initial rhythm assessment.

Category: Cardiovascular Emergencies/Cardiopulmonary arrest

Nursing Process: Intervention

References

American Heart Association. (2016). Effective high performance team dynamics. In *Advanced cardiovascular life support: Provider manual* (pp. 25–32). Dallas, TX: Author.

Kerber, R. E. (2008). "I'm clear, you're clear, everybody's clear": A tradition no longer necessary for defibrillation? *Circulation, 117*(19), 2435–2436. https://doi.org/10.1161/CIRCULATIONAHA.108.773721

---

9. A teenaged patient presents to triage stating that they have the sensation that their heart is jumping out of their chest for the past several hours. The patient denies routine drug use and states that they have been studying for end-of-the-semester final exams for the past 3 days and took a pill to help him study. You palpate a radial pulse that is 170 beats/minute and regular. Which of the following dysrhythmias would be suspected?

   A. Supraventricular tachycardia
   B. Ventricular tachycardia
   C. Atrial fibrillation
   D. Sinus rhythm with premature atrial complexes

Rationale

A. Supraventricular tachycardia (SVT) is common in young people with no history of organic heart disease and is frequently associated with the use of stimulants.

B. Ventricular tachycardia is associated with an underlying myocardial conduction disturbance or structural deficits. Sustained ventricular tachycardia is very rare without deteriorating into ventricular fibrillation.

C. Atrial fibrillation is characterized by an irregular heartbeat and is commonly associated with the presence of heart failure, atrial enlargement, hypertension, thyrotoxicosis, coronary artery disease, or rheumatic heart disease. The patient does not have any of these comorbidities, nor is their heart rate described as irregular, making it highly unlikely the patient is experiencing atrial fibrillation. The presence of SVT is more commonly associated with young people with no history of organic heart disease.

D. Premature atrial complexes are frequently associated with use of stimulants but would present with an irregular rhythm; this patient has a regular rhythm.

Category: Cardiovascular Emergencies/Dysrhythmias

Nursing Process: Analysis

Reference

Criddle, L. (2007). Cardiovascular emergencies. In K. S. Hoyt & J. Selfridge-Thomas (Eds.), *Emergency nursing core curriculum* (6th ed., pp. 187–248). St. Louis, MO: Saunders Elsevier.

---

10. The emergency nurse is participating in the treatment of a patient in cardiopulmonary arrest. Cardiopulmonary resuscitation is ongoing, an advanced airway is present, and vascular access has been obtained. The monitor shows an organized rhythm, but no palpable pulse is detected. In addition to evaluating the "Hs and Ts" as causes of pulseless electrical activity (PEA), the nurse anticipates the use of what device or procedure to better evaluate for potentially reversible causes of PEA?

A. Electrocardiogram
B. Point of care ultrasound
C. Bedside chest radiograph
D. Glucometer

Rationale

A. Although an electrocardiogram may give more detailed information about the rhythm compared with a bedside rhythm strip, it does not provide the detailed information about cardiac function and wall motion activity when compared with ultrasound.

B. Point of care ultrasound can quickly aid in identification of mechanical causes of PEA. A collapsed right ventricle suggests an inflow obstruction (i.e., tamponade, pneumothorax, or hyperinflation), whereas a dilated right ventricle indicates outflow obstruction (i.e., pulmonary embolism).

C. Although a bedside chest radiograph may show PEA causes such as tension pneumothorax or cardiac tamponade, it reveals no information about cardiac muscle function.

D. A glucometer may indicate the presence of hyperglycemia or hypoglycemia, which may contribute to a PEA scenario; however, the glucometer does not provide information regarding cardiac contractility and function.

Category: Cardiovascular Emergencies/Dysrhythmias

Nursing Process: Intervention

Reference

Littmann, L., Bustin, D. J., & Haley, M. W. (2014). A simplified and structured teaching tool for the evaluation and management of pulseless electrical activity. *Medical Principles and Practice, 23*, 1–6.

---

11. Echocardiography determines that a patient has infective endocarditis with bacterial or fungal growth isolated to the tricuspid valve. In addition to a heart murmur, what other pertinent signs or symptoms would the emergency department nurse include in the assessment related to this finding?

A. Blood-tinged frothy sputum
B. Jugular vein distension
C. Sharp, piercing chest pain that decreases when leaning forward
D. Severe chest pain radiating to the back, 20 mm Hg difference in blood pressure between arms

Rationale

A. Blood-tinged frothy sputum of left-sided heart failure. If the mitral valve were damaged because of infective endocarditis, the patient may exhibit these signs and symptoms.

B. The tricuspid valve is located on the right side of the heart and is most often the first to be damaged with infective endocarditis. Damage to this valve can lead to right-sided heart failure. Signs and symptoms of right-sided heart failure include shortness of breath, pedal edema, and jugular vein distension.

C. In addition to a friction rub, these are pertinent signs and symptoms for pericarditis.

D. These signs and symptoms are pertinent for the diagnosis of acute aortic dissection.

Category: Cardiovascular Emergencies/Endocarditis

Nursing Process: Assessment

References

Habib, G., Lancellotti, P., Antunes, M. J., Bongiorni, M. G., Casalta, J., Del Zotti, F., . . . Zamorano, J. L. (2015). 2015 ESC guidelines for the management of infective endocarditis: The Task Force for the Management of Infective Endocarditis of the European Society of Cardiology (ESC). *European Heart Journal, 36*, 3075–3123. https://doi.org/10.1093/eurheartj/ehv319

Hammond, B. B. (2013). Cardiovascular emergencies. In B. B. Hammond & P. G. Zimmermann (Eds.), *Sheehy's manual of emergency care* (7th ed., pp. 201–211). St. Louis, MO: Elsevier Mosby.

---

12. A dyspnic patient presents to the emergency department. Physical assessment reveals an S3 heart sound and auscultated bilateral crackles, in addition to an ultrasound finding of bilateral "B-lines" when scanning the anterior lung fields. The nurse suspects:

A. right-sided heart failure.
B. left-sided heart failure.
C. pneumonia.
D. pulmonary embolism.

Rationale

A. Right-sided heart failure signs and symptoms include peripheral edema, jugular venous distention, ascites, and nausea because of venous congestion.

B. Signs of left-sided heart failure include shortness of breath, dyspnea, an S3 heart sound, crackles and pulmonary edema. B-lines appear as vertical artifacts observed bilaterally on ultrasound examination of the anterior lungs and are present in acute decompensated heart failure (ADHF), indicating an excess of "lung water." The presence of (1) B-lines in the bilateral anterior lungs, (2) poor cardiac function, and (3) a nonrespirophasic (plethoric or large) inferior vena cava that does not collapse with respiration suggests a diagnosis of ADHF.

C. Signs and symptoms of pneumonia can include dyspnea, cough, wheezing, pleuritic chest pain, and coldlike symptoms. In pneumonia, ultrasound findings can include consolidations and B-lines that are usually unilateral.

D. Signs and symptoms of pulmonary embolism can include dyspnea with tachypnea and possible hemoptysis, pleuritic chest pain, tachycardia, anxiety, apprehension, restlessness, pleural friction rub, and clinical signs and symptoms of deep vein thrombosis.

Category: Cardiovascular Emergencies/Heart failure

Nursing Process: Assessment

References

Collins, S. P., Storrow, A. B., Levy, P. D., Alberet, N., Butler, J., Ezekowitz, J. A., . . . Lenihan, D. J. (2015). Early management of patients with acute heart failure: State of the art and future directions: A consensus document from the SAEM /HFSA Acute Heart Failure Working Group. *Academic Emergency Medicine, 22*(1), 94–112. https://doi.org/10.1111/acem.12538

Dresden, S., Mitchell, P., Rahimi, L., Leo, M., Rubin-Smith, J., Bibi, S., . . . Carmody, K. (2014). Right ventricular dilatation on bedside echocardiography performed by emergency physicians aids in the diagnosis of pulmonary embolism. *Annals of Emergency Medicine, 63*(1), 16–24. https://doi.org/10.1016/j.annemergmed.2013.08.016

Hammond, B. B. (2013). Cardiovascular emergencies. In B. B. Hammond & P. G. Zimmermann (Eds.), *Sheehy's manual of emergency care* (7th ed., pp. 201–211). St. Louis, MO: Elsevier Mosby.

Mantuani, D., Frazee, B. W., Famimi, J., & Nagdev, A. (2016). Point-of-care multi-organ ultrasound improves diagnostic accuracy in adults presenting to the emergency department with acute dyspnea. *Western Journal of Emergency Medicine, 17*(1), 46–53. https://doi.org/10.5811/westjem.2015.11.28525

Rihal, C. S., Naidu, S. S., Givertz, M. M., Szeto, W. Y., Burke, J. A., Kapur, N. K., . . . Tu, T. (2015). 2015 SCAI/ACC/HFSA/STS clinical expert consensus statement on the use of percutaneous mechanical circulatory support devices in cardiovascular care. *Journal of the American College of Cardiology, 65*(19), e7–e26.

Walsh, R. (2013). Respiratory emergencies. In B. B. Hammond & P. G. Zimmermann (Eds.), *Sheehy's manual of emergency care* (7th ed., pp. 185–199). St. Louis, MO: Elsevier Mosby.

Yancy, C. W., Jessup, M., Bozkurt, B., Butler, J., Casey, D. E., Colvin, M. M., . . . Westlake, C. (2016). 2016 ACC/AHA/HFSA focused update on new pharmacological therapy for heart failure: An update of the 2013 ACCF/AHA guideline for the management of heart failure. *Circulation, 134*. https://doi.org/10.1161/CIR.0000000000000435

Yancy, C. W., Jessup, B., Bozkurt, B., Butler, J., Casey, D. E., Drazner, M. H., . . . Wilkoff, B. L. (2013). 2013 ACCF/AHA guideline for the management of heart failure: Executive summary. *Journal of the American College of Cardiology, 62*(16),1495–1539.

---

13. Nitroprusside is ordered for a patient with a hypertensive emergency. This medication works to reduce blood pressure by:

A. decreasing heart rate and causing vasodilation.
B. inhibiting the influx of calcium ions.
C. relaxing vascular smooth muscle to reduce afterload and preload.
D. dilating arterioles.

Rationale

A. Labetalol (Normodyne) is a nonselective beta-blocker that reduces blood pressure by inhibiting alpha and beta receptors, causing both vasodilation and reduction of the sympathetic stimulation of the heart. Nitroprusside is not a beta-blocker.

B. Clevidipine (Cleviprex) is a calcium channel blocker that works to reduce blood pressure by inhibiting the transmembrane influx of extracellular calcium ions across membranes of myocardial cells and vascular smooth muscle cells without changing serum calcium concentrations. This results in inhibition of cardiac and vascular smooth muscle contraction, thereby dilating main coronary and systemic arteries. Nitroprusside does not inhibit the influx of calcium ions.

C. Nitroprusside is a vasodilator that works to reduce blood pressure by relaxing vascular smooth muscle, which reduces afterload and preload by producing nitrous oxide. It also dilates coronary arteries. Nitroprusside should be protected from light during administration.

D. Hydralazine (Apresoline) is a vasodilator that works by dilating arterioles with little effect on veins. It also decreases systemic resistance. Nitroprusside does not dilate the arterioles; it works to relax vascular smooth muscle.

Category: Cardiovascular Emergencies/Hypertension

Nursing Process: Analysis

References

PEPID LLC. (2016). *PEPID Emergency Medicine Platinum* (Version 17.1.1) [Mobile application software]. Retrieved from http://pepid.com

Salgado, D. R., Silva, E., & Vincent, J. L. (2013). Control of hypertension in the critically ill: A pathophysiological approach. *Annals of Intensive Care, 3*(17), 1–13.

---

14. Emergency medical services arrives with an elderly patient, the victim of a single-vehicle collision with a tree. The patient was not wearing a seat or shoulder restraint, was not ejected from the vehicle, and the airbag did not deploy. The patient has equal breath sounds and symmetrical chest rise and fall. The patient appears anxious and is complaining of sternal pain to palpation, although no crepitus is present. Vital signs: BP 128/74 mm Hg with the presence of a pulsus paradoxus of 15 mm Hg; HR 86 beats/minute; RR 28 breaths/minute. The emergency nurse anticipates that this patient will require the following intervention:

A. Needle thoracentesis
B. Pericardiocentesis
C. Administration of a 1000 mL warm 0.9% sodium chloride bolus
D. Endotracheal intubation

Rationale

A. Needle thoracentesis is used to relieve a tension pneumothorax, not a cardiac tamponade. The patient has equal breath sounds bilaterally.

B. Blunt chest trauma, especially in the geriatric population, puts the patient at greater risk to develop a pericardial effusion and tamponade. The lack of a seat or shoulder restraint, as demonstrated by the mechanism of injury places this patient at increased risk of striking their unprotected sternum against the steering column and developing a pulsus paradoxus greater than 10 mm Hg.

C. The patient's hypotension is most likely related to the presence of a cardiac tamponade, not hypovolemia. The administration of a 0.9% sodium chloride bolus is likely to exacerbate their condition, not improve it.

D. The patient does not exhibit any need for airway control or endotracheal intubation. The priority intervention is to perform a needle pericardiocentesis to relieve the patient's cardiac tamponade.

Category (Geriatric): Cardiovascular Emergencies/Pericardial tamponade

Nursing Process: Intervention

Reference

Everson, F. (2013). Chest trauma. In B. B. Hammond & P. G. Zimmermann (Eds.), *Sheehy's manual of emergency care* (7th ed., pp. 407–417). St. Louis, MO: Elsevier Mosby.

---

15. The definition of afterload is:

A. the amount of force needed by the ventricle walls during systole.
B. the amount of force needed by the atria during systole.
C. the volume of blood found within the venous system.
D. the volume of blood found within the arterial system.

Rationale

A. Afterload is the "load" that the ventricle must overcome to eject blood during systole and is related to the pressure within the aorta.

B. Afterload is the "load" that the ventricle, not the atria, must overcome to eject blood during systole and is related to the pressure in the aorta.

C. Afterload refers to pressure or force that must be exerted against the ventricle wall during systole in order to eject blood. Afterload does not refer to venous blood volume.

D. Afterload refers to pressure or force that must be exerted against the ventricle wall during systole in order to eject blood. Afterload does not refer to the arterial blood volume.

Category: Cardiovascular Emergencies/Shock (cardiogenic and obstructive)

Nursing Process: Assessment

References

Hall, J. E. (2016). Cardiac failure. In *Guyton and Hall textbook of medical physiology* (13th ed., pp. 271–282). Philadelphia, PA: Elsevier.

Hall, J. E. (2016). Cardiac output, venous return, and their regulation. In *Guyton and Hall textbook of medical physiology* (13th ed., pp. 245–258). Philadelphia, PA: Elsevier.

Hall, J. E. (2016). Muscle blood flow and cardiac output during exercise: The coronary circulation and ischemic heart disease. In *Guyton and Hall textbook of medical physiology* (13th ed., pp. 259–270). Philadelphia, PA: Elsevier.

---

16. A patient presents to the emergency department 2 weeks postoperative following a coronary artery bypass graft via an open sternotomy. The patient has a temperature of 37.8°C (100°F). The sternal wound is intact with no redness or drainage present. The patient describes a sudden onset of midsternal chest pain, increasing with inspiration. The emergency nurse auscultates a leathery grating sound with S1S2. The patient describes relief from the pain when leaning forward. The patient is describing symptoms associated with:

A. acute aortic dissection.
B. coronary artery occlusion.
C. wound infection.
D. pericarditis.

Rationale

A. A patient with an aortic dissection typically presents with severe tearing-like pain in the chest or across the back; this type of pain is associated with hypotension and tachycardia.

B. If a coronary artery were to occlude, chest pain would be more severe, and associated symptoms of a myocardial infarction would be present. A pericardial friction rub is not normally heard in the presence of a coronary artery occlusion.

C. The patient does not display signs and symptoms of a typical wound infection; the surgical site is described without redness or drainage present.

D. Inflammation of the pericardium, or pericarditis, can occur following open-heart surgery, acute myocardial infarction, or a viral illness. Symptoms include chest pain, low-grade fever, and a pericardial friction rub or leathery grating sound on auscultation. The pain or discomfort may be relieved by sitting up or leaning forward. Treatment options may include the administration of anti-inflammatory medications.

Category: Cardiovascular Emergencies/Pericarditis

Nursing Process: Assessment

Reference

Hammond, B. B. (2013). Cardiovascular emergencies. In B. B. Hammond & P. G. Zimmermann (Eds.), *Sheehy's manual of emergency care* (7th ed., pp. 201–211). St. Louis, MO: Elsevier Mosby.

---

17. A patient has been diagnosed with Raynaud's disease. Which of the following statements made by the patient would reflect an understanding of this disease?

A. "I developed this disease because I am female and live in a cold climate."
B. "I am fearful that I may require a liver transplant if the disease does not improve."
C. "If I take an antibiotic for a while, the disease should go away."
D. "I noticed the onset of the symptoms when I started coughing, usually at night."

Rationale

A. Raynaud's disease is a disorder of blood vessels that supply blood to the skin. Characteristics include intense vasospasms of the fingertips, pallor, and cool skin temperature. Women are affected more than men, and the fingers are the most common site. Cool environments are noted to enhance the disease.

B. Raynaud's disease is a circulatory disease affecting blood vessels of the skin. It generally causes throbbing pain to the fingers, along with pallor and coolness to touch. Raynaud's disease does not affect liver function.

C. Treatment for Raynaud's disease generally does not require antibiotic therapy unless an infectious process is also present. Chronic exacerbations may lead to skin thickening and possible development of gangrene in the affected fingers.

D. Nighttime coughs may indicate respiratory disease but are not associated with Raynaud's disease.

Category: Cardiovascular Emergencies/Peripheral vascular disease

Nursing Process: Evaluation

Reference

Criddle, L. (2007). Cardiovascular emergencies. In K. S. Hoyt & J. Selfridge-Thomas (Eds.), *Emergency nursing core curriculum* (6th ed., pp. 187–248). St. Louis, MO: Saunders Elsevier.

---

18. During the implementation of the massive transfusion protocol, the emergency nurse should observe for which of the following?

A. Hypercalcemia
B. Hyperkalemia
C. Acidosis
D. Hypercoagulopathy

Rationale

A. The anticoagulants, such as citrate, bind free calcium, resulting in hypocalcemia. During massive transfusion protocol (MTP), replacement calcium, such as calcium gluconate or calcium chloride, should be considered.

B. Potassium levels are noted to be elevated in banked blood because of potassium being released from lysed or broken red blood cell membranes. When MTP is being implemented, potassium levels should be monitored, along with cardiac monitoring for the presence of peaked T waves and dysrhythmias, which can indicate hyperkalemia.

C. The anticoagulant citrate is converted by the liver to bicarbonate, resulting in alkalosis. Citrate is used in banked blood to prevent clotting, so the patient's arterial pH should be monitored during implementation of MTP to assess for alkalosis.

D. Packed red cells do not contain clotting factors. As more packed cells are administered, coagulopathy issues occur with failure to clot. If hemodilution because of the infusion of excessive crystalloids has occurred, further coagulopathy issues will occur.

Category: Cardiovascular Emergencies/Trauma

Nursing Process: Assessment

Reference

Calder, S. (2013). Shock. In B. B. Hammond & P. G. Zimmermann (Eds.), *Sheehy's manual of emergency care* (7th ed., pp. 213–222). St. Louis, MO: Elsevier Mosby.

---

19. An obese patient presents to the emergency department complaining of leg pain. The patient relates no history of trauma. The lower leg appears swollen, slightly reddened, and painful to touch. When asked to dorsiflex the foot, the patient complains of increasing pain in the calf area of the leg. Based on this assessment, the emergency nurse would suspect which of the following?

A. Acute arthritis
B. Deep vein thrombosis
C. Chronic arterial occlusion
D. Raynaud's syndrome

Rationale

A. Although acute arthritis may cause painful joints and swelling, the pain is usually unchanged with dorsiflexion of the foot.

B. Patients at risk for developing a deep vein thrombosis include obese patients, those with limited use of the affected extremity, smokers, patients who have sustained extremity trauma (long-bone fractures), and those with long sedentary periods and limited mobility. Symptoms include a swollen, painful extremity that is warm to touch, and pain with dorsiflexion of the foot (Homen's sign) if the deep vein thrombosis is located in the lower extremity. Stasis of blood, damage to the vessel epithelium, and potential alterations in coagulation put a patient at risk for developing a deep vein thrombosis.

C. A chronic arterial occlusion would present with a painful extremity, usually swollen and discolored from a pale whitish to a bluish color. An arterial occlusion would also demonstrate decreased pulses distal to the occlusion.

D. Raynaud's syndrome affects the ears, nose, and fingertips, causing pale to bluish discoloration. Raynaud's syndrome is a peripheral vascular disease affecting blood vessels to the skin.

Category: Cardiovascular Emergencies/Thromboembolic disease

Nursing Process: Analysis

References

Criddle, L. (2007). Cardiovascular emergencies. In K. S. Hoyt & J. Selfridge-Thomas (Eds.), *Emergency nursing core curriculum* (6th ed., pp. 187–248). St. Louis, MO: Saunders Elsevier.

Williams, D. A. (2010). Cardiovascular emergencies. In P. K. Howard & R. A. Steinmann (Eds.), *Sheehy's emergency nursing: Principles and practice* (6th ed., pp. 411–444). St. Louis, MO: Mosby Elsevier.

---

20. Damage control resuscitation (DCR) is a principle of treating hemorrhage that focuses on prevention rather than intervention. Which of the following outcomes would demonstrate successful DCR?

A. Rapid infusion of isotonic crystalloid
B. Calcium chloride replacement
C. Hemostatic resuscitation
D. Autotransfusion

Rationale

A. Rapid infusion of isotonic crystalloid leads to excessive volumes of crystalloid, resulting in hemodilution, with fewer circulating red blood cells to carry oxygen; worsening acidosis; increased inflammatory response and potentially acute respiratory distress syndrome; abdominal compartment syndrome; and increased mortality. It is not damage control resuscitation.

B. Massive transfusions can cause hypocalcemia from the citrate added as a preservative. Citrates bind with calcium, rendering it inactive. Calcium is a vital part of the clotting cascade, so in a case of hemorrhage and massive transfusions, monitor calcium levels for replacement needs. This is not preventive; it is part of monitoring after intervention.

C. Goal-directed therapy is to optimize oxygenation and perfusion by preventing further losses through hemodilutional coagulopathy. Excessive use of isotonic crystalloids or replacement of whole blood loss with only packed red blood cells can produce a hemodilutional coagulopathy in which both platelets and clotting factors are significantly reduced. Hemorrhage control is optimized by giving component therapy using both packed red blood cells and frozen plasma at a 1:1 ratio. Platelets are added for a 1:1:1 ratio, resulting in a hemostatic resuscitation.

D. Autotransfusion is the collection and administration of the patient's own blood, usually through use of a chest tube collection chamber. It is not a part of the damage control resuscitation strategy.

Category: Cardiovascular Emergencies/Trauma

Nursing Process: Evaluation

Reference

Pentecost, D. A. (2014). Shock. In D. Gurney (Ed.), *Trauma Nursing Core Course: Provider manual* (7th ed., pp. 73–90). Des Plaines, IL: Emergency Nurses Association.

---

21. A patient who has been treated for an asthmatic attack is being discharged from the emergency department. The emergency nurse identifies that the patient requires additional instruction when they state:

A. "I will use my rescue inhaler if I become short of breath suddenly."
B. "I will avoid aggravating allergens."
C. "I will stop my corticosteroid therapy as soon as I feel better."
D. "In conjunction with my medications, I will use relaxation techniques and controlled breathing exercises when I begin to feel short of breath."

Rationale

A. Rescue inhalers, or short-acting beta-agonists, allow for bronchodilation and should be used at the first sign of shortness of breath in asthmatics.

B. Avoiding aggravating allergens is important to asthmatics when preventing exacerbations of their disease.

C. Corticosteroid therapy should never be stopped abruptly; it should be tapered off gradually as prescribed.

D. Relaxation and controlled breathing techniques, in conjunction with medications, are necessary teaching points to asthmatics to prevent future asthma exacerbations.

Category: Respiratory Emergencies/Asthma

Nursing Process: Evaluation

Reference

Selfridge-Thomas, J., & Hoyt, K. S. (2007). Respiratory emergencies. In K. S. Hoyt & J. Selfridge-Thomas (Eds.), *Emergency nursing core curriculum* (6th ed., pp. 685–720). St. Louis, MO: Saunders Elsevier.

---

22. Chronic obstructive pulmonary disease is diagnosed by:

A. arterial blood gas.
B. chest radiograph.
C. forced expiratory volume in 1 second per forced vital capacity by spirometry.
D. 6-minute walk test.

Rationale

A. An arterial blood gas may show mild hypoxemia in early stages of chronic obstructive pulmonary disease (COPD) but would most likely only be obtained during an acute exacerbation of the disease.

B. A chest radiograph is necessary to rule out other conditions such as lung cancer or pneumonia, but signs of COPD are generally not identified on chest radiograph until the advanced stages of the disease are present.

C. Forced expiratory volume (FEV1) is a measurement used to see how much air a person can exhale during a forced breath. The forced expiratory volume test is completed with multiple attempts at forced exhalation. Forced vital capacity (FVC) is the total amount of air exhaled during the FEV test. In a patient with symptoms of COPD, the presence of a FEV1 less than 70% following administration of a bronchodilator confirms the diagnosis of COPD.

D. The walk test measures exercise capacity and is used to help determine the stage of COPD the patient is experiencing.

Category: Respiratory Emergencies/Chronic obstructive pulmonary disease (COPD)

Nursing Process: Assessment

References

Hanania, N. A., & Sharafkhaneh, A. (2016). Chronic obstructive pulmonary disease. In E. T. Bope & R. D. Kellerman (Eds.), *Conn's current therapy 2016* (pp. 385–389). Philadelphia, PA: Elsevier.

Rastogi, S., Jain, A., Basu, S. K., & Rastogi, D. (2015). Current overview of COPD with special reference to emphysema. In M. Glass (Ed.), *Chronic obstructive pulmonary disease* (pp. 105–140). New York, NY: Hayle Medical.

---

23. A well-known patient with chronic obstructive pulmonary disease arrives to the emergency department with a history of increasing respiratory difficulty over the past several days. On assessment, the patient has diminished breath sounds bilaterally and is extremely anxious. The emergency provider orders an albuterol and atrovent nebulized treatment for this patient. The nurse anticipates which of the following responses to this intervention?

A. Increased respiratory rate
B. Auscultation of bilateral wheezing
C. Decreased heart rate
D. Increase in $PaCO_2$ level

Rationale

A. Following a nebulized treatment with albuterol and atrovent, airway passages should be relaxed and open, allowing for improved gas exchange and a decreased respiratory rate.

B. Following a nebulized treatment with albuterol and atrovent, airway passages should be relaxed and open, allowing for improved auscultation of breath sounds and the identification of bilateral wheezing in a patient which chronic obstructive pulmonary disease.

C. Following a nebulized treatment with albuterol and atrovent, heart rate will increase in response to the inhaled albuterol. A decrease in the patient's heart rate would indicate a deterioration in their condition.

D. Following the nebulized treatment, it would be anticipated that the patient would experience an opening of airway passages, allowing for improved gas exchange and resulting in a decrease in the patient's $PaCO_2$ level.

Category: Respiratory Emergencies/Chronic obstructive pulmonary disease (COPD)
Nursing Process: Evaluation

References

Selfridge-Thomas, J., & Hoyt, K. S. (2007). Respiratory emergencies. In K. S. Hoyt & J. Selfridge-Thomas (Eds.), *Emergency nursing core curriculum* (6th ed., pp. 685–720). St. Louis, MO: Saunders Elsevier.

Works, P., & Graunke, S. A. (2010). Respiratory emergencies. In P. K. Howard & R. A. Steinmann (Eds.), *Sheehy's emergency nursing: Principles and practice* (6th ed., pp. 395–310). St. Louis, MO: Mosby.

---

24. A patient with an endotracheal tube in place is at increased risk for the development of ventilator-associated pneumonia when which of the following occurs?

A. The endotracheal tube acts to impair the lungs' normal defense mechanism.
B. A silver-coated endotracheal tube is used for intubation.
C. The patient's subglottic secretions are removed frequently.
D. No leaks are present in the cuff of the endotracheal tube.

Rationale

A. The presence of an endotracheal tube prevents normal clearance of airway secretion by hindering the body's natural defense mechanism against organisms, thereby increasing the patient's risk for developing ventilator-associated pneumonia (VAP).

B. Endotracheal tubes that have been coated with silver properties have been shown to possibly reduce bacterial colonization, thereby reducing the incidence of VAP.

C. Frequent suctioning to remove subglottic secretions helps reduce the development of VAP. The principle behind this strategy is that secretions pool in the space between the laryngeal aperture and the endotracheal tube cuff, and removal of these secretions may prevent or minimize aspiration, tracheal colonization with bacteria, and, ultimately, the development of VAP.

D. A leak in the cuff of endotracheal tube increases the risk for infection. It is suggested that no leak be present with a cuffed endotracheal tube, thereby keeping secretions from entering the bronchial tree and preventing the development of VAP.

Category: Respiratory Emergencies/Infections

Nursing Process: Analysis

Reference

Stacy, K. M. (2014). Pulmonary therapeutic management. In L. D. Urden, K. M. Stacy, & M. E. Lough (Eds.), *Critical care nursing* (7th ed., pp. 549–586). Philadelphia, PA: Wolters Kluwer Health.

---

25. A person with acute bronchitis is most likely to have the presence of:

A. infiltrates on their chest radiograph.
B. a dry cough initially that develops into a productive cough.
C. wheezing on physical exam.
D. course crackles on physical exam.

Rationale

A. The presence of infiltrates on a chest radiograph is more indicative of pneumonia.

B. Acute bronchitis is usually brought on by a virus that results in airway irritation and inflammation. Patient presentation includes dyspnea, fever, pain, malaise, and an environmental history that involves either occupational exposures or smoking.

C. The presence of wheezing on physical exam is more indicative of asthma. Breath sounds on auscultation with a patient with acute bronchitis include the presence of rhonchi that may clear when the patient coughs.

D. Course crackles and bronchial sounds over the affected area are more indicative of the presence of pneumonia.

Category: Respiratory Emergencies/Infections

Nursing Process: Assessment

Reference

Works, P., & Graunke, S. A. (2010). Respiratory emergencies. In P. K. Howard & R. A. Steinmann (Eds.), *Sheehy's emergency nursing: Principles and practice* (6th ed., pp. 395–310). St. Louis, MO: Mosby.

26. A patient with a gastrostomy tube is diagnosed with aspiration pneumonia. Which of the following interventions would the emergency nurse perform last?

A. **Identifying the time of the patient's last tube feeding**
B. Suctioning the patient's oropharyngeal area
C. Initiating mechanical ventilation if indicated
D. Administering oxygen

Rationale

A. The protection of the patient's airway is most important. Determining the time of the last tube feeding is not a priority.

B. A patient care priority is the maintaining of a patent airway; therefore, suctioning is an important function to perform.

C. A patient with aspiration pneumonia may require support with mechanical ventilation, but the first priority of care would be to suction the patient's airway.

D. A patient with aspiration pneumonia has impaired gas exchange and therefore will require supplemental oxygen to be delivered.

Category: Respiratory Emergencies/Infections

Nursing Process: Intervention

Reference

Stacy, K. M. (2014). Pulmonary therapeutic management. In L. D. Urden, K. M. Stacy, & M. E. Lough (Eds.), *Critical care nursing* (7th ed., pp. 549–586). Philadelphia, PA: Wolters Kluwer Health.

---

27. A patient arrives at the emergency department via emergency medical services. The patient has sustained burns to the face, neck, and chest from a fire. The patient is alert and has a productive cough of carbonaceous sputum. The priority intervention for the emergency nurse to perform is to:

A. **prepare for intubation.**
B. obtain a full set of vital signs.
C. place the patient on continuous pulse oximetry.
D. remove all clothing and jewelry.

Rationale

A. Carbonaceous sputum is a sign of possible inhalation injury, and the patient will likely need intubation because of progressive airway edema caused by thermal burns.

B. Although assessing the patient's vitals are an important assessment for the patient's respiratory status, this is not the priority. Carbonaceous sputum is a sign of possible inhalation injury, and the patient will likely need intubation because of progressive airway edema caused by thermal burns.

C. Although assessing the patient's pulse oximetry is an important assessment for the patient's respiratory status, this is not the priority. Carbonaceous sputum is a sign of possible inhalation injury, and the patient will likely need intubation because of progressive airway edema caused by thermal burns.

D. It is important to assess the entire patient for additional thermal burns and to stop the burning process from clothing and jewelry in contact with the skin. However, the priority is always to assess the airway first, especially when early intubation is a consideration.

Category: Respiratory Emergencies/Inhalation injuries

Nursing Process: Intervention

Reference

Ribbens, K. A., & DeVries, M. (2013). Burns. In B. B. Hammond & P. G. Zimmermann (Eds.), *Sheehy's manual of emergency care* (7th ed., pp. 453–462). St. Louis, MO: Elsevier Mosby.

---

28. A young patient presents to the emergency department with difficulty swallowing, drooling, inspiratory stridor, and an elevated temperature of 39.2°C (102.6°F). The physician suspects the patient may have acute epiglottitis. What is the priority intervention that the emergency nurse should anticipate for this patient?

A. Administer high-flow humidified oxygen
B. Establish intravenous access
C. Prepare for endotracheal intubation
D. Attempt to visualize the oropharynx using a tongue blade

Rationale

A. In a patient with acute epiglottitis, you want to provide the patient with as much supplemental oxygen as the patient will tolerate; however, the priority is to stabilize the airway and prepare for endotracheal intubation.

B. In a patient with acute epiglottitis, it is important to establish intravenous access; however, the priority is to maintain airway patency.

C. Hallmark signs of epiglottitis are an abrupt onset of symptoms, muffled voice, inspiratory stridor, and sore throat. Epiglottitis, or inflammation of the epiglottitis, places a patient at severe risk for airway obstruction. Endotracheal intubation is performed to protect the patient's airway patency.

D. Stimulation to the oropharynx can cause laryngospasm, leading to complete airway obstruction. Therefore, it is important to avoid any unnecessary stimulation of the patient's airway that could lead to airway obstruction.

Category (Pediatric): Respiratory Emergencies/Obstruction

Nursing Process: Intervention

Reference

Andreoni, C. (2013). Pediatric considerations in emergency nursing. In B. B. Hammond & P. G. Zimmermann (Eds.), *Sheehy's manual of emergency care* (7th ed., pp. 547–570). St. Louis, MO: Elsevier Mosby.

---

29. A patient arrives at the emergency department complaining of mild pleuritic chest pain and a productive cough. The nurse notes the presence of a pleural friction rub. What plan of care would be most appropriate for this patient?

A. Prepare for hospital admission
B. Provide comfort measures
C. Obtain blood cultures and administer antibiotics
D. Identify underlying disease process

Rationale

A. Chest pain, productive cough, and pleural friction rub are indicative of both pleural effusion and pneumonia. Identification of the underlying disease process is necessary to determine the plan of care.

B. Identification of the underlying disease process is necessary before determining proper management of symptoms.

C. Chest pain, productive cough, and pleural friction rub are indicative of both pleural effusion and pneumonia. Identification of the underlying disease process is initially the priority because multiple disease processes may cause pleural effusions that could mimic the symptoms of pneumonia.

D. Chest pain, productive cough, and pleural friction rub are indicative of both pleural effusion and pneumonia. However, pleural effusions are a clinical manifestation of an underlying problem and can be caused by multiple disease processes, including pneumonia. Identification of the underlying disease process is necessary to determine proper disease management.

Category: Respiratory Emergencies/Pleural effusion

Nursing Process: Analysis

Reference

Walsh, R. (2013). Respiratory emergencies. In B. B. Hammond & P. G. Zimmermann (Eds.), *Sheehy's manual of emergency care* (7th ed., pp. 185–199). St. Louis, MO: Elsevier Mosby.

---

30. Which of the following is the leading risk factor for the development of a spontaneous pneumothorax?

A. Cigarette smoking
B. Barotrauma
C. Rupture of bleb
D. Chronic obstructive pulmonary disease

Rationale

A. Smoking, even in the absence of emphysema or other underlying pulmonary disease, increases the occurrence of developing blebs, thus putting the individual at risk of developing a spontaneous pneumothorax. However, chronic obstructive pulmonary disease (COPD) is the leading risk factor for spontaneous pneumothorax.

B. Barotrauma is known as the damage to body tissue caused by the difference in pressure between a gas space and the surrounding fluid. In the hospital setting, this translates into lung injury caused by increased alveolar pressures during mechanical ventilation. Air can escape through the damaged tissue and travel into the pleura, causing a spontaneous pneumothorax. Because of this complication, any patient receiving mechanical ventilation, invasive or noninvasive, should be closely monitored for a pneumothorax and developing tension pneumothorax. Patients with a history of COPD are at an even greater risk for developing a pneumothorax when receiving mechanical ventilation because of an increased need for positive end-expiratory pressure to maintain alveolar gas exchange and underlying damaged lung tissue.

C. A bleb is an air-filled sac that forms on the lung, typically on the apex. These can develop in otherwise healthy individuals and are typically found in young men who are taller than average. When a bleb ruptures, air is allowed into the pleural space, resulting in a spontaneous pneumothorax. However, this occurrence is less common than a pneumothorax caused by COPD.

D. A pneumothorax occurs when air accumulates in the pleural space, resulting in increased pressure, or a loss of negative pressure, causing a partial or complete collapsed lung. In the absence of trauma, this is referred to as a spontaneous pneumothorax. The presence of damaged lung tissue found in underlying pulmonary disease puts patients at risk for developing spontaneous pneumothorax. COPD is the leading risk factor for spontaneous pneumothorax, accounting for approximately 70% of cases.

Category: Respiratory Emergencies/Pneumothorax

Nursing Process: Assessment

References

O'Neal, J. V. (2013). Airway management. In B. B. Hammond & P. G. Zimmermann (Eds.), *Sheehy's manual of emergency care* (7th ed., pp. 77–88). St. Louis, MO: Elsevier Mosby.

Sedlak, K. (2013). Environmental emergencies. In B. B. Hammond & P. G. Zimmermann (Eds.), *Sheehy's manual of emergency care* (7th ed., pp. 333–343). St. Louis, MO: Elsevier Mosby.

Walsh, R. (2013). Respiratory emergencies. In B. B. Hammond & P. G. Zimmermann (Eds.), *Sheehy's manual of emergency care* (7th ed., pp. 185–199). St. Louis, MO: Elsevier Mosby.

---

31. An unresponsive patient arrives via emergency medical services following a motor vehicle collision. Patient assessment reveals absent breath sounds and bruising on the left side of the chest, a deviated trachea, and the appearance of sudden cyanosis. The emergency nurse suspects the patient has developed a:

A. tension pneumothorax.
B. rupture of the diaphragm.
C. flail chest.
D. right mainstem bronchial intubation.

Rationale

A. A tension pneumothorax is a life-threatening emergency that occurs when air enters the pleural space during inspiration and is unable to escape during exhalation. The increasing intrathoracic pressure compresses the lungs, heart, and great vessels, resulting in markedly decreased cardiac output. Noted signs and symptoms include severe respiratory distress, decreased or absent breath sounds to the affected side, tachycardia, hypotension, and poor tissue perfusion. As intrathoracic pressure increases, chest cavity contents are compressed and shift to the unaffected side, and tracheal deviation will occur.

B. Rupture of the diaphragm occurs when blunt or penetrating trauma causes a tear in the diaphragm, allowing abdominal contents to herniate into the chest cavity. Signs and symptoms include dyspnea, dysphagia, decreased breath sounds on the affected side (most commonly the left), and bowel sounds in the thoracic cavity.

C. Flail chest occurs when two or more adjacent ribs are fractured in two or more places or when the sternum is detached, causing the flail segment to respond to changes in intrathoracic pressure in a paradoxical manner. Flail chest may lead to respiratory distress and respiratory failure as pulmonary mechanics are disrupted. A pneumothorax or hemothorax may accompany a flail chest.

D. Advancement of the endotracheal tube too far during intubation will most often cause a malposition of the tube into the right mainstem, leading to atelectasis of the left lung. Breath sounds will be absent on the left, and inadequate ventilation will occur; however, a right mainstem bronchial intubation will not cause tracheal deviation.

Category: Respiratory Emergencies/Pneumothorax

Nursing Process: Analysis

References

Everson, F. (2013). Chest trauma. In B. B. Hammond & P. G. Zimmermann (Eds.), *Sheehy's manual of emergency care* (7th ed., pp. 407–417). St. Louis, MO: Elsevier Mosby.

O'Neal, J. V. (2013). Airway management. In B. B. Hammond & P. G. Zimmermann (Eds.), *Sheehy's manual of emergency care* (7th ed., pp. 77–88). St. Louis, MO: Elsevier Mosby.

---

32. The emergency nurse is caring for the victim of a motor vehicle collision. The patient has experienced a large pneumothorax on the right side, and a chest tube has been inserted. The emergency nurse anticipates this treatment has been effective when the patient has which of the following responses?

A. Sucking sound heard with respiration
B. Increase in heart rate
C. Absence of fluctuation in water seal chamber
D. Decreasing respiratory rate

Rationale

A. The presence of a sucking chest sound is an indication of an open pneumothorax. This patient has a closed pneumothorax with a chest tube inserted. In the presence of a closed pneumothorax, a sucking chest sound is an indication of an air leak. It is important to ensure that the dressing is secure around the insertion site and that all chest tube connections are secure. If left untreated, the presence of the sucking chest sound can lead to the development of a tension pneumothorax.

B. With any respiratory difficulty, patients become anxious, tachycardic, and tachypneic. As oxygenation improves, the patient's heart rate, respiratory rate, and feelings of anxiety should decrease.

C. Water seal level should fluctuate with the patient's respiration as air escapes from the pneumothorax, resulting in the water seal level rising with inspiration and falling with expiration. This is an indication of chest tube patency and function. Once the affected lung has expanded, this fluctuation will be absent in the water seal chamber.

D. As the pneumothorax resolves, the patient will experience increasing lung capacity with increased gas exchange, resulting in a decrease in the patient's respiratory rate and effort.

Category: Respiratory Emergencies/Pneumothorax

Nursing Process: Evaluation

References

Day, M. W. (2014). Thoractic and neck trauma. In D. Gurney (Ed.), *Trauma Nursing Core Course: Provider manual* (7th ed., pp. 137–150). Des Plaines, IL: Emergency Nurses Association.

Denke, N. (2010). Thoracic trauma. In P. K. Howard & R. A. Steinmann (Eds.), *Sheehy's emergency nursing: Principles and practice* (6th ed., pp. 285–300). St. Louis, MO: Mosby Elsevier.

---

33. A patient presents to triage with chest wall pain and worsening cough after cliff-diving 90 feet into the water below. The patient complains of pink, frothy sputum when coughing. Based on the patient's history, the emergency nurse is concerned this patient may have which of the following?

A. Pulmonary embolism
B. Pulmonary edema
C. Asthma
D. Pleural effusion

Rationale

A. The presence of pink, frothy sputum when coughing is a sign of pulmonary edema, not a pulmonary embolus. The signs and symptoms of a pulmonary embolism include dyspnea, hypoxia, feelings of anxiety, and chest pain. Risk factors for a pulmonary embolism include venous stasis, recent trauma, obesity, pregnancy, use of oral contraceptives, and a history of thrombosis.

B. The presence of frothy, pink sputum is indicative of pulmonary edema. A patient with a history of diving 90 feet into water is at risk for possible drowning injuries related to impact. When a human is submerged, there is initial panic, followed by breath holding and hyperventilation; this results in aspiration and swallowing of fluid, which leads to hypoxia and pulmonary injury.

C. The presence of pink, frothy sputum when coughing is a sign of pulmonary edema, not asthma. The signs and symptoms of asthma include tachypnea, wheezing, anxiety, and dyspnea.

D. The presence of pink, frothy sputum when coughing is a sign of pulmonary edema, not pleural effusion. The signs and symptoms of a pleural effusion include chest pain, dyspnea, and a dry, nonproductive cough.

Category: Respiratory Emergencies/Pulmonary edema, noncardiac
Nursing Process: Analysis

Reference

Walsh, R. (2013). Respiratory emergencies. In B. B. Hammond & P. G. Zimmermann (Eds.), *Sheehy's manual of emergency care* (7th ed., pp. 185–199). St. Louis, MO: Elsevier Mosby.

---

34. A patient presents with increased shortness of breath. Vital signs: BP 128/72 mm Hg; HR 115 beats/minute; RR 20 breaths/minute; SpO_2 88% room air; T 37.1°C (98.9°F). The patient reports recently having been a passenger on a transcontinental airline flight. The emergency nurse would use which of the following anatomical areas to initiate an intravenous line prior to a computerized tomography scan?

A. Exterior jugular vein
B. Cephalic vein
C. Dorsal metacarpal veins
D. Median cubital vein

Rationale

A. Although this site can be used, it is not the preferred site because of risk for infiltration of computerized tomography (CT) intravenous (IV) contrast from the pressurized syringe and rapid infusion of the delivery system.

B. The IV must be within 1 inch of the median cubital vein because of the pressure used to infuse the IV contrast; CT personnel will not infuse the contrast required through an IV inserted into the cephalic vein.

C. IV insertion must be within 1 inch of the median cubital vein because of the pressure used to infuse the IV contrast; CT personnel will not infuse the contrast required through an IV inserted into a dorsal metacarpal vein.

D. This is the ideal IV site for a CT angiogram because the vein is large enough to handle the pressure of the contrast infusion that will be needed to evaluate the lungs for the presence of a pulmonary embolism.

Category: Respiratory Emergencies/Pulmonary embolus

Nursing Process: Intervention

Reference

Walsh, R. (2013). Respiratory emergencies. In B. B. Hammond & P. G. Zimmermann (Eds.), *Sheehy's manual of emergency care* (7th ed., pp. 185–199). St. Louis, MO: Elsevier Mosby.

---

35. A patient arrives complaining of dyspnea and mild right-sided chest pain that began last evening and now increases with exertion. The patient states that 3 days ago, they sustained an injury to their right lower leg. The patient has a previous history of deep vein thrombosis that occurred 15 years ago. The emergency nurse is aware that the laboratory test that is most specific for the presence of a pulmonary embolus is:

A. complete blood count.
B. D-dimer.
C. complete metabolic panel.
D. B-type natriuretic peptide.

Rationale

A. This test is useful in ruling out pneumonia and an infection process but does not directly indicate the presence of a pulmonary embolism.

B. Based on the patient's chief complaint and history, the nurse should be concerned for a deep vein thrombosis and a pulmonary embolism on this patient. The specific test for fibrin split products is a D-dimer test; results elevated above 500 indicate the presence of a pulmonary embolism.

C. This test is useful in providing information about electrolyte imbalances but does not directly indicate a pulmonary embolism.

D. This test is useful in evaluating and identifying the presence of congestive heart failure but does not indicate the presence of a pulmonary embolism.

Category: Respiratory Emergencies/Pulmonary embolus

Nursing Process: Assessment

Reference

Walsh, R. (2013). Respiratory emergencies. In B. B. Hammond & P. G. Zimmermann (Eds.), *Sheehy's manual of emergency care* (7th ed., pp. 185–199). St. Louis, MO: Elsevier Mosby.

36. Extracorporeal membrane oxygenation may be used in the treatment of a patient with severe acute respiratory distress syndrome in order to:

A. circumvent the damaging effects of mechanical ventilation.
B. maintain the patient's oxygen levels while allowing the lungs to rest.
C. provide hemodynamic support.
D. prevent respiratory failure.

Rationale

A. Preventing further lung damage is a benefit of extracorporeal membrane oxygenation (ECMO), but it is not a reason to use ECMO for a particular patient (or not).

B. ECMO can be used in patients with severe refractory hypoxemia in conjunction with lung protective mechanical ventilation to provide gas exchange while decreasing stress on the lungs. ECMO is often a last resort treatment because of its complexity and cost, and the specialized knowledge needed to care for the patient.

C. ECMO may be used for hemodynamic support in some circumstances. However, in the treatment of acute respiratory distress syndrome (ARDS), ECMO is used for respiratory support of the patient. Using ECMO will ease stress on the lungs caused by ARDS and may assist the patient in achieving improved hemodynamic stability.

D. A patient with ARDS is already experiencing the signs and symptoms of respiratory failure.

Category: Respiratory Emergencies/Respiratory distress syndrome
Nursing Process: Analysis

Reference

Gibbons, C. (2015). Acute respiratory distress syndrome. *Radiologic Technology*, *86*(4), 419–436.

---

37. An elderly male with dementia is brought to the emergency department by his family, who state, "We just can't handle him at home anymore." The patient frequently attempts to get out of bed, and the emergency nurse is afraid the patient will fall. Which intervention is most appropriate to prevent falls in this patient?

A. Place the patient in a vest restraint
B. Provide the patient with the call light
C. Have family remain with the patient
D. Place the patient in a geriatric chair near the nurse's station

Rationale

A. This restraint can be used to prevent falls; however, it can also restrict the patient, creating unneeded distress and agitation. The application of restraints would also require frequent monitoring and restraint documentation.

B. Although this is a best practice, the patient with dementia will frequently forget to use the call light, and they may try to get out of the emergency gurney or bed and potentially fall.

C. Family are known faces to this patient. They can remain at bedside and remind the patient to ask for assistance to get out of bed, or notify staff if the patient has any needs.

D. A geriatric (Geri) chair can be used to prevent falls; however, it can also restrict the patient, creating distress and agitation, and a patient placed in a Geri chair would require restraint monitoring. In addition, the emergency nursing station is busy and noisy, potentially leading to a further increase in the patient's confusion and agitation.

Category (Geriatric): Neurological Emergencies/Alzheimer's disease/dementia

Nursing Process: Analysis

Reference

Clevenger, C. K., Chu, T. A., Yang, Z., & Hepburn, K. W. (2012). Clinical care of persons with dementia in the emergency department: A review of the literature and agenda for research. *Journal of the American Geriatrics Society, 60*(9), 1742–1748. https://doi.org/10.1111/j.1532-5415.2012.04108.x

---

38. A young mother presents to triage with her 6-week-old infant. The mother states the infant has a had a fever and "acts funny." While drawing blood, the emergency nurse observes the infant to rapidly move her right leg in a bicycling fashion. The emergency nurse is concerned that this behavior indicates which of the following?

A. Intracerebral bleeding
B. A temper tantrum
C. Seizure
D. Electrolyte imbalance

Rationale

A. Although the infant's movement may be related to intracranial trauma, the infant presents with a fever, indicting a possible infection; therefore, the most likely cause is related to meningitis and increased intracranial pressure.

B. This is not developmentally appropriate for a 6-week-old infant.

C. Meningitis causes signs and symptoms of seizures and of increased intracranial pressure. Any infant younger than 60 days of age with a fever or a subnormal temperature must be evaluated for the presence of meningitis. Meningitis is a syndrome involving inflammation and infection of the brain.

D. Although electrolyte imbalances, especially abnormal sodium levels, can precipitate seizure activity, the most likely cause in this patient is an infectious process.

Category (Pediatric): Neurological Emergencies/Meningitis

Nursing Process: Analysis

Reference

Richard, G. C., & Lepe, M. (2013). Meningitis in children: Diagnosis and treatment for the emergency clinician. *Clinical Pediatric Emergency Medicine, 14*(2), 146–156. https://doi.org/10.1016/j.cpem.2013.04.008

---

39. A patient who is 26 weeks pregnant arrives at the emergency department exhibiting left-sided weakness and slurred speech that began 20 minutes before arrival. The computed tomography scan comes back negative for cerebral hemorrhage. Which intervention should the emergency team prepare for next?

A. Induction of labor
B. Administration of fibrinolytics
C. Emergency cesarean section
D. Transfer to a labor and delivery unit

Rationale

A. The induction of labor delays treatment of the patient with a stroke. At 26 weeks' gestation, the goal is to keep the fetus in utero and maintain placenta perfusion for as long as possible.

B. The priority intervention for stroke is the administration of fibrinolytics. Fibrinolytics do not cross the placenta, thereby minimizing risk to the fetus. Risks associated with the administration of fibrinolytics to the pregnant patient are similar to those of any other patient.

C. An emergency cesarean section increases risk of bleeding and delays proper intervention for the mother.

D. Transferring the patient to labor and delivery will further delay the administration of fibrinolytics for the mother, which is the priority for a patient with an ischemic stroke.

Category: Neurological Emergencies/Stroke (ischemic or hemorrhagic)

Nursing Process: Intervention

References

Demchuck, A. (2013). Yes, intravenous thrombolysis should be administered in pregnancy when other clinical and imaging factors are favorable. *Stroke, 44*(3), 864–865. https://doi.org/10.1161/STROKEAHA.111.000134

Tassi, R., Acampa, M., Marotta, G., Cioni, S., Guideri, F., Rossi, S., . . . Martini, G. (2013). Systemic thrombolysis for stroke in pregnancy. *American Journal of Emergency Medicine*, *31*(2), 448.e1–448.e3. https://doi.org/10.1016/j.ajem.2012.05.040

---

40. An elderly patient arrives at the emergency department via emergency medical services from an assisted living facility with a history of a "brain shunt" and contractures. Recent history indicates that the patient is "less interactive than usual," has been "sleepy," and has had no bowel movement for 3 days. The computed tomography scan exam reveals evidence of hydrocephalus, and the abdominal radiograph shows a large amount of feces, causing the ventriculoperitoneal shunt to kink. The emergency nurse anticipates which intervention for this patient?

A. An enema to clear feces from the bowel
B. Immediate transfer of the patient to an ICU
C. Preparing the patient for surgery to replace the shunt
D. Performing a digital rectal exam

Rationale

A. Severe constipation can cause bowel edema, which can result in an occlusion, or kink, forming in the bowel, resulting in a blockage of the ventriculoperitoneal (VP) shunt. The subsequent VP shunt blockage can result in hydrocephalus, leading the patient to demonstrate signs of increased intracranial pressure, including an altered level of consciousness.

B. This action does not address the problem of the patient's nonfunctioning VP shunt; it merely transfers the patient to another location.

C. Replacement of the shunt will correct the problem but will not address the underlying pathophysiology of excessive feces in the bowel.

D. A digital rectal exam may be used to determine if there is a fecal impaction, however, performing a disimpaction will not address the problem of profound constipation, nor will it address the issue of the kink in the VP shunt.

Category (Geriatric): Neurological Emergencies/Shunt dysfunctions

Nursing Process: Intervention

References

Cohen, J. S., Jamal, N., Dawes, C., Chamberlain, J. M., & Atabaki, S. M. (2014). Cranial computed tomography utilization for suspected ventriculoperitoneal shunt malfunction in a pediatric emergency department. *Journal of Emergency Medicine, 46*(4), 449–455. https://doi.org/10.1016/j.jemermed.2013.08.137

Mater, A., Shroff, M., Al-Farsi, S., Drake, J., & Goldman, R. D. (2008). Test characteristics of neuroimaging in the emergency department evaluation of children for cerebrospinal fluid shunt malfunction. *CJEM: Canadian Journal of Emergency Medicine, 10*(2), 131–135.

---

41. A patient presents to triage complaining that they have experienced increasing difficulty walking. The patient has an uneven gait and feels "unsteady" when standing. Speech is clear, and vital signs are stable. Which assessment criteria would the emergency nurse use to evaluate the patient for the presence of cerebellar dysfunction?

A. Extraocular eye movements
B. Appropriate decision making
C. Finger-to-nose coordination
D. Visual acuity assessment

Rationale

A. Extraocular eye movements are used to evaluate the function of cranial nerve III, cranial nerve IV, and cranial nerve VI.

B. Decision making is a complex function that uses the frontal lobe of the brain, not the cerebellum.

C. Finger-to-nose coordination is assessed by having the patient place their finger to the examiner's finger, and then returning their finger to their nose; these movements are repeated quickly, over and over. The cerebellum is responsible for coordinated movement and balance. The function of the cerebellum is assessed via finger-to-nose coordinated movement or by the heel-to-shin coordinated movement.

D. Visual acuity assesses cranial nerve II or the optic nerve, which is essential for vision.

Category: Neurological Emergencies/Chronic neurological disorders

Nursing Process: Evaluation

Reference

Bickley, L. (2017). *Bates guide to physical examination and history taking* (12th ed.). Philadelphia, PA: Wolters Kluwer Health-Lippincott Williams & Wilkins.

---

42. The emergency nurse is preparing to discharge a patient who has been treated for a migraine headache. The patient asks how similar headaches in the future can be prevented. The most appropriate response by the emergency nurse would be:

A. "Maintaining a headache diary to identify what triggers your headache is often helpful in preventing similar episodes in the future."
B. "Reducing stress levels will reduce the incidence of migraine headaches."
C. "Avoid foods that contain tyramine, such as aged cheeses, pickled food, and red wine."
D. "Herbal products such as butterbur or feverfew are helpful."

Rationale

A. Identifying triggers by maintaining a headache diary can help patients track and identify migraine triggers. The information can then be shared with the healthcare provider.

B. Reducing stress levels aids some patients but may not help all patients to reduce the incidence of their migraine headaches.

C. These foods have been identified as triggers in some patients who experience migraine headaches. Keeping a headache dairy will help the patient identify if these foods are a potential headache trigger.

D. These products should only be used under the direction of a healthcare provider. These products may be helpful for some patients in controlling the frequency and/or intensity of their migraine headaches.

Category: Neurological Emergencies/Headache
Nursing Process: Intervention

Reference

D'Arcy, Y. (2014). Migraine headache prevention. *Nursing, 44*(1), 58–61.

---

43. The emergency nurse understands that the purpose of the Glasgow Coma Scale is to:

A. allow the provider to predict outcomes for the trauma patient.
B. assess the level of consciousness in all patients.
C. identify interventions to improve outcomes for unconscious patients.
D. assess the level of consciousness in head-injured patients.

Rationale

A. The Glasgow Coma Scale (GCS) assesses level of consciousness and severity of brain injury in patients with a head injury. The GCS further provides assessment data, which allows for early identification of neurological changes, thereby facilitating prompt interventions; it does not predict patient outcomes.

B. The GCS assesses level of consciousness and severity of brain injury in patients who have sustained a head injury. The GCS is not used to assess level of consciousness in all patients.

C. The GCS assesses level of consciousness and severity of brain injury in patients with a head injury. The GCS further provides assessment data, which allows for early identification of neurological changes, thereby facilitating prompt interventions. The GCS does not identify the interventions that need to be performed.

D. The GCS assesses level of consciousness and severity of brain injury in patients with a head injury. The GCS further provides assessment data, which allows for early identification of neurological changes, thereby facilitating prompt interventions. The GCS is the gold standard of neurological assessment for head-injured patients.

Category: Neurological Emergencies/Trauma

Nursing Process: Assessment

Reference

Hansen, B., Quick, J., Sinkovits, E., & Smith, J. (2014). Glasgow coma scale: How to improve and enhance documentation. *Journal of Trauma Nursing, 21*(3), 122–124. https://doi.org/10.1097/JTN.0000000000000044

---

44. The emergency nurse is preparing to discharge a child who has been diagnosed with epilepsy. Which information is essential for the child's parents and caregivers to understand regarding this diagnosis?

A. The types of surgery available for patients with epilepsy
B. Completion of a cardiopulmonary resuscitation course
C. How to find an epilepsy support group
D. Basic first aid for epilepsy

Rationale

A. Surgical options in the treatment for epilepsy are available, but information regarding these procedures is not essential for the parents and caregivers at the time of their child's discharge.

B. Although it is helpful for the parents and caregivers to be cardiopulmonary resuscitation (CPR) certified, it is not essential. Knowledge of CPR will not provide knowledge of care of the child during or following a seizure.

C. It will be helpful to discuss concerns and issues with parents and caregivers, but it is not essential information for the parents at the time of discharge.

D. Parents and caregivers must know how to safely care for the patient during the active seizure and during the postictal phase, which follows the seizure.

Category (Pediatric): Neurological Emergencies/Seizure disorders

Nursing Process: Evaluation

Reference

Smith, G., Wagner, J., & Edwards, J. (2015). Epilepsy update: Nursing care and evidence-based treatment. *American Journal of Nursing, 115*(6), 34–44.

---

45. The emergency nurse is caring for a patient with increased intracranial pressure following a traumatic head injury. Which of the following vital signs should the nurse immediately report to the physician?

A. Heart rate 94 beats/minute
B. Temperature of 38.5°C (101.3°F)
C. Capnography of 30 mm Hg
D. Mean arterial pressure 70 mm Hg

Rationale

A. This heart rate is within normal physiological parameters.

B. Fever in a patient with a traumatic brain injury is associated with poorer outcomes. Aggressive treatment in the presence of a fever is very important for optimal patient outcome.

C. This is a normal reading indicating adequate respiratory effort and gas exchange.

D. A mean arterial pressure of 70 indicates that the brain is receiving adequate perfusion.

Category: Neurological Emergencies/Trauma

Nursing Process: Evaluation

Reference

Madden, L., & DeVon, H. (2015). A systematic review of the effects of body temperature on outcomes after adult traumatic brain injury. *Journal of Neuroscience Nursing, 47*(4), 190–203. https://doi.org/10.1097/jnn.0000000000000142

---

46. The emergency nurse is preparing to administer intranasal midazolam to a patient in status epilepticus. The nurse is aware of which of the following regarding intranasal administration of midazolam?

A. Onset of the drug action may be delayed.
B. Onset of action is similar to the doses administered intramuscularly.
C. The drug rapidly crosses the blood–brain barrier.
D. The dose is given in one nostril.

Rationale

A. The administration of medications via nasal, buccal, rectal, and oral routes requires the medication to enter the enteric circulation, where the drug is metabolized by the liver before reaching the systemic circulation; this results in a delay in the onset of action.

B. The intramuscular route bypasses the liver metabolism; therefore, the onset of action will be faster than the intranasal route.

C. All benzodiazepines cross the blood–brain barrier, but only after they have reached the systemic circulation.

D. It is important to split the dose between the two nostrils, with half being administered in each. The maximum amount that can be administered in each nostril is 1 mL.

Category: Neurological Emergencies/Seizure disorders

Nursing Process: Assessment

Reference

Rogalski, R., & Rogalski, A. (2015). Benzodiazepine selection in the management of status epilepticus: A review. *Advanced Emergency Nursing Journal, 37*(2), 83–94.

---

47. A patient presents to the emergency department with a headache, and the diagnosis of subarachnoid hemorrhage is confirmed. When reviewing the patient's presenting chief complaint, the emergency nurse would expect to find:

A. a report of a recent traumatic injury to the head.
B. a sudden, brief loss of consciousness followed by a period of lucidity.
C. an insidious onset of headache with progressive worsening.
D. a report of the worst headache of the patient's life.

Rationale

A. A report of a recent traumatic injury to the head is most consistent with an epidural hematoma or subdural hematoma. The most common cause of a subarachnoid hemorrhage is an aneurysm rupture, not a traumatic head injury.

B. A sudden loss of consciousness followed by a period of lucidity is most consistent with an epidural hematoma.

C. An insidious onset of headache with progressive worsening is most consistent with a subdural hematoma.

D. The patient's report of the "worst headache of my life" would be the most likely presenting complaint associated with a subarachnoid hemorrhage. The headache associated with a subarachnoid hemorrhage is typically described as a sudden, severe onset and is commonly referred to as the "thunderclap" headache.

Category: Neurological Emergencies/Headache

Nursing Process: Assessment

References

Bajsarowicz, P., Prakash, I., Lamoureux, J., Saluja, R. S., Feyz, M., Maleki, M., & Marcoux, J. (2015). Nonsurgical acute traumatic subdural hematoma: What is the risk? *Journal of Neurosurgery, 123*(5), 1176–1183. https://doi.org/10.3171/2014.10.jns141728

Specogna, A. V. (2014). Subarachnoid hemorrhage diagnosis. *Journal of the American Medical Association, 311*(2), 201. https://doi.org/10.1001/jama.2013.284318

Tsai, J., Chen, T., & Yang, S. (2014). Depressed skull fracture and epidural hematoma resulted from pin-type head holder for craniotomy in children. *Journal of Medical Sciences, 34*(5), 238. https://doi.org/10.4103/1011-4564.143654

---

48. A patient presents to the emergency department following an all-terrain vehicle collision. During the neurological assessment, the emergency nurse notes motor paralysis and a loss of pain and temperature sensation below the level of T2. However, proprioception, touch, and vibratory sense are preserved. What is the most likely spinal cord injury associated with this clinical presentation?

A. Anterior cord syndrome
B. Brown-Sequard syndrome
C. Posterior cord syndrome
D. Central cord syndrome

Rationale

A. The correct answer to this question is anterior cord syndrome. A diagnosis of anterior cord syndrome is consistent with motor paralysis and a loss of pain and temperature sensation below the level of the injury, with a preservation of proprioception, touch, and vibratory sense.

B. Brown-Sequard syndrome is consistent with hemiparaplegia (weakness or paralysis) on the same side as the cord injury, and hemianesthesia (loss of sensation) on the opposite side of the cord injury but below the level of injury.

C. Posterior cord syndrome is consistent with preserved motor function below the level of the injury, with a loss of sensory function.

D. Central cord syndrome results from a cervical spine injury and is consistent with more pronounced motor impairment in the upper body, as compared with the lower body, with variable sensory loss below the level of the injury.

Category: Neurological Emergencies/Spinal cord injuries

Nursing Process: Assessment

References

Aarabi, B., Alexander, M., Mirvis, S. E., Shanmuganathan, K., Chesler, D., Maulucci, C., . . . Blacklock, T. (2011). Predictors of outcome in acute traumatic central cord syndrome due to spinal stenosis: Clinical article. *Journal of Neurosurgery: Spine, 14*(1), 122–130. https://doi.org/10.3171/2010.9.spine09922

Diabira, S., Henaux, P. L., Riffaud, L., Hamlat, A., Brassier, G., & Morandi, X. (2011). Brown-Sequard syndrome revealing intradural thoracic disc herniation. *European Spine Journal, 20*(1), 65–70. https://doi.org/10.1007/s00586-010-1498-3

Kirshblum, S. C., Burns, S. P., Biering-Sorensen, F., Donovan, W., Graves, D. E., Jha, A., . . . Schmidt-Read, M. (2011). International standards for neurological classification of spinal cord injury. *Journal of Spinal Cord Medicine, 34*(6), 535–546. https://doi.org/10.1007/978-0-387-79948-3_5034

Markandaya, M., Stein, D. M., & Menaker, J. (2012). Acute treatment options for spinal cord injury. *Current Treatment Options in Neurology, 14*(2), 175–187. https://doi.org/10.1007/s11940-011-0162-5

---

49. Which of the following assessment findings would represent increased intracranial pressure according to the Cushing reflex?

A. Narrowing pulse pressure
B. Hypotension
C. Tachycardia
D. Cheyne–Stokes respirations

Rationale

A. Widening pulse pressure, not narrowing pulse pressure, is a sign of increased intracranial pressure. The three components of Cushing's triad are (1) bradycardia, (2) widening pulse pressure because of a rise in the systolic blood pressure, and (3) irregular or absent respirations.

B. Hypotension is not associated with the presence of Cushing's triad. Components of the Cushing's triad are (1) bradycardia, (2) widening pulse pressure because of a rise in the systolic blood pressure, and (3) irregular or absent respirations.

C. Bradycardia, not tachycardia, is a sign of increased intracranial pressure. Components of Cushing's triad are (1) bradycardia, (2) widening pulse pressure because of a rise in the systolic blood pressure, and (3) irregular or absent respirations.

D. Signs of intracranial pressure include the presence of Cushing's triad: (1) bradycardia, (2) widening pulse pressure because of a rise in the systolic blood pressure, and (3) irregular or absent respirations.

Category: Neurological Emergencies/Increased intracranial pressure (ICP)

Nursing Process: Assessment

Reference

Marino, P. (2013). *The ICU book.* Philadelphia, PA: Lippincott Williams & Wilkins.

---

50. A patient presents to the emergency department complaining of a headache for the past 10 hours after being tackled and kicked in the head during a football game the previous day. A concussion is suspected without the presence of any neurological deficits. While continuing to evaluate the patient, which of the following would indicate to the emergency nurse the need for a computed tomography scan of the head?

A. Presence of cervical spine pain
B. Continued report of a headache
C. A Glasgow Coma Scale score of 12
D. Intermittent amnesia of the event

Rationale

A. A patient with cervical spine pain would require a computed tomography (CT) scan of the cervical spine, but not a head CT scan.

B. CT scan of the head is indicated in any patient with suspected concussion with the following: Glasgow Coma Scale (GCS) score is $<$ 15 2 hours after the event, suspected skull fracture, repeated episodes of vomiting, if the patient is over 65 years of age, drug/alcohol intoxication, or persistent anterograde amnesia. In addition, if the mechanism of injury is significant, a headache may persist for a few days to weeks postconcussion. Amnesia may be present for 24–48 hours after the event.

C. CT scan of the head is indicated in any patient with suspected concussion with the following: GCS score is $<$ 15 2 hours after the event, suspected skull fracture, repeated episodes of vomiting, if the patient is over 65 years of age, drug/alcohol intoxication, or persistent anterograde amnesia. In addition, if the mechanism of injury is significant, a headache may persist for a few days to weeks postconcussion. Amnesia may be present for 24–48 hours after the event.

D. A patient with intermittent amnesia would require reorientation and observation. Amnesia may be present for 24–48 hours after the event.

Category: Neurological Emergencies/Trauma

Nursing Process: Analysis

Reference

Bhat, P., Dretler, A., Gdowski, M., Ramgopal, R., & Williams, D. (2016). *The Washington manual of medical therapeutics* (35th ed.). Philadelphia, PA: Wolters Kluwer.

---

51. A patient presents to the emergency department via emergency medical services with a cervical collar in place following an altercation in the nearby pub. The patient reports being struck in the head, torso, and pelvic region numerous times with a bar stool. On assessment, the emergency nurse observes an obvious deformity of the left upper extremity, tenderness to the chest on palpation, and multiple abrasions and contusions to the face and head. The patient is able to move all extremities but has no recollection of the event and is oriented to person only. The presence of right otorrhea is also observed. Vital signs: BP 110/60 mm Hg; HR 106 beats/minute; RR 20 breaths/minute; SpO_2 98% on 4 L nasal cannula. The most appropriate intervention to be performed for this patient is which of the following?

A. Removal of the cervical collar
B. Computed tomography scan of the neck
C. Application of a long spine board
D. Obtain blood alcohol level

Rationale

A. The National Emergency X-radiography Utilization Study (NEXUS) low-risk criteria include (1) no midline cervical tenderness, (2) no focal neurologic deficit, (3) normal alertness and level of consciousness, (4) absence of intoxication, and (5) no painful, distracting injury. This patient does not meet these criteria and therefore warrants computed tomography (CT) scanning of the neck. The cervical collar should remain in place until the CT scan has been completed and reviewed by the provider.

B. The National Emergency X-radiography Utilization Study (NEXUS) low-risk criteria include (1) no midline cervical tenderness, (2) no focal neurologic deficit, (3) normal alertness and level of consciousness, (4) absence of intoxication, and (5) no painful, distracting injury. This patient does not meet the NEXUS low-risk criteria and therefore warrants CT scanning of the neck. Based on the patient's assessment, the patient will also require a CT scan of the head.

C. Use of a long spine board facilitates transport of the patient. Maintaining the patient in alignment in a supine position is adequate and will reduce complications associated with long board use, such as pressure sore development.

D. Assessing the blood alcohol level (BAL) may be appropriate. However, assessing intoxication solely on a BAL is not necessary. The patient already meets other NEXUS exclusion criteria.

Category: Neurological Emergencies/Spinal cord injuries

Nursing Process: Intervention

References

EMS Spinal Precautions and the Use of the Long Backboard: Position Statement of the National Association of EMS Physicians and the American College of Surgeons Committee on Trauma. (2012). Retrieved from https://www.facs.org/~/media/files/quality%20programs/trauma/vrc%20resources/9_backboardpositionpaper%20final%20approved_2012.ashx

Everson, F. P. (2013). Spinal cord and neck trauma. In B. B. Hammond & P. G. Zimmermann (Eds.), *Sheehy's manual of emergency care* (7th ed., pp. 395–406). St. Louis, MO: Elsevier Mosby.

---

52. A patient presents to the emergency department with a history of a prior cerebrovascular infarction. The family reports that the patient was functioning independently before suddenly becoming confused, screaming, and throwing things at home. The nurse recognizes these symptoms are an indication of which of the following?

A. Delirium
B. Dementia
C. Lacunar stroke
D. Hyperoxia

Rationale

A. Delirium is defined as an acute and sudden onset of a change in behavior, resulting in a potentially reversible state of confusion, lack of attention, and change in cognition and perception that can be precipitated by a medical condition. It is more common in patients who are elderly or suffer comorbid conditions.

B. Dementia represents a chronic progressive loss of independent functioning and memory. Dementia onset is slow; the patient's attention is initially normal with clear consciousness, whereas the patient's orientation is often impaired.

C. Symptoms commonly associated with lacunar syndrome include numbness and/or tingling on one side of the body, and occasionally patients complain of pain, burning, or another unpleasant sensation.

D. Hyperoxia is the overabundance of oxygen in tissue. The presence of hyperoxia typically does not result in a patient developing confusion, lack of attention, or changes in cognition.

Category: Neurological Emergencies/Stroke (ischemic or hemorrhagic)

Nursing Process: Analysis

References

Agranoff, A. (2017). Lacunar stroke. *Medscape*. Retrieved from http://emedicine.medscape.com/article/322992-overview

Dunphy, L., Winland-Brown, J., Porter, B., & Thomas, D. (2015). *Primary care: The art and science of advanced practice nursing* (4th ed.) Philadelphia, PA: F. A. Davis.

Rice, K. L., & Albright, M. (2013). Geriatric considerations in emergency nursing. In B. B. Hammond & P. G. Zimmermann (Eds.), *Sheehy's manual of emergency care* (7th ed., pp. 571–592). St. Louis, MO: Elsevier Mosby.

---

53. A patient presents to the emergency department with complaints of bright red blood with clots in their stool for the past 2 weeks. The patient is in no apparent distress and has normal vital signs, and laboratory values are within normal limits. The emergency nurse suspects the source of the bleeding is:

A. ulcerative colitis.
B. esophageal varices.
C. hemorrhoids.
D. Mallory–Weiss syndrome

Rationale

A. The symptoms of ulcerative colitis include bloody diarrhea with cramping abdominal pain, fever, and tachycardia. The patient's current vital signs are not abnormal, so an inflammatory bowel etiology such as ulcerative colitis is not likely.

B. Bleeding from esophageal varices results in vomiting of bright red blood. Blood that travels through the gastrointestinal tract will become darker and results in the passage of dark red or black tarry stools.

C. The patient's symptoms suggest bleeding that originates from the lower gastrointestinal area. Bleeding from hemorrhoids, located closer to the rectum, is more likely to be bright red and contain clots.

D. Mallory–Weiss syndrome occurs as the result of mucosal tears in the gastroesophageal junction because of violent retching or vomiting. The patient is in no distress, and vital signs do not suggest fluid loss from vomiting.

Category: Gastrointestinal, Genitourinary, Gynecology, and Obstetrical Emergencies/Gastrointestinal/Bleeding

Nursing Process: Analysis

Reference

Wolf, L., & Zimmermann, P. G. (2013). Abdominal pain and emergencies. In B. B. Hammond & P. G. Zimmermann (Eds.), *Sheehy's manual of emergency care* (7th ed., pp. 291–301). St. Louis, MO: Elsevier Mosby.

---

54. A patient with recent history of gastric bypass surgery presents to the emergency department with a 3-day history of right upper quadrant pain that radiates to the right shoulder. The emergency nurse suspects these symptoms are associated with:

A. pyelonephritis.
B. pancreatitis.
C. appendicitis.
D. cholecystitis.

Rationale

A. The pain associated with a kidney infection or pyleonephritis usually is experienced in the flank area over the costovertebral angle. The pain does not radiate into the abdomen or to the shoulder area.

B. The presence of gallstones can result in the development of pancreatitis; however, pancreatitis would cause the patient to experience epigastric pain that radiates through to the back.

C. The pain associated with an inflamed appendix typically begins in the periumbilical area and then localizes to the right lower quadrant.

D. The rapid weight loss associated with bariatric surgery is a risk factor for the development of gallstones, which can lead to cholecystitis. Right upper quadrant pain radiating to the right shoulder area is a typical presentation for cholecystitis.

Category: Gastrointestinal, Genitourinary, Gynecology, and Obstetrical Emergencies/Gastrointestinal/Cholecystitis

Nursing Process: Assessment

References

Herrington, A. (2010). Gastrointestinal emergencies. In P. K. Howard & R. A. Steinmann (Eds.), *Sheehy's emergency nursing: Principles and practice* (6th ed., pp. 467–477). St. Louis, MO: Mosby Elsevier.

Quallich, S. (2013). Genitourinary emergencies. In B. B. Hammond & P. G. Zimmermann (Eds.), *Sheehy's manual of emergency care* (7th ed., pp. 353–360). St. Louis, MO: Elsevier Mosby.

Quesada, B. M., Kohan, G., Roff, H. E., Canullán, C. M., & Porras, L. T. C. (2010). Management of gallstones and gallbladder disease in patients undergoing gastric bypass. *World Journal of Gastroenterology, 16*(17), 2075–2079. http://doi.org/10.3748/wjg.v16.i17.2075

---

55. A patient with a history of cirrhosis presents to the emergency department stating that they are "spitting up bright red blood." The patient's abdomen is severely distended, with numerous bruises in various stages of healing. The emergency nurse suspects the source of the patient's bleeding is most likely which of the following?

A. Tuberculosis
B. Intraoral abscess
C. Esophageal varices
D. Peptic ulcer disease

Rationale

A. Hemoptysis is a symptom associated with tuberculosis, however, the patient's history of cirrhosis, distended abdomen, and bruises are more suggestive of ascites and portal hypertension as a result of hepatic disease.

B. Necrotizing ulcerative gingivitis is an intraoral bacterial infection associated with a debilitating illness, immunosuppression, and nutritional deficiencies. The patient may develop intraoral ulcerations and bleeding gums but would also exhibit intraoral pain, fever > 38.3°C (101°F), cervical adenopathy, and cervical lymph node enlargement.

C. Esophageal varices often develop as a result of portal hypertension secondary to liver cirrhosis. Bleeding esophageal varices are a frequent cause of death in patients with hepatic disease.

D. Peptic ulcers can cause upper gastrointestinal bleeding, and the nurse should consider this etiology as a source of the patient's symptoms; however, the patient's history of cirrhosis, distended abdomen, and evidence of bruising suggest a coagulopathy along with portal hypertension. Esophageal varices are the most likely source of the patient's symptoms.

Category: Gastrointestinal, Genitourinary, Gynecology, and Obstetrical Emergencies/Gastrointestinal/Esophageal varices

Nursing Process: Analysis

References

Almeida, S. (2010). Communicable diseases. In P. K. Howard & R. A. Steinmann (Eds.), *Sheehy's emergency nursing: Principles and practice* (6th ed., pp. 513–524). St. Louis, MO: Mosby Elsevier.

Herrington, A. (2010). Gastrointestinal emergencies. In P. K. Howard & R. A. Steinmann (Eds.), *Sheehy's emergency nursing: Principles and practice* (6th ed., pp. 467–477). St. Louis, MO: Mosby Elsevier.

Wolf, L., & Zimmermann, P. G. (2013). Abdominal pain and emergencies. In B. B. Hammond & P. G. Zimmermann (Eds.), *Sheehy's manual of emergency care* (7th ed., pp. 291–301). St. Louis, MO: Elsevier Mosby.

---

56. A patient with a diagnosis of esophagitis secondary to gastroesophageal reflux disease is treated in the emergency department and prepared for discharge. Which statement, made by the patient, indicates a correct understanding of the discharge instructions?

A. "I should take only small sips of water with any of my pills."
B. "I should lie on my left side after I eat to aid in my digestion."
C. "I should eat several small meals a day instead of three large meals."
D. "I should follow a gluten-free diet."

Rationale

A. Medications can be a source of irritation to the esophagus, especially if swallowed with only a small amount of fluid.

B. Lying down after eating or taking medications will worsen symptoms of esophagitis. The patient should be instructed to sit upright after eating or taking medication.

C. Esophageal irritation and inflammation frequently result from acid reflux in patients with a history of gastroesophageal reflux disease. Making lifestyle modifications, such as eating several small meals per day instead of three large meals, will reduce symptoms.

D. There is no current evidence to suggest that a gluten-free diet is beneficial to reduce the symptoms of reflux in patients who do not have celiac disease.

Category: Gastrointestinal, Genitourinary, Gynecology, and Obstetrical Emergencies/Gastrointestinal/Gastritis

Nursing Process: Evaluation

References

Russoll, L. W. (2007). Abdominal emergencies. In K. S. Hoyt & J. Selfridge-Thomas (Eds.), *Emergency nursing core curriculum* (6th ed., pp. 159–186). St. Louis, MO: Saunders Elsevier.

Wolf, L., & Zimmermann, P. G. (2013). Abdominal pain and emergencies. In B. B. Hammond & P. G. Zimmermann (Eds.), *Sheehy's manual of emergency care* (7th ed., pp. 291–301). St. Louis, MO: Elsevier Mosby.

---

57. A patient presents to the emergency department with complaints of a burning, gnawing type pain in the left upper quadrant, and epigastrium that is associated with nausea and vomiting. The patient is diagnosed with acute gastritis. Based on the patient's symptoms, the nurse would expect which diagnostic test to yield abnormal results?

A. Serum creatinine
B. Liver enzymes
C. Serum electrolytes
D. Serum lipase

Rationale

A. Serum creatinine is a measurement of renal function and will be increased in renal failure. Prolonged dehydration as a result of vomiting may lead to acute renal injury, but the patient has no evidence of this at this time.

B. Liver enzymes should remain normal in a patient with gastritis.

C. Potassium is found in gastric juices and can be lost through vomiting; therefore, the patient may have a decreased potassium level or hypokalemia.

D. The patient's serum amylase and serum lipase would be elevated in acute pancreatitis. This diagnostic testing would not be abnormal in the presence of gastritis.

Category: Gastrointestinal, Genitourinary, Gynecology, and Obstetrical Emergencies/Gastrointestinal/Gastroenteritis

Nursing Process: Analysis

References

Kuiper, B. L. (2007). Fluid and electrolyte emergencies. In K. S. Hoyt & J. Selfridge-Thomas (Eds.), *Emergency nursing core curriculum* (6th ed., pp. 361–386). St. Louis, MO: Saunders Elsevier.

Wolf, L., & Zimmermann, P. G. (2013). Abdominal pain and emergencies. In B. B. Hammond & P. G. Zimmermann (Eds.), *Sheehy's manual of emergency care* (7th ed., pp. 291–301). St. Louis, MO: Elsevier Mosby.

---

58. A patient presents to the emergency department complaining of fatigue, joint pain, and anorexia for the past 3 months. On assessment, the patient has an elevated temperature, yellowed sclera, and tenderness in the right upper quadrant. The patient admits to intravenous drug use. The emergency nurse would anticipate a positive result to which diagnostic test?

A. Hepatitis B antigen
B. Hepatitis A antigen
C. Human immunodeficiency virus immunoassay
D. Enzyme-linked immunosorbent assay test

Rationale

A. The patient's symptoms of right upper quadrant tenderness, anorexia, and jaundice are consistent with hepatic disease, and the patient's history of intravenous (IV) drug use suggests hepatitis B as the source. Presence of the hepatitis B antigen indicates that the patient has an acute hepatitis B infection.

B. The patient's symptoms are consistent with hepatic disease, and the patient's s admission of previous IV drug use suggests an infection with the hepatitis B virus. Hepatitis A is spread through contact with contaminated food or water.

C. A patient with a history of IV drug abuse is at risk for contracting human immunodeficiency virus; however, this patient's clinical presentation is consistent with hepatic disease, most likely as a result of hepatitis B contracted through IV drug use.

D. The enzyme-linked immunosorbent assay (ELISA) test is used to identify antibodies in the blood and is used in the diagnosis of diseases such as Lyme disease, Rocky Mountain spotted fever, and varicella zoster. ELISA is not a test used to diagnose hepatitis B.

Category: Gastrointestinal, Genitourinary, Gynecology, and Obstetrical Emergencies/Gastrointestinal/Hepatitis

Nursing Process: Assessment

Reference

U.S. Department of Health and Human Services. (2016). *Viral hepatitis: Hepatitis B information*. Centers for Disease Control and Prevention, Atlanta, GA. Retrieved from https://www.cdc.gov/hepatitis/hbv/bfaq.htm

---

59. An elderly male presents to triage complaining of intense pain in his lower abdomen. The patient states it started as a mild ache but has become more severe over the past week. The emergency nurse palpates the area and feels a mass in the mid-abdominal area. The emergency nurse suspects which of the following conditions?

A. Abdominal aortic aneurysm
B. Hernia
C. Appendicitis
D. Small bowel obstruction

Rationale

A. An aneurysm is caused by a weakening in the arterial wall, resulting in a dilated area of the artery. The onset of symptoms is rapid when the aneurysm begins to dissect; signs and symptoms experienced by the patient are dependent on the location of the aneurysm.

B. Hernia results from a weak spot in the fascia that allows a portion of the bowel to become entrapped, resulting in dull or sharp pain that is slow in onset.

C. Appendicitis is caused by an obstruction and distention of the lumen of the appendix, resulting in ischemia and bacterial invasion of the appendix. As the inflammation progresses, the appendix becomes nonviable until it ruptures, emptying infectious material into the abdominal cavity.

D. A small bowel obstruction can result from either a twisting of the bowel or a mechanical obstruction; the patient experiences cramping and severe bloating because the bowel is unable to move contents forward.

Category: Gastrointestinal, Genitourinary, Gynecology, and Obstetrical Emergencies/Gastrointestinal/Hernia

Nursing Process: Assessment

References

Williams, D. A. (2010). Cardiovascular emergencies. In P. K. Howard & R. A. Steinmann (Eds.), *Sheehy's emergency nursing: Principles and practice* (6th ed., pp. 411–444). St. Louis, MO: Mosby Elsevier.

Wolf, L., & Zimmermann, P. G. (2013). Abdominal pain and emergencies. In B. B. Hammond & P. G. Zimmermann (Eds.), *Sheehy's manual of emergency care* (7th ed., pp. 291–301). St. Louis, MO: Elsevier Mosby.

---

60. A patient presents to the emergency department complaining of the feeling that something is caught in their throat. It began after the patient swallowed a piece of meat. After assessing that the patient's airway is not compromised, the nurse would anticipate the intravenous administration of what medication?

A. Omeprazole (Prilosec)
B. Glucagon
C. Metoclopramide (Reglan)
D. Nitroglycerin

Rationale

A. Omeprazole is a proton pump inhibitor, which decreases gastric acid secretion. It has no effect on facilitating the movement of a food bolus through the esophagus.

B. Glucagon relaxes esophageal smooth muscle and the lower esophageal sphincter, which helps to move the impacted food bolus through the esophagus to the stomach. Glucagon also acts to increase blood glucose in patients who are hypoglycemic.

C. Metoclopramide is indicated as a treatment for gastric paresis. It stimulates gastric motility and increases the tone of the lower esophageal sphincter, which would make passage of an impacted esophageal food bolus more difficult.

D. Nitrates may relax the gastrointestinal muscles; however, there is a substantial risk of producing hypotension in the patient, so its use is not recommended.

Category: Gastrointestinal, Genitourinary, Gynecology, and Obstetrical Emergencies/Gastrointestinal/Obstructions

Nursing Process: Intervention

References

Ko, H. H., & Enns, R. (2008). Review of food bolus management. *Canadian Journal of Gastroenterology*, *22*(10), 805–808.

Munter, D. W. (2014). Gastrointestinal foreign bodies: Treatment and management. *Medscape*. Retrieved from http://emedicine.medscape.com/article/776566-treatment#d11

Smith, D. A. (2007). Dental, ear, nose, and throat emergencies. In K. S. Hoyt & J. Selfridge-Thomas (Eds.), *Emergency nursing core curriculum* (6th ed., pp. 249–289). St. Louis, MO: Saunders Elsevier.

---

61. The most common cause of acute pancreatitis is:

A. **alcohol abuse.**
B. abdominal trauma.
C. endoscopic retrograde cholangiopancreatography.
D. diabetes mellitus.

Rationale

A. Between 50% and 75% of cases of acute pancreatitis are attributable to alcoholism or the presence of gallstones in the common bile duct.

B. Acute pancreatitis can develop following an acute pancreatic injury, however, it is not the most common cause.

C. Pancreatitis may be a complication following an endoscopic retrograde cholangiopancreatography, but it is not the most common cause. An endoscopic retrograde cholangiopancreatography is performed to treat problems associated with the common bile or pancreatic duct.

D. Pancreatitis may cause an alteration in serum glucose levels, but diabetes mellitus is not a causative factor associated with acute pancreatitis.

Category: Gastrointestinal, Genitourinary, Gynecology, and Obstetrical Emergencies/Gastrointestinal/Pancreatitis

Nursing Process: Assessment

References

Russoll, L. W. (2007). Abdominal emergencies. In K. S. Hoyt & J. Selfridge-Thomas (Eds.), *Emergency nursing core curriculum* (6th ed., pp. 159–186). St. Louis, MO: Saunders Elsevier.

Wolf, L., & Zimmermann, P. G. (2013). Abdominal pain and emergencies. In B. B. Hammond & P. G. Zimmermann (Eds.), *Sheehy's manual of emergency care* (7th ed., pp. 291–301). St. Louis, MO: Elsevier Mosby.

---

62. A patient presents to the emergency department complaining of recurrent "stomach" pain that occurs before meals and is relieved by eating. The patient has no significant medical history and takes 200 mg ibuprofen daily for chronic shoulder pain. Based on this information, the nurse suspects the patient's symptoms are most likely the result of:

A. gastroesophageal reflux disease.
B. gastric ulcer.
C. **duodenal ulcer.**
D. Mallory–Weiss syndrome.

Rationale

A. The pain associated with gastroesophageal reflux disease is typically described as a burning or squeezing in the upper chest, which may mimic cardiac-related chest pain. Symptom onset usually occurs after the ingestion of irritating foods or medications.

B. The pain associated with a gastric ulcer is typically experienced after eating. This is an important assessment finding that assists in differentiating between a duodenal ulcer and a gastric ulcer.

C. The pain associated with duodenal ulcers is typically worse when the stomach is empty and is relieved when there is food in the stomach. Duodenal ulcers occur most commonly in persons between 30 and 55 years of age. A patient's risk of developing a duodenal ulcer is elevated with chronic ingestion of irritants such as nonsteroidal anti-inflammatory drugs.

D. Mallory–Weiss syndrome is the development of tears in the gastroesophageal mucosa as a result of violent retching. Upper gastrointestinal bleeding may result from a Mallory–Weiss tear. Persistent vomiting, not pain, is the presenting symptom of this syndrome.

Category: Gastrointestinal, Genitourinary, Gynecology, and Obstetrical Emergencies/Gastrointestinal/Ulcers

Nursing Process: Analysis

References

Herrington, A. (2010). Gastrointestinal emergencies. In P. K. Howard & R. A. Steinmann (Eds.), *Sheehy's emergency nursing: Principles and practice* (6th ed., pp. 467–477). St. Louis, MO: Mosby Elsevier.

Wolf, L., & Zimmermann, P. G. (2013). Abdominal pain and emergencies. In B. B. Hammond & P. G. Zimmermann (Eds.), *Sheehy's manual of emergency care* (7th ed., pp. 291–301). St. Louis, MO: Elsevier Mosby.

---

63. A patient is being discharged home with a diagnosis of renal calculi. Which of the following statements by the patient indicates the need for further education regarding the discharged instructions?

A. "I may still see some blood in my urine until the stone passes."
B. "Once the pain is relieved, I should strain my urine and check the filter for stones."
C. "I will need to increase my intake of fluids, especially water."
D. "If I should experience any pain tonight, I should return to the emergency department immediately."

Rationale

A. Gross or microscopic hematuria, including the presence of small clots, is a common finding and may still be noted by the patient as the calculus moves through the ureter.

B. Urine should be strained for up to 72 hours *after* pain relief in order to retrieve calculi for chemical analysis. If the patient is experiencing pain, the calculus is most likely still in the ureter. Once the patient experiences no further pain, the calculus has most likely passed into the urinary bladder.

C. This statement is correct; if the stone causes a blockage, an emergency procedure may be required to remove the kidney stone.

D. The pain associated with renal calculi may continue as the calculus passes through the ureter. The patient should be instructed to return to the emergency department if they experience increasing pain, vomiting, fever or chills.

Category: Gastrointestinal, Genitourinary, Gynecology, and Obstetrical Emergencies/Genitourinary/Renal calculi

Nursing Process: Evaluation

References

Baxter, C. S. (2010). Renal and genitourinary emergencies. In P. K. Howard & R. A. Steinmann (Eds.), *Sheehy's emergency nursing: Principles and practice* (6th ed., pp. 478–489). St. Louis, MO: Mosby Elsevier.

Preminger, G. M., Curhan, G. C., Goldfarb, S., O'Leary, M. P., Lam, A. Q. (2016). Patient information: Kidney stones in adults (beyond the basics). *UpToDate.* Retrieved from http://www.uptodate.com/contents/kidney-stones-in-adults-beyond-the-basics

Quallich, S. (2013). Genitourinary emergencies. In B. B. Hammond & P. G. Zimmermann (Eds.), *Sheehy's manual of emergency care* (7th ed., pp. 353–360). St. Louis, MO: Elsevier Mosby.

---

64. Which of the following conditions is caused by a sexually transmitted infection?

A. Priapism
B. Epididymitis
C. Prostatitis
D. Testicular torsion

Rationale

A. Priapism is a painful and sustained erection not associated with sexual arousal.

B. Epididymitis is frequently caused by inflammation of the epididymis and is the result of a sexually transmitted infection commonly caused by *C. trachomatis* or *N. gonorrhoeae.*

C. Prostatitis is an inflammation of the prostate that is commonly the result of an E. coli infection and frequently related to the presence of a urinary tract infection.

D. Testicular torsion occurs because of a sudden twisting of spermatic cord, resulting in vascular compromise to the male testis. If left untreated, testicular torsion will result in male sterility.

Category: Gastrointestinal, Genitourinary, Gynecology, and Obstetrical Emergencies/Genitourinary/Infection

Nursing Process: Assessment

Reference

Baxter, C. S. (2010). Renal and genitourinary emergencies. In P. K. Howard & R. A. Steinmann (Eds.), *Sheehy's emergency nursing: Principles and practice* (6th ed., pp. 478–489). St. Louis, MO: Mosby Elsevier.

---

65. The emergency nurse anticipates that the treatment for a patient with the diagnosis of vaginitis would most likely include the administration of:

A. antimicrobial medications.
B. probiotic medications.
C. antiviral medications.
D. immune-response modifier medications.

Rationale

A. The most common causes of vaginitis include bacterial vaginosis, *Candida albicans* and *Trichomonas vaginitis.* Antibiotics or antifungal agents are required to eradicate these organisms.

B. Although there is evidence to support the benefit of probiotics in the prevention and treatment of bacterial vaginosis, probiotics are not effective in the treatment of *Candida albicans* or *Trichomonas vaginalis.*

C. Antiviral medications are effective in the management of gynecological viral infections such as the herpes simplex virus; they are not indicated for the treatment of infections caused by bacterial or fungal organisms.

D. Immune-response modifiers are an effective treatment for genital condylomas (warts) that do not respond to other treatments. They are not indicated for the treatment of vaginitis.

Category: Gastrointestinal, Genitourinary, Gynecology, and Obstetrical Emergencies/Gynecology/Infection

Nursing Process: Intervention

References

Egging, D. (2013). Sexually transmitted infections. In B. B. Hammond & P. G. Zimmermann (Eds.), *Sheehy's manual of emergency care* (7th ed., pp. 361–366). St. Louis, MO: Elsevier Mosby.

Homayouni, A., Bastani, P., Ziyadi, S., Mohammad-Alizadeh-Charandabi, S., Ghalibaf, M., Mortazavian, A. M., & Mehrabany, E. V. (2014). Effects of probiotics on the recurrence of bacterial vaginosis: A review. *Journal of Lower Genitourinary Tract Diseases, 18*(1), 79–86. https://doi.org/10.1097/LGT.0b013e31829156ec

Jordan, K. S. (2007). Obstetric and gynecologic emergences. In K. S. Hoyt & J. Selfridge-Thomas (Eds.), *Emergency nursing core curriculum* (6th ed., pp. 536–570). St. Louis, MO: Saunders Elsevier.

---

66. A woman with a history of ovarian cysts presents to the emergency department complaining of severe lower abdominal pain. Which of the following diagnostic testing would best confirm the presence of an ovarian cyst?

A. Serum beta HCG
B. Pelvic examination
C. Pelvic ultrasound
D. Clean-catch urine specimen

Rationale

A. A urine or serum beta-HCG test may be done to rule out pregnancy but will neither identify the presence of, nor verify the absence of, an ovarian cyst.

B. A pelvic examination would identify tenderness of the uterus, fallopian tubes, or cervix but would not identify or rule out the presence of an ovarian cyst.

C. The definitive diagnosis of an ovarian cyst is best made through a pelvic ultrasound.

D. A clean-catch urine specimen would be helpful to identify a urinary cause for the abdominal pain but would not identify the presence of, nor verify the absence of, an ovarian cyst.

Category: Gastrointestinal, Genitourinary, Gynecology, and Obstetrical Emergencies/Gynecology/Ovarian cyst

Nursing Process: Analysis

Reference

Jordan, K. S. (2007). Obstetric and gynecologic emergences. In K. S. Hoyt & J. Selfridge-Thomas (Eds.), *Emergency nursing core curriculum* (6th ed., pp. 536–570). St. Louis, MO: Saunders Elsevier.

67. A patient with sudden onset of severe testicular pain is diagnosed with testicular torsion. The next appropriate intervention for the emergency nurse to perform is to:

A. elevate the scrotum.
B. insert an indwelling urinary catheter.
C. administer an antibiotic.
D. prepare the patient for emergency surgery.

Rationale

A. Elevation of the scrotum in testicular torsion may cause intense pain and therefore should be avoided.

B. Urinary retention is not associated with testicular torsion; therefore, the insertion of an indwelling urinary catheter is not indicated.

C. Testicular torsion is a mechanical twisting of the spermatic cord. It does not have an infectious etiology, so the administration of an antibiotic is not indicated.

D. Testicular torsion is a true emergency. If surgery is not performed within 6–8 hours from the onset of the torsion, the affected testicle's blood supply is compromised, and the testicle may become necrotic.

Category: Gastrointestinal, Genitourinary, Gynecology, and Obstetrical Emergencies/Genitourinary/Testicular torsion

Nursing Process: Intervention

References

Quallich, S. (2013). Genitourinary emergencies. In B. B. Hammond & P. G. Zimmermann (Eds.), *Sheehy's manual of emergency care* (7th ed., pp. 353–360). St. Louis, MO: Elsevier Mosby.

Shenot, P. J. (2017). Testicular torsion. *Merck Manual online*. Retrieved from http://www.merckmanuals.com/professional/genitourinary-disorders/penile-and-scrotal-disorders/testicular-torsion

---

68. If left untreated, a male who experiences a penile fracture resulting from the rupture of the tunica albuginea may develop which complication?

A. Erectile difficulties
B. Impaired urinary function
C. Penile ischemia
D. Infertility

Rationale

A. If treatment is delayed for rupture of the tunica albuginea or if it is left untreated, erectile difficulties may develop.

B. A penile fracture resulting from a rupture of the tunica albuginea will not impair urinary function.

C. Penile ecchymosis, which may be significant to distort the penile shaft, can occur but will eventually resolve and will not result in penile ischemia.

D. A fractured penis as the result of a rupture of the tunica albuginea does not affect the production of sperm.

Category: Gastrointestinal, Genitourinary, Gynecology, and Obstetrical Emergencies/Genitourinary/Trauma

Nursing Process: Analysis

Reference

Quallich, S. (2013). Genitourinary emergencies. In B. B. Hammond & P. G. Zimmermann (Eds.), *Sheehy's manual of emergency care* (7th ed., pp. 353–360). St. Louis, MO: Elsevier Mosby.

---

69. A patient with bacterial vaginosis is prescribed clindamycin vaginal cream. It is important to include which information in the patient's discharge instructions for the use of this antibiotic?

A. Clindamycin cream should be applied immediately on arising in the morning.
B. Clindamycin cream may weaken a condom.
C. Clindamycin is the only medication needed to treat this infection.
D. Continue to use the medication until your symptoms are no longer present.

Rationale

A. Clindamycin cream should be applied at bedtime.

B. Clindamycin cream contains mineral oil, which can weaken latex condoms, so an alternative form of birth control should be used for 72 hours following the use of clindamycin vaginal cream.

C. Metronidazole (Flagyl) is frequently administered concurrently with clindamycin to treat bacterial vaginosis.

D. The patient should continue to take the medication as directed until the prescription is completed. This is especially important because a patient with bacterial vaginosis may be asymptomatic.

Category: Gastrointestinal, Genitourinary, Gynecology, and Obstetrical Emergencies/Gynecology/Infection

Nursing Process: Intervention

References

Kelly, L. (2013). Gynecological emergencies. In B. B. Hammond & P. G. Zimmermann (Eds.), *Sheehy's manual of emergency care* (7th ed., pp. 497–503). St. Louis, MO: Elsevier Mosby.
Pfizer. (2015). *Clindamycin*. Retrieved from http://labeling.pfizer.com/showlabeling.aspx?id=627

---

70. A 40-year-old female in the first trimester of her pregnancy presents to the emergency department complaining of severe left-sided abdominal tenderness with vaginal bleeding. The patient is lethargic, pale, hypotensive, and tachycardic. The emergency nurse recognizes the priority intervention for this patient is to:

A. prepare the patient for a transvaginal ultrasound.
B. prepare for the administration of a methotrexate injection.
C. prepare the patient for surgery.
D. obtain a serum beta human chorionic gonadotropin level.

Rationale

A. Transvaginal ultrasound can accurately identify the intrauterine gestational sac and is effective for diagnosis, particularly before a tubal rupture. However, the clinical presentation of this patient suggests a ruptured ectopic pregnancy, and because she is hemodynamically unstable, surgical intervention—not additional diagnostic testing—is the priority.

B. Methotrexate is a cytotoxic agent that interferes with cell multiplication. It is indicated for use in patients with an unruptured tubal ectopic pregnancy who are hemodynamically stable and have minimal symptoms.

C. Ectopic pregnancy is a considerable cause of maternal morbidity, causing pelvic pain and vaginal bleeding. A ruptured ectopic pregnancy should be strongly suspected in a patient between 6 and 10 weeks' gestation who presents with syncope and signs of shock, including tachycardia, pallor, and collapse. Decompensation with shock is suggestive of tubal rupture with an intraperitoneal bleeding. Immediate surgical intervention is indicated.

D. An elevated beta human chorionic gonadotropin (B-hCG) concentration will indicate that the patient is pregnant but will not identify the pregnancy as being an ectopic pregnancy (not implanted within the uterus). An initial B-hCG level may be beneficial for baseline determination, but resuscitation and surgical intervention take priority.

Category: Gastrointestinal, Genitourinary, Gynecology, and Obstetrical Emergencies/Obstetrical/Ectopic pregnancy

Nursing Process: Intervention

References

Poole, J. H., & Thompson, J. E. (2013). Obstetric emergencies. In B. B. Hammond & P. G. Zimmermann (Eds.), *Sheehy's manual of emergency care* (7th ed., pp. 483–495). St. Louis, MO: Elsevier Mosby.

Sivalingam, V. N., Duncan, W. C., Kirk, E., Shephard, L. A., & Horne, A. W. (2011). Diagnosis and management of ectopic pregnancy. *Journal of Family Planning Reproductive Health Care, 37*(4), 231–240. https://doi.org/10.1136/jfprhc-2011-0073

---

71. The recommended method of performing chest compressions on a neonate is:

A. **cardiac compression using two thumbs with the fingers encircling the chest and supporting the back.**
B. cardiac compressions with two fingers and the opposite hand supporting the back.
C. compressions with the heel of one hand depressing the sternum not more than 4 cm (1.5 in).
D. five back blows followed by five chest thrust compressions.

Rationale

A. This is the preferred method because the two-thumb encircling technique generates higher blood pressure and coronary perfusion pressure with less rescuer fatigue.

B. Compressions using the two-thumb technique were found to be superior to compressions using the two-finger technique; not only did the two-thumb technique generate a higher blood pressure and improved cardiac perfusion, but users of the two-thumb technique demonstrated more accurate placement on the chest, more consistency in compressions, and less fatigue over time.

C. Delivering chest compressions with the heel of the hand on the center of the chest is the recommended method for a child over the age of 1 year and should not be used for a neonate.

D. Five sharp back blows followed by five chest thrusts is the American Heart Association recommended sequence for relieving an obstructed airway in an infant.

Category (Pediatric): Gastrointestinal, Genitourinary, Gynecology, and Obstetrical Emergencies/Obstetrical/Neonatal resuscitation

Nursing Process: Intervention

Reference

Wyckoff, M. H., Aziz, K., Escobedo, M. B., Kapadia, V. S., Kattwinkel, J., Perlman, J. M., . . . Zaichkin, J. G. (2015). Part 13: Neonatal resuscitation: 2015 American Heart Association guidelines update for cardiopulmonary resuscitation and emergency cardiovascular care. *Circulation, 132*(18), S543–S560. https://doi.org/10.1161/CIR.0000000000000267

---

72. Following the delivery of a full-term neonate in the emergency department, the emergency nurse administers a dose of intravenous pitocin to the mother. The nurse can expect which of the following outcomes from the administration of this medication?

A. Facilitated delivery of the placenta
B. Reduction of postpartum bleeding
C. Stimulated breast milk production
D. Prevention of Rh incompatibility between the mother and the fetus

Rationale

A. Placental delivery occurs naturally up to 30 minutes after delivery. The process should be allowed to occur naturally. Fundal massage can assist in the separation of the placenta from the uterine wall.

B. The most common cause of postpartum hemorrhage is uterine atony. Administration of intravenous pitocin will promote and maintain uterine contractility.

C. Pitocin has no effect on the mother's production of breast milk.

D. Rh immune globulin is the drug indicated for the prevention of Rh incompatibility.

Category: Gastrointestinal, Genitourinary, Gynecology, and Obstetrical Emergencies/Obstetrical/Hemorrhage

Nursing Process: Evaluation

References

Jordan, K. S. (2007). Obstetric and gynecologic emergences. In K. S. Hoyt & J. Selfridge-Thomas (Eds.), *Emergency nursing core curriculum* (6th ed., pp. 536–570). St. Louis, MO: Saunders Elsevier.

Vallerand, A. H., Sanoski, C. A., & Deglin, J. H. (2011). *Davis's drug guide for nurses* (13th ed.). Philadelphia, PA: F. A. Davis.

---

73. A 36-week-pregnant female presents to the emergency department with a sudden onset of painless, bright red vaginal bleeding. Placenta previa is suspected. The emergency nurse should prepare this patient for which procedure?

A. Manual pelvic examination
B. Assessment of fetal heart tones
C. Immediate cesarean delivery
D. Pelvic ultrasound.

Rationale

A. If the placenta is covering the cervical os, the insertion of the provider's hand or a speculum can result in an unintentional placental perforation, resulting in hemorrhage. Therefore, the pelvic examination is contraindicated until the exact location of the placenta is identified.

B. Assessment of fetal heart tones is an important component of the nursing assessment; however, a change in fetal heart tones can only verify fetal distress, but it does not identify the cause. Determining the origin of the vaginal bleeding is critical to ensure the hemodynamic stability of the mother and baby.

C. If a diagnosis of placenta previa is confirmed, an immediate cesarean delivery may be indicated, depending on the gestational age of the fetus, extent of the bleeding, and hemodynamic status of the mother.

D. The transabdominal (pelvic) ultrasound is indicated as the initial procedure test to diagnose placenta previa and identify the specific location of the placenta.

Category: Gastrointestinal, Genitourinary, Gynecology, and Obstetrical Emergencies/Obstetrical/Placenta previa

Nursing Process: Analysis

References

Benrubi, G. (2010). *Handbook of obstetric and gynecologic emergencies* (4th ed.). Philadelphia, PA: Lippincott Williams & Wilkins.

Jordan, K. S. (2007). Obstetric and gynecologic emergences. In K. S. Hoyt & J. Selfridge-Thomas (Eds.), *Emergency nursing core curriculum* (6th ed., pp. 536–570). St. Louis, MO: Saunders Elsevier.

Mason, D. (2010). Obstetric emergencies. In P. K. Howard & R. A. Steinmann (Eds.), *Sheehy's emergency nursing: Principles and practice* (6th ed., pp. 619–629). St. Louis, MO: Mosby Elsevier.

Poole, J. H., & Thompson, J. E. (2013). Obstetric emergencies. In B. B. Hammond & P. G. Zimmermann (Eds.), *Sheehy's manual of emergency care* (7th ed., pp. 483–495). St. Louis, MO: Elsevier Mosby.

---

74. The triage nurse suspects a patient may be the victim of intimate partner violence. The primary survey is within normal limits, and there is no visible acute injury. Which of the following is a priority intervention for this patient?

A. Ask hospital security personnel to sit with the patient during the triage interview
B. Provide a private area for the assessment interview
C. Allow the patient to remain dressed in their own clothing during the provider examination
D. Document the name of the suspected offender in the patient record

Rationale

A. Bringing security personnel into the triage area may create undue patient anxiety and may call attention to the patient's situation.

B. Victims of intimate partner violence need to feel safe, and their privacy must be respected. The patient should be moved to a safe and private area to complete the screening and assessment process.

C. Allowing the patient to remain in their own clothing during the provider examination will prevent the inspection of possible hidden injuries. Patients should be instructed to change into a hospital gown for the physical examination.

D. The nurse may document statements made by the patient regarding the offender, but this is a task usually reserved for the police report. The priority is to ensure that the patient feels safe.

Category: Psychosocial and Medical Emergencies/Psychosocial/Abuse and neglect

Nursing Process: Intervention

Reference

Cohen, S. (2013). Intimate partner violence. In B. B. Hammond & P. G. Zimmermann (Eds.), *Sheehy's manual of emergency care* (7th ed., pp. 531–536). St. Louis, MO: Elsevier Mosby.

---

75. The nurse considers which statement regarding pediatric posttraumatic stress disorder (PTSD) to be *false*?

A. Children under the age of 3 do not exhibit signs of pediatric PTSD.
B. School-aged children typically do not have "flashbacks" of the traumatic event.
C. How a parent responds to an infant's needs after a traumatic event has an effect on the child.
D. Teenagers may be expected to be hypervigilant and exhibit impulsive behaviors.

Rationale

A. Signs and symptoms of PTSD may occur at any age following a traumatic event. The presentation varies according to developmental age of the child. Children under the age of 3 can experience PTSD, and symptoms in this age group may include inability to soothe, nightmares, sleep disturbances, or regression from previous developmental milestones.

B. This age group may exhibit hypervigilant behavior to prevent another traumatic event. Their recall of the event may not be accurate, but they typically do not experience flashbacks of the actual event.

C. Infants express their unease by crying. Comforting of the infant by the parent can increase the level of attachment that the infant experiences.

D. It is common for adolescent patients to feel anxiety and to be hypervigilant. The adolescent will exhibit symptoms of a stress response, including increased heart rate, sleep disturbances, and frightening thoughts.

Category (Pediatric): Psychosocial and Medical Emergencies/Psychosocial/Situational crisis

Nursing Process: Assessment

Reference

Rideout, L. C., & Normandin, P. A. (2015). Pediatric post-traumatic stress disorder. *Journal of Emergency Nursing, 41*(6), 531–532.

---

76. The acting out of the emotions of fear or anger is a definition of which of the following?

A. Anxiety
B. Paranoia
C. Violence
D. Panic

Rationale

A. Anxiety is the feeling of fear, worry, and apprehension, often accompanied by physical symptoms.

B. Paranoia is the loss of reality through a delusional thought system. The person believes that someone is out to "get" them.

C. Violence is the acting out of the emotions of fear or anger. This behavior is found in individuals who are paranoid, manic, acutely intoxicated, or sociopathic.

D. Panic is the feeling of intense fear, accompanied by chest pain, shortness of breath, dizziness, and other somatic complaints that often begins without notice.

Category: Psychosocial and Medical Emergencies/Psychosocial/Aggressive/violent behavior

Nursing Process: Assessment

References

Gagnon, L. (2007). Psychiatric/psychosocial emergencies. In K. S. Hoyt & J. Selfridge-Thomas (Eds.), *Emergency nursing core curriculum* (6th ed., pp. 659–684). St. Louis, MO: Saunders Elsevier.

Gagnon, L. (2010). Behavioral health emergencies. In P. K. Howard & R. A. Steinmann (Eds.), *Sheehy's emergency nursing: Principles and practice* (6th ed., pp. 677–688). St. Louis, MO: Mosby Elsevier.

Manton, A. (2013). Mental health emergencies. In B. B. Hammond & P. G. Zimmermann (Eds.), *Sheehy's manual of emergency care* (7th ed., pp. 505–520). St. Louis, MO: Elsevier Mosby.

---

77. A patient presents to the emergency department hyperventilating. On further assessment, the emergency nurse determines that the patient is having a panic attack and encourages the patient to use slow, regular breathing. Which of the following interventions would next be most effective in assisting this patient?

A. Teach the patient the correct way to deal with anxiety
B. Assure the patient that things are going to be OK
C. Listen to the patient with empathy and concern
D. Tell the patient that the emergency team is in control, and everything will be fine.

Rationale

A. It is important to first build a trusting relationship and acknowledge the patient's anxiety. The emergency nurse should then help the patient to identify the precipitating event and what previous coping mechanisms have been effective.

B. It is not therapeutic to offer false or excessive reassurance. Instead, the nurse should acknowledge the patient's anxiety and assure the patient that they are in a safe environment.

C. It is important for the emergency nurse to build a trusting relationship and assure the patient that they are safe.

D. It would be most therapeutic to allow the patient to have some control over the situation and to assist the patient to identify the precipitating event and what previous coping mechanisms have been effective. Offering false reassurance is not effective.

Category: Psychosocial and Medical Emergencies/Psychosocial/Anxiety/panic

Nursing Process: Intervention

References

Gagnon, L. (2007). Psychiatric/psychosocial emergencies. In K. S. Hoyt & J. Selfridge-Thomas (Eds.), *Emergency nursing core curriculum* (6th ed., pp. 659–683). St. Louis, MO: Saunders Elsevier.

Gagnon, L. (2010). Behavioral health emergencies. In P. K. Howard & R. A. Steinmann (Eds.), *Sheehy's emergency nursing: Principles and practice* (6th ed., pp. 677–688). St. Louis, MO: Mosby Elsevier.

Manton, A. (2013). Mental health emergencies. In B. B. Hammond & P. G. Zimmermann (Eds.), *Sheehy's manual of emergency care* (7th ed., pp. 505–520). St. Louis, MO: Elsevier Mosby.

---

78. A teenaged patient presents to the emergency department reporting recent suicidal thoughts. The patient has never experienced these thoughts in the past. The patient's only history is anxiety, which began several months ago for which the family physician recently prescribed some medication. The emergency nurse is aware that which of the following medications can lead to possible suicidal ideation and actions?

A. Benzodiazepine
B. Beta-blocker
C. Selective serotonin reuptake inhibitor
D. Tricyclic antidepressant

Rationale

A. Benzodiazepines are used to treat acute anxiety; however, they are typically not associated with causing suicidal thoughts in pediatric patients.

B. The beta-blocker propranolol (Inderal) is sometimes used to treat anxiety; however, the drug typically does not cause the patient to experience suicidal thoughts. An off-label use for propranolol is the treatment of migraine headaches in children.

C. Selective serotonin reuptake inhibitors (SSRIs) are commonly prescribed for social anxiety disorder and generalized anxiety disorder. SSRIs and serotonin norepinephrine reuptake inhibitors (SNRIs) have both been found to cause suicidal thoughts and actions, especially in teenagers and patients in their early 20s and in patients for whom depression is a comorbid condition. Patients and family members must be informed to watch for signs of suicidal ideation and actions and react immediately if they occur.

D. Tricyclic antidepressants (TCAs) are not the first-line treatment for anxiety, but they may be used in place of other treatments that have failed. Therefore, it is unlikely that a TCA would be a first-line medication prescribed in the treatment of anxiety.

Category: Psychosocial and Medical Emergencies/Psychosocial/Anxiety/panic

Nursing Process: Analysis

References

DeSelm, T. M. (2016). Mood and anxiety disorders. In J. E. Tintinalli, J. Stapczynski, O. Ma, D. M.Yealy, G. D. Meckler, & D. M. Cline (Eds.), *Tintinalli's emergency medicine: A comprehensive study guide* (8th ed.). Retrieved from http://accessemergencymedicine.mhmedical.com/content.aspx?bookid=1658&Sectionid=109448311

Wagers, B., Hariharan, S., Wagers, B., & Hariharan, S. (2014). Psychiatric emergencies. In C. Stone, R. L. Humphries, D. Drigalla, & M. Stephan (Eds.), *CURRENT diagnosis & treatment: Pediatric emergency medicine.* Retrieved from http://accessemergencymedicine.mhmedical.com/content.aspx?bookid=1175&Sectionid=65115102

---

79. A female adolescent presents to triage accompanied by her father. The patient has a deep linear abrasion with yellow drainage surrounded by a reddened area on her forearm. The emergency nurse observes numerous linear abrasions and scars in various stages of healing on both arms. The patient denies suicidal thoughts or attempts. The patient's father states he recently obtained custody of the patient after her mother was arrested, and his daughter has been diagnosed with depression. He asks the nurse why his daughter is cutting herself. What is the best explanation for the emergency nurse to provide for this behavior?

A. "When people cut themselves, they are seeking attention."
B. "Patients who report feeling numb from their depression induce physical pain, which allows them to 'feel something.'"
C. "Your daughter attempted suicide by cutting herself."
D. "Your daughter is seeking pain medication."

Rationale

A. The patient has been diagnosed with depression and has visible signs of depression while in the emergency department (ED). Self-harm is a behavior closely associated with depression and mental illness and should never be ignored.

B. It is important for the patient's father to understand that the patient's self-harming behavior is a symptom of her depression. Self-harm, including cutting and burning, is often seen in patients suffering from depression; it is a coping mechanism for their emotional pain, intense anger, and frustration. It is important for the parent to ensure that the patient receives and complies with treatment for her illness. The family should be instructed to return immediately to the ED if the patient reports thoughts of suicide, if the patient attempts suicide, or if the patient cutting herself causes a serious injury.

C. Self-harm, such as cutting, is typically not meant as a suicide attempt. Some patients use cutting as a coping mechanism for their depression, but others may escalate their self-harm as their condition worsens. It is important for the patient's father to be vigilant while monitoring his daughter's condition and to seek help for any suicidal ideation or attempt immediately.

D. Although some patients do inflict injury on themselves to attempt to obtain pain medication, this is likely not the case with this patient; she is diagnosed with depression, not reporting pain in the ED, and appears to have a history of cutting (based on the scars on her arms).

Category (Pediatric): Psychosocial and Medical Emergencies/Psychosocial/Depression

Nursing Process: Intervention

References

Self-injury/cutting. (2015). *MayoClinic.org*. Retrieved from http://www.mayoclinic.org/diseases-conditions/self-injury/home/ovc-20165425

Teen depression. (2016). *MayoClinic.org*. Retrieved from http://www.mayoclinic.org/diseases-conditions/teen-depression/symptoms-causes/dxc-20164556

---

80. A patient arrives to the emergency department via emergency medical services after being found "passed out in a park." The patient is now awake, smells of alcohol, appears to be intoxicated, and states, "Go away and leave me alone." The patient's spouse reports that the patient has been suffering from depression since their son died a few years ago but believed he had recently been improving. The patient had cleaned out the garage and given items away to friends, and the previous evening, he had spoken of making a will and "getting things in order." This morning, a large amount of alcohol and sleeping pills were found in the home with a letter telling the family "goodbye." Once medically cleared, the emergency nurse anticipates the next step in the patient's treatments will be:

A. to discharge the patient home once he is less intoxicated.
B. to admit the patient to a psychiatric facility.
C. to provide the patient and family with resources for help with alcoholism.
D. to contact adult protective services because the patient was found intoxicated in a park.

Rationale

A. The patient should not be allowed to return home until he is no longer intoxicated and has had a psychiatric evaluation. Returning home at this point could put the patient, his wife, and others in a dangerous situation.

B. The patient's history of depression, coupled with his recent actions, strongly indicates that he was attempting or planning to attempt suicide in the near future. Heavy alcohol use, risky behavior, giving away personal belongings, saying goodbye to family members, wanting to make a will, stockpiling alcohol and sleeping pills, and the goodbye letter (likely a suicide note) to his wife all indicate that the patient needs further evaluation and long-term psychiatric treatment.

C. Although alcohol may play a role in his depression, based on his wife's interview, alcohol was not the root cause of his problems. The patient needs psychiatric treatment for depression and suicidal ideation.

D. Although the patient is making poor decisions, the situation indicates that they are suffering from mental illness rather than incompetence to manage his affairs. There is nothing in the situation that indicates that the patient's wife is an inappropriate caregiver or that there are problems in his home environment. At this time, the patient appears to have an adequate support system but is in need of more intense psychiatric treatment.

Category: Psychosocial and Medical Emergencies/Psychosocial/Suicidal ideation

Nursing Process: Analysis

Reference

MayoClinic. (2015). *Suicide and suicidal thoughts.* Retrieved from https://www.mayoclinic.org/diseases-conditions/suicide/symptoms-causes/syc-20378048

---

81. A patient has just been treated for an allergic reaction to a bee sting. On discharge, the patient is given a prescription for an epinephrine auto injector (EpiPen). What education should the emergency nurse provide to the patient regarding their condition and the use of the EpiPen?

A. If symptoms resolve after use of the EpiPen, the patient does not need to seek further care in the emergency department (ED).

B. The patient must administer the EpiPen at the onset of symptoms following a bee sting and then proceed to the nearest ED immediately after use.

C. The EpiPen should be stored in a safe place at home so the patient always knows where it is located.

D. Because the patient has had one severe anaphylactic reaction, they will likely not experience another similar episode.

Rationale

A. Follow-up in the ED is still necessary after using an EpiPen.

B. Anaphylaxis is a life-threatening condition in which the progression of symptoms can occur rapidly. Patients should have the EpiPen with them at all times and should seek follow-up care in the ED for further evaluation following its use.

C. The patient should have the EpiPen with them when they are away from home. The patient may experience an allergic reaction away from home and may not have enough time to return home for the EpiPen before allergic symptoms begin to appear.

D. Allergic reactions tend to become more severe with each exposure to the antigen trigger. Therefore, the patient is at risk for a more severe reaction the next time they are stung by a bee.

Category: Psychosocial and Medical Emergencies/Medical/Allergic reactions and anaphylaxis

Nursing Process: Intervention

Reference

Yunker, N. S., & Wagner, B. J. (2014). A pharmacologic review of anaphylaxis. *Plastic Surgical Nursing, 34*(4), 183–189. https://doi.org/10.1097/PSN.0000000000000072

---

82. A patient with a history of bipolar disorder presents to the emergency department complaining of increased thirst, excessive urination, a headache, and vision changes. The emergency nurse identifies that which of the following medications is the most likely cause of the patient's symptoms?

A. Ziprasidone (Geodon)
B. Haloperidol (Haldol)
C. Lithium
D. Carbamazepine (Tegretol)

Rationale

A. Ziprasidone is a second-generation antipsychotic. Side effects include anticholinergic and extrapyramidal symptoms, but the risk is lower than with the first-generation medications such as haloperidol. Medications in this class can cause QT prolongation and hyperglycemia.

B. Haloperidol is a first-generation antipsychotic. Side effects include the development of anticholinergic effects and extrapyramidal symptoms, including akathisia (increased agitation and restlessness), QT prolongation, and lowering of the seizure threshold.

C. Lithium, a heavy metal and antimanic mood stabilizer, is a medication used for patients with bipolar disorder. Chronic use of this medication can lead to nephrogenic diabetes insipidus. Patients will experience polyuria, dehydration, headaches, vision changes, and, in severe cases, seizures. Hypernatremia, hypercalcemia, and hypokalemia are common electrolyte alterations.

D. Carbamazepine is an antiepileptic medication. Side effects include vision changes, and chronic use can lead to syndrome of inappropriate antidiuretic hormone. Because of the increased release of antidiuretic hormone, there is increased water reabsorption. The patient can experience weight gain and dilutional hyponatremia, leading to altered mental status and seizures.

Category: Psychosocial and Medical Emergencies/Psychosocial/Bipolar disorder

Nursing Process: Evaluation

References

Meltzer, H. (2012). Antipsychotic agents and lithium. In B. G. Katzung, S. B. Masters, & A. J. Trevor (Eds.), *Basic and clinical pharmacology* (12th ed., pp. 501–520). New York, NY: McGraw-Hill Lange.

White, M. H., & Overman, C. M. (2015). Diabetes insipidus. In J. J. Schaider, A. Z. Barkin, R. M. Barkin, P. Shayne, R. E. Wolfe, S. R. Hayden, & P. Rosen, (Eds.), *Rosen and Barkin's 5-minute emergency medicine consult* (5th ed., pp. 306–307). Philadelphia, PA: Wolters Kluwer.

---

83. What is the most common physical complaint exhibited by children being evaluated in the emergency department that is symptomatic of both depression and mood disorders?

A. Increased fatigue
B. Recent change in the child's weight
C. Changes in sleep
D. Frequent unexplained "stomach pains"

Rationale

A. Complaints of fatigue and changes in sleep patterns may be signs of depression, but the most common physical complaint is stomach pains, followed by a complaint of headaches.

B. Weight loss or gain may be experienced with depression or mood disorders, but the most common physical complaint is stomach pains, followed by a complaint of headaches.

C. Changes in sleep or inability to sleep may be signs of depression; the most common physical complaint is stomach pains, followed by a complaint of headaches.

D. The most common physical complaint of children being evaluated in the emergency department that is symptomatic of both depression and mood disorders is frequent stomach pains. This is followed by complaints of headaches. A loss of interest in school and poor school performance may also be reported. Parents will often keep their children out of school or have them evaluated by their provider numerous times without physiologic findings for the child's symptoms.

Category (Pediatric): Psychosocial and Medical Emergencies/Psychosocial/Depression

Nursing Process: Assessment

References

Gagnon, L. (2010). Behavioral health emergencies. In P. K. Howard & R. A. Steinmann (Eds.), *Sheehy's emergency nursing: Principles and practice* (6th ed., pp. 677–688). St. Louis, MO: Mosby Elsevier.

Hart, B. (2012). Behavioral emergencies. In *Emergency Nursing Pediatric Course: Provider manual* (4th ed., pp. 317–328). Des Plaines, IL: Emergency Nurses Association.

Manton, A. (2013). Mental health emergencies. In B. B. Hammond & P. G. Zimmermann (Eds.), *Sheehy's manual of emergency care* (7th ed., pp. 505–520). St. Louis, MO: Elsevier Mosby.

---

84. A schizophrenic patient who has been hearing voices telling them to kill their children is presently in a manic state after receiving haloperidol (Haldol) in the emergency department for their aggressive behavior. The emergency nurse should be prepared to administer which of the following medications if the patient should develop side effects related to haloperidol?

A. Lorazepam (Ativan)
B. Diphenhydramine (Benadryl)
C. Promethazine (Phenergan)
D. Ziprasidone (Geodon)

Rationale

A. Lorazepam is a benzodiazepine used in conjunction with haloperidol to treat the symptoms of aggressive behavior. Lorazepam will not reverse the dystonic effects of haloperidol.

B. Individuals receiving the antipsychotic medication haloperidol can experience dystonic reactions, such as tightening of the neck muscles and repetitive uncontrollable extruding of the tongue through the oral cavity. Diphenhydramine and benztropine are used to reverse the dystonic effects of haloperidol.

C. Promethazine is an antihistamine and antiemetic. Promethazine will not reverse the dystonic effects of haloperidol.

D. Ziprasidone is another antipsychotic medication. It is not used to treat the dystonic reaction related to the administration of haloperidol.

Category: Psychosocial and Medical Emergencies/Psychosocial/Homicidal ideation

Nursing Process: Intervention

References

Citrome, L. (2015). Aggression. *Medscape Drugs, Diseases, and Procedures.* Retrieved from http://emedicine.medscape.com/article/288689-overview#a4

Haldol. (2016). *RxList.* Retrieved from http://www.rxlist.com/haldol-drug/patient-images-side-effects.htm

---

85. Which of the following medications would be administered to manage a patient's severe agitation in the emergency department?

A. Ketamine
B. Haloperidol (Haldol)
C. Lorazepam (Ativan)
D. Fentanyl (Duragesic)

Rationale

A. Ketamine produces sedative dissociation and analgesia. Some research supports its use for rapid take-down in patients who are an imminent danger to themselves or others, but at present, it is not routinely recommended in the use of acute psychotic symptoms.

B. Haloperidol is an antipsychotic agent that may be used to treat acute psychosis, but it takes longer to act than lorazepam. It does have potential side effects, such as dystonia, dysrhythmias, and hyperpyrexia.

C. Lorazepam is a sedative-hypnotic that can be administered orally, by intravenous, or by intramuscular injection. It has a relatively rapid onset and a shorter half-life than other medications. It is also used to treat anxiety and alcohol withdrawal that can also appear to be a psychotic episode.

D. Fentanyl is a potent opioid medication that can provide sedation and analgesia. It has severe side effects, including respiratory depression. It is currently not recommended as a medication for psychotic agitation.

Category: Psychosocial and Medical Emergencies/Psychosocial/Psychosis

Nursing Process: Intervention

Reference

Deal, N., & Matorin, A. (2015). Stabilization and management of the acutely agitated or psychotic patient. *Emergency Medicine Clinics of North America, 33*, 739–752.

---

86. Hemorrhagic signs that indicate the presence of disseminated intravascular coagulation include:

A. purpura.
B. gangrene of the fingers.
C. bowel infarction.
D. renal failure.

Rationale

A. Two mechanisms cause the signs and symptoms of disseminated intravascular coagulation. Hemorrhagic signs result from the inability of the blood to clot, leading to the presence of petechiae, purpura, hemoptysis, and hematuria.

B. Gangrene of the digits results from the second mechanism, which is thrombosis that occurs in the microcirculation. In this case, circulation is compromised to the fingers, resulting in gangrene and necrosis.

C. Bowel infarction results from the second mechanism, which is thrombosis that occurs in the microcirculation. In this case, circulation is compromised because of thrombosis to the mesentery, resulting in an infarction of the bowel.

D. Renal failure results from the second mechanism, which is thrombosis that occurs in the microcirculation. In this case, circulation is compromised because of thrombosis to the kidneys, resulting in renal failure.

Category: Psychosocial and Medical Emergencies/Medical/Disseminated intravascular coagulation (DIC)

Nursing Process: Assessment

Reference

Smith, D. A. (2010). Hematologic and oncologic emergencies. In P. K. Howard & R. A. Steinmann (Eds.), *Sheehy's emergency nursing: Principles and practice* (6th ed., pp. 554–563). St. Louis, MO: Mosby Elsevier.

---

87. The emergency nurse is caring for a patient who states they are receiving chemotherapy for breast cancer. The patient lives alone and has a pet. Which type of pet would be most concerning as a possible source of infection for this patient?

A. Fish
B. Cat
C. Dog
D. Ant farm

Rationale

A. Aquarium fish typically do not transmit diseases to humans.

B. Toxoplasmosis is caused by the one-celled protozoan parasite *Toxoplasma gondii*. Humans may acquire toxsoplasmosis in several ways, including contact with animal excrement, specifically via cleaning a cat litter box. Cats that go outside are more likely to be carriers of the parasite than cats kept exclusively indoors. Toxoplasmosis is an opportunistic infection seen in those who are immunocompromised.

C. If the dog is house trained, the patient should not have frequent contact with fecal matter. If they walk the dog and must clean up bowel movements, they should be encouraged to wear gloves and a mask and wash their hands frequently.

D. Ant farms are contained. It is unlikely the patient will contact an infection from the ants.

Category: Psychosocial and Medical Emergencies/Medical/Immunocompromise
Nursing Process: Analysis

Reference

Centers for Disease Control and Prevention. (2018). Toxoplasmosis. Retrieved from https://www.cdc.gov/parasites/toxoplasmosis/

---

88. Which of the following diagnostic interventions would have the highest priority to be performed in a patient with hemophilia who presents to the emergency department with altered mental status following a fall?

A. Cervical spine radiograph
B. Serum coagulation studies
C. Computed tomography scan of the head
D. Blood gas

Rationale

A. Imaging of the cervical spine is indicated in patients who have sustained a fall, but when the patient also has an altered mental status, a computed tomography (CT) scan of the head to assess for intracranial hemorrhage is the most important diagnostic test. A CT scan of the spine is preferred to radiographs in most trauma patients.

B. Serum coagulation studies are indicated in the hemophilic trauma patient; however, when the patient has an altered mental status, a CT scan of the head to assess for intracranial hemorrhage has the highest priority.

C. In the hemophilic trauma patient with altered mental status, a CT scan of the head is the most important diagnostic test to assess for the presence of an intracranial hemorrhage.

D. A blood gas would help evaluate for the presence of hypoxia as the possible cause of altered mental status in a trauma patient. However, in the hemophilic trauma patient with altered mental status, a CT scan of the head to assess for intracranial hemorrhage has the highest priority.

Category: Psychosocial and Medical Emergencies/Medical/Blood dyscrasias: Hemophilia
Nursing Process: Intervention

References

Bowman, S. H., & Georgopoulos, C. H. (2015). Hemophilia. In J. J. Schaider, R. M. Barkin, S. R. Hayden, R. E Wolfe, A. Z. Barkin, P. Shayne, & P. Rosen. (Eds.), *Rosen and Barkin's 5-minute emergency medicine consult* (5th ed., pp. 502–503). Philadelphia, PA: Wolters Kluwer.

Croteau, S. E., Fleegler, E. W., & Brett-Fleegler, M. (2016). Hematologic emergencies. In K. N. Shaw & R. G. Bachur (Eds.), *Fleisher and Ludwig's textbook of pediatric emergency medicine* (7th ed., pp. 804–837). Philadelphia, PA: Wolters Kluwer.

---

89. Which of the following skin conditions is most closely associated with leukemia?

A. Petechiae
B. Skin bronzing
C. Jaundice
D. Erythematous rash

Rationale

A. Petechiae and ecchymoses are often seen in patients with leukemia related to the presence of thrombocytopenia.

B. Skin bronzing and hyperpigmentation is closely associated with hemochromatosis, the buildup of excessive iron in the body.

C. Jaundice may eventually occur in patients with leukemia, but it is more commonly associated with patients who have liver disease.

D. Erythematous rash is not commonly associated with leukemia. This type of rash is present in patients with rubella or rubeola.

Category: Psychosocial and Medical Emergencies/Medical/Blood dyscrasias: Leukemia

Nursing Process: Assessment

Reference

Bickley, L. S., & Szilagyi, P. G. (Eds.). (2013). The skin, hair, and nails. In *Bates' guide to physical examination and history* (11th ed., pp. 171–204). Philadelphia, PA: Wolters Kluwer/Lippincott Williams & Wilkins.

---

90. A patient presents to triage with a history of increasing fatigue and extreme pallor. The patient is suspected of having undiagnosed leukemia. Which of the following interventions should the emergency nurse prepare for?

A. Lumbar puncture
B. Initiation of the first dose of chemotherapy
C. Administration of nonsteroidal anti-inflammatory drugs
D. Bone marrow aspiration

Rationale

A. Lumbar punctures are commonly performed in the emergency department (ED) and are part of a comprehensive work-up. The definitive diagnosis of leukemia is usually done after consultation with a hematologist or oncologist. Once the type of leukemia is identified, a treatment plan is initiated.

B. Definitive treatment such as chemotherapy will be initiated in a stable, controlled inpatient setting after confirmative diagnostic evaluation occurs. Chemotherapy is not initiated in the ED unless by a nurse specially trained in the administration of chemotherapy.

C. Acetaminophen may be administered and is preferred over nonsteroidal anti-inflammatory drugs (NSAIDs) such as ibuprofen. Ibuprofen should be avoided in patients with thrombocytopenia because of the increased risk of bleeding with the administration of NSAIDs.

D. Bone marrow aspiration is a confirmative diagnostic test for leukemia, but this test is not typically completed in the ED. It will typically be performed following consultation with a hematologist or oncologist.

Category: Psychosocial and Medical Emergencies/Medical/Blood dyscrasias: Leukemia

Nursing Process: Intervention

References

Carringer, C. J., & Hammond, B. B. (2013). Hematologic and immunologic emergencies. In B. B. Hammond & P. G. Zimmermann (Eds.), *Sheehy's manual of emergency care* (7th ed., pp. 245–254). St. Louis, MO: Elsevier Mosby.

Hunt, S. (2007). Hematologic/oncologic emergencies. In K. S. Hoyt & J. Selfridge-Thomas (Eds.), *Emergency nursing core curriculum* (6th ed., pp. 409–437). St. Louis, MO: Saunders Elsevier.

---

91. A major trauma victim has received multiple transfusions of blood products. Which of the following electrolytes has the highest priority for the emergency nurse to monitor?

A. Serum calcium
B. Serum glucose
C. Serum sodium
D. Serum phosphate

Rationale

A. The anticoagulant often used in banked blood products is citrate, which can bind to serum calcium, resulting in the patient developing hypocalcemia.

B. Monitoring serum glucose in a critically ill or injured patient is important, however, blood glucose levels are not typically affected by the administration of blood products.

C. Monitoring of all electrolytes is important in a critically ill or injured patient, but sodium levels are not typically affected by the administration of blood products.

D. Monitoring of all electrolytes is important in a critically ill or injured patient, but phosphate levels are not typically affected by the administration of blood products.

Category: Psychosocial and Medical Emergencies/Medical/Electrolyte/fluid imbalance

Nursing Process: Analysis

References

Calder, S. (2013). Shock. In B. B. Hammond & P. G. Zimmermann (Eds.), *Sheehy's manual of emergency care* (7th ed., pp. 213–222). St. Louis, MO: Elsevier Mosby.

Pentecost, D. A., & Smith, S. G. (2014). Shock. In D. Gurney (Ed.), *Trauma Nursing Core Course: Provider manual* (7th ed., pp. 73–90). Des Plaines, IL: Emergency Nurses Association.

---

92. A patient presents to the emergency department and states they are experiencing a sickle cell episode. The nurse knows that a pathophysiologic change occurs in a sickle cell episode when:

A. leukocytes assume a sickled shape and clump together in the micro vasculature.
B. platelets assume a sickled shape and clump together in the micro vasculature.
C. red blood cells assume a sickled shape and clump together in the micro vasculature.
D. neutrophils assume a sickled shape and clump together in the microvasculature.

Rationale

A. It is the red blood cells (RBCs) in sickle cell disease that become sickled in shape and clump together, causing vaso-occlusive crisis and pain. The leukocytes do not assume a sickle shape, nor do they clump together.

B. In sickle cell disease, the RBCs become sickled in shape and clump together, causing vaso-occlusive crisis and pain. In a sickle cell episode, the platelets do not assume a sickle shape, nor do they clump together.

C. In sickle cell disease, RBCs contain abnormal hemoglobin (HbS) that precipitates into long crystals when exposed to cold temperatures, low O_2, dehydration, infection, or strenuous exercise. This causes the RBCs to assume a sickle shape, resulting in the cells clumping together.

D. It is the RBCs in sickle cell disease that become sickled in shape and clump together, causing vaso-occlusive crisis and pain. Neutrophils do not assume a sickle shape, nor do they clump together.

Category: Psychosocial and Medical Emergencies/Medical/Blood dyscrasias/Sickle cell crisis

Nursing Process: Assessment

Reference

Smith, D. A. (2010). Hematologic and oncologic emergencies. In P. K. Howard & R. A. Steinmann (Eds.), *Sheehy's emergency nursing: Principles and practice* (6th ed., pp. 554–563). St. Louis, MO: Mosby Elsevier.

---

93. Which medication does the emergency nurse anticipate to be administered to a patient who is being treated for an adrenal crisis because of the lack of aldosterone?

A. Spironolactone (Aldactone)
B. Metoprolol (Lopressor)
C. Dexamethasone (Decadron)
D. Nicardipine (Cardene)

Rationale

A. Fludrocortisone is a synthetic mineralocorticoid that would be appropriate to administer to the patient who is experiencing an adrenal crisis. The drug causes reabsorption of sodium and excretion of potassium and hydrogen ions from the distal renal tubules.

B. Metoprolol is a beta-blocker and would not correct the patient's lack of aldosterone.

C. Dexamethasone is the drug of choice for adrenal crisis because it does not interfere with plasma cortisol measurements. Hydrocortisone may be used for patients with known adrenal insufficiency.

D. Nicardipine is a calcium channel blocker and would not correct the patient's lack of aldosterone.

Category: Psychosocial and Medical Emergencies/Medical/Endocrine conditions: Adrenal

Nursing Process: Intervention

References

Sommers, M. S., & Fannin, E. (2015). *Diseases and disorders: A nursing therapeutics manual* (5th ed.). Philadelphia, PA: F. A. Davis Company.

Vallerand, A. H., Sanoski, C. A., & Deglin, J. H. (2017). *Davis's drug guide for nurses* (15th ed.). Philadelphia, PA: F. A. Davis Company.

94. The emergency nurse is caring for a patient with diabetic ketoacidosis. Which of the following values would *best* indicate that this patient is improving?

A. Respiratory rate of 16 breaths/minute
B. Pulse rate of 108 beats/minute
C. Blood pressure 138/72
D. Pulse oximetry 98%

Rationale

A. A patient being treated for diabetic ketoacidosis (DKA) will demonstrate improvement by the normalization in the patient's respiratory rate. An increased respiratory rate in a patient with diabetes is an indicator of the DKA disease process.

B. A patient experiencing DKA will demonstrate tachycardia (heart rate greater than 100 beats/minute) secondary to the presence of dehydration. A heart rate of 108 beats/minute indicates that the patient continues to be dehydrated.

C. Patients with DKA do not usually have variances in their blood pressure reading; therefore, the patient's blood pressure value is not the best indicator that the patient's condition is improving.

D. The PaO_2 of a patient with DKA is usually within normal range. Thus, the pulse oximetry reading would be normal even though a pathophysiological state is occurring. Therefore, oxygen saturation is not the best indicator of patient improvement.

Category: Psychosocial and Medical Emergencies/Medical/Endocrine conditions: Glucose-related conditions

Nursing Process: Analysis

References

Marett, B. E. (2013). Metabolic emergencies. In B. B. Hammond & P. G. Zimmermann (Eds.), *Sheehy's manual of emergency care* (7th ed., pp. 303–318). St. Louis, MO: Elsevier Mosby.
Morey, C. M. (2010). Endocrine emergencies. In P. K. Howard & R. A. Steinmann (Eds.), *Sheehy's emergency nursing: Principles and practice* (6th ed., pp. 499–512). St. Louis, MO: Mosby Elsevier.

---

95. Which of the following statements made by the patient reveals to the emergency nurse an understanding of the discharge instructions regarding how to avoid further episodes of hypoglycemia?

A. "As long as I check my glucose daily, I will not have further hypoglycemic reactions."
B. "I will keep a couple of pieces of candy with me at all times."
C. "I will eat small, frequent meals throughout the day and monitor my blood glucose before meals and at bedtime."
D. "I will keep my glucose oral gel with me at work, at school, and when I play sports."

Rationale

A. Patients with frequent episodes of hypoglycemia should check their blood glucose throughout the day, on arising in the morning, before meals, and again at bedtime.

B. In patients with frequent hypoglycemic reactions, candy may not provide enough carbohydrates to adequately treat their hypoglycemia.

C. Eating 4–6 small meals that contain at least 15 g of carbohydrates and monitoring their blood glucose at least 4 times daily is recommended for patients who experience frequent episodes of hypoglycemia.

D. Oral glucose gel should only be administered to a conscious, alert patient who is hypoglycemic. However, the administration of the glucose gel may not be enough to increase the patient's blood glucose levels. Therefore, following the administration of oral glucose gel, at least an additional 15 g of carbohydrate should also be offered to the patient.

Category: Psychosocial and Medical Emergencies/Medical/Endocrine conditions: Glucose-related conditions

Nursing Process: Evaluation

References

Marett, B. E. (2013). Metabolic emergencies. In B. B. Hammond & P. G. Zimmermann (Eds.), *Sheehy's manual of emergency care* (7th ed., pp. 303–318). St. Louis, MO: Elsevier Mosby.

Morey, C. M. (2010). Endocrine emergencies. In P. K. Howard & R. A. Steinmann (Eds.), *Sheehy's emergency nursing: Principles and practice* (6th ed., pp. 499–512). St. Louis, MO: Mosby Elsevier.

---

96. A patient with elevated T3 and T4 levels has a temperature of 40.1°C (104.3°F). Which medication should be avoided to control this patient's fever?

A. Ibuprofen (Motrin)
B. Acetaminophen (Tylenol)
C. Naproxen (Naprosyn)
D. Aspirin (acetylsalicylic acid)

Rationale

A. Ibuprofen is a nonsteroidal anti-inflammatory drug that may assist with lowering temperature, decreasing pain, and alleviating inflammation, but it is not the primary antipyretic of choice.

B. Tylenol does not displace the thyroid hormone from binding sites and will assist with fever reduction.

C. Naproxen is a nonsteroidal anti-inflammatory drug that will assist in the management of inflammation and pain. Its primary action is not to lower body temperature as an antipyretic medication would.

D. Aspirin should be avoided because it may further increase T4 levels by displacing the thyroid hormones from and interfering with protein-binding sites. Increased thyroxine levels will lead to a worsening of the patient's clinical condition.

Category: Psychosocial and Medical Emergencies/Medical/Endocrine conditions: Thyroid

Nursing Process: Analysis

References

Marett, B. E. (2013). Metabolic emergencies. In B. B. Hammond & P. G. Zimmermann (Eds.), *Sheehy's manual of emergency care* (7th ed., pp. 303–318). St. Louis, MO: Elsevier Mosby.

Morey, C. M. (2010). Endocrine emergencies. In P. K. Howard & R. A. Steinmann (Eds.), *Sheehy's emergency nursing: Principles and practice* (6th ed., pp. 499–512). St. Louis, MO: Mosby Elsevier.

97. Which of the following assessment findings should the emergency nurse be most concerned about in a patient who presents with a fever of unknown origin?

A. **Altered mental status**
B. Tachycardia
C. Nasal congestion
D. Rash

Rationale

A. Altered mental status in any patient is very concerning. In a patient who also presents with fever, the emergency nurse should be concerned about the possibility of a life-threatening problem such as a central nervous system infection, which could lead to seizures and potential loss of the patient's airway.

B. Tachycardia is an expected finding in the patient with a fever. This increase in heart rate usually is not serious and resolves as the fever resolves. Other assessment findings, such as an altered mental status, are more concerning.

C. Nasal congestion is often experienced with upper respiratory infections, but this rarely causes a serious airway problem. The patient should be monitored for airway compromise. Other assessment findings, such as altered mental status, are more concerning.

D. A rash in the presence of fever can be associated with certain viral and bacterial infections. However, neurologic findings, such as altered mental status, are more concerning.

Category: Psychosocial and Medical Emergencies/Medical/Fever

Nursing Process: Analysis

References

Lazear, S. E., & Roberts, A. (2007). Medical emergencies. In K. S. Hoyt & J. Selfridge-Thomas (Eds.), *Emergency nursing core curriculum* (6th ed., pp. 483–508). St. Louis, MO: Saunders Elsevier.

Sterling, S. A., & Jones, A. E. (2015). Fever. In A. B. Wolfson (Ed.), *Harwood-Nuss' clinical practice of emergency medicine* (6th ed., pp. 74–79). Philadelphia, PA: Wolters Kluwer.

---

98. A patient presents to the emergency department complaining of swollen lymph nodes, generalized aches and pains, and a headache. The patient has recently been receiving chemotherapy for breast cancer. The patient states they live alone, and their only companion is their pet cat. In providing education to the patient, the emergency nurse acknowledges the patient's understanding of the cause of the infection when they makes the following statement:

A. "I should have had someone clean my fish tank for me, instead of doing it myself."
B. **"I should have had someone clean the cat litter box for me."**
C. "I'll have to have someone help me by walking my dog."
D. "I'll have to get rid of the ant farm that I maintain for work."

Rationale

A. Aquarium fish typically do not transmit diseases to humans.

B. Toxoplasmosis is caused by the one-celled protozoan parasite *Toxoplasma gondii*. Humans may acquire toxoplasmosis through contact with undercooked meat, contaminated water, and animal excrement, specifically cleaning a cat litter box. Cats that are allowed to go outside are more likely to be carriers of the parasite than cats kept exclusively indoors. Toxoplasmosis is an opportunistic infection seen in those who are immunocompromised.

C. The patient should not have contact with the dog's fecal matter, but walking the dog is not contraindicated. If they have to clean up the dog's bowel movements, the patient should wear gloves and a mask, and wash their hands frequently.

D. Ant farms are contained. It is unlikely that the patient will contract an infection from the ants.

Category: Psychosocial and Medical Emergencies/Medical/Immunocompromise

Nursing Process: Evaluation

Reference

Beddoe, A. E., & Lawrence, P. (2016). Toxoplasmosis, cerebral. *CINAHL nursing guide.* Ipswich, MA: EBSCO Publishing.

---

99. A patient has unintentionally amputated the distal end of their middle finger. The emergency department nurse is aware that the proper care of the amputated part is to perform which of the following?

A. **Rinse the amputated part in normal saline, wrap in saline moistened gauze, secure it in a plastic bag, and then place it on a bed of ice.**
B. Place the amputated part directly in ice water.
C. Immediately rinse the amputated part with distilled water to remove dirt and debris, place it back onto the injury site, and secure it with a sterile gauze dressing.
D. Place the amputated part in a sterile dressing and then place it into a cold milk solution.

Rationale

A. The amputated part is preserved for reimplantation by wrapping it in saline-moistened gauze and placing it in a plastic bag or container. The sealed container is then placed on top of crushed ice and water. This cools the part without causing direct damage to tissue.

B. If the amputated part is placed directly in water or on ice, cells can be damaged by water moving across the cellular membranes, including cellular freezing and cell death.

C. Distilled water is not used because of its deleterious effect on tissue. The amputated part needs to be cooled. Placing the amputated part back onto the injury site will not cool the amputated digit and will damage the tissue.

D. A cold milk solution is indicated for tooth avulsions, but it is not indicated for the treatment of an amputated limb.

Category: Maxillofacial, Ocular, Orthopedic, and Wound Emergencies/Orthopedic/Amputation

Nursing Process: Intervention

Reference

Cerepani, M. J. (2010). Orthopedic and neurovascular trauma. In P. K. Howard & R. A. Steinmann (Eds.), *Sheehy's emergency nursing: Principles and practice* (6th ed., pp. 313–339). St. Louis, MO: Mosby Elsevier.

---

100. An elderly male presents to the emergency department complaining of a swollen left knee that is reddened and warm to touch. Bursitis of the knee is diagnosed, and the emergency provider performs a knee aspiration in order to:

A. administer prophylactic antibiotics directly into the joint space.
B. obtain a gram stain and culture of the synovial fluid.
C. remove the knee cyst.
D. prevent further infection.

Rationale

A. Oral antibiotics are indicated after a bursa is aspirated and the cause of the infection is identified. Antibiotics are not injected directly into the joint space.

B. Bursitis is inflammation of a bursa, a saclike structure that covers the bony prominence among bones, muscles, and tendons. The bursa contains only a small amount of viscous (synovial) fluid. It is important to determine whether the bursitis is the result of inflammation or infection, because the definitive therapy will differ depending on the cause of the bursitis.

C. Inflammation of a bursa is the result of trauma (e.g., a direct blow or a chronic injury associated with prolonged, repetitive use) or infection (bacterial or fungal).

D. Oral antibiotics are indicated after the fluid in the bursa is aspirated and the cause of the infection is identified.

Category (Geriatric): Maxillofacial, Ocular, Orthopedic, and Wound Emergencies/Orthopedic/Inflammatory conditions

Nursing Process: Analysis

Reference

Cerepani, M. J., & Ramponi, D. R. (2007). Orthopedic emergencies. In K. S. Hoyt & J. Selfridge-Thomas (Eds.), *Emergency nursing core curriculum* (6th ed., pp. 585–603). St Louis, MO: Saunders Elsevier.

101. A patient has sustained a forearm fracture. Following the application of a short-arm cast, the emergency nurse will assess sensation and motion of the patient's fingers. Numbness and tingling at the tips of the index and middle fingers may indicate compromise of which nerve?

A. Radial nerve
B. Peroneal nerve
C. Median nerve
D. Ulnar nerve

Rationale

A. Check for sensation and motor function at the dorsum of the hand from the thumb to the middle of the ring finger.

B. The peroneal nerve is a division of the sciatic nerve. Check for sensation at the web space between the first and second toes and for sensation of the lateral area of the lower leg and the dorsum of the foot.

C. To assess for motor function of the median nerve, oppose the thumb to the other fingers. Check for sensation at the palmar aspect of the hand, from midthumb to the middle of the ring finger, and the tips of the index, long, and ring fingers.

D. Check for sensation and motor function at the dorsum of the hand in the middle of the ring finger and small finger.

Category: Maxillofacial, Ocular, Orthopedic, and Wound Emergencies/Orthopedic/Fractures/dislocations

Nursing Process: Assessment

Reference

Halpern, J. S. (2013). Musculoskeletal trauma. In B. B. Hammond & P. G. Zimmermann (Eds.), *Sheehy's manual of emergency care* (7th ed., pp. 427–438). St. Louis, MO: Elsevier Mosby.

---

102. Which of the following assessment findings would lead the emergency nurse to suspect that a patient with a fracture of the left femur may be developing a fat embolus?

A. Acute dyspnea
B. Numbness and tingling of the left leg
C. Clusterlike headaches
D. Muscle spasms of the left leg

Rationale

A. Respiratory distress, including dyspnea and hypoxia, is a classic presentation associated with the presence of fat emboli syndrome.

B. Numbness, tingling, or loss of sensation may occur as nerves and blood vessels are compressed, such as with compartment syndrome. These symptoms are not associated with the presence of a fat embolus.

C. Clusterlike headaches are not an assessment finding in patients who are developing a fat embolus. Symptoms of fat embolus are often nonspecific and may mimic other conditions—including pleuritic chest pain, myocardial infarction, and panic attacks—but not headaches. Anxiety, apprehension, and restlessness are common signs and symptoms of a fat embolus.

D. Numbness, tingling, or loss of sensation may occur as nerves and blood vessels are compressed. With loss of sensation, there may be a relief of pain. This is indicative of a worsening perfusion, not an improvement.

Category: Maxillofacial, Ocular, Orthopedic, and Wound Emergencies/Orthopedic/Trauma

Nursing Process: Assessment

Reference

Walsh, R. (2013). Respiratory emergencies. In B. B. Hammond & P. G. Zimmermann (Eds.), *Sheehy's manual of emergency care* (7th ed., pp. 185–199). St. Louis, MO: Elsevier Mosby.

---

103. The emergency nurse is caring for a patient who presented with increasing arm pain following a long-arm splint application 2 days ago for an olecranon fracture. Assessment of the affected extremity reveals +1 radial pulse, a pale hand, and inability to wiggle or move the fingers. The patient is requesting pain medication. The emergency nurse identifies that the priority intervention for this patient is to:

A. apply ice to the extremity.
B. administer pain medication to the patient.
C. remove or loosen the long-arm splint.
D. elevate the extremity.

Rationale

A. Applying ice to the injured extremity causes vasoconstriction of the vessels, which can further limit circulation within the affected arm.

B. The patient may require pain medication, but the first priority intervention is to remove the splint.

C. The patient is experiencing compartment syndrome. The splint may be increasing the intracompartmental pressure and should be removed or loosened immediately. Signs and symptoms of compartment syndrome are pain, pallor, pulselessness, paresthesia paralysis, and pressure.

D. Elevating the extremity can decrease arterial blood flow, thereby limiting tissue perfusion to the extremity. The extremity should not be raised above the level of the heart.

Category: Maxillofacial, Ocular, Orthopedic, and Wound Emergencies/Orthopedic/Compartment syndrome

Nursing Process: Intervention

Reference

Cerepani, M. J., & Ramponi, D. R. (2007). Orthopedic emergencies. In K. S. Hoyt & J. Selfridge-Thomas (Eds.), *Emergency nursing core curriculum* (6th ed., pp. 891–928). St. Louis, MO: Saunders Elsevier.

---

104. A patient presents to the emergency department following blunt trauma to the right upper leg and is diagnosed with a contusion. On receiving discharge instructions, the emergency nurse identifies the patient's understanding when they state:

A. "I will apply heat and ice to my leg and keep a loose gauze dressing over the injured area."
B. "I will apply heat to my leg, have my leg dangle, and leave the wound open to air."
C. "I will apply ice to the bruise on my leg, make sure the ace wrap is secure around my leg, and keep my leg elevated."
D. "I will let the leg dangle, and I will apply loose gauze directly over the injured area."

Rationale

A. Heat can cause vasodilatation, which will increase swelling, and so should be avoided. A loose gauze dressing will not provide any benefit to the injured area. Keeping the leg elevated is a correct intervention for this patient's injury.

B. Applying heat to the contusion can promote vasodilation, which can increase swelling and will not aid in tissue healing. Allowing the leg to be dependent and not keeping it elevated may promote additional swelling. The application of a compression or pressure type dressing can act to decrease swelling at the site.

C. Applying ice to the injured area will cause vasoconstriction, which will reduce the amount of swelling and possible bleeding. Using compression or pressure dressings and keeping the injured leg elevated also act to reduce bleeding and swelling in the injured area.

D. Ice will help decrease swelling because it causes vasoconstriction. Keeping the leg dependent and not elevated may promote further swelling of the injured area; applying a pressure dressing such as an ACE bandage may help decrease swelling.

Category: Maxillofacial, Ocular, Orthopedic, and Wound Emergencies/Orthopedic/Contusions
Nursing Process: Evaluation

Reference

Cerepani, M. J., & Ramponi, D. R. (2007). Orthopedic emergencies. In K. S. Hoyt & J. Selfridge-Thomas (Eds.), *Emergency nursing core curriculum* (6th ed., pp. 891–928). St. Louis, MO: Saunders Elsevier.

---

105. A patient presents to the emergency department after falling and sustaining multiple contusions to their trunk, right upper extremity, and right lower extremity. On reviewing the patient's list of current prescribed medications, the emergency nurse identifies that the patient is at risk for complications from their multiple contusions related to which of the following?

A. Hydroxychloroquine (Plaquenil)
B. Clopidogrel (Plavix)
C. Ciprofloxacin (Cipro)
D. Acetaminophen (Tylenol)

Rationale

A. Hydroxychloroquine is an antimalarial/antiprotozoal medication that is also used to treat inflammation for autoimmune diseases like lupus. This medication would not place the patient at risk for complications related to contusion.

B. Plavix is an antiplatelet medication that can increase risk of bleeding/hemorrhage. In addition, there is an increased risk for compartment syndrome because of bleeding and swelling in the extremity. Other medications that can place a patient at increased risk for complications related to contusions include warfarin, rivaroxaban, and aspirin.

C. Ciprofloxacin is an antibiotic that has an increased risk of tendon rupture associated with its administration. There is no known risk of complications related to the presence of contusions when taking ciprofloxacin.

D. Acetaminophen is a nonnarcotic analgesic and is not associated with an increased risk of complications in the presence of a contusion.

Category: Maxillofacial, Ocular, Orthopedic, and Wound Emergencies/Orthopedic/Contusions
Nursing Process: Assessment

References

Cerepani, M. J., & Ramponi, D. R. (2007). Orthopedic emergencies. In K. S. Hoyt & J. Selfridge-Thomas (Eds.), *Emergency nursing core curriculum* (6th ed., pp. 891–928). St. Louis, MO: Saunders Elsevier.
Skidmore-Roth, L. (2015). *Mosby's 2016 nursing drug reference* (29th ed.). St. Louis, MO: Mosby.

---

106. A patient presents to triage with a complaint of chest pain. The patient has a recent history of upper respiratory infection and a prescription for an antitussive medication that is taken as indicated. Vital signs: BP 150/88 mm Hg; HR 92 beats/minute; RR 20 breaths/minute; SpO_2 95%; T 38.1°C (100.6°F). The chest pain increases with deep inspiration, and the area around the patient's sternum is tender to palpation. An electrocardiogram shows regular sinus rhythm; a chest radiograph and serum troponins are normal. What is the most likely cause of this patient's chest pain?

A. Pleurisy
B. Myocardial infarction
C. Costochondritis
D. Pulmonary embolism

Rationale

A. Pleurisy is caused by swelling and inflammation around the lungs that usually feels sharp and often increases in intensity when taking a deep breath.

B. Myocardial infarction pain is often characterized as tightness, crushing, and squeezing, and radiating to the arm, jaw, or back. Electrocardiogram may show changes indicating an acute myocardial event, and/or laboratory studies may indicate an abnormal rise in cardiac enzymes.

C. Costochondritis is the inflammation of cartilage that connects the ribs to the sternum. Causes may include recent chest injury, heavy lifting, respiratory infection, and strain from repeated coughing. Symptoms include point tenderness with palpation to the chest wall and pain that varies with respiration.

D. Pulmonary embolism is a blood clot in the lungs. Common signs and symptoms include shortness of breath that is often worse with exertion; cough; and chest pain that often worsens with respirations, cough, or change in positions but does not go away with rest. Other symptoms include fever, leg pain/swelling, cyanosis, dizziness, and rapid or irregular heartbeat.

Category: Maxillofacial, Ocular, Orthopedic, and Wound Emergencies/Orthopedic/Costochondritis
Nursing Process: Analysis

Reference

Chen, M. A. (2014). Chest pain. *MedlinePlus.* Retrieved from http://www.nlm.nih.gov/medlineplus/ency/article/003079.htm

---

107. Numerous patients arrive to the emergency department with multiple lacerations over their entire bodies following a suspected pipe bomb that was detonated into a crowd. The emergency nurse anticipates that these injuries are the result of which category of blast injury?

A. Primary
B. Secondary
C. Tertiary
D. Quaternary

Rationale

A. Primary blast injury is the result of the overpressurization wave moving across an area. Gas-filled structures such as the lungs, middle ear, and gastrointestinal tract are most susceptible to primary blast injuries.

B. Secondary injuries are caused by projectiles from the area near the blast and/or the device. The nurse should anticipate that multiple foreign bodies could be present in the wounds.

C. Tertiary injuries occur when a victim is thrown into a stationary object. Fractures, amputations, and open or closed head/scalp wounds are examples of tertiary injuries.

D. Quaternary injuries are all explosion-related injuries, illnesses, or diseases that are not directly related to primary, secondary, or tertiary mechanisms.

Category: Maxillofacial, Ocular, Orthopedic, and Wound Emergencies/Orthopedic/Trauma

Nursing Process: Analysis

Reference

Wolff, A. (2014). Biomechanics, kinematics, and mechanisms of injury. In D. Gurney (Ed.), *Trauma Nursing Core Course: Provider manual* (7th ed., pp. 25–37). Des Plaines, IL: Emergency Nurses Association.

---

108. Which of the following findings would the emergency nurse expect to assess in a patient who had received procedural sedation before the reduction of a right radius and ulna fracture?

A. The patient is unarousable.
B. There is purposeful response following repeated painful stimulation.
C. There is a purposeful response to verbal/tactile stimulus.
D. The patient is awake, tracking the team.

Rationale

A. General anesthesia results in an unarousable patient even with painful stimuli; airway and ventilation management is required.

B. Deep sedation results in a purposeful response following repeated painful stimulation, and airway interventions may be required to maintain adequate ventilation.

C. Moderate sedation, also known as procedural sedation, results in a purposeful response to verbal or tactile stimulation. Normally, no airway intervention is required in the presence of procedural sedation, and the patient is able to maintain adequate ventilation.

D. Anxiolysis results in awake patients with normal responses. Pain control would not be adequate for a patient experiencing anxiolysis.

Category: Maxillofacial, Ocular, Orthopedic, and Wound Emergencies/Orthopedic/Fracture/dislocations

Nursing Process: Evaluation

Reference

Metzner, J., & Domino, K. B. (2015). Moderate sedation: A primer for perioperative nurses. *AORN Journal, 102*(5), 526–535.

---

109. An elderly patient presents to the emergency department after being found on the floor for an unknown period of time. The patient is awake and responsive. Head trauma has been ruled out, and the patient has been diagnosed with rhabdomyolysis. The patient has received a total of five liters of intravenous crystalloid solution. The emergency nurse identifies that the treatment has been effective when:

A. the urine output is 80 mL/hour.
B. the patient's urine appears clear.
C. the blood urea nitrogen approaches 35 mg/dL.
D. the serum creatinine approaches 3.0 mg/dL.

Rationale

A. It is recommended that the urinary output be maintained at 100 mL/hour until myoglobin is cleared.

B. Myoglobin causes the urine to turn dark red or brown. Aggressive fluid resuscitation is necessary to flush out the myoglobin and prevent renal failure.

C. A blood urea nitrogen (BUN) value of 35 mg/dL is an indication of renal injury. An elevated BUN increases the risk of renal failure and indicates ineffectiveness of treatment; normal value is 8–21 mg/dL.

D. An elevated serum creatinine is an indication of renal injury. An elevated serum creatinine increases the risk of renal failure and indicates ineffectiveness of treatment. Normal serum creatinine value is 0.5–1.2 mg/dL.

Category: Maxillofacial, Ocular, Orthopedic, and Wound Emergencies/Orthopedic/Trauma

Nursing Process: Evaluation

References

Bhavsar, P., Rathod, K. J., Rathod, D., & Chamania, C. S. (2013). Utility of serum creatinine, creatine kinase and urinary myoglobin in detecting acute renal failure due to rhabdomyolysis in trauma and electrical burns patients. *Indian Journal of Surgery*, *75*(1), 17–21. http://doi.org/10.1007/s12262-012-0451-6

Bratcher, C. M. (2014). Musculoskeletal trauma. In D. Gurney (Ed.), *Trauma Nursing Core Course: Provider manual* (7th ed., pp. 193–203). Des Plaines, IL: Emergency Nurses Association.

Van Leeuwen, A. M, Poelhuis-Leth, D., & Bladh, M. L. (2011). *Davis comprehensive handbook of laboratory diagnostic tests with nursing implications* (4th ed., pp. 531–535). Philadelphia, PA: F. A. Davis.

Van Leeuwen, A. M, Poelhuis-Leth, D., & Bladh, M. L. (2011). *Davis comprehensive handbook of laboratory diagnostic tests with nursing implications* (4th ed., pp. 1296–1299). Philadelphia, PA: F. A. Davis.

110. An elderly male patient is complaining of severe back pain that began 2 days ago and has increasingly gotten worse. The patient has no prior history of a similar episode. Unable to walk unassisted because of a loss of sensation in the groin area, the patient presents to the exam room in a wheelchair. The patient does not recall any heavy lifting, pushing, or pulling. When performing the patient assessment, the emergency nurse would be most concerned regarding the presence of:

A. positive left straight leg raise.
B. patellar and Achilles reflex +3 bilaterally.
C. a distended bladder on abdominal exam.
D. monofilament test 3/10 bilaterally.

Rationale

A. Straight leg raise is used to assess for the presence of a disc herniation, which, if found, is not usually emergent and is treated with conservative measures such as administration of anti-inflammatory medications and physical therapy.

B. Although these reflex findings are considered stronger than average, it is not necessarily an emergent finding by itself that requires an intervention at this time.

C. The patient may be experiencing urinary retention, indicating the possibility of a more serious medical problem such as cauda equina or conus medullaris syndrome. This finding needs to be further evaluated, especially if the patient is complaining of loss of sensation in the groin area (saddle paresthesia), is unable to start urinary stream, or has the sensation of the bladder being full. Either syndrome requires immediate treatment.

D. The monofilament test is used to assess for peripheral neuropathy in the feet usually caused by diabetes. This patient does not have a complaint of decreased sensation, so this test is not indicated.

Category (Geriatric): Maxillofacial, Ocular, Orthopedic, and Wound Emergencies/Orthopedic/Low back pain

Nursing Process: Analysis

References

Bickley, L. S. (2012). *Bates' guide to physical assessment and history taking* (11th ed.). Philadelphia, PA: Lippincott Williams & Wilkins.

Cerepani, M. J., & Ramponi, D. R. (2007). Orthopedic emergencies. In K. S. Hoyt & J. Selfridge-Thomas (Eds.), *Emergency nursing core curriculum* (6th ed., pp. 891–928). St. Louis, MO: Saunders Elsevier.

---

111. A patient presents to the emergency department complaining of pain in their nondominant hand after being bitten by their cat 3 days previously. On assessment of the hand, it is noted to be red, swollen, and warm to touch. The nurse suspects the patient may have:

A. pasteurellosis.
B. rabies.
C. wound botulism.
D. gas gangrene.

Rationale

A. Pasteurellosis is a bacterial infection caused by the *Pasteurella* bacteria. The infection results in tissue necrosis and is linked to animal bites, with cat bites being the most common cause.

B. It is possible to contract rabies from a cat bite if the cat is infected with rabies; however, pasteurellosis is the most common infection resulting from a cat bite.

C. Wound botulism results from a significant traumatic or crush injury, when dirt or debris enters the wound. Wound botulism is not associated with animal bites. Pasteurellosis is the most common organism associated with a cat bite.

D. An infection related to gas gangrene is attributed to *Clostridium perfringens* organisms found in the intestine or gallbladder. The presence of gas gangrene in a wound is not associated with animal bites.

Category: Maxillofacial, Ocular, Orthopedic, and Wound Emergencies/Wound/Infections

Nursing Process: Analysis

References

Centers for Disease Control and Prevention. (2017). *Rabies: Domestic Animals: Cats, dogs and ferrets.* Retrieved from http://www.cdc.gov/rabies/exposure/animals/domestic.html

Ramirez, E. G. (2007). Wounds and wound management. In K. S. Hoyt & J. Selfridge-Thomas (Eds.), *Emergency nursing core curriculum* (6th ed., pp. 738–759). St. Louis, MO: Saunders Elsevier.

---

112. The emergency nurse is conducting discharge teaching for a patient with a forehead laceration that has been closed with adhesive wound glue. The patient acknowledges understanding of discharge instructions when stating the following:

A. "I need to avoid showering for 24 hours."
B. "It is important for me to apply a thin layer of antibiotic ointment to the laceration every day after showering."
C. "I will be sure to wear sunscreen over the area."
D. "I must return to the emergency department for removal of adhesive glue in 3 days."

Rationale

A. Patients may shower without risk of removing the adhesive wound glue.

B. An ointment that has a petroleum jelly base will result in the adhesive wound glue coming away from the newly closed wound.

C. Abraded skin is sensitized, and hyperpigmentation can occur after sun exposure. Patients should be instructed to use sunscreen over any area that has been recently abraded or injured.

D. Adhesive wound glue will gradually slough off in 5–10 days from the area of application.

Category: Maxillofacial, Ocular, Orthopedic, and Wound Emergencies/Wound/Lacerations
Nursing Process: Evaluation

Reference

Herr, R. D. (2013). Wound management. In B. B. Hammond & P. G. Zimmermann (Eds.), *Sheehy's manual of emergency care* (7th ed., pp. 147–160). St. Louis, MO: Elsevier Mosby.

---

113. A patient presents to the emergency department with a human bite to the hand. The patient states they were the victim of an assault. What is the emergency nurse's priority in the care of this patient?

A. Assess the wound for the presence of exudate
B. Determine the source of the bite
C. Ask the patient when the bite occurred
D. Treatment of the bite before arrival

Rationale

A. The presence of exudate may indicate a possible wound infection.

B. Determining the source of the bite is not the priority in the care of the patient.

C. Finding out when the injury occurred is important in determining when and if wound closure should take place, but it is not the priority in the care of the patient.

D. The treatment of the injury before arrival is important to determine further wound treatment, but the treatment of the injury is not the priority in the care of the patient.

Category: Maxillofacial, Ocular, Orthopedic, and Wound Emergencies/Wound/Puncture wounds

Nursing Process: Assessment

Reference

Herr, R. D. (2013). Wound management. In B. B. Hammond & P. G. Zimmermann (Eds.), *Sheehy's manual of emergency care* (7th ed., pp. 147–160). St. Louis, MO: Elsevier Mosby.

---

114. A patient arrives to the emergency department from an extended care facility. The emergency nurse is assessing the sacrum of the patient and notes an area of nonblanching erythema. What intervention would be most appropriate to protect the patient's skin from further pressure injury?

A. Place the patient in the Trendelenburg position
B. Insert an indwelling urinary catheter
C. Place the patient in a left lateral recumbent position
D. Calculate a Braden score

Rationale

A. Placing the patient in a Trendelenburg position would not remove pressure from the sacrum.

B. An indwelling urinary catheter is not indicated at this time. Pressure on the sacral area would continue even if a catheter was inserted. Repositioning the patient to protect the area from further injury is the priority intervention at this time.

C. Repositioning is the priority to protect the patient's skin from further injury.

D. Calculating a Braden score is indicated for this patient to determine the risk for further skin breakdown, however, this will not protect the patient from further skin injury. Repositioning the patient to protect the area from further injury is the priority intervention.

Category: Maxillofacial, Ocular, Orthopedic, and Wound Emergencies/Wound/Pressure ulcer

Nursing Process: Intervention

Reference

National Pressure Ulcer Advisory Panel, European Pressure Ulcer Advisory Panel and Pan Pacific Pressure Injury Alliance. (2014). *Prevention and treatment of pressure ulcers: Quick reference guide.* Emily Haesler (Ed.). Osborne Park, Australia: Cambridge Media. Retrieved from http://www.npuap.org/wp-content/uploads/2014/08/Updated-10-16-14-Quick-Reference-Guide-DIGITAL-NPUAP-EPUAP-PPPIA-16Oct2014.pdf

---

115. The patient presents to triage with a complaint of a persistent toothache for over 1 week. The patient has been traveling and has been unable to see a dentist. On assessment, the emergency nurse observes that the affected tooth is loose, with marked edema and inflammation in the surrounding gum. The emergency nurse anticipates that the patient will require which of the following from the emergency provider?

A. Acetaminophen (Tylenol) for the pain control
B. Tooth extraction
C. Antibiotic
D. Referral to a dentist

Rationale

A. Dental pain does not usually resolve with the administration of acetaminophen; however, it is indicated for the treatment of any associated fever. Nonsteroidal anti-inflammatory medications such as ibuprofen are preferred for the treatment of dental pain.

B. Tooth extraction is not indicated for a dental abscess unless it is unresponsive to therapy. All efforts should be made to salvage the tooth once the infection has resolved.

C. The patient most likely has a dental abscess. A dental abscess results in swelling and inflammation in the tissue surrounding the affected tooth, resulting in the tooth being loose within the dental socket. The administration of an antibiotic will help to relieve the swelling and inflammation associated with the infection.

D. Referral to a dentist within 24–48 hours is necessary for definitive care.

Category: Maxillofacial, Ocular, Orthopedic, and Wound Emergencies/Maxillofacial/Dental conditions

Nursing Process: Intervention

References

Goolsby, M. (2015). Ear, nose, mouth, and throat. In M. Goolsby & L. Gruggs, *Advanced assessment* (3rd ed., pp. 123–162). Philadelphia, PA: F. A. Davis.

Nolan, E. G. (2010). Dental, ear, nose, throat, and facial emergencies. In P. K. Howard & R. A. Steinmann (Eds.), *Sheehy's emergency nursing: Principles and practice* (6th ed., pp. 590–601). St. Louis, MO: Mosby Elsevier.

Smith, D. A. (2007). Dental, ear, nose, and throat emergencies. In K. S. Hoyt & J. Selfridge-Thomas (Eds.), *Emergency nursing core curriculum* (6th ed., pp. 249–289). St. Louis, MO: Saunders Elsevier.

---

116. A patient presents to the emergency department complaining of severe, stabbing pain in the right side of the cheek and jaw after shoveling snow. The patient reports prior episodes of severe pain while eating. The nurse suspects a disorder of which cranial nerve?

A. Cranial nerve V
B. Cranial nerve VII
C. Cranial nerve IX
D. Cranial nerve XII

Rationale

A. Severe, stabbing pain in the cheek and jaw are common signs and symptoms of trigeminal neuralgia, which involves the fifth cranial nerve. The trigeminal nerve controls muscles involved in chewing and carries sensory information from the face to the brain. Exposure to extreme cold, shaving, eating, and washing the face often lead to exacerbations.

B. Cranial nerve VII, or the facial nerve, is responsible for moving the facial muscles, allows the tongue to detect taste, and stimulates production within the salivary glands. Bell's palsy, a sudden weakness or paralysis of one side of the face, is caused by a problem with the function of cranial nerve VII.

C. The glossopharyngeal nerve, or cranial nerve IX, moves the muscles of the throat and communicates information from the tongue and throat to the brain. Glossopharyngeal neuralgia causes severe pain to one side of the tongue, throat, or ear.

D. Disorders of the hypoglossal nerve, or cranial nerve XII, result in difficulty speaking, chewing, or swallowing and are characterized by atrophy or weakness of the tongue on one side. Cranial nerve XII disorders may be caused by a stroke, brain stem infection, or brain tumor.

Category: Maxillofacial, Ocular, Orthopedic, and Wound Emergencies/Maxillofacial/Facial nerve disorders

Nursing Process: Analysis

References

Daniels, J. H. (2007). Facial emergencies. In K. S. Hoyt & J. Selfridge-Thomas (Eds.), *Emergency nursing core curriculum* (6th ed., pp. 349–360). St. Louis, MO: Saunders Elsevier.

Gisness, C. M. (2010). Maxillofacial trauma. In P. K. Howard & R. A. Steinmann (Ed.), *Sheehy's emergency nursing: Principles and practice* (6th ed., pp. 355–363). St. Louis, MO: Mosby Elsevier.

---

117. The presence of labyrinthitis is associated with which of the following signs and symptoms?

A. Periauricular cellulitis
B. Pain with movement of the tragus
C. Headache
D. History of recent infective process

Rationale

A. Periauricular cellulitis is found in the presence of otitis externa but is not a symptom of labyrinthitis.

B. Pain is associated with movement of the tragus in the presence of otitis media.

C. The presence of a headache is associated with mastoiditis but is not commonly associated with labyrinthitis.

D. Labyrinthitis is associated with the presence of a recent viral infection, such as measles, mumps, rubella, Epstein Barr virus, herpes, or influenza.

Category: Maxillofacial, Ocular, Orthopedic, and Wound Emergencies/Maxillofacial/Acute vestibular dysfunction

Nursing Process: Assessment

Reference

Egging, D. (2013). Facial, ENT, and dental emergencies. In B. B. Hammond & P. G. Zimmermann (Eds.), *Sheehy's manual of emergency care* (7th ed., pp. 275–284). St. Louis, MO: Elsevier Mosby.

---

118. An elderly patient presents to triage stating, "I can't see out of my right eye." The patient states the vision began to change when it appeared that a shade was lowering over the eye, and vision began to deteriorate. The patient denies pain in the right eye and has a history of diabetes and hypertension. The right pupil is dilated. The immediate intervention of the emergency nurse is to:

A. advise the patient that the loss of their vision is painless and a benign event, and assign the patient an Emergency Severity Index category 3.
B. perform a 12-lead electrocardiogram immediately.
C. contact the emergency provider and initiate an emergent consult with an ophthalmologist immediately.
D. perform a Snellen visual acuity assessment.

Rationale

A. Blood flow to the retinal artery must be reestablished within 60–90 minutes to prevent permanent loss of vision in the affected eye. This patient should be assigned an Emergency Severity Index category 1.

B. A 12-lead electrocardiogram (ECG) may diagnose atrial fibrillation or other cardiac dysrhythmia, which may assist in determining the cause of the patient's sudden loss of vision, but the12-lead ECG will not assist in restoring the patient's eyesight. The immediate intervention is to restore the patient's eyesight.

C. Sudden painless loss of monocular vision is a sign of central artery occlusion and is an ophthalmology emergency. This patient requires the immediate lowering of intraocular pressure using medical management of timolol, acetazolamide, or mannitol, ocular massage, and anterior chamber paracentesis. The immediate lowering of intraocular pressure is associated with increased vision recovery.

D. The results of a Snellen visual acuity test will not aid in the patient's diagnosis and will not alter the necessary treatment that is required. The sudden loss of vision is a medical emergency and must be assessed and treated immediately to prevent permanent loss of vision, which can occur in 60–90 minutes if left untreated.

Category: Maxillofacial, Ocular, Orthopedic, and Wound Emergencies/Ocular/Retinal artery occlusion
Nursing Process: Intervention

Reference

Egging, D. (2013). Ocular emergencies. In B. B. Hammond & P. G. Zimmerman (Eds.), *Sheehy's manual of emergency care*, (7th ed., pp. 285–289). St. Louis, MO: Elsevier Mosby.

---

119. A patient presents to the emergency department for treatment of a laceration to their eyelid. What is the priority assessment for the emergency nurse to perform?

A. Assessment of cranial nerve II and cranial nerve III.
B. Assessment of cranial nerve I and cranial nerve II
C. Assessment of cranial nerve V and cranial nerve VII
D. Assessment of cranial nerve III and cranial nerve VII.

Rationale

A. The eye should be assessed for direct trauma and potential impact on visual acuity. Cranial nerve II is optic, responsible for the patient's vision and cranial nerve III is the oculomotor, which regulates pupil size, accommodation, and extraocular movement.

B. Cranial nerve I is the olfactory nerve and is responsible for the sense of smell. This patient's injury should not have affected the olfactory nerve. Cranial nerve II is the optic nerve and is responsible for the patient's vision.

C. Cranial nerve V if the trigeminal nerve and is responsible for controlling facial sensation and mastication. Cranial nerve VII is the facial nerve that is responsible for facial movement, taste, lacrimation, and salivation.

D. Cranial nerve III is the oculomotor, which regulates pupil size, accommodation, and extraocular movement. Cranial nerve VII is the facial nerve that is responsible for facial movement, taste, lacrimation, and salivation.

Category: Maxillofacial, Ocular, Orthopedic, and Wound Emergencies/Wound/Lacerations

Nursing Process: Assessment

Reference

Walsh, R. (2013). Respiratory emergencies. In B. B. Hammond & P. G. Zimmermann (Eds.), *Sheehy's manual of emergency care* (7th ed., pp. 185–199). St. Louis, MO: Elsevier Mosby.

---

120. An adult patient presents to the emergency department with thermal burns to the face, chest, bilateral arms, and groin. Primary assessment reveals that the patient is alert, agitated, and having difficulty speaking. The patient has blisters around their mouth, and decreased breath sounds are noted auscultation. Vital signs: BP 180/120 mm Hg; HR 140 beats/minute; RR 36 breaths/minute; T 35.8°C (96.4°F); SpO_2 85% on 6 L/minute via mask; pain 10/10. The priority intervention for this patient is to:

A. administer pain medication.
B. establish intravenous access.
C. maintain a patent airway.
D. adhere to universal precautions to prevent infection.

Rationale

A. Pain management is an important part of the immediate plan of care for this patient; however, the priority intervention is managing the patient's airway.

B. This patient is at risk for fluid volume deficit, and this requires intervention; however, securing a patent airway would take priority.

C. The patient has signs of respiratory distress and of burn injury to the airway. The management of this patient's airway is the priority for care, and early intubation should be considered.

D. The potential for infection is an important consideration in the patient's plan of care; however, securing a patent airway would take priority.

Category: Environment and Toxicology Emergencies, and Communicable Diseases/Environment/Burns

Nursing Process: Intervention

References

Ribbens, K. A., & DeVries, M. (2013). Burns. In B. B. Hammond & P. G. Zimmermann (Eds.), *Sheehy's manual of emergency care* (7th ed., pp. 453–462). St. Louis, MO: Elsevier Mosby.

Wraa, C. (2007). Burn trauma. In K. S. Hoyt & J. Selfridge-Thomas (Eds.), *Emergency nursing core curriculum* (6th ed., pp. 803–819). St. Louis, MO: Saunders Elsevier.

---

121. A patient with suspected *Escherichia coli* food poisoning is at risk for developing which potentially life-threatening complication?

A. Central nervous system syndrome
B. Disseminated intravascular coagulation
C. Toxoplasmosis
D. Hemolytic uremic syndrome

Rationale

A. Central nervous system syndrome is associated with radiation exposure, not *Escherichia coli (E. coli)* exposure.

B. DIC is not associated with *E. coli* exposure.

C. Toxoplasmosis is associated with exposure to the parasite *Toxoplasma gondii*, not *E. coli.*

D. Approximately 5–10% of patients diagnosed with *E. coli* infections will develop hemolytic uremic syndrome. Symptoms include abdominal pain, vomiting, fever, and bloody or watery diarrhea. Hemolytic uremic syndrome occurs when an immune reaction causes low platelet and red blood cell counts and kidney injury.

Category: Environment and Toxicology Emergencies, and Communicable Diseases/Environment/Food poisoning

Nursing Process: Analysis

Reference

Centers for Disease Control and Prevention. (n.d.). E. coli *and food safety*. Retrieved from http://www.cdc.gov/features/ecoliinfection/

---

122. The hospital is notified that two victims of radiation exposure are en route from the nearby nuclear power plant. What is the priority of care for these patients on arrival to the hospital?

A. Notifying law enforcement
B. Decontamination
C. Medical stabilization
D. Consulting the hospital radiation safety officer

Rationale

A. Notification of law enforcement is not a priority for these patients.

B. Decontamination is appropriate following medical stabilization. Avoiding contamination must be considered during resuscitation efforts.

C. Stabilization of the patent is the top priority. The patient must have a patent airway, with breathing and adequate circulation assessed immediately. Once life-threatening priorities are corrected, decontamination can occur.

D. Consultation with the hospital radiation officer is appropriate but not the priority of care for these patients.

Category: Environment and Toxicology Emergencies, and Communicable Diseases/Environment/Radiation exposure

Nursing Process: Intervention

Reference

Flarity, K. (2010). Environmental emergencies. In P. K. Howard & R. A. Steinmann (Eds.), *Sheehy's emergency nursing: Principles and practice* (6th ed., pp. 535–553). St. Louis, MO: Mosby Elsevier.

---

123. A patient is brought into the emergency department via ambulance after participating in 8 hours of intense outdoor physical training. The patient is combative and confused. Vital signs: BP 80/48 mm Hg; HR 166 beats/minute; RR 30 breaths/minute and shallow; T 41°C (105.8°F) core temperature; SpO_2 90% on room air. The priority nursing intervention for this patient is to:

A. administer supplemental oxygen by the most appropriate method for the patient's level of consciousness.
B. administer 1–2 L of 0.9% sodium chloride over the first 4 hours.
C. apply cooling blankets and continuously monitor the patient's core temperature.
D. place the patient on the cardiac monitor and observe for signs of high-output cardiac failure.

Rationale

A. Support of airway, breathing, and circulation is crucial for patient recovery and is a priority of care.

B. Although fluid volume is depleted in most victims of hyperthermia, the priority of care is for airway support.

C. Cooling blankets are a recommended treatment for heat stroke, however, the initial priority of care is airway support.

D. Cardiac monitoring for high-output cardiac failure is recommended for heat stroke, but the initial priority of care for this patient is airway support.

Category: Environment and Toxicology Emergencies, and Communicable Diseases/Environment/Temperature-related emergencies

Nursing Process: Intervention

Reference

Sedlak, K. (2013). Environmental emergencies. In B. B. Hammond & P. G. Zimmermann (Eds.), *Sheehy's manual of emergency care* (7th ed., pp. 333–343). St. Louis, MO: Elsevier Mosby.

---

124. After providing discharge instructions to the mother of a child diagnosed with head lice, the nurse acknowledges the mother understands the instructions when she states:

A. "I will apply the pyrethrins 0.33%/piperonyl butoxide 4% (RID®) shampoo to dry hair."
B. "I will take my child to the barber to have his head shaved, which will remove the lice."
C. "I will shampoo my child's hair in hot soapy water to kill the lice."
D. "I will apply bleach to my child's head to kill the lice."

Rationale

A. Pyrethrins 0.33%/piperonyl butoxide 4% (RID®) shampoo is to be applied to dry hair and washed off after 5 minutes. The hair should be combed with a fine-tooth comb, and the procedure should be repeated in 7 days.

B. Shaving the head may further spread the nits and aid in lice growth. The recommended treatment is using pyrethrins 0.33%/piperonyl butoxide 4% (RID®) shampoo.

C. Hot soapy water has not been proved to kill lice nits.

D. This application would be dangerous to the child and is not effective in killing the nits.

Category (Pediatric): Environment and Toxicology Emergencies, and Communicable Diseases/Environment/Parasite and fungal infestations

Nursing Process: Evaluation

References

Habif, T. (2004). *Clinical dermatology* (4th ed.). Philadelphia, PA: Mosby.

Peard, A. S. (2007). Communicable and infectious disease emergencies. In K. S. Hoyt & J. Selfridge-Thomas (Eds.), *Emergency nursing core curriculum* (6th ed., pp. 439–482). St. Louis, MO: Saunders Elsevier.

---

125. A patient presents to the emergency department requesting post exposure rabies prophylaxis after being bitten by a fox. The patient has open wounds on the right buttock and right forearm. The patient reports having previously not received rabies vaccines. The site that would be the most appropriate for the nurse to administer the rabies vaccine is:

A. any large muscle used for intramuscular injections.
B. left deltoid.
C. right buttock.
D. right deltoid.

Rationale

A. The administration of the vaccine near sites where the rabies immune globulin has been administered may cause suppression of antibody production. Therefore, not all intramuscular sites are appropriate for administration.

B. A patient who has never been vaccinated for rabies requires both rabies immune globulin and the rabies vaccine for the first rabies postexposure prophylaxis. The rabies immune globulin is administered once into and around the wounds when anatomically feasible. The vaccine should be administered to a site distal to where the rabies immune globulin was administered because rabies immune globulin may partially suppress antibody production from the vaccine.

C. The right buttock would be proximal to where the immune globulin is administered, running the risk of suppression of antibody production; therefore, this site should not be used.

D. The right deltoid is more proximal to the site where rabies immune globulin is administered, running the risk of antibody suppression; therefore, this site should not be used.

Category: Environment and Toxicology Emergencies, and Communicable Diseases/Environment/Vector-borne illnesses: Rabies

Nursing Process: Assessment

Reference

U.S. Department of Health and Human Services, Centers for Disease Control and Prevention. (2010). Use of a reduced (4-dose) vaccine schedule for post exposure prophylaxis to prevent human rabies. *Morbidity and Mortality Weekly Report*, *59*, 1–9. Retrieved from https://www.cdc.gov/mmwr/preview/mmwrhtml/rr5902a1.htm

---

126. A patient presents to triage complaining of fever, muscle pain, headache, and a small, flat, pink rash on the palms, wrists, forearms, soles, and ankles. The patient reports that the symptoms began a few days after returning home from a camping trip. The triage nurse suspects that the patient has which of the following disorders?

A. Rocky Mountain spotted fever
B. Lyme disease
C. Tularemia
D. Colorado tick fever

Rationale

A. This patient is presenting with early signs and symptoms of Rocky Mountain spotted fever. Patients will often develop a fever, headache, and rash in the first 10 days following a tick bite.

B. The signs and symptoms in this case do not match Lyme disease. The patient is not complaining of fatigue or malaise. Headache would be a common symptom of Rocky Mountain spotted fever, but it is also common in many disorders.

C. Tularemia usually presents with a single lesion.

D. Patients with Colorado tick fever will have signs of malaise, fever, and headache; however, it typically resolves in 2–3 days.

Category: Environment and Toxicology Emergencies, and Communicable Diseases/Environment/Vector-borne illnesses: Tick-borne illness

Nursing Process: Assessment

References

Centers for Disease Control and Prevention. (2016). *Ticks*. Retrieved from http://www.cdc.gov/ticks/index.html

Sedlak, S. K. (2013). Bite and sting emergencies. In B. B. Hammond & P. G. Zimmermann (Eds.), *Sheehy's manual of emergency care* (7th ed., pp. 345–352). St. Louis, MO: Elsevier Mosby.

---

127. A toddler is brought to triage with general malaise, fever, and a pruritic rash on the face and trunk that has progressed from macules to vesicles over the past several days. The nurse should plan to implement which of the following precautions?

A. Droplet precautions
B. Standard precautions
C. Contact precautions
D. Airborne precautions

Rationale

A. This patient is most likely presenting with varicella (chickenpox), which would require airborne precautions. Droplet precautions are not sufficient to prevent the spread of infection.

B. Emergency nurses should use standard precautions with all patients. This patient is most likely presenting with varicella (chickenpox), which would require airborne precautions.

C. This patient is most likely presenting with varicella (chickenpox), which would require airborne precautions. Contact precautions would not be sufficient to prevent the spread of this infection.

D. This patient is most likely presenting with varicella (chickenpox), which would require airborne precautions.

Category (Pediatric): Environment and Toxicology Emergencies, and Communicable Diseases/ Communicable Diseases/Childhood diseases

Nursing Process: Analysis

Reference

Centers for Disease Control and Prevention. (2016). *Preventing varicella in health care settings.* Retrieved from http://www.cdc.gov/chickenpox/hcp/healthcare-setting.html

---

128. A firefighter presents to the emergency department with seizures, hypotension, and hypoxia after fighting a house fire. Which substance may the firefighter have been exposed to that is causing these symptoms?

A. Iron
B. Pesticides
C. Petroleum distillates
D. Cyanide

Rationale

A. Iron toxicity is most commonly a result of iron supplement ingestion. Signs and symptoms may include gastrointestinal disturbances, hematemesis, coagulopathy, or shock.

B. Patients with pesticide toxicity present with muscarinic effects of sweating, wheezing, or urinary incontinence, and nicotinic effects of tachycardia, hypertension, anxiety, restlessness, or cramps.

C. Exposure to petroleum distillates can produce signs and symptoms of respiratory difficulty, infiltrates on chest radiographs, abnormal arterial blood gases, or dysrhythmias.

D. The patient presents with signs and symptoms of cyanide toxicity, secondary to exposure to smoke from the fire. Exposure to cyanide can occur from the combustion of polyurethane, wood, cotton, and nylon. Even minute amounts of cyanide exposure can lead to severe lactate acidosis; therefore, cyanide poisoning must be considered in a patient with an elevated lactate level and minimal difference between arterial and venous oxygen saturation levels.

Category: Environment and Toxicology Emergencies, and Communicable Diseases/Toxicology/Cyanide

Nursing Process: Analysis

References

Andress, K. (2010). Nuclear, biologic, and chemical agents of mass destruction. In P. K. Howard & R. A. Steinmann (Eds.), *Sheehy's emergency nursing: Principles and practice* (6th ed., pp. 198–210). St. Louis, MO: Mosby Elsevier.
Badillo, R.B., Hovseth, K., & Schaffer S. (2012). Toxicologic emergencies. In B. B. Hammond & P. G. Zimmermann (Eds.), *Sheehy's manual of emergency care* (7th ed., pp. 319–332). Philadelphia, PA: Elsevier Mosby.

---

129. Treatment is initiated for a patient who presents to the emergency department with signs and symptoms of an acute digoxin (Lanoxin) overdose. Which of the following changes in the patient's status would indicate to the nurse that the treatment is having its intended effect?

A. Hypoglycemia
B. Bradycardia
C. Potassium level within normal limits (3.5–5.0 mEq/L)
D. Signs and symptoms of hypovolemia

Rationale

A. Patients with digoxin overdose may present with signs and symptoms of hypoglycemia, so a treatment goal would be to increase the patent's serum glucose level to normal values.

B. Bradycardia can occur as a result of digoxin toxicity, so an increase in the patient's heart rate is indicative of a positive treatment goal.

C. Patients with digoxin overdose may present with hyperkalemia, so a decreasing potassium level within normal limits will indicate that the treatment is having the intended effect.

D. Hypovolemia may result from digoxin overdose, so the provider would want to correct hypovolemia by increasing circulating fluid volume to maintain adequate blood pressure.

Category: Environment and Toxicology Emergencies, and Communicable Diseases/Toxicology/Overdose and ingestions

Nursing Process: Evaluation

Reference

Badillo, R. B., Hovseth, K., & Schaffer S. (2012). Toxicologic emergencies. In B. B. Hammond & P. G. Zimmermann (Eds.), *Sheehy's manual of emergency care* (7th ed., pp. 319–332). Philadelphia, PA: Elsevier Mosby.

---

130. A patient with a history of alcohol abuse is being admitted to the hospital for pneumonia. Which early sign of alcohol withdrawal should the emergency nurse observe for in this patient?

A. Hallucinations
B. Tremulousness
C. Delirium
D. Low-grade fever

Rationale

A. Hallucinations can occur 12–48 hours after the last drink was consumed. This is also referred to as alcoholic hallucinosis.

B. Tremulousness can occur within 6–8 hours of when the last drink was consumed. The patient may also exhibit anxiety and restlessness.

C. Delirium tremens is a late sign of alcohol withdrawal, and it can occur 48–96 hours after the last drink was taken. The risk of delirium increases in patients over the age of 30 and in those with a prolonged drinking history.

D. A low-grade fever is a late sign of alcohol withdrawal and can occur in the presence of delirium tremens.

Category: Environment and Toxicology Emergencies, and Communicable Diseases/Toxicology/Withdrawal syndrome

Nursing Process: Assessment

Reference

Williamson, D. (2013). Alcohol abuse. In B. B. Hammond & P. G. Zimmermann (Eds.), *Sheehy's manual of emergency care* (7th ed., pp. 137–146). St. Louis, MO: Elsevier Mosby.

---

131. A patient presents to the emergency department suspected of ingesting an overdose of acetaminophen. The emergency nurse should anticipate to administer which medication as the appropriate antidote for acetaminophen overdose?

A. N-acetylcysteine (Mucomyst)
B. Flumazenil (Romazicon)
C. Octreotide (Sandostatin)
D. Diphenhydramine (Benadryl)

Rationale

A. Toxic doses of acetaminophen destroy liver cells, resulting in permanent liver damage. N-acetylcysteine binds to the acetaminophen, allowing it to be removed from the body, reducing the toxic effects. N-acetylcysteine should be administered within 8 hours of acetaminophen ingestion to minimize liver damage.

B. Flumazenil is administered in cases of benzodiazepine overdoses; it is not indicated in the treatment of acetaminophen overdose.

C. Octreotide is the antidote for sulfonylurea overdose.

D. Diphenhydramine is given for patients who have overdosed by taking phenothiazines.

Category: Environment and Toxicology Emergencies, and Communicable Diseases/Toxicology/Overdose and ingestions

Nursing Process: Intervention

Reference

Badillo, R. B., Hovseth, K., & Schaffer S. (2012). Toxicologic emergencies. In B. B. Hammond & P. G. Zimmermann (Eds.), *Sheehy's manual of emergency care* (7th ed., pp. 319–332). Philadelphia, PA: Elsevier Mosby.

---

132. A patient is discharged from the emergency department with a prescription for doxycycline monohydrate (Doxycycline). Which statement made by the patient to the emergency nurse demonstrates an understanding of the side effects of this medication?

A. "I must stay out of the sun while taking this medicine."
B. "I must take calcium carbonate (Maalox) with my medication to avoid diarrhea."
C. "This medication is safe while I am breastfeeding."
D. "This medication may discolor my teeth."

Rationale

A. Tetracyclines such as doxycycline monohydrate have two common adverse effects. Photosensitivity reactions, especially to direct sunlight, may be severe, and gastrointestinal disturbances, including diarrhea, nausea, and vomiting, can occur. Instructions should be shared with patients concerning avoiding sunlight and to make them aware of the possible gastrointestinal issues.

B. Calcium carbonate (Maalox) should not be taken within 2–4 hours of doxycycline monohydrate. Antacids containing aluminum and magnesium may interact with the doxycycline monohydrate, decreasing the amount of the doxycycline monohydrate absorbed by the body.

C. Doxycycline monohydrate is contraindicated in breastfeeding patients because the medication appears in the breast milk and can be transmitted to the infant.

D. Tetracyclines such as doxycycline monohydrate may cause teeth discoloration during teeth formation years, generally in children younger than 8 years of age. Children younger than 8 should not have tetracyclines prescribed because of possible permanent teeth discoloration, enamel hypoplasia, and a decrease in calcification of the bone.

Category: Environment and Toxicology Emergencies, and Communicable Diseases/Toxicology/Drug interaction

Nursing Process: Evaluation

Reference

Wolters Kluwer. (2017). Tetracyclines. In *Nursing 2017 drug handbook* (pp. 62–63). Philadelphia, PA: Author.

---

133. A 16-year-old patient presents to the emergency department after being tackled early in a football game. The patient is complaining of left shoulder pain. History reveals the patient just returned to school following an extended absence related to infectious mononucleosis. The patient's vital signs: BP 96/48 mm Hg; HR 104/beats minute; RR 22 breaths/minute; SpO_2 97%; T 37.2°C (99.0°F); Wt 86.3 kg. What is the most likely cause of the patient's vital signs?

A. Hypovolemia related to splenic injury
B. Recurrence of the infectious mononucleosis
C. Dehydration related to physical activity
D. The patient's vital signs are within normal limits and intervention isn't necessary

Rationale

A. The patient just returned to school from infectious mononucleosis, which can cause an enlarged spleen. The patient's left shoulder pain is referred pain from irritation of the phrenic nerve to the diaphragm caused by bleeding from the spleen. A splenic injury can result in hypovolemia and tachycardia.

B. The patient is afebrile and has no other symptoms of recurrence of the disease, including extreme fatigue, sore throat, head and body aches, swollen lymph nodes in the neck or armpits, or rash.

C. The patient was tackled early in the game. Because they have a history of infectious mononucleosis and is complaining of left shoulder pain, a spleen injury is the more likely cause of the patient's symptoms.

D. The patient is experiencing hypotension and tachycardia. Given the patient's recent history and probability of a splenic injury, interventions for hypovolemia are necessary.

Category: Environment and Toxicology Emergencies, and Communicable Diseases/Communicable Disease/Mononucleosis

Nursing Process: Analysis

References

Centers for Disease Control and Prevention. (2016). *About infectious mononucleosis.* Retrieved from http://www.cdc.gov/epstein-barr/about-mono.html

Peard, A. S. (2007). Communicable and infectious disease emergencies. In K. S. Hoyt & J. Selfridge-Thomas (Eds.), *Emergency nursing core curriculum* (6th ed., pp. 438–482). St. Louis, MO: Saunders Elsevier.

---

134. The patient reports a history of having been diagnosed with tuberculosis. Which of the following would indicate that the patient is no longer infectious?

A. Patient has been compliant taking the prescribed medications for 1 week.
B. Patient had two consecutive negative sputum cultures for acid-fast bacillus.
C. Patient reports less coughing at night, and temperature is 37.7°C (99.9°F).
D. Patient's earlier tuberculin skin test induration diameter is less than 10 mm.

Rationale

A. The patient is generally considered infectious for the first 2 weeks after starting treatment. In addition, having two consecutive negative cultures is the requirement for a patient not to be considered infectious.

B. Two consecutive negative sputum cultures are required to declare a patient no longer infectious.

C. A history of less coughing and a temperature less than 100°F could indicate improvement, but negative sputum cultures for acid-fast bacillus are required to indicate that a patient is no longer infectious.

D. The tuberculin skin test (Mantoux test) using purified protein derivative is a standard to screen for M tuberculosis exposure. A positive result (greater than 10 mm in a healthy adult) then requires additional testing. The size/appearance is not indicative of whether the patient is infectious or responding to any prescribed medications for treatment.

Category: Environment and Toxicology Emergencies, and Communicable Diseases/Communicable Disease/Multi-drug resistant organisms

Nursing Process: Assessment

Reference

Mondor, E. E. (2016). Lower respiratory problems. In S. L. Lewis, L. Bucher, M. M. Heitkemper, & M. M. Harding, (Eds.), *Medical-surgical nursing* (10th ed., pp. 499–537). St. Louis: Elsevier.

---

135. The development of secondary traumatic stress (STS) can occur as the result of caring for those who are exposed to suffering or traumatic events. Symptoms of STS include which of the following signs and symptoms?

A. Emotional exhaustion
B. The repeated reliving of disturbing events
C. Difficulty making decisions
D. Presence of reduced empathy toward patients or their families

Rationale

A. Emotional exhaustion is an example of a symptom associated with burnout, not with STS.

B. The repeated reliving of disturbing events is a symptom of intrusion. Intrusion is one of the three categories associated with STS; the other categories are avoidance and arousal.

C. Repeated difficulty in making decisions is an associated symptom of a response to a traumatic event.

D. A symptom of compassion fatigue is lack of empathy toward patients or families; it is not associated with STS.

Category: Professional Issues/Nurse/Critical Incident Stress Management

Cognitive Level: Application

Reference

Healy, M. M., & Gurney, D. (2014). Psychosocial aspects of trauma care. In D. Gurney (Ed.), *Trauma Nursing Core Course: Provider manual* (7th ed., pp. 295–310). Des Plaines, IL: Emergency Nurses Association.

---

136. A patient with terminal cancer arrives at the emergency department in septic shock. The patient refuses to have any life-sustaining interventions initiated. The emergency nurse states they cannot morally care for this patient because it is against their beliefs. What document supports transferring the care of this patient to another nurse?

A. Emergency Nurses position statement: Patient handoff/transfer
B. The patient's bill of rights
C. The Patient Self-Determination Act
D. American Nurses Association code of ethics

Rationale

A. The Emergency Nurses Association position statement: Patient handoff/transfer supports the development and use of standardized tools to improve handoff communication between caregivers. It does not address circumstances under which a transfer of care would or should occur.

B. The patient's bill of rights was developed by the American Hospital Association and outlines the services that should be offered to the patient and directs the hospital and practitioners to provide fair and ethical treatment. Transferring the care of this patient to another nurse preserves the patient's rights.

C. This act requires all facilities that receive Medicare and Medicaid funds to provide all patients with written information and counseling on advance directives and the institution's policy governing them.

D. The American Nurses Association code of ethics states that a nurse is justified in refusing to participate in the care of a patient based on moral (but not prejudiced or biased) grounds. The nurse may not abandon the patient and can only cease to provide care when nursing care to the individual is assured.

Category: Professional Issues/Nurse/Ethical dilemmas

Cognitive Level: Analysis

References

American Nurses Association. (2015). *Code of ethics for nurses with interpretive statements.* Silver Spring, MD: Author. Retrieved from http://nursingworld.org/DocumentVault/Ethics-1/Code-of-Ethics-for-Nurses.html

Emergency Nurses Association. (2013). *Patient handoff and transfers (position statement).* Des Plaines, IL: Author. Retrieved from https://www.ena.org/docs/default-source/resource-library/practice-resources/position-statements/patienthandofftransfer.pdf?sfvrsn=e2c42cb6_16

LeMoyne, P., Burke, K., & Bauldoff, G. (2011). *Medical-surgical nursing: Critical thinking in patient care* (5th ed.). Boston, MA: Pearson.

---

137. Along with identifying the best available research and their clinical expertise, emergency nurses incorporate which other component to make evidence-based practice decisions in the clinical area?

A. Education level of nursing staff
B. Administrative support
C. Traditional practices
D. Patient preferences

Rationale

A. The education level of nursing staff is not a component of the evidence-based practice decision-making process.

B. Administrative support is important to the development and implementation of evidence-based practice changes, but it is not a component of the individual patient care decision-making process.

C. Traditional practices frequently provide the basis for evidence-based practice change, but these practices are not incorporated into the individual patient care decision-making process.

D. Evidence-based practice incorporates the best available research with knowledge gained through clinical experience, and individual patient preferences are used to drive decision making in patient care.

Category: Professional Issues/Nurse/Evidence-based practice

Cognitive Level: Application

References

Keough, V. A. (2010). Evidence-based practice. (2010). In P. K. Howard & R. A. Steinmann (Eds.), *Sheehy's emergency nursing: Principles and practice* (6th ed., pp. 35–44). St. Louis, MO: Mosby Elsevier.

Melnyk, B. M., & Fineout-Overholt, E. (2011). Making the case for evidence-based practice and cultivating a spirit of inquiry. In *Evidence-based practice in nursing and healthcare: A guide to best practices* (pp. 3–24). Philadelphia, PA: Wolters Kluwer/Lippincott Williams & Wilkins.

---

138. The emergency nurse is aware that a patient with which of the following preexisting medical conditions is not eligible to donate organs or tissues for transplantation?

A. Diabetes mellitus
B. History of cancer
C. Human immunodeficiency virus
D. Coronary artery disease

Rationale

A. A patient with diabetes is eligible to donate organs and tissue for transplantation.

B. A patient with a metastatic cancer is usually not eligible for organ or tissue donation.

C. Although a medical evaluation is conducted to determine organ viability on a case-by-case basis, patients with human immunodeficiency virus do not normally meet criteria for organ donation.

D. A patient with coronary artery disease may donate organs and tissue for transplantation.

Category: Professional Issues/Patient/End-of-life issues: Organ and tissue donation

Cognitive Level: Recall

References

Gift of Life Donor Program (n.d.). *Who can become a donor?* Retrieved from http://www.donors1.org/learn2/faqs/#9

Missouri Department of Health and Senior Services (n.d.). *Myths & misconceptions.* Retrieved from http://health.mo.gov/living/organdonor/myths.php

---

139. A patient with end-stage lung cancer is brought to the emergency department with progressive dyspnea. The patient is diagnosed with a pleural effusion secondary to the lung malignancy. Which of the following interventions is appropriate and consistent with the patient's palliative care management at home?

A. Administer intravenous antibiotics
B. Perform chest physiotherapy
C. Prepare the patient for a paracentesis
D. Prepare the patient for a thoracentesis

Rationale

A. Infections such as tuberculosis and pneumonia can cause a pleural effusion; however, the etiology of this patient's effusion is the malignancy, so antibiotics would not be initially indicated.

B. Chest physiotherapy is indicated when the patient is dyspneic because of an inability to mobilize secretions. The patient's symptoms are related to a pleural effusion, and a thoracentesis is the indicated medical intervention.

C. A paracentesis may be indicated if the patient's dyspnea is related to ascites. This patient's symptoms are related to excess fluid in the pleural cavity, not the abdominal cavity.

D. The intent of palliative care in end-stage disease is to relieve symptoms. This patient's breathing difficulty is because of an increase of fluid in the pleural space, which limits lung expansion. A thoracentesis will remove the excess fluid, allowing the lung to expand and relieve the patient's dyspnea.

Category: Professional Issues/Patient/End-of-life issues: Withholding, withdrawing, and palliative care

Cognitive Level: Application

References

Chan, G. K. (2007). End-of-life issues in the emergency department. In K. S. Hoyt & J. Selfridge-Thomas (Eds.), *Emergency nursing core curriculum* (6th ed., pp. 86–110). St. Louis, MO: Saunders Elsevier.

Selfridge-Thomas, J., & Hoyt, K. S. (2007). Respiratory emergencies. In K. S. Hoyt & J. Selfridge-Thomas (Eds.), *Emergency nursing core curriculum* (6th ed., pp. 685–720). St. Louis, MO: Saunders Elsevier.

---

140. The victim of multiple gunshot wounds arrives to the emergency department via emergency medical services. The emergency nurse is aware that a key principle of preserving clothing evidence of the victim of a violent crime is to perform which of the following actions?

A. Place each piece of clothing in an individual paper bag; label, seal with tape, and include appropriate patient identification.
B. Place the clothing in a plastic bag because of saturation of blood on the clothing.
C. Cut the clothing off immediately to expose the patient as quickly as possible; because it is a trauma patient, you may cut through bullet holes, tears, rips, or holes.
D. Place all the clothing in a large paper bag; label, seal with tape, and include appropriate patient identification.

Rationale

A. Use of paper bags for each piece of clothing is the best way to preserve evidence and prevent cross-contamination if clothing is placed together in the same bag.

B. Moisture can collect within the plastic bag and alter the clothing evidence.

C. In the primary assessment of the trauma patient, exposure is important, but to preserve evidence, care should be taken to *not* cut through any bullet holes, tears, rips, or stains on the clothing if possible. It is important to preserve the integrity of the evidence as much as possible.

D. Placing all the clothes together in one large paper bag may lead to possible cross-contamination of evidence from one piece of clothing to the other.

Category: Professional Issues/Patient/Forensic evidence collection

Cognitive Level: Application

References

Eckes-Roper, J. (2013). Forensics. In B. B. Hammond & P. G. Zimmermann (Eds.), *Sheehy's manual of emergency care* (7th ed., pp. 49–58). St. Louis, MO: Elsevier Mosby.

Sheridan, D., Nash, K., & Bresee, H. (2010). Forensic nursing in the emergency department. In P. K. Howard & R. A. Steinmann (Eds.), *Sheehy's emergency nursing: Principles and practice* (6th ed., pp. 176–186). St. Louis, MO: Mosby Elsevier.

---

141. Which agent administered intravenously before procedural sedation has the shortest duration of action?

A. Ketalar (Ketamine)
B. Midazolam (Versed)
C. Propofol (Diprivan)
D. Fentanyl (Sublimaze)

Rationale

A. Intravenous (IV) ketamine has a rapid onset and peak, with a duration of action of 5–10 minutes.

B. IV midazolam has a rapid onset and peak, with a duration of action of 2–6 hours.

C. IV propofol has a rapid onset and peak, with a duration of action of 3–5 minutes.

D. IV fentanyl has a rapid onset and peak, with a duration of action of 30 minutes to 1 hour.

Category: Professional Issues/Patient/Pain management and procedural sedation

Cognitive Level: Recall

References

Amidate. (2018). *Epocrates.* Retrieved from https://online.epocrates.com/drugs/1968/Amidate

Ketalar. (2018). *Epocrates.* Retrieved from https://online.epocrates.com/drugs/197007/Ketalar/Pharmacology

Valium. (2018). *Epocrates.* Retrieved from https://online.epocrates.com/drugs/136507/Valium/Pharmacology

Vallerand, A. H., Sanoski, C.A., & Deglin, J. H. (2016). *Davis's drug guide for nurses.* Philadelphia, PA: F. A. Davis. http://www.fadavis.com/

Versed. (2018). *Epocrates.* Retrieved from https://online.epocrates.com/drugs/175307/Versed/Pharmacology

142. Research has demonstrated that patients who report satisfaction with the care they received in an emergency department (ED) are more likely to perform which of the following actions?

A. Frequently access the ED
B. Use the ED as a source for primary care
C. Require hospital admission
D. Adhere to their treatment plan

Rationale

A. Duplicate patient satisfaction surveys are typically not sent to patients who are seen more than once within a specific time frame.

B. Use of the ED as a provider of primary care is more closely associated with ease of access than satisfaction with a previous experience.

C. The majority of healthcare surveys are sent to a random population of individuals who were seen in the ED within a particular period of time. Most do not differentiate between patients who were admitted to the hospital and those who were discharged.

D. Patients who report satisfaction with the care they received in the ED are found to be more likely to follow their treatment plan and experience improved outcomes.

Category: Professional Issues/Patient/Patient satisfaction

Cognitive Level: Recall

References

Emergency Nurses Association. (2014). *Patient experience/satisfaction in the emergency care setting.* Des Plaines, IL: Author.

Welch, S. J. (2010). Twenty years of patient satisfaction research applied to the emergency department: A qualitative review. *American Journal of Medical Quality, 25*(1), 64–72.

---

143. Studies have shown that patients report increased satisfaction with the care they received during their emergency department (ED) visit when they are provided with which of the following?

A. The ability to fill the prescription provided at discharge in the hospital pharmacy
B. Distraction devices such as televisions or laptop computers
C. Frequent interactions with the ED registered nurse
D. Additional blankets and pillows

Rationale

A. Drivers of increased patient satisfaction in the ED include shorter wait times, receiving accurate information regarding care, and clear discharge instructions. Patients do not report being inconvenienced by having to fill prescriptions at an outside pharmacy.

B. The patient perception of their ED wait time is a significant driver of patient satisfaction. Providing distractions such as magazines, television, and Wi-Fi Internet access reduces the patient's idle time, making the wait seem shorter. A perceived shorter wait time leads to increased patient satisfaction.

C. Frequent interactions with ED personnel is an important element leading to increased patient satisfaction, however, this includes registration staff, greeters, technicians, and physicians as well as the registered nurse.

D. Patients appreciate comfort measures, but increased patient satisfaction in the ED is more closely associated with experiences such as shorter wait times, receiving accurate information regarding their care, and clear discharge instructions.

Category: Professional Issues/Patient/Patient satisfaction

Cognitive Level: Application

References

Emergency Nurses Association. (2014). *Patient experience/satisfaction in the emergency care setting.* Retrieved from https://www.ena.org/practice-resources/resource-library/position-statements

Soremekun, O. A., Takayesu, J. K., & Bohan, S. J. (2011). Framework for analyzing wait times and other factors that impact patient satisfaction in the emergency department. *Journal of Emergency Medicine, 41*(6), 686–692. https://doi.org/10.1016/j.jemermed.2011.01.018

---

144. When using a certified translator to communicate with a non-English-speaking patient, the emergency nurse should direct questions to which participant in the conversation?

A. The patient
B. The certified translator
C. The patient's oldest male family member
D. The patient's designated family spokesperson

Rationale

A. When using an interpreter, the nurse should speak directly to the patient, phrasing questions in the first and second person ("I" and "you" questions) and avoid the use of the third person ("tell her" or "ask him").

B. Questions and statements should be directed to the patient. The certified translator should serve only as a facilitator of the conversation that takes place between the nurse and the patient.

C. In some cultures, the oldest male family member may be the decision maker; however, for reasons of accuracy and privacy, the conversation must occur between the patient and the nurse, with the certified translator serving as the facilitator of the conversation.

D. For reasons of accuracy and privacy, the conversation should occur between the patient and the nurse, with the certified translator serving as the facilitator of the conversation.

Category: Professional Issues/Patient/Cultural considerations

Cognitive Level: Application

References

Juckett, G., & Unger, K. (2014). Appropriate use of medical interpreters. *American Family Physician, 90*(7), 476–480.

Newnum, G. (2017, December 14). Fact & Fiction: What Do Joint Commission Standards Say About Healthcare Interpretation? (Blog entry). Retrieved from http://blog.cyracom.com/new-joint-commission-standards-healthcare-interpreting

Ruiz-Contreras, A. (2010). Approaching diversity. (2010). In P. K. Howard & R. A. Steinmann (Eds.), *Sheehy's emergency nursing: Principles and practice* (6th ed., pp. 27–32). St. Louis, MO: Mosby Elsevier.

145. The Five Rights of Delegation are: right task, right circumstances, right person, right direction and communication, and which of the following?

A. Right equipment and supplies
B. Right documentation
C. Right supervision and evaluation
D. Right assessment and reassessment

Rationale

A. The registered nurse, under right supervision and evaluation, would be assessing if the assistive personnel is using the right equipment and supplies.

B. The registered nurse would be assessing that the proper direction and communication have taken place, however, right documentation completed is not a component of the five rights of delegation. Proper documentation is the responsibility of the registered nurse.

C. Right supervision and evaluation is the fifth right of delegation.

D. The registered nurse is accountable for the ongoing monitoring of the outcomes of nursing care.

Category: Professional Issues/System/Delegation of tasks to assistive personnel

Cognitive Level: Recall

Reference

Bonulami, N. M., & King, D. (2007). Professionalism and leadership. In K. S. Hoyt & J. Selfridge-Thomas (Eds.), *Emergency nursing core curriculum* (6th ed., pp. 1046–1056). St. Louis, MO: Saunders Elsevier.

---

146. A nurse leaves a patient's chart open on a portable work station. A patient's family member is observed looking at the open chart on the work station. This action by the nurse is considered a violation of the:

A. patient's bill of rights.
B. Emergency Medical Treatment and Active Labor Act.
C. Health Insurance Portability and Accountability Act.
D. Patient Self-Determination Act.

Rationale

A. Typically a patient's bill of rights includes autonomy over medical decisions, fair treatment, and other guarantees while receiving medical care.

B. Emergency Medical Treatment and Active Labor Act (EMTALA) requires the medical screening of individuals seeking emergency care to determine whether an emergency condition exists and, if so, stabilizing the patient to the best of the hospital's capabilities before discharge or transfer. EMTALA does not address issues of unprotected health information.

C. Leaving health information unprotected is considered a violation of Health Insurance Portability and Accountability Act (HIPAA). HIPAA states that a patient's protected health information cannot be used or shared without the consent of the patient unless it is for treatment, payment, and other healthcare operation activities.

D. The Patient Self-Determination Act is a federal law that provides hospitalized patients with information regarding advance directives; it does not address the issues of unprotected health information.

Category: Professional Issues/System/Federal regulations

Cognitive Level: Application

Reference

Jagim, M. (2007). Legal and regulatory issues. In K. S. Hoyt & J. Selfridge-Thomas (Eds.), *Emergency nursing core curriculum* (6th ed., pp. 1033–1045). St. Louis, MO: Saunders Elsevier.

---

147. A terminally ill patient is admitted to the emergency department (ED). The patient informs the and nurse that they have a living will (advance directive) with a Do Not Resuscitate (DNR) order. The emergency nurse would:

A. make the patient a full code because nothing will likely happen while in the ED.

B. document in the chart that the patient is a DNR and ask the patient for a copy of their living will and DNR to place in their medical record.

C. ask the patient's family members what lifesaving interventions they would like performed in the event of a cardiopulmonary arrest.

D. take no action, because the advance directive and the DNR only apply once the patient is admitted to the hospital.

Rationale

A. A living will is a legal document that states a person's wishes regarding medical care should they become terminally ill and incompetent or unable to communicate. It should be honored and noted despite the patient's current condition or expected outcome of the admission.

B. A living will is an advance care document that states a person's wishes regarding medical care should they become terminally ill and incompetent or unable to communicate. Because of the Patient Self-Determination Act, all patients must be asked during the admission phase whether they have an advance directive (living will) in place. If so, copies must be placed in the medical record. Interactions about advance directives must be documented in the medical record.

C. If the patient already has a living will and DNR, the patient's wishes regarding medical care should be honored. The family members' opinions may vary; following the advance directive will honor the patient's wishes.

D. Because of the Patient Self-Determination Act, all patients must be asked during the admission phase whether they have an advance directive in place. If so, copies must be placed in the medical record. Interactions about advance directives must be documented in the medical record. Asking about advance directives is a part of the ED nurse's admission responsibilities. Also noting that the patient is a DNR while they remain in the ED is important in the event that the patient's condition deteriorates before being admitted.

Category: Professional Issues/System/Patient consent for treatment

Cognitive Level: Analysis

Reference

Jagim, M. (2007). Legal and regulatory issues. In K. S. Hoyt & J. Selfridge-Thomas (Eds.), *Emergency nursing core curriculum* (6th ed., pp. 1033–1045). St. Louis, MO: Saunders Elsevier.

---

148. The emergency department provider directs the nurse who is caring for a patient to suture the patient's forearm laceration. The nurse should do which of the following on receiving this order?

A. Do not perform the procedure
B. Perform the procedure
C. Perform the procedure with a physician assistant present
D. Delegate the task to assistive personnel

Rationale

A. Suturing would be outside the scope of practice for a registered nurse. Emergency nurses are accountable to, and expected to practice within, the Nurse Practice Act guidelines in their state and follow the policies and procedures developed within their place of employment.

B. Suturing would be outside the scope of practice for a registered nurse. Emergency nurses are accountable to, and expected to practice within, the Nurse Practice Act guidelines in their state and follow the policies and procedures developed within their place of employment.

C. Suturing would be outside the scope of practice for a registered nurse. Emergency nurses are accountable to, and expected to practice within, the Nurse Practice Act guidelines in their state and follow the policies and procedures developed within their place of employment. It would, however, be within the scope of practice for a physician assistant to suture the patient's laceration.

D. Emergency nurses are accountable to, and expected to practice within, the Nurse Practice Act guidelines in their state and follow the policies and procedures developed within their place of employment. Suturing would be outside the scope of practice for a registered nurse and could not be delegated to unlicensed assistive personnel.

Category: Professional Issues/System/Risk management
Cognitive Level: Application

Reference

National Council of State Boards of Nursing. (2015). Nurse practice act, rules & regulations. Retrieved from https://www.ncsbn.org/1455.htm/1455.htm

149. A child is transported to the emergency department following a mass casualty incident. The child is unable to ambulate, has spontaneous respirations of 32 breaths/minute, has a palpable pulse, and is alert. Which JumpSTART triage category should be assigned to this child?

A. Yellow (delayed)
B. Red (immediate)
C. Black (expectant)
D. Green (minor)

Rationale

A. A child who is not able to ambulate but has spontaneous respirations at a rate greater than 15 and less than 45 breaths per minute with a palpable pulse and who is alert or responsive to verbal stimuli falls in the yellow (delayed) JumpSTART triage category.

B. An adult patient would meet criteria to be placed in the red (immediate) category because of the respiratory rate of 32. Children are physiologically different from adults, and the respiratory parameters are greater than 15 and less than 30. This child does not ambulate but meets all other JumpSTART triage criteria and therefore would be placed into the yellow (delayed) category.

C. Although this patient is not able to ambulate, the child does have spontaneous respirations and a palpable pulse. This would move the patient into a higher level within the JumpSTART categories than the black (expectant) category.

D. The green (minor) category is assigned to those patients who are able to walk. This child is not ambulatory and would need to be further triaged to determine the triage level. Because this child meets all other triage criteria—respiratory rate greater than 15 and less than 45, a palpable pulse, and alert or responding to verbal stimuli—the triage category would be yellow (delayed).

Category (Pediatric): Professional Issues/System/Disaster management

Cognitive Level: Analysis

Reference

Upton, L. A. (2012). Disaster. In *Emergency Nursing Pediatric Course: Provider manual* (4th ed., pp. 365–382.). Des Plaines IL: Emergency Nurses Association.

---

150. A pediatric traumatic cardiopulmonary arrest is in progress when the charge nurse comes to assist the primary emergency department nurse with the resuscitation. At first glance, the patient looks similar to the son the charge nurse recently loss due to a terminal illness. The charge nurse is unable to stay focused on the necessary resuscitation tasks for this patient. Upon debriefing, the code team discusses the charge nurse's challenges. The best response to encourage resiliency is which of the following?

A. "This experience should help you get you back to the bedside. You are a "super nurse." You can take care of anyone that rolls through those doors."

B. "This is a tough place to work. Management didn't give you enough time off to grieve, staff members don't take initiative to help, and you are tired and overworked. Have you considered looking to work somewhere else that will support you in a better way?"

C. "Don't forget, we are a team and you are part of our team. Some of us want to pray with you at the end of the shift and join you when you go to visit your son's grave site."

D. "We need more situation awareness from this team. If one us is not able to step up, we need to speak up and get someone else in who can do the job. We cannot risk patient safety."

Rationale

A. Hospital cultures that implicitly or explicitly encourage staff members to be emotionally tough and convey the opinion that they should be able to handle anything may exacerbate the stressors already present and further predispose staff to or accelerate secondary traumatic stress (STS) and compassion fatigue.

B. Trauma nurses with higher levels of burnout have a significantly higher variability in STS. Identifying factors that support the nurse's burnout will exacerbate the STS.

C. STS, burnout, and compassion satisfaction have a high correlation with such coping strategies as coworker support, a sense of personal accomplishment in your work, meditation and exercise, and decreasing hours of exposure to traumatic events. This leads to the development of compassion satisfaction and resiliency.

D. Although recognizing the dynamics of the code response was subpar is necessary, the delivery of the message should be reworded with consideration of the charge nurse's STS experience. Perhaps a different forum could be considered for process improvement.

Category: Professional Issues/Nurse/Critical Incident Stress Management

Cognitive Level: Application

References

Flarity, K. F., Gentry, J. E., & Mesnikoff, N. (2013). The effectiveness of an educational program on preventing and treating compassion fatigue in emergency nurses. *Advanced Emergency Nursing Journal, 35*(3), 247–258.

Hinderer, K. A., VonReuden, K. T., Friedmann, E., McQuillan, K. A., Gilmore, R., Kramer, B., & Murray, M. (2014). Burnout, compassion fatigue, compassion satisfaction, and secondary traumatic stress in trauma nurses. *Journal of Trauma Nursing, 21*(4), 160–169.

Li, A., Early, S. F., Mahrer, N. E., Klaristenfeld, J. L., & Gold, J. I. (2014). Group cohesion and organizational commitment: protective factors for nurse residents' job satisfaction, compassion fatigue, compassion satisfaction, and burnout. *Journal of Professional Nursing, 30*(1), 89–99.

SELF-DIAGNOSTIC PROFILE

How to Use the Self-Assessment Worksheet

1. Indicate on your answer sheet whether your answers are correct or incorrect.
2. Note the items you answered incorrectly.
3. Count the total number of items you answered incorrectly in each category.
4. Compare the total number of items you answered incorrectly in each category with the total number of items per category. This information will give you an idea of where you will need to focus your continued study.

Content Category	Questions Answered Incorrectly	Total Number of Questions Answered Incorrectly in Each Category	Total Number of Questions in Each CEN Content Category
Cardiovascular Emergencies			20
Respiratory Emergencies			16
Neurological Emergencies			16
Gastrointestinal, Genitourinary, Gynecology, and Obstetrical Emergencies			21
Psychosocial and Medical Emergencies			25
Maxillofacial, Ocular, Orthopedic, and Wound Emergencies			21
Environment and Toxicology Emergencies, and Communicable Diseases			15
Professional Issues			16

CHAPTER 10

Practice Examination 5

PART 1

1. A patient presents to the emergency department experiencing an anterior ST segment elevation myocardial infarction. The patient's vital signs are normal. The hospital is not equipped with a cardiac catheterization laboratory. The patient can be transferred to a cardiac catheterization lab within 60 minutes. Which of the following would you anticipate for this patient?
   A. A bolus of tissue plasminogen activator, followed by an infusion for fibrinolytic therapy
   B. Immediate transfer to the hospital with a cardiac catheterization lab for percutaneous coronary intervention
   C. A single bolus of tenecteplase (TNKase) for fibrinolytic therapy
   D. A bolus of reteplase (Retavase), followed by a second bolus of reteplase (Retavase) 30 minutes later for fibrinolytic therapy

2. An anxious patient arrives by ambulance following an acute onset of difficulty breathing. The patient is diaphoretic and denies chest pain. High-flow oxygen by nonrebreather mask has been applied. Vital signs: BP 210/140 mm Hg; HR 130 beats/minute; RR 32 breaths/minute; SpO_2 88%. In addition to initiating noninvasive ventilation to treat the patient's difficulty breathing, the nurse anticipates the administration of which medication to further treat the patient's symptoms?
   A. Morphine (morphine sulfate)
   B. Furosemide (Lasix)
   C. Initiation of a continuous nitroglycerin infusion
   D. Acetylsalicylic acid (aspirin)

3. An unrestrained driver is brought to the emergency department following a motor vehicle collision. The patient reports hitting their chest on the steering wheel and is complaining of chest pain across the front of their chest. There are no vital sign abnormalities and no other complaints of pain. The diagnosis of blunt cardiac injury is considered. The nurse anticipates an order for which of the following?
   A. Electrocardiogram
   B. Cardiac marker evaluation (creatine kinase and/or troponin)
   C. Cardiac monitoring
   D. Chest radiograph

4. Which of the following is a form of distributive shock?
   A. Neurogenic
   B. Metabolic
   C. Respiratory
   D. Obstructive

5. A patient presents following an acute onset of chest pain, dyspnea, and severe diaphoresis, with near syncope. Assessment shows a patient in severe distress, with HR 110 beats/minute; BP 60/40 mm Hg; and RR 36 breaths/minute and bilateral rales. An electrocardiogram reveals ST segment elevation across the precordial leads. A diagnosis of acute myocardial infarction with cardiogenic shock is made, and the patient is being prepared for transfer to the cardiac catheterization lab. The vasopressor of choice, based on this patient's degree of hypotension, is:
   A. norepinephrine (Levophed).
   B. dopamine (Intropin).
   C. dobutamine (Dobutrex).
   D. vasopressin (Pitressin).

6. A patient presents with complaints of chest pain that radiates to the jaw, stating the pain is a 6 on a 0–10 scale. Other symptoms include nausea, dizziness, shortness of breath with clear lung sounds, and a sense of impending doom. The pain started 40 minutes before arrival. Vital signs: BP 116/58 mm Hg; HR 98 beats/minute; RR 20 breaths/minute; SpO_2 94%; T 37°C (98.6°F). The 12-lead electrocardiogram (ECG) shows an inferior wall myocardial injury pattern. Which clinical presentations indicate the need to complete a right sided 12-lead ECG?
   A. Shortness of breath with clear lung sounds
   B. Nausea and dizziness
   C. Chest pain with radiation to jaw
   D. Sense of impending doom

7. Following the successful resuscitation of a patient in a cardiac arrest, which of the following findings is the best indicator of high-quality cardiopulmonary resuscitation (CPR)?
   A. A compression depth of 1 ½ inches
   B. Palpable pulses with the performance of chest compressions during CPR
   C. A decrease of skin and mucus membrane cyanosis
   D. An increasing end-tidal carbon dioxide level

8. During transcutaneous pacing for a patient in third-degree heart block, there is a loss of ventricular capture. Which is a significant physiological reason for loss of pacemaker capture?
   A. Metabolic alkalosis
   B. Hypomagnesemia
   C. Lactic acidosis
   D. Hypokalemia

9. A patient presents with complaints of lightheadedness, weakness, and near syncope. The patient's 12-lead electrocardiogram reveals the presence of 2:1 atrial flutter. The most appropriate intervention for this presentation with an atrial flutter rhythm is to perform:
   A. synchronized cardioversion at 50 joules.
   B. unsynchronized cardioversion at 120 joules.
   C. unsynchronized cardioversion at 50 joules.
   D. synchronized cardioversion at 120 joules.

10. In preparing to discharge a patient who has been given a prescription for nitroglycerin tablets 0.4 mg SL PRN, the emergency nurse acknowledges that the patient teaching has been effective when the patient states:

A. "I am to take the tablets at least every 2–3 minutes when I experience chest pain."
B. "I will call my doctor every time I need to take a tablet for my chest pain."
C. "I should keep the tablets on my window sill in the kitchen so I can find them easily."
D. "If my chest pain has not gone away after I have taken 2 tablets, I will come to the hospital."

11. Which of the following findings would the emergency nurse anticipate in a patient experiencing signs and symptoms of cardiac tamponade following successful aspiration of fluid from the pericardial sac?

A. Presence of electrical alternans
B. Increase in the patient's heart rate
C. Decrease in the patient's blood pressure
D. Increase in the patient's blood pressure

12. Initial interventions for a patient diagnosed with acute aortic dissection include two large-caliber intravenous lines, oxygen, and aortic wall pressure control with beta blocker administration. Maintaining which assessment finding is a priority for determining end organ perfusion?

A. Heart rate below 60 beats/minute
B. Systolic blood pressure above 120 mm Hg
C. Normal mental status
D. Urinary output above 30 mL/hour

13. A 5-year-old child weighing 33 pounds (15 kg) presents to the emergency department in cardiac arrest. The child remains in ventricular tachycardia despite having been defibrillated three times, having received epinephrine 0.15 mg intraosseous (IO), and receiving good-quality cardiopulmonary resuscitation. Which drug should be administered next?

A. Amiodarone (Cordarone) 75 mg IO
B. Atropine 0.3 mg IO
C. Calcium chloride 1.0 mL intravenous (IV)
D. Lidocaine (Xylocaine) 50 mg IV

14. The emergency nurse is caring for a patient with a permanent pacemaker and observes that the patient has a paced rhythm with an occasional normal beat (patient's own intrinsic beat) without the presence of a pacemaker spike. The emergency nurse would interpret this rhythm as:

A. paced rhythm with capture.
B. paced rhythm with failure to sense.
C. paced rhythm with sensing.
D. malfunctioning pacemaker.

15. A female patient presents to the emergency department complaining of numb fingertips and throbbing pain. The fingertips of both hands are noted to be pale to light blue in color and are cool to touch. The patient denies both trauma and any recent exposure to a cold environment. The patient is a two-pack-per-day smoker and has a history of hypertension. Based on the assessment findings, the emergency nurse suspects the patient has which condition?

A. Raynaud's disease
B. Buerger's disease
C. Thrombocytopenia
D. Inflammatory arthritis

16. Which condition places a patient at the highest risk for infective endocarditis due to a dental procedure?
   A. Prosthetic cardiac valve
   B. Diabetes
   C. Congestive heart failure
   D. Rheumatoid arthritis

17. A clevidipine (Cleviprex) infusion is ordered for a symptomatic patient with severe hypertension. The nurse is aware that this medication would be contraindicated in a patient with which history?
   A. Soybean or egg allergy
   B. Asthma
   C. Sinus bradycardia
   D. Recent use of Sildenafil (Viagra)

18. A patient is brought into the emergency department by ambulance with chest pain, a low-grade fever of 37.89°C (100.2°F), cough, shortness of breath, and a 1–3 mm ST segment elevation on their 12-lead electrocardiogram in all leads except aVR and V_1. The nurse recognizes that the patient's symptoms are associated with the presence of:
   A. congestive heart failure.
   B. ST segment elevation myocardial infarction.
   C. pericarditis.
   D. acute coronary syndrome.

19. A patient recently discharged from the hospital following a 3-week hospitalization for a right femur fracture with internal fixator repair returns to the emergency department with a sudden onset of right calf pain. The nurse notes swelling and redness to the right calf. The nurse realizes that the patient is exhibiting signs and symptoms of what disorder?
   A. Phlebitis of the right leg
   B. Postoperative infection
   C. Deep vein thrombosis
   D. Compartment syndrome

20. The definition of preload is:
   A. end systolic volume.
   B. end diastolic volume.
   C. systolic blood pressure.
   D. mean arterial pressure.

21. A patient with a history of asthma has audible wheezing, tachypnea, and pale, cool skin that persists following the administration of an albuterol nebulizer breathing treatment. What medication would the emergency nurse anticipate giving next to this patient?
   A. Etomidate via intravenous (IV) push
   B. Oral prednisone
   C. Magnesium sulfate via IV infusion
   D. Oral ibuprofen

22. To limit the recurrence of chronic obstructive pulmonary disease exacerbations, it is important that patients should perform which intervention?

A. Stop smoking
B. Exercise
C. Take all medications as directed
D. Get immunized against pneumonia

23. A patient is receiving an enteral feeding. Which of the following statements indicates that the nurse understands the importance of keeping the head of the patient's bed elevated?

A. "The head of the bed is elevated to increase patient comfort when sitting up in bed and eating."
B. "The head of the bed is elevated to facilitate the tube feeding formula getting to the patient faster, thereby helping to reduce a negative nitrogen balance from lack of nutrition."
C. "Keeping the head of the bed elevated helps to prevent aspiration pneumonia."
D. "Keeping the head of the bed elevated prevents the feeding tube from becoming occluded as the tube feeding flows into the stomach."

24. Patients with chronic obstructive pulmonary disease (COPD) should receive influenza and pneumococcal vaccines:

A. so they will not get sick during flu season.
B. because these vaccines prevent the need for long-acting beta agonists.
C. because these vaccines will prevent them from acquiring pneumonia.
D. because viral and bacterial infections play a major role in COPD exacerbations.

25. A patient with no past medical history arrives to triage with the complaint of fever, malaise, cough, and crackles that do not clear with coughing. The emergency nurse anticipates that the patient will most likely will be treated for which of the following?

A. Chronic obstructive pulmonary disease exacerbation
B. Acute bronchitis
C. Acute asthma exacerbation
D. Pneumonia

26. A patient has just been intubated and placed on mechanical ventilation. What measure can the emergency nurse initiate to reduce the risk of ventilator-associated pneumonia?

A. Only suction the patient once a shift to allow oral secretions to pool in the oral cavity and prevent irritation to the oral mucosa from frequent suctioning
B. Keep the patient supine
C. Verify that the endotracheal tube cuff is deflated
D. Elevate the head of the bed

27. A patient is admitted to the emergency department via emergency medical services following the detection of carbon monoxide in their home. The patient is alert to verbal stimuli but is demonstrating intermittent snoring-type respirations. After opening the patient's airway and administering supplemental oxygen via a nonrebreather mask, what assessment finding would indicate that the patient is receiving adequate oxygenation?

A. A pCO_2 level of 70 mm Hg
B. A continuous pulse oximetry reading of 100%
C. Alertness to verbal stimuli
D. The patient's level of consciousness returning to their normal level of alertness

28. A patient presents to triage with complaints of throat pain, hoarseness, and difficulty swallowing after sustaining a "clothesline" injury. The patient is having difficulty speaking and tolerating oral secretions, and there is ecchymosis to the anterior neck. The emergency nurse suspects that the patient may have a fractured larynx and provides appropriate instructions. The patient demonstrates understanding when:
    A. the patient requests ice chips for comfort.
    B. the patient communicates by writing on a piece of paper.
    C. the patient opens their mouth wide and sticks their tongue out for the nurse to inspect.
    D. the patient states a detailed description of the injury.

29. A patient arrives by ambulance unresponsive after falling off a bicycle. The patient was not wearing a helmet at the time of injury. Cervical spine immobilization is in place. During the primary assessment, the emergency nurse observes loose teeth and vomitus in the mouth. To properly suction the patient, the emergency nurse should:
    A. open the airway using jaw thrust maneuver.
    B. open the airway using the head tilt chin lift maneuver.
    C. insert an appropriately sized nasopharyngeal airway.
    D. place the patient in the "sniffing position" with neck and chin extended.

30. A toddler presents to the emergency department triage with their parents. The child is sitting in a tripod position, drooling with stridorous respirations, and diaphoretic. The parent states that the child was playing when they suddenly heard the child coughing. The parent denies recent illness or ill contacts, past medical history is negative for similar episodes or chronic illnesses, and immunizations are up to date. The emergency nurse recognizes that the child is most likely experiencing:
    A. foreign body aspiration.
    B. acute asthma exacerbation.
    C. acute epiglottitis.
    D. acute laryngotracheobronchitis (croup).

31. A patient with end-stage renal failure is complaining of increasing shortness of breath and exercise intolerance. The emergency nurse auscultates muffled breath sounds on assessment and anticipates that the patient is at risk for developing which respiratory complication?
    A. Unstable airway
    B. Pulmonary embolism
    C. Pleural effusion
    D. Pulmonary edema

32. A tension pneumothorax leading to inadequate tissue perfusion is considered to be which type of shock?
    A. Obstructive
    B. Hypovolemic
    C. Distributive
    D. Cardiogenic

33. A patient presents to the emergency department complaining of sudden onset of wheezing and difficulty breathing. The patient states that they sustained an acute myocardial infarction 1 month ago. On auscultation of bilateral lung fields, scattered wheezing and bibasilar crackles are heard. As the emergency nurse, which order from the provider would you question?

A. Give the patient 125 mg methylprednisolone (Solu-Medrol) intravenously
B. Place the patient on oxygen via a nonrebreather mask
C. Give the patient 2.5 mg albuterol via nebulizer
D. Give the patient 1000 mL 0.9% sodium chloride bolus over 30 minutes

34. A 34-week-pregnant female arrives to triage complaining of dyspnea with exertion and right-sided chest pain since the previous evening. She admits to smoking a half-pack of cigarettes per day. Vital signs: BP 135/90 mm Hg; HR 125 beats/minute; RR 32 breaths/minute; SpO_2 85% on room air; T 37.5°C (99.5°F). The emergency nurse knows that these signs and symptoms are consistent with which of the following?

A. Pneumonia
B. HELLP syndrome
C. Pulmonary embolism
D. Asthma exacerbation

35. Which disease process is characterized by the presence of foreign material occluding one or more pulmonary blood vessels?

A. Pulmonary embolism
B. Pulmonary edema
C. Pneumothorax
D. Pulmonary effusion

36. The emergency nurse is caring for a patient with apparent ligature marks on the neck. The patient is experiencing dyspnea, hoarseness, and subcutaneous emphysema in the neck and face. The priority intervention for this patient is to:

A. prepare for laryngoscopy.
B. prepare for intubation.
C. prepare for bronchoscopy.
D. administer oxygen via mask with an oxygen reservoir (nonrebreather mask).

37. A young adult presents to triage with fever, severe headache, and stiff neck. The emergency provider diagnoses the patient with meningitis. The emergency nurse is aware that the priority for this patient is the administration of:

A. antibiotics.
B. acetaminophen (Tylenol).
C. morphine sulfate.
D. osmitrol (Mannitol).

38. A young adult presents to triage with dry mouth, blurred vision, profound fatigue, and constipation. The patient was recently diagnosed with multiple sclerosis and has begun taking a selective serotonin reuptake inhibitor (SSRI). The emergency nurse anticipates that the most likely cause of the patient's symptoms is:

A. new onset of diabetes.
B. progression of multiple sclerosis.
C. side effects related to the SSRI.
D. a hemorrhagic stroke.

39. Which assessment parameter should be performed on a 26-week-pregnant female who presents with a tonic–clonic seizure?

A. Continuous electronic fetal heart monitoring
B. Measurement of abdominal girth
C. Pelvic ultrasound
D. Measurement of fundal height

40. What is the least important information for the emergency nurse to obtain from a patient who has experienced a tonic–clonic seizure?

A. History of febrile seizures as a child
B. History of current medications, alcohol use, and illicit drug use
C. Pregnancy status
D. Family history of a seizure disorder

41. Assessment of a patient who was thrown from a horse 1 hour before arrival in the emergency department reveals the patient is able to move their right leg but cannot feel pain or touch. They are unable to move their left leg but can feel pain and touch. The emergency nurse is aware that this assessment finding is consistent with the following spinal cord syndrome:

A. central cord syndrome.
B. cauda equina syndrome.
C. Brown–Sequard syndrome
D. anterior cord syndrome.

42. A patient has been receiving an intravenous infusion of norepinephrine (Levophed) for the treatment of hypotension related to the presence of spinal shock following a fracture of thoracic vertebrae 4 and accompanying spinal cord injury. Which of the following clinical signs would suggest that this intervention has had the desired effect?

A. The patient becoming less responsive
B. Capillary refill time of 4 seconds
C. A systolic blood pressure of 100
D. Urine output of 20 mL/hour and 25 mL/hour over each of the past 2 hours

43. The emergency nurse is caring for a patient with a subdural hematoma. Which of the following assessment findings would indicate the presence of an early increase in intracranial pressure?

A. Dilated, nonreactive pupils
B. Headache
C. Bradycardia
D. Decreased respiratory effort

44. The emergency department nurse is preparing to administer tissue plasminogen activator to a stroke patient. What percentage of the total dose should the nurse first administer to this patient as a bolus dose?

A. 1%
B. 5%
C. 10%
D. 15%

45. Which of the following assessment findings best describes the presence of a Le Fort II fracture?

A. A pyramidal maxillary bone fracture involving the midface
B. A transverse maxillary bone fracture occurring above the level of the teeth
C. A complete craniofacial separation, including the maxilla, zygoma, and orbits
D. A fracture of the base of the skull resulting in cerebrospinal fluid leakage

46. On arrival to triage, a patient states they have experienced facial numbness and slurred speech, although the symptoms disappeared just before arrival. The patient states that they no longer wish to be seen by the emergency provider. In formulating a response to the patient's wish to leave the department, the emergency nurse should state the following to the patient:

A. "You have likely experienced a transient ischemic attack and therefore should be evaluated by the provider for appropriate care and follow-up."
B. "You should be evaluated by the provider since your symptoms will return in less than 24 hours."
C. "You are experiencing a lacunar stroke and should immediately be evaluated by the provider."
D. "A hemorrhagic stroke is the likely cause of your symptoms, and you will deteriorate rapidly."

47. A patient with cerebral edema has received 1 g/kg mannitol intravenously. Which of the following clinical signs would indicate that this intervention has had the desired effect?

A. Systolic blood pressure of 80
B. Intracranial pressure reading of 60
C. A cerebral perfusion pressure decreased to 30
D. Urinary output of 500 mL in the last hour

48. A patient arrives to the emergency department accompanied by her husband. The husband states that the patient has a history of Alzheimer's disease, and he is concerned that she has experienced a stroke. While evaluating his understanding of his wife's disease, the emergency nurse suspects he requires additional education when he states:

A. "She forgot the word for *oven* but remembered it in the car."
B. "I know she can't die from Alzheimer's disease, but I got worried that she was really having a stroke. Her mother died of a stroke."
C. "She takes her medication every day and has always been able to take care of herself."
D. "She wasn't able to make a cake today because she couldn't follow the recipe."

49. A young male presents to the emergency triage stating that he felt a "pop" in his head after lifting heavy weights. The patient now complains of a right-sided headache that he rates as a 10 out of 10 on the pain scale. The emergency nurse notes that the patient's right pupil is oval and sluggishly reactive to light. The emergency triage nurse will next:

A. proceed with immediate bedding.
B. place the patient in fast track.
C. place the patient in the waiting room until a room becomes available.
D. complete the medical screening exam in triage.

50. The emergency nurse is caring for a patient with increased intracranial pressure due to a subarachnoid hemorrhage. The provider has ordered a bolus administration of intravenous mannitol. Which of the following would indicate that this medication has had the desired effect?

A. A decrease in level of consciousness
B. A partial pressure of carbon dioxide between 35 and 40 mm Hg
C. An increase in serum sodium level above 145 mEq
D. An increase in urinary output

51. Following a motor vehicle collision, an unresponsive male patient is received in the emergency department. On patient assessment, priapism is noted. Based on this finding, what intervention should the emergency nurse perform first?

A. Ensure full spinal immobilization
B. Insert a urinary drainage catheter
C. Prepare the patient for an abdominal ultrasound
D. Obtain intravenous access and begin fluid resuscitation

52. An elderly female presents to the emergency department for evaluation of headache and vomiting. The family reports that the patient sustained a fall 2 days ago, during which she struck her head. The patient's medications include lisinopril, atorvastatin, and warfarin. The emergency nurse anticipates this patient may have experienced which of the following?

A. Intraparenchymal hemorrhage
B. Epidural hematoma
C. Subdural hematoma
D. Subarachnoid hemorrhage

53. When assessing a patient with suspected appendicitis, the emergency nurse would expect the patient to demonstrate rebound tenderness in which area of the abdomen?

A. Right lower quadrant
B. Left lower quadrant
C. Right upper quadrant
D. Periumbilical area

54. When assessing a patient who presents to the emergency department complaining of bright red rectal bleeding, what question regarding the patient's history is most important for the nurse to ask the patient?

A. "Are you diabetic?"
B. "Do you have atrial fibrillation?"
C. "Do you take nonsteroidal anti-inflammatory drugs?"
D. "Do you take iron supplements?"

55. A 28-year-old female presents to the emergency department with a sudden onset of epigastric pain that radiates to the right upper quadrant. The patient is nauseated and has vomited. While obtaining the patient's medical history, the nurse also notes that the patient is 3 months postpartum. Which of the following conditions is most consistent with the patient's presenting symptoms?

A. Pancreatitis
B. Esophagitis
C. Acute gastroenteritis
D. Cholecystitis

56. A patient presents to the emergency department with restlessness, severe right flank pain, nausea, and diaphoresis. The emergency nurse should anticipate preparing the patient for which diagnostic test?
   A. Kidneys, ureters, and bladder radiograph
   B. Intravenous pyelogram
   C. Renal ultrasound
   D. Helical computed tomography scan

57. A patient is being treated in the emergency department for chronic liver disease related to cirrhosis. The emergency nurse knows that the most common cause of cirrhosis is:
   A. nonalcoholic or fatty liver disease.
   B. chronic hepatitis B.
   C. excessive alcohol consumption.
   D. end-stage cardiac disease.

58. The emergency nurse has administered lactulose to a patient with hepatic encephalopathy. The nurse is able to determine that the medication has been effective if the patient exhibits which of the following?
   A. Decreased pain
   B. Increased urine output
   C. Improved mental status
   D. Diminished deep tendon reflexes

59. A patient presents with left-sided abdominal pain and is diagnosed with diverticulitis. The emergency nurse would anticipate administering which medication to manage the patient's symptoms?
   A. A proton pump inhibitor
   B. An anticholinergic medication
   C. An antiemetic medication
   D. An antidiarrheal agent

60. Which of the following is a priority intervention for a patient with bleeding esophageal varices?
   A. Administer 2 units of whole blood
   B. Establish intravenous (IV) access with two large-caliber IV catheters
   C. Secure the patient's airway
   D. Administer high-flow oxygen via nonrebreather mask

61. A patient presents to the emergency department with a 72-hour history of vomiting and diarrhea. The patient's heart rate is elevated, skin is pale, and the patient is hard to arouse. The emergency nurse is aware that the priority management for this patient is to perform which of the following?
   A. Obtain a stool sample
   B. Establish intravenous access for administration of crystalloid fluids
   C. Administer antiemetics
   D. Maintain airway, breathing, and circulation

62. A 65-year-old patient has been diagnosed with hepatitis C. After receiving patient education regarding this diagnosis, which of the following statements made by the patient indicates their correct understanding of the disease?

A. "I'll separate my eating and drinking utensils from those used by other family members."
B. "I never used intravenous drugs or had unprotected sex with multiple partners, even when I was much younger."
C. "My partner will need to be vaccinated so they won't become infected too."
D. "I know I can be infected even though I don't have any symptoms."

63. Following the insertion of a large-caliber gastric tube, which of the following nursing measures would best assist the nurse in initially determining that the gastric tube has been properly positioned in the gastrointestinal system?

A. Assessment of the pH of the gastric aspirate
B. Auscultation of instilled air over the epigastrium
C. Determination of the carbon dioxide level within the gastric tube
D. Assessing the patient for signs of respiratory distress

64. A patient presents to the emergency department with complaints of upper left quadrant pain radiating to the back for the past week. The patient's serum amylase level is normal, but the serum lipase is elevated. The nurse suspects that the patient may have which of the following disease processes?

A. Peptic ulcer
B. Pyelonephritis
C. Cholecystitis
D. Pancreatitis

65. The emergency nurse would anticipate hospital admission for a patient newly diagnosed with renal calculi (renal stones) if the patient demonstrated which of the following?

A. Renal calculi size greater than 3 mm
B. Inability to tolerate oral fluids
C. Pain
D. Hematuria

66. A bicyclist is brought to the emergency department after crashing into a wall and flying over the handlebars. The patient is awake and alert and is complaining of left-sided abdominal pain with nausea. Vital signs: BP 124/60 mm Hg; HR 80 beats/minute; RR 16 breaths/minute; SpO_2 98%; T 36.4°C (97.6°F). The emergency nurse would anticipate which diagnostic test to assess for possible intra-abdominal injury?

A. Diagnostic peritoneal lavage
B. Exploratory laparotomy
C. Computed tomography scan of the abdomen and pelvis with contrast
D. A focused assessment with sonography for trauma

67. Following the incision and drainage of a Bartholin's gland abscess, the patient's discharge teaching instructions should include which of the following?

A. Your sexual partners will not need to be treated for this infection.
B. Take a sitz bath or soak in a bathtub with warm water several times a day.
C. You should follow up with your healthcare provider to have the drainage (Word) catheter removed in 24 hours.
D. Having an intrauterine device puts you at greater risk for developing a Bartholin's gland abscess.

68. A female patient presents to the emergency department with complaints of right lower abdominal pain and is diagnosed as having an unruptured ectopic pregnancy in the right fallopian tube. The patient's vital signs are stable, and the ectopic pregnancy is estimated to be 3.0 cm in size. A nonsurgical treatment to terminate the ectopic pregnancy is recommended. The nurse anticipates that the patient will receive which medication?

A. Rh_o(D) immune globulin
B. Oxytocin (Pitocin)
C. Methotrexate
D. Medroxyprogesterone (Provera)

69. While treating a patient with postpartum hemorrhage, the nurse administers 20 units of oxytocin per 1000 mL of Ringer's lactate solution. The nurse recognizes that the desired effect of this medication has occurred when:

A. the patient's blood pressure has decreased.
B. there is decreased vaginal bleeding.
C. the patient experiences a decrease in abdominal discomfort.
D. there is a softening of the uterus.

70. A woman who is 39-weeks-pregnant presents to the emergency department. Which of the following findings would alert the emergency nurse that a vaginal delivery is imminent?

A. The patient states that her contractions are 3 minutes apart and lasting a long time.
B. The patient reports an urge to push.
C. The patient reports feeling "gush of water" 1 hour ago.
D. A pulsating umbilical cord is felt in the vagina.

71. The most characteristic clinical finding in a patient with placenta previa is:

A. elevated blood pressure.
B. painless bright red vaginal bleeding.
C. vaginal discharge of blood-tinged mucus.
D. vaginal passing of tissue.

72. Following a precipitous delivery of a full-term infant in the emergency department, the infant is successfully intubated and adequately ventilated. The emergency nurse would begin chest compressions if the infant's heart rate is below which of the following?

A. 60–80 beats/minute
B. 90–100 beats/minute
C. 110–120 beats/minute
D. 130–150 beats/minute

73. A 25-year-old female presents to the emergency department 4 days postpartum. She has a high fever and rigors following a vaginal delivery with an episiotomy and a left sulcus laceration. On examination, the vaginal area is edematous and tender to touch, with a purpuric discoloration from the left labia that extends to the buttocks unilaterally and the presence of a “foul smelling” liquid discharge from the episiotomy site. The patient is tachycardic and tachypneic. The emergency nurse suspects this patient may have:

A. septic thrombophlebitis.
B. endometritis.
C. pelvic abscess.
D. necrotizing fasciitis.

74. An adolescent is being evaluated for abdominal pain. When the mother leaves the exam room to make a phone call, the patient reveals to the emergency nurse that they are being sexually fondled at school by a teacher. The priority nursing intervention for this patient is to:

A. notify the appropriate child protective services or law enforcement agency.
B. obtain consent from the mother to report the abuse to the appropriate agency.
C. report the name of the alleged abuser to law enforcement immediately.
D. discuss birth control and sexually transmitted infection prevention with the patient.

75. When caring for a patient who has been recently diagnosed with leukemia, the emergency nurse should consider which assessment variation in this patient?

A. The sudden onset of initial symptoms is related to thrombocytosis.
B. Hepatomegaly and splenomegaly are common assessment findings in a patient with leukemia.
C. Leukemia is a nonmalignant neoplasm.
D. Early symptoms of fatigue may be related to the presence of thrombocytopenia.

76. A patient presents to triage, extremely tearful and visibly trembling. The patient states, “I can’t take it anymore... this new medication the doctor gave me is not working! I have been taking this medication for 5 days, and I feel even more depressed than I did before!” The emergency nurse begins the patient assessment by completing the medication reconciliation and identifies that the new medication the patient has been prescribed is fluoxetine (Prozac). What intervention by the nurse would have the greatest impact for this patient?

A. Provide the patient with a benzodiazepine such as lorazepam (Ativan) to calm the patient’s nerves.
B. Inform the patient that the provider will likely change the medication given that symptoms are worsening.
C. Instruct the patient to stop the medication immediately.
D. Reassure the patient that fluoxetine requires at least 1–4 weeks before a noticeable improvement in depression symptoms is evident.

77. A young child presents to the emergency department with signs and symptoms of diabetic ketoacidosis. The emergency nurse anticipates the need to correct the child’s dehydration by administering which of the following intravenous (IV) fluids?

A. 10–20 mL/kg of 0.9% sodium chloride IV over 1–2 hours
B. 20 mL/kg of 0.9% sodium chloride rapid IV push over 15 minutes
C. 30 mL/kg bolus of 0.9% sodium chloride IV administered over 1 hour
D. 10–20 mL/kg dextrose 5% with 0.9% sodium chloride IV over 2 hours

78. A patient with myxedema coma is most likely to seek care in an emergency department in which season of the year?

A. Winter
B. Fall
C. Spring
D. Summer

79. During the assessment of a young nonambulatory child, the emergency nurse identifies the presence of a possible spiral leg fracture. The parents state that the child rolled off a bed onto the floor. Based on this assessment, the emergency nurse prepares for which of the following?

A. Separate the parents and ask each what event led to the child's leg injury
B. Do not permit the parents to hold the child
C. Record all verbal interactions between the parents and emergency providers
D. Report suspicion of child maltreatment to the child protective services agency

80. A patient is brought to the emergency department from an outpatient clinic following increasing agitation and the verbal and physical abuse of a staff member after being denied narcotics. The patient is speaking loudly and threatening to "blow the place up" if narcotics are not ordered to be given to him. The nurse has called for the rapid response team. Which of the following indicates an initial desired patient response to the rapid response team intervention? The patient:

A. requests removal from physical restraints.
B. follows verbal instruction.
C. requires intramuscular injection of an antianxiolytic medication.
D. tolerates being placed in seclusion.

81. A patient was involved in a severe motor vehicle collision 2 months ago. Although the patient's injuries are healing appropriately, the patient has been treated in the emergency department 6 times for a variety of complaints since the incident. The patient reports trouble sleeping because of nightmares, fear when driving or riding in cars, and frequent thoughts of the incident. What mental health disorder should the nurse consider when assessing this patient?

A. Agoraphobia
B. Depression
C. Bipolar disorder
D. Posttraumatic stress disorder

82. A patient who was diagnosed with terminal cancer 2 days previously presents to the emergency department (ED). Since receiving their diagnosis, the patient has repeatedly verbalized a desire to commit suicide, making such statements as, "I will just get my shotgun when things get bad," and "You can't stop me from driving my pickup into a tree." They are angry that their family has brought them to the ED and is continually yelling at their family members. What is the priority intervention the emergency nurse should take in this situation?

A. Explain to the family that the patient is experiencing the normal reaction of anger
B. Reassure the patient that they will be provided with resources such as hospice care
C. Recommend that the patient follow up with their primary care provider for antidepressants
D. Call for extra staff to assist

83. A patient presents to the emergency department with severe swelling around their eyes and lips (angioedema). They deny any known allergies and states that they are currently taking only one medication for a recent diagnosis of hypertension. The emergency nurse recognizes that the most likely cause of the patient's angioedema is related to which of the following?

A. Midodrine (ProAmatine)
B. Losartan (Cozaar)
C. Diltiazem (Cardizem)
D. Lisinopril (Zestril)

84. A patient from a skilled nursing facility is transported to the emergency department (ED) after sustaining a minor hand laceration; the bleeding has been controlled. The patient has recently been receiving high-dose chemotherapy for treatment of non-Hodgkin's lymphoma. The most appropriate area in the ED for the patient to receive treatment is in which of the following?

A. The waiting room
B. An ED room with reverse isolation precautions
C. Any available ED room
D. A quick care or rapid care minor treatment area

85. Which of the following assessment findings would the emergency nurse be most concerned about in a hemophiliac patient with hemarthrosis?

A. Skin breakdown
B. Severe pain
C. Paresthesias
D. Impaired range of motion

86. Which of the following interventions would the emergency nurse expect to implement first in the patient who has developed signs of neuroleptic malignant syndrome?

A. Application of a cooling blanket
B. Administration of a benzodiazepine
C. Administration of a dopamine agonist
D. Insertion of a urinary catheter

87. The emergency nurse has provided discharge education to the parents of a child who experienced a febrile seizure. Which of the following statements made by the parents indicates to the emergency nurse that the teaching has been effective?

A. "Axillary temperature measurement is the preferred route for temperature measurement because it is the most accurate."
B. "Aspirin and acetaminophen (Tylenol) are the preferred medications for reducing a fever."
C. "Febrile seizures occur most often in children over the age of 2."
D. "Febrile seizures most often occur because of a rapid rise in the body's temperature."

88. A patient is brought to the emergency department by law enforcement after attempting to kill their brother with a knife. Presently the patient is calm, cooperative, and following directions. When performing the patient's initial assessment, which of the following would be the highest priority for the emergency nurse?

A. Offer the patient food or drink as soon as possible
B. Approach the patient early with a display of a power attitude
C. Have the patient undress completely
D. Physically restrain the patient with soft restraints

89. A patient who has sustained a 4-inch laceration to the left anterior thigh arrives in the emergency department via emergency medical services. The wound had previously been bleeding profusely, however, direct pressure to the wound has reduced the blood flow. The patient is anxious and continually states, "I am a bleeder! I know I will need some factor VIII! Get it quick!" The emergency nurse is aware that this patient most likely has which of the following coagulopathies?

A. Hemophilia B
B. Hemophilia A
C. Von Willebrand disease
D. Christmas disease

90. Which of the following statements made by a patient being treated for diabetic ketoacidosis would increase the emergency nurse's suspicion that an untoward effect was occurring during the treatment phase?

A. "I seem to have developed a pretty serious headache in the past hour."
B. "I feel like I need to urinate very badly."
C. "Can I have something for this back pain that has been getting worse?"
D. "I feel like I am aching all over."

91. Which laboratory test would indicate that a patient's psychotic symptoms may be related to a medical condition and not a psychiatric condition?

A. A sodium level of 145 mg/dL
B. A potassium level of 4.0 mEq/L
C. A blood glucose level of 20 mg/dL
D. A calcium level of 10 mg/dL

92. Which of the following laboratory trends does the emergency nurse expect to be present in a patient diagnosed with disseminated intravascular coagulation?

A. Decreased platelet count, elevated D-dimer, and prolonged prothrombin time
B. Increased platelet count, elevated D-dimer, and prolonged prothrombin time
C. Decreased platelet count, increased fibrinogen, and decreased D-dimer
D. Increased platelet count, decreased D-dimer, and prolonged prothrombin

93. After receiving fluid resuscitation with an isotonic crystalloid solution, an emergency department patient diagnosed with septic shock remains hypotensive. Which of the following would be initiated to assist in maintaining the patient's blood pressure?

A. Transfuse hydroxyethyl starches to maintain a mean arterial pressure (MAP) of 65 mm Hg or higher
B. Addition of albumin to the current crystalloid solution to maintain a MAP of 65 mm Hg or higher
C. Transfuse packed red blood cells to maintain a MAP of 65 mm Hg or higher
D. Vasopressor to maintain a MAP of 65 mm Hg or higher

94. An emergency patient has been diagnosed with thrombocytopenia. The emergency nurse is aware the following laboratory value has confirmed this diagnosis:

A. White blood cell count of 8000 uL
B. Platelet count of 5000 uL
C. Platelet count of 900,000 uL
D. White blood cell count of 26,000 uL

95. A patient presents to the emergency department with a swollen abdomen. The patient's arms and legs are very thin, their face is round, their skin is very thin, and there is a buffalo hump between their shoulders. Pink stretch marks are noted on the abdomen. The patient has a history of long-term dexamethasone (Prednisone) use for urticaria. Vital signs include: BP 200/100 mm Hg. The emergency nurse suspects that this patient has which of the following?

A. Hashimoto disease
B. Thyrotoxicosis
C. Syndrome of inappropriate antidiuretic hormone
D. Cushing's syndrome

96. A patient presents to triage complaining of nausea, weakness, and fatigue. The patient appears anorexic and has hyperpigmentation to the knuckles and creases of the hands. The patient's medical history includes the presence of Addison's disease, and the provider orders a dose of hydrocortisone to be administered. The emergency nurse anticipates which of the following outcomes as a result of this medication?

A. Increase in blood pressure
B. Decrease in sodium
C. Decrease in glucose
D. Weight gain

97. The emergency nurse is assessing a patient with a history of sickle cell disease (SCD). The patient tells the nurse that he is experiencing wheezing, fever, and shortness of breath. Which high-morbidity complication of SCD would the emergency nurse suspect this patient is experiencing?

A. Priapism
B. Acute chest syndrome
C. Cholecystitis
D. Splenic sequestration

98. Which of the following conditions is a rare, life-threatening, and serious complication of hypothyroidism?

A. Adrenal crisis
B. Myxedema coma
C. Thyroid storm
D. Cushing's syndrome

99. Parents arrive to triage with their toddler, whose hand was caught in the car door, resulting in amputation of the index finger. The amputated part has been wrapped in gauze, which is presented to the triage nurse. The emergency nurse is aware that the proper way to care for the amputated part is to:

A. wrap the amputated part with sterile gauze soaked in tap water, place in a sealed bag, place the sealed bag in another bag, and place in tepid water.
B. wrap the amputated part in sterile gauze soaked with hibiclens and saline, place the part in a sealed bag, place the sealed bag in another bag, and place in ice water.
C. wrap the amputated part with dry sterile gauze, place in a sealed bag, place the sealed bag in another bag, and place in tepid water.
D. wrap the amputated part in sterile gauze moistened by saline, place the part in a sealed bag, place the sealed bag in another bag, and place in ice water.

100. When caring for a variety of patients, the emergency nurse is knowledgeable that the patient with the least risk for developing compartment syndrome would be a patient with which of the following injuries?

A. A patient with a venomous snake bite to the forearm
B. A crush injury to the shaft of the femur
C. A patient with a circumferential full thickness burn to the calf
D. A nondisplaced fracture to the medial malleolus

101. The emergency nurse is discharging a patient who developed back pain 1 week ago after bending over to pick up a young child. The emergency nurse determines that patient teaching has been effective when the patient states which of the following?

A. "Nonsteroidal anti-inflammatory drugs and acetaminophen (Tylenol) are not effective in relieving my back pain."
B. "I need to limit my activity and rest my back as much as possible."
C. "It is important that I stop smoking so that I will heal faster."
D. "I should only use ice and heat during the first 24 hours of my back pain."

102. A patient presents to the emergency department by emergency medical services (EMS) in complete cervical spine immobilization. The patient is intoxicated, and EMS reports that the patient had been drinking and jumped off the second floor of a parking garage and landed on their heels. The patient is found to have bilateral calcaneal fractures. The emergency nurse also anticipates the patient may have experienced which of the following injuries?

A. Spinous process fracture of thoracic vertebrae 6 (T6)
B. Spiral fracture of the femur
C. Bilateral bipartite patella
D. Burst fracture of lumbar vertebrae 1 (L1)

103. A patient is being discharged from the emergency department with a lower leg cast. The patient is concerned about how they will be able to walk up and down the steps with crutches at home. The emergency nurse will instruct the patient that the proper technique to go up and down stairs is:

A. up with the "bad" leg and down with the "good" leg.
B. up with the "bad" leg and down with the "bad" leg.
C. up with the "good" leg and down with the "bad" leg.
D. up with the "good" leg and down with the "good" leg.

104. The emergency nurse is caring for a patient with a pelvic fracture. At the beginning of the assessment, the nurse notes the presence of distal pulses with good motor and sensory function of the lower extremities. However, during ongoing assessments, the nurse is no longer able to palpate distal pulses, and the patient has an altered mental status. Which of the following could be responsible for this change in the patient's status?

A. Fat embolism
B. Hemorrhage
C. Compartment syndrome
D. Neurogenic shock

105. The emergency nurse is aware that patients with gout will experience periodic exacerbation of painful joint inflammation, resulting in acute painful episodes to be treated with the following medication:

A. allopurinol.
B. antibiotics.
C. nonsteroidal anti-inflammatory medications.
D. bisphosphonates.

106. A patient arrives by emergency medical services (EMS) to the emergency department. EMS reports that the patient jumped from a third-story balcony when the support structure gave way. The patient landed on both feet and has been found to have a compression fracture of the lumbar spine with significant pain. Neurological assessment indicates the spine is intact, and the patient has no other complaints of pain. Glasgow Coma Scale score is 15, with no reported loss of consciousness. In addition to the compression fracture of the lumbar spine, this patient should also be evaluated for the presence of a:

A. hidden foreign body impalement.
B. femur fracture.
C. subdural hematoma.
D. calcaneus fracture.

107. A young patient presents to triage with complaints of left ankle pain. The patient reports that while playing basketball, they lost their balance and landed hard on their left foot; a "popping" sound in the ankle followed. The ankle is swollen and painful, and the patient is unable to bear weight on the left foot. The patient is exhibiting signs and symptoms of what type of ankle injury?

A. Avulsion fracture
B. Sprain
C. Dislocation
D. Strain

108. A patient with a laceration to the middle phalanx of the palmar side of the index finger from a kitchen knife presents to triage. Bleeding has been controlled. After examining the patient for possible tendon injury, the emergency nurse anticipates preparing the patient for wound closure by first:

A. cleansing the wound.
B. administering antibiotics.
C. providing anesthesia with lidocaine and epinephrine into the affected finger.
D. administering an opioid analgesia.

109. A patient presents to the emergency department with a shortened, deformed, and outwardly rotated right leg. The patient requires the application of a traction splint. The splint has been appropriately applied when:

A. the affected limb begins to swell.
B. the patient reports an increase in pain.
C. the dorsalis pedis pulse is faint.
D. the patient reports a decrease in pain.

110. A college student presents to triage complaining of a constant buzzing sound in their ear. On examination, an insect is seen in the ear canal. The physician has instilled viscous lidocaine in the ear of the patient. The emergency nurse identifies that this treatment has been effective when the patient states which of the following?

A. "My ear feels numb."
B. "I no longer hear the buzzing sound in my ear, I don't think the insect is moving."
C. "My ear no longer hurts."
D. "My hearing has improved in that ear now."

111. A patient presents to the emergency department complaining of decreased vision, an intense headache, and the appearance of halos around lights with photophobia. The emergency nurse identifies these symptoms as being consistent with the development of which of the following?

A. Central retinal artery occlusion
B. Glaucoma
C. Corneal abrasion
D. Iritis

112. The emergency nurse is preparing to dress a stage 2 pressure injury on the shoulder of a patient. Which solution would be most appropriate to cleanse the wound bed with?

A. Ringer's lactate solution
B. Povidone iodine (Betadine)
C. Hydrogen peroxide
D. Tap water

113. Which patient would be least likely to require a tetanus booster shot?

A. The 70-year-old patient with burns on the leg
B. The 13-year-old patient with a facial laceration
C. The 24-year-old patient who stepped on a nail
D. The 35-year-old pregnant female who sustained a laceration to the hand

114. A patient presents with complaints of generalized muscle spasms, pain, and headache. The patient reports stepping on a nail 2 days ago. Which bacterial organism does the emergency nurse anticipate to be the cause of the patient's symptoms?

A. Group A streptococcus
B. *Clostridium tetani*
C. *Staphylococcus aureus*
D. *Clostridium perfringens*

115. A patient arrives to the emergency department complaining of sudden onset of severe jaw pain that radiates to their ear. The patient states that they are having difficulty speaking because of the excessive pain. The pain started as they were biting into a large sandwich. The emergency nurse anticipates that this patient has which of the following?

A. Angina
B. Trigeminal neuralgia
C. Dental pain
D. Temporomandibular joint syndrome

116. A patient presents to triage with the complaint of a foreign body sensation and excessive pain to their left eye but denies any recent change to their vision. The patient states they were treated earlier in the week for conjunctivitis. The emergency nurse anticipates that this patient is experiencing which of the following conditions?

A. Uveitis
B. Subconjunctival hemorrhage
C. Keratitis
D. Episcleritis

117. A patient rushes into triage and stating that there is something in their eye. A large sliver of wood is noted to be impaled in the patient's right eye. Following completion of the visual acuity (Snellen) exam, what is the next intervention that the emergency nurse should perform for this patient?

A. Instill a topical ophthalmic anesthetic
B. Irrigate the eye as soon as possible
C. Apply a cotton patch to the unaffected eye
D. Place a rigid eye shield over the affected orbit

118. A patient presents to the emergency department with a history of blunt force trauma to their face. The patient relates falling down and striking their face on the floor. There is periorbital bruising and edema around the left eye, and the patient is complaining of diplopia. Which of the following assessment findings would confirm a diagnosis of an orbital rim fracture with entrapment of extraocular muscles?

A. Decreased ability to look upward
B. Teardrop shape of their left pupil
C. Presence of blood in the anterior chamber
D. Complaint of halos around lights

119. While at triage, the emergency nurse assesses a patient who presents with a complaint of increasing difficulty speaking. The patient's voice is muffled, they are drooling, and the left side of their face is markedly swollen. The patient's tongue is protruding slightly through their lips. The patient indicates that they were recently assaulted. The emergency nurse anticipates that this patient has which of the following?

A. Pharyngitis
B. Peritonsillar abscess
C. Ludwig's angina
D. Tonsillitis

120. A patient with burns to their anterior trunk and both arms from a camp fire presents to the emergency department. Based on the "rule of nines," the patient's estimated total body surface area burned is:

A. 36%.
B. 18%.
C. 45%.
D. 40%.

121. A patient was brought into the emergency department following a house fire that was believed to have started as a result of a gas leak. The patient's skin is flushed, they are not oriented to time, place, or person, and they are complaining of nausea associated with a severe headache. What should be performed first to properly care for this patient?

A. Obtain a carboxyhemoglobin level
B. Provide continuous pulse oximetry
C. Obtain an arterial blood gas test
D. Provide continuous capnography

122. After unintentionally being sprayed by a crop duster, a patient presents to the emergency department with excessive tearing, salivation, nausea, vomiting, and bradycardia. The emergency nurse should anticipate the administration of which intravenous medication to this patient?

A. Naloxone (Narcan)
B. Atropine (atropine sulfate)
C. Sodium nitrite
D. Flumazenil (Romazicon)

123. The most important factor in the survival of a drowning victim is:

A. immediate cardiopulmonary resuscitation.
B. the speed of rewarming the victim while in the emergency department.
C. the type of water (saltwater or freshwater) that the victim was found in.
D. an initial Glasgow Coma Score of 3 or greater.

124. A patient arrives at the emergency department after a sudden onset of severe pain to the left calf area while playing tennis. The provider performs a Thompson test on the patient's left calf, which is positive and indicates an Achilles tendon injury. The patient reports that they were recently taking an antibiotic. The emergency nurse is aware that the following antibiotic is associated with the development of an Achilles tendon injury:

A. ciprofloxacin (Cipro).
B. cephalexin (Keflex).
C. azithromycin (Zithromax).
D. amoxicillin (Amoxil).

125. The emergency nurse is caring for a child who presents with a red ring-shaped rash to the right leg. The nurse anticipates that the provider will prescribe which of the following treatments?

A. Oral antifungal medication
B. Topical antibiotic medication
C. Oral antibiotic medication
D. Topical antifungal medication

126. An adult patient who has been diagnosed with Lyme disease presents to the emergency department with a complaint of left-sided facial weakness for 2 days. On assessment, the nurse notes unilateral facial drooping on the left side, and drooling. The patient is alert and oriented. Gait is normal, and strength is equal in both arms and legs. Vital signs: BP 140/78 mm Hg; HR 92 beats/minute; RR 20 breaths/minute; SpO_2 99%; T 36.8°C (98.2°F). Which of the following is the most likely cause of this patient's signs and symptoms?

A. Bell's palsy
B. Transient ischemic attack
C. Allergic reaction
D. Ischemic stroke

127. The emergency nurse is caring for a child who has been diagnosed with rubeola (measles). The nurse anticipates that the patient will require which of the following interventions?

A. Measles, mumps, rubella vaccination
B. Intravenous antibiotics
C. Isolation with standard and droplet precautions
D. Vitamin K injection

128. A patient is brought to the emergency department after cleaning solution is unintentionally splashed over the patient's face and eyes. Irrigation is currently in progress. Which of the following would indicate to the emergency nurse that effective eye irrigation has occurred?

A. 1.0 L of dextrose and water has been used for irrigation
B. Eye pH of 7.25 after irrigation
C. Clear sclera after irrigation
D. Visual acuity of 20/20 after irrigation

129. The emergency nurse is aware that the cyanide antidote kit contains:

A. acetylcysteine.
B. dimercaprol.
C. amyl nitrite.
D. sodium polystyrene sulfonate.

130. A patient presents to the emergency department after taking an overdose of beta blocker medication. Which of the following signs and/or symptoms indicate that the treatment has been effective?

A. Increasing glucose level
B. Lowering blood pressure
C. Decreasing heart rate
D. Decreasing level of consciousness

131. A patient arrives to emergency department following recent ingestion of cocaine. Which of the following symptoms being exhibited by the patient would cause the nurse the greatest concern?

A. Auditory hallucinations
B. Fever
C. Poor appetite
D. Abdominal pain

132. A patient presents to the emergency department in acute alcohol withdrawal. The alcohol withdrawal treatment protocol is initiated for this patient. Which change in the patient's condition would indicate to the nurse that the treatment is having its intended effect?

A. Increased blood pressure
B. Decreased heart rate
C. Increased temperature
D. Increased motor activity

133. You are caring for a patient who has presented directly from their primary care provider for hydration therapy secondary to 2 days of watery diarrhea and the presence of blood in their stool. Which of the following statements by the patient would be concerning for a *Clostridium difficile* infection?

A. "I work at a daycare with toddlers all day."
B. "I've been taking penicillin for this infection in my leg for several weeks."
C. "I work on a farm around cattle and livestock every day."
D. "I just returned from traveling in Africa for 2 weeks."

134. The nurse is caring for a patient who presents with a fracture of the radius. The patient provides a history of having human immunodeficiency virus and is taking multiple medications for tuberculosis. Which physical finding should the nurse assess for that is related to potential complications from the tuberculosis medications?

A. Urine is orange colored.
B. Skin has a yellow tinge.
C. Patient reports having diarrhea.
D. Patient reports presence of tinnitus.

135. Following introduction of the participants, which of the following statements would be used at the beginning of a critical incident stress debriefing?

A. "Can you tell me what you think should have been done differently?"
B. "Can you provide me with a brief description of what happened during the situation from your viewpoint?"
C. "Can you tell us what you perceive to be the positive outcomes of this event?"
D. "Can you describe how you are feeling after going through this event?"

136. A patient with a known history of alcohol abuse was found lying on the sidewalk and brought to the emergency department by emergency medical services. The patient is confused, speech is slurred, and there is a strong smell of alcohol on the patient's breath. After placing the patient in a treatment area, what is the next action performed by the emergency nurse?

A. Request an evaluation by the physician
B. Request a blood alcohol level to be drawn
C. Initiate intravenous (IV) access and begin an infusion of a thiamine-containing IV fluid
D. Begin the process for referral to a detoxification unit

137. When caring for a patient who has experienced an act of interpersonal violence, it is important the emergency nurse perform which of the following?

A. Use only fluorescent lights when photographing injuries
B. Document patient statements using proper medical terminology
C. Label bullet wounds as "entrance" and "exit"
D. Recognize items that may have forensic value

138. Nursing staff in the emergency department voice a concern that blood culture contamination rates are high. What is the initial step the nurses should complete to develop a new, evidence-based blood-drawing protocol?

A. Collect the evidence
B. Develop the clinical question
C. Evaluate the hierarchy of evidence
D. Identify patient preferences and values

139. The emergency nurse is caring for a 10-year-old trauma patient who is unresponsive and hemodynamically unstable because of severe internal hemorrhage. The trauma surgeon has ordered that the massive transfusion protocol (MTP) be initiated for this patient. The family is refusing the blood transfusion because of their religious beliefs. Although the patient's family is refusing to consent to the MTP treatment, the nurse should plan to:

A. initiate the transfusion protocol.
B. provide comfort measures only.
C. ask the family to sign a Do Not Resuscitate form.
D. complete an incident report for not initiating the transfusion protocol.

140. Which of the following is the most effective method for an emergency nurse to reinforce a patient's understanding of their discharge instructions?

A. Assist the patient in scheduling a follow-up appointment with their primary care provider
B. Provide written discharge instructions
C. Arrange for a follow-up phone call
D. Demonstrate all procedures before discharge

141. Hospital staff who access the medical record of a patient whom they have no responsibility to care for would be in violation of which federal regulation?

A. Reportable conditions
B. Emergency Medical Treatment and Active Labor Act
C. Health Insurance Portability and Accountability Act
D. Advance directives

142. Following the death of a patient in the emergency department, who determines if the patient's organs and tissues are suitable for donation?

A. The local medical examiner
B. The emergency physician
C. A representative of the organ procurement organization
D. The patient's legal next-of-kin

143. The emergency department is notified that a patient will soon be arriving via emergency medical services. The patient was involved in a possible shooting, and the police are requesting that the patient's hands be "bagged." The emergency nurse is aware that the police are requesting that which of the following actions be performed when the patient arrives?

A. Place a sterile drape over each hand and secure at the wrist.
B. Place a clear plastic bag over each hand and secure at the wrist.
C. Place a paper bag over each hand and secure at the wrist.
D. Wrap each hand in a towel and secure at the wrist.

144. The emergency nurse is preparing a treatment room for procedural sedation. Review of the preprocedure checklist identifies that the patient's ASA (American Society of Anesthesiologists) physical status classification is a level 3. The nurse should perform which of the following actions?

A. Refuse to do the procedure and call the nursing supervisor.
B. Continue to set up the treatment room for the procedure as indicated and ensure that end-tidal CO_2 capnography is readily available.
C. Discuss with the patient's physician that an ASA class 3 indicates that the patient has a history of severe systemic disease and therefore may require an anesthesia consult, or the procedure may be performed more safely in the operating room.
D. Request that the emergency department charge nurse immediately notify the on-call anesthesiologist of the procedure.

145. A nationwide initiative being used in emergency departments to increase patient safety during nurses' change-of-shift report is to perform a:

A. uninterrupted report.
B. bedside report.
C. designated timed report.
D. taped report.

146. There are five mission areas of emergency response according to the Federal Emergency Management Agency. The five phases are prevention, protection, response, recovery, and:
A. education.
B. management.
C. evacuation.
D. mitigation.

147. An emergency department guideline being used to improve patient safety is to weigh all children in:
A. grains.
B. pounds.
C. ounces.
D. kilograms.

148. A patient arrives by ambulance to the emergency department demonstrating delusions, hallucinations, and suicidal ideation. The patient refuses all medical treatment. The emergency nurse is aware that the healthcare team can legally treat the patient based on which type of consent?
A. Express consent
B. Involuntary consent
C. Implied consent
D. Informed consent

149. Which of the following is a mandatory reportable disease to the Centers for Disease Control and Prevention?
A. Urinary tract infections
B. Pneumonia
C. Hand, foot, and mouth disease
D. Measles (rubeola)

150. While working in triage, the emergency nurse is speaking on the phone to an individual who is seeking medical advice for abdominal pain. What is the appropriate response for the emergency triage nurse to give to this patient?
A. "It sounds like you have a viral infection. Be sure to increase your fluids and avoid dairy products."
B. "I will call you back after I speak to the emergency provider. Can you tell me more about the pain that you are experiencing?"
C. "It is very busy here right now; I think you should just wait and be seen by your physician tomorrow."
D. "I cannot answer your question over the phone; the emergency department is open 24 hours a day, and we can evaluate you here in person if you wish to be seen."

PART 2

1. A patient presents to the emergency department experiencing an anterior ST segment elevation myocardial infarction. The patient's vital signs are normal. The hospital is not equipped with a cardiac catheterization laboratory. The patient can be transferred to a cardiac catheterization lab within 60 minutes. Which of the following would you anticipate for this patient?

   A. A bolus of tissue plasminogen activator, followed by an infusion for fibrinolytic therapy
   B. Immediate transfer to the hospital with a cardiac catheterization lab for percutaneous coronary intervention
   C. A single bolus of tenecteplase (TNKase) for fibrinolytic therapy
   D. A bolus of reteplase (Retavase), followed by a second bolus of reteplase (Retavase) 30 minutes later for fibrinolytic therapy

Rationale

A. When ST segment elevation myocardial infarction (STEMI) patients cannot be transferred to a percutaneous intervention (PCI)-capable hospital in a timely manner, fibrinolytic therapy with routine transfer for angiography may be an acceptable alternative to immediate transfer to PPCI (Class IIb, LOE C-LD).

B. In adult patients presenting with STEMI to the emergency department of a hospital that does not have PCI capability, it is recommended that the patient be transferred immediately without fibrinolysis to a PCI center, instead of immediate fibrinolysis at the initial hospital with transfer only for ischemia-driven PCI (Class I, LOE B-R). When STEMI patients cannot be transferred to a PCI-capable hospital in a timely manner, fibrinolytic therapy with routine transfer for angiography may be an acceptable alternative to immediate transfer to PPCI (Class IIb, LOE C-LD).

C. Although treatment of STEMI may include the use of fibrinolytic agents, it is preferred that the patient be transferred for immediate PCI if it can be accomplished in a timely fashion.

D. The preferred treatment of STEMI is PCI; fibrinolytic therapy should only be considered if transfer to a PCI-capable facility cannot be performed in a timely fashion.

Category: Cardiovascular Emergencies/Acute coronary syndrome
Nursing Process: Intervention

Reference

O'Connor, R. E., Al Ali, A. S., Brady, W. J., Ghaemmaghami, C. A., Menon, V., Welsford, M., & Shuster, M. (2015). Part 9: Acute coronary syndromes: 2015 American Heart Association guidelines update for cardiopulmonary resuscitation and emergency cardiovascular care. *Circulation, 132*(Suppl. 2), S483–S500.

2. An anxious patient arrives by ambulance following an acute onset of difficulty breathing. The patient is diaphoretic and denies chest pain. High-flow oxygen by nonrebreather mask has been applied. Vital signs: BP 210/140 mm Hg; HR 130 beats/minute; RR 32 breaths/minute; SpO_2 88%. In addition to initiating noninvasive ventilation to treat the patient's difficulty breathing, the nurse anticipates the administration of which medication to further treat the patient's symptoms?

   A. Morphine (morphine sulfate)
   B. Furosemide (Lasix)
   C. Initiation of a continuous nitroglycerin infusion
   D. Acetylsalicylic acid (aspirin)

Rationale

A. Morphine (morphine sulfate), in the treatment algorithm for acute pulmonary edema, is not effective in afterload reduction and has been shown in observational and retrospective studies to increase morbidity and mortality. It should no longer be part of the acute pulmonary edema treatment package.

B. Loop diuretics should not be used early in treatment; 50% of patients do not have significant volume overload. Increased cardiac filling pressure results from shifts in fluid instead of fluid retention. Additionally, many of the patients who are volume overloaded have end-stage renal disease, and loop diuretics will not be useful. Finally, small studies have shown that an initial increase in preload resulting from loop diuretic administration can potentially lead to worse patient outcomes.

C. Patients who present with acute pulmonary edema are typically markedly hypertensive and in acute respiratory distress. Rapid initiation of appropriate treatment is vital to reversing the neurohormonal surge and rescuing patients from respiratory and complete cardiac failure. Immediate interventions should focus on reduction of afterload and preload, as well as respiratory support. Nitroglycerin (NTG) is the most important first-line medication in treatment of acute pulmonary edema and respiratory distress. The initiation of a continuous NTG infusion at low doses acts as a vasodilator, leading to decreased preload; at higher doses (> 100 mcg/minute), it acts as a potent afterload reducer.

D. Although acetylsalicylic acid (aspirin) may have a role in this patient if acute coronary syndrome or acute myocardial infarction is suspected or confirmed, it provides no immediate effect in the treatment of acute pulmonary edema to reduce afterload.

Category: Cardiovascular Emergencies/Heart failure
Nursing Process: Intervention

References

Bryant, W. (2014). Acute pulmonary edema "answers." *EM Lyceum*. Retrieved from https://emlyceum.com/2011/07/25/acute-pulmonary-edema-answers/

Swaminathan, A. (2014). Furosemide in the treatment of acute pulmonary edema. *emDocs*. Retrieved from http://www.emdocs.net/furosemide-treatment-acute-pulmonary-edema

---

3. An unrestrained driver is brought to the emergency department following a motor vehicle collision. The patient reports hitting their chest on the steering wheel and is complaining of chest pain across the front of their chest. There are no vital sign abnormalities and no other complaints of pain. The diagnosis of blunt cardiac injury is considered. The nurse anticipates an order for which of the following?

   A. Electrocardiogram
   B. Cardiac marker evaluation (creatine kinase and/or troponin)
   C. Cardiac monitoring
   D. Chest radiograph

Rationale

A. An electrocardiogram evaluated for dysrhythmias, heart block, or ischemia is part of the initial evaluation for blunt cardiac injury.

B. Not all trauma patients with blunt cardiac injury will have acute alterations in cardiac markers, and other organ injury may cause release of creatine kinase and confound the diagnosis of blunt cardiac injury.

C. Continuous cardiac monitoring evaluating for dysrhythmias should be included in the initial evaluation for blunt cardiac injury.

D. A chest radiograph is part of the initial evaluation for blunt cardiac injury.

Category: Cardiovascular Emergencies/Trauma

Nursing Process: Intervention

Reference

Carden, L. O., Gibbs, M. A., MacVane, C. Z, & Stafford, P. W. (2012). Penetrating and blunt cardiac trauma. *Trauma Reports, 13*(2).

---

4. Which of the following is a form of distributive shock?
   A. Neurogenic
   B. Metabolic
   C. Respiratory
   D. Obstructive

Rationale

A. Neurogenic is a form of distributive shock.

B. Metabolic is not an identified form of shock

C. Respiratory is not an identified form of shock.

D. Obstructive shock results from inadequate circulating volume due to the presence of pulmonary embolus, pericardial tamponade, or a tension pneumothorax.

Category: Cardiovascular Emergencies/Shock (cardiogenic and obstructive)

Nursing Process: Assessment

Reference

Richards, J. B., & Wilcox, R. (2014). Diagnosis and management of shock in the emergency department. *Emergency Medicine Practice, 16*(3), 1–22. Retrieved from http://europepmc.org/abstract/med/24883457

5. A patient presents following an acute onset of chest pain, dyspnea, and severe diaphoresis, with near syncope. Assessment shows a patient in severe distress, with HR 110 beats/minute; BP 60/40 mm Hg; and RR 36 breaths/minute and bilateral rales. An electrocardiogram reveals ST segment elevation across the precordial leads. A diagnosis of acute myocardial infarction with cardiogenic shock is made, and the patient is being prepared for transfer to the cardiac catheterization lab. The vasopressor of choice, based on this patient's degree of hypotension, is:

   A. norepinephrine (Levophed).
   B. dopamine (Intropin).
   C. dobutamine (Dobutrex).
   D. vasopressin (Pitressin).

Rationale

A. The initial use of norepinephrine (Levophed) for marked hypotension, < 70 mm Hg systolic, is the current recommendation from the American Heart Association and the American College of Cardiology.

B. Dopamine (Intropin) has been associated with a higher risk of death and arrhythmia in the setting of hypotensive cardiogenic shock.

C. Dobutamine (Dobutrex) is a positive inotrope, but its vasodilatory effects may make its use limited in hypotensive cardiogenic shock.

D. Vasopressin (Pitressin) is a useful adjunctive drug along with norepinephrine in the setting of refractory hypotensive cardiogenic shock.

Category: Cardiovascular Emergencies/Shock (cardiogenic and obstructive)

Nursing Process: Intervention

Reference

Dargin, J., Dhokarh, R., & Grgurich, P. E. (2013). The use of vasoactive agents in the management of circulatory shock. *EM Critical Care, 3*(5). Retrieved from https://www.ebmedicine.net/topics.php?paction=showTopic&topic_id=384

---

6. A patient presents with complaints of chest pain that radiates to the jaw, stating the pain is a 6 on a 0–10 scale. Other symptoms include nausea, dizziness, shortness of breath with clear lung sounds, and a sense of impending doom. The pain started 40 minutes before arrival. Vital signs: BP 116/58 mm Hg; HR 98 beats/minute; RR 20 breaths/minute; SpO_2 94%; T 37°C (98.6°F). The 12-lead electrocardiogram (ECG) shows an inferior wall myocardial injury pattern. Which clinical presentations indicate the need to complete a right sided 12-lead ECG?

   A. Shortness of breath with clear lung sounds
   B. Nausea and dizziness
   C. Chest pain with radiation to jaw
   D. Sense of impending doom

Rationale

A. Classic right ventricular infarcts are associated with absence of pulmonary congestion.

B. Classical acute coronary syndrome clinical presentation may include nausea and dizziness, but it does not serve to localize the area of myocardial infarction.

C. Classical acute coronary syndrome clinical presentation includes chest pain with radiation to the jaw.

D. Patients experiencing acute coronary syndrome may have a sense of impending doom.

Category: Cardiovascular Emergencies/Acute coronary syndrome

Nursing Process: Analysis

Reference

Hammond, B. B. (2013). Cardiovascular emergencies. In B. B. Hammond & P. G. Zimmermann (Eds.), *Sheehy's manual of emergency care* (7th ed., pp. 201–211). St. Louis, MO: Elsevier Mosby.

---

7. Following the successful resuscitation of a patient in a cardiac arrest, which of the following findings is the best indicator of high-quality cardiopulmonary resuscitation (CPR)?

A. A compression depth of 1 ½ inches
B. Palpable pulses with the performance of chest compressions during CPR
C. A decrease of skin and mucus membrane cyanosis
D. An increasing end-tidal carbon dioxide level

Rationale

A. High-performance CPR requires compression depth of 1 ½ to 2 inches for optimal outcomes.

B. Pulses should be palpable during effective CPR, but it is not the best indicator of high-quality CPR.

C. Cyanosis is the result of poor tissue oxygenation, however, an improvement in tissue color does not indicate an increase in end cellular perfusion.

D. An increasing end-tidal carbon dioxide level indicates increasing cellular perfusion with effective CPR or return of spontaneous circulation.

Category: Cardiovascular Emergencies/Cardiopulmonary arrest

Nursing Process: Evaluation

Reference

American Heart Association. (2016). The ACLs cases: Cardiac arrest: VF/pulseless VT. In *Advanced cardiovascular life support: Provider manual* (p. 94). Dallas, TX: American Heart Association.

---

8. During transcutaneous pacing for a patient in third-degree heart block, there is a loss of ventricular capture. Which is a significant physiological reason for loss of pacemaker capture?

A. Metabolic alkalosis
B. Hypomagnesemia
C. Lactic acidosis
D. Hypokalemia

Rationale

A. Metabolic alkalosis may present with atrial tachycardia and can be related to hypotension as a result of excessive fluid loss related to gastrointestinal losses or diuretic abuse.

B. Hypomagnesemia may present with torsades de pointes, ventricular tachycardia, and/or ventricular fibrillation, but it is not associated with loss of pacemaker capture.

C. Lactic acidosis alters the contractility of the myocardium, leading to decreased ability to gain ventricular capture; this results in a lack of tissue perfusion.

D. Hypokalemia presents with the presence of U waves on the electrocardiogram, ventricular dysrhythmias, or pulseless electrical activity, but it is not associated with loss of pacemaker capture.

Category: Cardiovascular Emergencies/Dysrhythmias

Nursing Process: Analysis

References

Kuiper, B. (2010). Fluids & electrolytes. In P. K. Howard & R. A. Steinmann (Eds.), *Sheehy's emergency nursing: Principles and practice* (6th ed., pp. 490–498). St. Louis, MO: Mosby Elsevier.

Williams, D. (2010). Cardiovascular emergencies. In P. K. Howard & R. A. Steinmann (Eds.), *Sheehy's emergency nursing: Principles and practice* (6th ed., pp. 411–444). St. Louis, MO: Mosby Elsevier.

---

9. A patient presents with complaints of lightheadedness, weakness, and near syncope. The patient's 12-lead electrocardiogram reveals the presence of 2:1 atrial flutter. The most appropriate intervention for this presentation with an atrial flutter rhythm is to perform:

A. synchronized cardioversion at 50 joules.
B. unsynchronized cardioversion at 120 joules.
C. unsynchronized cardioversion at 50 joules.
D. synchronized cardioversion at 120 joules.

Rationale

A. Synchronized cardioversion is recommended for rhythms with a normal width QRS complex. A patient with new onset of atrial flutter who is experiencing chest pain, shortness of breath, or other symptoms of instability should be considered for cardioversion. Atrial flutter requires less energy to cardiovert than other dysrhythmias.

B. Unsynchronized cardioversion will result in the electrical impulse to occur randomly during the cardiac cycle, which could cause a life-threatening dysrhythmia; therefore, its use should be limited to patients who are pulseless or deteriorating.

C. Unsynchronized cardioversion will result in the electrical impulse to occur randomly during the cardiac cycle, which could cause a life-threatening dysrhythmia; therefore, its use should be limited to patients who are pulseless or deteriorating.

D. Synchronized cardioversion requires less energy, with energy doses commonly between 50 and 100 joules for patients experiencing atrial flutter.

Category: Cardiovascular Emergencies/Dysrhythmias

Nursing Process: Intervention

Reference

American Heart Association. (2016). The ACLS cases: Tachycardia, stable and unstable. In *Advanced cardiovascular life support: Provider manual* (pp. 136–137). Dallas, TX: Author.

---

10. In preparing to discharge a patient who has been given a prescription for nitroglycerin tablets 0.4 mg SL PRN, the emergency nurse acknowledges that the patient teaching has been effective when the patient states:

A. “I am to take the tablets at least every 2–3 minutes when I experience chest pain.”

B. “I will call my doctor every time I need to take a tablet for my chest pain.”

C. “I should keep the tablets on my window sill in the kitchen so I can find them easily.”

D. “If my chest pain has not gone away after I have taken 2 tablets, I will come to the hospital.”

Rationale

A. Patients are instructed to take 1 nitroglycerin (NTG) tablet every 5 minutes. The onset of action of NTG is 1–3 minutes after administration. Taking the medication more frequently can result in excessive vasodilatation, which can lead to an altered level of consciousness and hypotension.

B. It is not appropriate to call the physician each time a NTG tablet is taken. Many patients can experience relief of their chest discomfort following only 1 NTG tablet.

C. NTG should be kept in a small, dark bottle a cool, dark place to enhance the longevity of the medication. Extra or excess tablets can be kept in the refrigerator to increase longevity.

D. Nitroglycerin should result in vasodilatation of the coronary arteries, leading to improved blood flow and a decrease in the patient’s chest discomfort. Patients are instructed to seek further medical care if their chest pain has not subsided after taking 2–3 NTG tablets 5 minutes apart.

Category: Cardiovascular Emergencies/Acute coronary syndrome

Nursing Process: Evaluation

References

Karch, A. M. (2017). *Focus on nursing pharmacology* (7th ed., pp. 789–795). Philadelphia, PA: Wolters Kluwer.

Vallerand, A. H., Sanoski, C. A., & Deglin, J. H. (2015). Nitroglycerin. In *Davis drug guide for nurses* (14th ed., pp. 906–909). Philadelphia, PA: F. A. Davis.

---

11. Which of the following findings would the emergency nurse anticipate in a patient experiencing signs and symptoms of cardiac tamponade following successful aspiration of fluid from the pericardial sac?

A. Presence of electrical alternans
B. Increase in the patient’s heart rate
C. Decrease in the patient’s blood pressure
D. Increase in the patient’s blood pressure

Rationale

A. Electrical alternans is a finding in the presence of cardiac tamponade and is characterized by the alternating amplitude of each QRS complex. This is a diagnostic finding in the presence of cardiac tamponade and should not be present after the tamponade has been eliminated.

B. An elevated or increased heart rate would be evident in the presence of pericardial tamponade because of decreased cardiac filling, however, following removal of fluid from the pericardial sac, the heart rate should lower.

C. With an increase in cardiac function, the patient's blood pressure should increase following a pericardiocentesis.

D. Following removal of fluid from the pericardial sac, the patient's central venous pressure should decrease, allowing for increased preload and an increase in the patient's blood pressure.

Category: Cardiovascular Emergencies/Pericardial tamponade

Nursing Process: Evaluation

Reference

Everson, F. (2013). Chest trauma. In B. B. Hammond & P. G. Zimmermann (Eds.), *Sheehy's manual of emergency care* (7th ed., pp. 407–417). St. Louis, MO: Elsevier Mosby.

---

12. Initial interventions for a patient diagnosed with acute aortic dissection include two large-caliber intravenous lines, oxygen, and aortic wall pressure control with beta blocker administration. Maintaining which assessment finding is a priority for determining end organ perfusion?

A. Heart rate below 60 beats/minute
B. Systolic blood pressure above 120 mm Hg
C. Normal mental status
D. Urinary output above 30 mL/hour

Rationale

A. The target heart rate to manage aortic wall pressure is 60–80 beats/minute, but it is not a direct evaluation of end organ perfusion.

B. The target systolic blood pressure to manage adequate aortic wall pressure is between 100 and 120 mm Hg, but it is not a direct evaluation of end organ perfusion.

C. Determining the patient's mental status is an important finding in determining adequate end organ perfusion. Balancing the risks of pressure on the aortic wall versus the benefits of acceptable end organ perfusion can be difficult. Clinically, the patient must be assessed frequently for hemodynamic compromise, mental status changes, neurologic or peripheral vascular changes, and development or progression of carotid, brachial, and femoral bruits to establish the presence of continued adequate organ perfusion.

D. Urinary output is an important parameter to evaluate fluid resuscitation with hypovolemic shock, but it is not a priority for evaluating end organ perfusion in the presence of aortic dissection.

Category: Cardiovascular Emergencies/Aneurysm/dissection

Nursing Process: Evaluation

Reference

Wiesenfarth, J. M. (2015). Acute aortic dissection. *Medscape.* Retrieved from http://emedicine.medscape.com/article/756835-overview#a3

---

13. A 5-year-old child weighing 33 pounds (15 kg) presents to the emergency department in cardiac arrest. The child remains in ventricular tachycardia despite having been defibrillated three times, having received epinephrine 0.15 mg intraosseous (IO), and receiving good-quality cardiopulmonary resuscitation. Which drug should be administered next?

A. Amiodarone (Cordarone) 75 mg IO
B. Atropine 0.3 mg IO
C. Calcium chloride 1.0 mL intravenous (IV)
D. Lidocaine (Xylocaine) 50 mg IV

Rationale

A. Amiodarone would be the next drug used in a patient with pulseless ventricular tachycardia after defibrillation and epinephrine. Amiodarone dosing is 5 mg/kg, or 75 mg, for this patient. The patient should receive continued good-quality cardiopulmonary resuscitation, be reevaluated every 2 minutes, and be defibrillated as indicated.

B. Atropine is not indicted for a patient in ventricular tachycardia. Atropine is used in the treatment of symptomatic bradycardia.

C. Although calcium may be indicated for hypocalcemia, it is not considered primary treatment for pulseless ventricular tachycardia.

D. Lidocaine may be used for the treatment of pulseless ventricular tachycardia, however, administering 50 mg of lidocaine far exceeds the recommended dose of 1 mg/kg for this child.

Category (Pediatric): Cardiovascular Emergencies/Dysrhythmias

Nursing Process: Intervention

Reference

American Heart Association. (2016). Recognition and management of cardiac arrest. In *Pediatric advanced life support: Provider manual* (pp. 88–94). Dallas, TX: Author.

---

14. The emergency nurse is caring for a patient with a permanent pacemaker and observes that the patient has a paced rhythm with an occasional normal beat (patient's own intrinsic beat) without the presence of a pacemaker spike. The emergency nurse would interpret this rhythm as:

A. paced rhythm with capture.
B. paced rhythm with failure to sense.
C. paced rhythm with sensing.
D. malfunctioning pacemaker.

Rationale

A. A paced rhythm with capture would display a complex pattern immediately after the pacemaker spike. The pacemaker spike would occur with either a P wave (atrial pacing) or a QRS (ventricular pacing), or both (dual chamber or atrial/ventricular pacing).

B. Sensing is noted when the pacemaker recognizes the patient's own intrinsic cardiac rhythm and does not fire, allowing the patient's own cardiac cycle to occur. If the pacemaker discharges during the patient's own cardiac cycle, a serious cardiac dysrhythmia could occur. Sensing is a safety feature for a pacemaker. The heart may only require the pacemaker intermittently, when the heart rate decreases below a predetermined rate. As the patient's heart rate increases, a pacemaker can be programmed to sense the patient's own cardiac rhythm and not emit an impulse.

C. A pacemaker can have the capability of sensing an intrinsic beat or intrinsic rhythm and ceasing to fire. This is a safety feature to prevent a demand pacemaker from firing during a cardiac cycle, possibly causing a lethal dysrhythmia. Emergency pacing using a transcutaneous pacemaker does not have this sensing capability.

D. If the pacemaker recognizes a cardiac cycle and does not discharge, the pacemaker is sensing and functioning normally. A malfunction occurs when the pacemaker fails to recognize the patient's own intrinsic rhythm and continues to emit an impulse or pacer spike that has the potential to occur on the patient's own T wave, resulting in ventricular fibrillation.

Category: Cardiovascular Emergencies/Dysrhythmias
Nursing Process: Analysis

Reference

Dubin, D. (2000). *Rapid interpretation of EKG's* (6th ed., pp. 268–272). Tampa, FL: Cover Publishing.

---

15. A female patient presents to the emergency department complaining of numb fingertips and throbbing pain. The fingertips of both hands are noted to be pale to light blue in color and are cool to touch. The patient denies both trauma and any recent exposure to a cold environment. The patient is a two-pack-per-day smoker and has a history of hypertension. Based on the assessment findings, the emergency nurse suspects the patient has which condition?

A. Raynaud's disease
B. Buerger's disease
C. Thrombocytopenia
D. Inflammatory arthritis

Rationale

A. Raynaud's disease is a blood vessel disease affecting the skin. Symptoms include numbness and pallor to the fingertips, nose, and ears. Light bluish color discoloration can also be present. Smoking, being a female, and having hypertension are noted to be predisposing factors, along with living in a cold environment.

B. Buerger's disease, or thromboangiitis obliterans, is an uncommon peripheral vascular disease that affects the distal arms and legs. The disease decreases blood flow to the extremities, causing ischemia to the tissue.

C. Thrombocytopenia is a decrease in the number of platelets available in the blood, resulting in a high risk for both internal and external bleeding, such as epistaxis (nosebleeds). It is diagnosed with laboratory testing for a complete blood cell count.

D. Arthritis symptoms include pain and swelling in joints. Arthritis does not result in numbness of the fingertips or skin discoloration.

Category: Cardiovascular Emergencies/Peripheral vascular disease

Nursing Process: Assessment

References

Criddle, L. (2007). Cardiovascular emergencies. In K. S. Hoyt & J. Selfridge-Thomas (Eds.), *Emergency nursing core curriculum* (6th ed., pp. 187–248). St. Louis, MO: Saunders Elsevier.

Hunt, S. (2007). Hematologic/oncologic emergencies. In K. S. Hoyt & J. Selfridge-Thomas (Eds.), *Emergency nursing core curriculum* (6th ed., pp. 409–437). St. Louis, MO: Saunders Elsevier.

---

16. Which condition places a patient at the highest risk for infective endocarditis due to a dental procedure?

A. Prosthetic cardiac valve

B. Diabetes

C. Congestive heart failure

D. Rheumatoid arthritis

Rationale

A. To reduce the incidence of infective endocarditis, it is recommended that patients with prosthetic valves, a previous history of infective endocarditis, or congenital heart disease receive antibiotic prophylaxis before dental procedures. Dental procedures that place this high-risk group of patients at risk for infective endocarditis include manipulation of gingival tissue, periapical region of the teeth, or perforation of the oral mucosa (Class IIa recommendation). Antibiotic prophylaxis is not recommended for local anesthetic injections in noninfected tissues, treatment of superficial caries, removal of sutures, dental radiographs, placement or adjustment of removable prosthodontic or orthodontic appliances or braces, or following the shedding of deciduous teeth or trauma to the lips and oral mucosa (Class III recommendation).

B. Diabetes is not considered a high-risk condition for endocarditis.

C. Congestive heart failure is not considered a high-risk condition for endocarditis.

D. Rheumatoid arthritis is not considered a high-risk condition for endocarditis.

Category: Cardiovascular Emergencies/Endocarditis

Nursing Process: Assessment

References

Habib, G., Lancellotti, P., Antunes, M. J., Bongiorni, M. G., Casalta, J., Del Zotti, F., . . . Zamorano, J. L. (2015). 2015 ESC guidelines for the management of infective endocarditis: The task force for the management of infective endocarditis of the European Society of Cardiology (ESC). *European Heart Journal, 36*, 3075–3123. https://doi.org/10.1093/eurheartj/ehv319

Hammond, B. B. (2013). Cardiovascular emergencies. In B. B. Hammond & P. G. Zimmermann (Eds.), *Sheehy's manual of emergency care* (7th ed., pp. 201–211). St. Louis, MO: Elsevier Mosby.

Nishimura, R. A., Otto, C. M., Bonow, R. O., Carabello, B. A., Erwin, J. P., Guyton, R. A., . . . Thomas, J. D. (2014). 2014 AHA/ACC guideline for the management of patients with valvular heart disease: A report of the American College of Cardiology/American Heart Association Task Force on Practice Guidelines. *Journal of Thoracic and Cardiovascular Surgery, 148*(1), e1–e132. https://doi.org/10.1016/j.jtcvs.2014.05.014

---

17. A clevidipine (Cleviprex) infusion is ordered for a symptomatic patient with severe hypertension. The nurse is aware that this medication would be contraindicated in a patient with which history?

A. Soybean or egg allergy
B. Asthma
C. Sinus bradycardia
D. Recent use of Sildenafil (Viagra)

Rationale

A. Clevidipine is a calcium channel blocker used for blood pressure reduction. It is a lipid emulsion and is contraindicated in patients with allergies to soybeans, soy products, eggs, or egg products. Defective lipid metabolism is another contraindication. Strict aseptic technique should be followed, and unused medication should be discarded within 12 hours of puncturing the stopper.

B. Asthma is a contraindication for labetalol (Normodyne) administration, but not for the administration of clevidipine.

C. Sinus bradycardia is a contraindication for esmolol (Brevibloc) and labetalol (Normodyne) administration, but not for the administration of clevidipine.

D. Recent (last 24 hours) use of sildenafil is a contraindication for nitroglycerine administration, but not for the administration of clevidipine.

Category: Cardiovascular Emergencies/Hypertension

Nursing Process: Assessment

References

Center for Drug Evaluation and Research. (2008). Labeling. http://www.accessdata.fda.gov/drugsatfda_docs/nda/2008/022156s000_Lbl.pdf

Chiesi Farmaceutici S.p.A. (2016). *Cleviprex (clevidipine) injectable emulsion: Important safety information*. Retrieved from http://www.cleviprex.com/

PEPID LLC. (2016). *PEPID Emergency Medicine Platinum* (version 17.1.1) [Mobile application software]. Retrieved from http://pepid.com

---

18. A patient is brought into the emergency department by ambulance with chest pain, a low-grade fever of 37.89°C (100.2°F), cough, shortness of breath, and a 1–3 mm ST segment elevation on their 12-lead electrocardiogram in all leads except aVR and V_1. The nurse recognizes that the patient's symptoms are associated with the presence of:

A. congestive heart failure.
B. ST segment elevation myocardial infarction.
C. pericarditis.
D. acute coronary syndrome.

Rationale

A. Shortness of breath and cough alone do not indicate the presence of congestive heart failure.

B. ST segment elevation in all leads except aVR and V_1 is indicative of pericarditis.

C. Fever, chest pain, shortness of breath, and ST segment elevation in all leads except aVR and V_1 are indicative of pericarditis.

D. The patient's symptoms of fever, chest pain, and shortness of breath are not consistent with acute coronary syndrome.

Category: Cardiovascular Emergencies/Pericarditis

Nursing Process: Analysis

Reference

Hammond, B. B. (2013). Cardiovascular emergencies. In B. B. Hammond & P. G. Zimmermann (Eds.), *Sheehy's manual of emergency care* (7th ed., pp. 201–211). St. Louis, MO: Elsevier Mosby.

---

19. A patient recently discharged from the hospital following a 3-week hospitalization for a right femur fracture with internal fixator repair returns to the emergency department with a sudden onset of right calf pain. The nurse notes swelling and redness to the right calf. The nurse realizes that the patient is exhibiting signs and symptoms of what disorder?

A. Phlebitis of the right leg
B. Postoperative infection
C. Deep vein thrombosis
D. Compartment syndrome

Rationale

A. Phlebitis is associated with superficial veins. Given the history of this patient, phlebitis is not likely.

B. The patient reports redness and swelling to the calf, which is not the site of the surgical intervention. The leg is not warm to touch, which would indicate a possible infection.

C. Swelling, pain, and redness, as well as a recent fracture with an extended period of immobilization, indicate that the patient is most likely exhibiting signs of a deep vein thrombosis.

D. Compartment syndrome occurs 6–8 hours, and in some cases, up to 96 hours, after the injury has occurred. This patient's injury occurred more than 3 weeks earlier. Compartment syndrome is associated with closed traumatic injuries. Because the injury for this patient was a femur fracture, compartment syndrome of the calf is unlikely.

Category: Cardiovascular Emergencies/Thromboembolic disease

Nursing Process: Analysis

References

Centers for Disease Control and Prevention. (n.d.). *Venous thromboembolism (blood clots)*. Retrieved from http://www.cdc.gov/ncbddd/dvt/facts.html

Cerepani, M. J. (2010). Orthopedic and neurovascular trauma. In P. K. Howard & R. A. Steinmann (Eds.), *Sheehy's emergency nursing: Principles and practice* (6th ed., pp. 313–339). St. Louis, MO: Mosby Elsevier.

---

20. The definition of preload is:
   A. end systolic volume.
   B. end diastolic volume.
   C. systolic blood pressure.
   D. mean arterial pressure.

Rationale

A. Preload is the stretch the heart must do to accept blood before contraction of the heart chambers.

B. Preload is the amount of blood within the left ventricle at the end of diastole, or left ventricular end diastolic pressure. The amount of blood within the ventricle at the end of diastole is related to venous return, total blood volume, and "atrial kick."

C. Systolic blood pressure represents the ventricular volume of blood ejected and the response to the blood ejected by the arterial system.

D. Mean arterial pressure (MAP) represents the body's perfusion pressure. MAP is calculated by adding the systolic blood pressure to twice the diastolic pressure and dividing that number by 3. Preload is the amount of blood within the left ventricle at the end of diastole. The amount of blood within the ventricle at the end of diastole is related to venous return, total blood volume, and "atrial kick."

Category: Cardiovascular Emergencies/Shock (cardiogenic and obstructive)

Nursing Process: Assessment

References

Hall, J. E. (2016). Cardiac failure. In *Guyton and Hall textbook of medical physiology* (13th ed., pp. 271–282). Philadelphia, PA: Elsevier.

Hall, J. E. (2016). Cardiac output, venous return, and their regulation. *Guyton and Hall textbook of medical physiology* (13th ed., pp. 245–258). Philadelphia, PA: Elsevier.

Hall, J. E. (2016). Muscle blood flow and cardiac output during exercise: The coronary circulation and ischemic heart disease. *Guyton and Hall textbook of medical physiology* (13th ed., pp. 259–270). Philadelphia, PA: Elsevier.

---

21. A patient with a history of asthma has audible wheezing, tachypnea, and pale, cool skin that persists following the administration of an albuterol nebulizer breathing treatment. What medication would the emergency nurse anticipate giving next to this patient?
   A. Etomidate via intravenous (IV) push
   B. Oral prednisone
   C. Magnesium sulfate via IV infusion
   D. Oral ibuprofen

Rationale

A. Etomidate is used as an induction agent for rapid sequence intubation (RSI). Patients with respiratory compromise, or status asthmaticus, may require RSI. However, at this time, there is no indication that the patient requires RSI.

B. Oral prednisone is a corticosteroid that decreases inflammation in the bronchi. Although a corticosteroid would be anticipated in an acute asthma exacerbation treatment, when a patient is having a severe asthma exacerbation that is unresponsive to first-line treatments, the nurse would anticipate that a corticosteroid be administered intravenously rather than being given orally.

C. Magnesium sulfate inhibits calcium influx into airway smooth muscle cells, thus allowing for bronchodilation. Magnesium sulfate is used in the treatment of acute severe asthma exacerbations for patients who are not responsive to conventional treatments.

D. Ibuprofen is a nonsteroidal anti-inflammatory that has no indication in the treatment of acute asthma.

Category: Respiratory Emergencies/Asthma

Nursing Process: Intervention

Reference

Hoyt, K. S., & Selfridge-Thomas, J. (2007). Respiratory emergencies. In K. S. Hoyt & J. Selfridge-Thomas (Eds.), *Emergency nursing core curriculum* (6th ed., pp. 685–720). St. Louis, MO: Saunders Elsevier.

---

22. To limit the recurrence of chronic obstructive pulmonary disease exacerbations, it is important that patients should perform which intervention?

A. Stop smoking
B. Exercise
C. Take all medications as directed
D. Get immunized against pneumonia

Rationale

A. Smoking irritates lung tissue, causing pulmonary inflammation, and damages the alveoli. Continuous irritation decreases the lungs' ability to function normally. Not smoking is the most important way to prevent further lung damage and to limit the recurrence of chronic obstructive pulmonary disease (COPD) exacerbations.

B. Exercise can help by increasing a patient's physical stamina and lung capacity. Pulmonary rehabilitation also addresses related issues such as depression and nutrition. However, exercise and pulmonary rehabilitation will not prevent recurrence of COPD exacerbations.

C. Taking prescribed medications such as bronchodilators when symptoms are mild may prevent airway constriction from worsening, but it will not limit the frequency of exacerbations.

D. Patients with COPD are at greater risk of complications from secondary illnesses, such as pneumonia. However, receiving the pneumonia vaccine will not decrease the frequency of exacerbations.

Category: Respiratory Emergencies/Chronic obstructive pulmonary disease (COPD)

Nursing Process: Assessment

Reference

Hanania, N. A., & Sharafkhaneh, A. (2016). Chronic obstructive pulmonary disease. In E. T. Bope & R. D. Kellerman (Eds.), *Conn's current therapy 2016* (pp. 385–389). Philadelphia, PA: Elsevier.

---

23. A patient is receiving an enteral feeding. Which of the following statements indicates that the nurse understands the importance of keeping the head of the patient's bed elevated?

A. "The head of the bed is elevated to increase patient comfort when sitting up in bed and eating."
B. "The head of the bed is elevated to facilitate the tube feeding formula getting to the patient faster, thereby helping to reduce a negative nitrogen balance from lack of nutrition."
C. "Keeping the head of the bed elevated helps to prevent aspiration pneumonia."
D. "Keeping the head of the bed elevated prevents the feeding tube from becoming occluded as the tube feeding flows into the stomach."

Rationale

A. If no contraindications exist, the head of the patient's bed should be elevated to minimize the risk of aspiration. A patient who is immobile should also be turned every 2 hours to prevent the development of pressure ulcers.

B. Lying supine increases the risk of aspiration while receiving enteral formula; having the head of the bed raised will not increase the rate of nutrition absorption.

C. Maintaining the patient in a supine position during enteral feedings can result in reflux and subsequent aspiration, leading to pneumonia. Therefore, all patients who are receiving an enteral feeding should be in a semi-Fowler's position to minimize the risk of aspiration pneumonia.

D. The head of the bed is elevated to prevent any aspiration of the formula into the lungs, which could result in pneumonia. An enteral feeding should be placed on a pump to prevent the patient from receiving formula too fast.

Category: Respiratory Emergencies/Infections
Nursing Process: Evaluation

Reference

Urden, L., Stacy, K., & Lough, M. (Eds.). (2014). *Critical care nursing* (7th ed.). Philadelphia, PA: Mosby.

---

24. Patients with chronic obstructive pulmonary disease (COPD) should receive influenza and pneumococcal vaccines:

A. so they will not get sick during flu season.
B. because these vaccines prevent the need for long-acting beta agonists.
C. because these vaccines will prevent them from acquiring pneumonia.
D. because viral and bacterial infections play a major role in COPD exacerbations.

Rationale

A. The influenza vaccine only protects against the influenza virus, not other viruses.

B. Long-acting beta agonists are used for the treatment of COPD; receiving immunizations will not prevent the progression of COPD or reduce the need for long-acting beta agonists.

C. Patients can still get pneumonia even if they received an influenza and a pneumococcal immunization. Several organisms that are not a part of the pneumococcal vaccine can cause pneumonia.

D. This is a preventive measure to help reduce morbidity and mortality in patients with COPD. Patients with COPD should be educated on medication compliance that includes the use of inhalers and nebulizers, as well as the need to receive pneumococcal and influenza immunizations.

Category: Respiratory Emergencies/Infections

Nursing Process: Assessment

Reference

Works, P., & Graunke, S. (2010). Respiratory emergencies. In P. K. Howard & R. A. Steinmann. *Sheehy's Emergency nursing: Principles and practice* (6th ed., pp. 395–410). St. Louis, MO: Mosby.

---

25. A patient with no past medical history arrives to triage with the complaint of fever, malaise, cough, and crackles that do not clear with coughing. The emergency nurse anticipates that the patient will most likely will be treated for which of the following?

A. Chronic obstructive pulmonary disease exacerbation
B. Acute bronchitis
C. Acute asthma exacerbation
D. Pneumonia

Rationale

A. This patient has no past medical history noted. Patients with chronic obstructive pulmonary disease have causative factors in developing this disease, such as smoking, environmental pollution, occupational exposure, and heredity.

B. Although acute bronchitis can produce fever, cough, and malaise, adventitious breath sounds in a person with acute bronchitis will clear when the patient coughs.

C. A person with asthma is more likely to have wheezing on auscultation, and dyspnea, cough, and restlessness. This patient has no history of asthma.

D. This patient meets clinical diagnostic criteria for pneumonia, with fever, malaise, cough, and crackles that do not clear with coughing.

Category: Respiratory Emergencies/Infections

Nursing Process: Analysis

Reference

Works, P., & Graunke, S. (2010). Respiratory emergencies. In P. K. Howard & R. A. Steinmann (Eds.), *Sheehy's emergency nursing: Principles and practice* (6th ed., pp. 395–410). St. Louis, MO: Mosby.

---

26. A patient has just been intubated and placed on mechanical ventilation. What measure can the emergency nurse initiate to reduce the risk of ventilator-associated pneumonia?

A. Only suction the patient once a shift to allow oral secretions to pool in the oral cavity and prevent irritation to the oral mucosa from frequent suctioning
B. Keep the patient supine
C. Verify that the endotracheal tube cuff is deflated
D. Elevate the head of the bed

Rationale

A. A patient should be suctioned whenever there are oral secretions present to prevent aspiration of the secretions, which allows bacteria to enter the respiratory tract, leading to ventilator-associated pneumonia (VAP).

B. An intubated patient should not remain supine unless contraindicated; a supine position increases the risk of aspiration and VAP. Keeping the patient in a semirecumbent position with the head of the bed between 30 and 45 degrees aids in reducing the incidence of gastroesophageal reflux and the potential for aspiration, which leads to VAP.

C. An intubated patient who requires mechanical ventilation should have the endotracheal (ET) tube cuff inflated to minimize the risk of aspiration. Oral secretions as well as gastric secretions from reflux can enter the trachea, leading to aspiration pneumonia if the ET tube cuff is not inflated.

D. Elevation of the head of the bed and oral care with chlorhexidine are measures to assist in preventing VAP.

Category: Respiratory Emergencies/Infections

Nursing Process: Intervention

Reference

Urden, L., Stacy, K., & Lough, M. (Eds.). (2014). *Critical care nursing* (7th ed.). Philadelphia, PA: Mosby.

---

27. A patient is admitted to the emergency department via emergency medical services following the detection of carbon monoxide in their home. The patient is alert to verbal stimuli but is demonstrating intermittent snoring-type respirations. After opening the patient's airway and administering supplemental oxygen via a nonrebreather mask, what assessment finding would indicate that the patient is receiving adequate oxygenation?

A. A pCO_2 level of 70 mm Hg
B. A continuous pulse oximetry reading of 100%
C. Alertness to verbal stimuli
D. The patient's level of consciousness returning to their normal level of alertness

Rationale

A. The normal pCO_2 level is 35–45 mm Hg. A pCO_2 of 70 mm Hg, an elevated pCO_2 level, is an indication of poor ventilation with severe retention of carbon dioxide.

B. This is a possible false reading. The oximeter cannot distinguish between the amount of oxygen and carbon monoxide that is attached to the hemoglobin molecule. Pulse oximetry only detects saturated hemoglobin and does not differentiate between oxygen and carbon monoxide, so the pulse oximetry reading is not a reliable indicator of oxygen delivery to tissue.

C. A patient who responds to verbal stimuli is indicating a deteriorating level of alertness.

D. A patient who is at their normal level of consciousness and level of alertness is the correct finding for adequate oxygenation and ventilation of a patient with a patent airway.

Category: Respiratory Emergencies/Inhalation injuries

Nursing Process: Evaluation

Reference

Gurney, D., & Westergard, A. M. (2014). Initial assessment. In D. Gurney (Ed.), *Trauma Nursing Core Course: Provider manual* (7th ed., pp. 39–54). Des Plaines, IL: Emergency Nurses Association.

28. A patient presents to triage with complaints of throat pain, hoarseness, and difficulty swallowing after sustaining a "clothesline" injury. The patient is having difficulty speaking and tolerating oral secretions, and there is ecchymosis to the anterior neck. The emergency nurse suspects that the patient may have a fractured larynx and provides appropriate instructions. The patient demonstrates understanding when:

A. the patient requests ice chips for comfort.
B. the patient communicates by writing on a piece of paper.
C. the patient opens their mouth wide and sticks their tongue out for the nurse to inspect.
D. the patient states a detailed description of the injury.

Rationale

A. The patient should be instructed not to eat or drink anything to prevent any further airway inflammation and edema. The patient may also require surgical correction of their laryngeal injury, and therefore should have nothing to eat or drink until further testing is completed.

B. Resting the voice will increase the patient's comfort and reduce swelling and inflammation to the airway.

C. This action may cause the patient to gag and result in further airway obstruction due to inflammation and edema.

D. Resting the voice is imperative because it will increase the comfort of the patient and reduce swelling and inflammation to the airway.

Category: Respiratory Emergencies/Obstruction
Nursing Process: Evaluation

Reference

Everson, F. (2013). Spinal cord and neck trauma. In B. B. Hammond & P. G. Zimmermann (Eds.), *Sheehy's manual of emergency care* (7th ed., pp. 395–406). St. Louis, MO: Elsevier Mosby.

---

29. A patient arrives by ambulance unresponsive after falling off a bicycle. The patient was not wearing a helmet at the time of injury. Cervical spine immobilization is in place. During the primary assessment, the emergency nurse observes loose teeth and vomitus in the mouth. To properly suction the patient, the emergency nurse should:

A. open the airway using jaw thrust maneuver.
B. open the airway using the head tilt chin lift maneuver.
C. insert an appropriately sized nasopharyngeal airway.
D. place the patient in the "sniffing position" with neck and chin extended.

Rationale

A. When a cervical spine injury is suspected, the jaw thrust maneuver is the safest method to use in order to maintain cervical spine protection while a second person is suctioning the airway.

B. The head tilt chin lift maneuver should never be used to open the airway in a patient with suspected cervical trauma because the use of this maneuver can result in further damage to the cervical spine in patients with a spinal injury.

C. The insertion of a nasopharyngeal airway is contraindicated in patients with suspected facial trauma or basilar skull fractures.

D. The sniffing position is contraindicated when cervical spine immobilization must be maintained. The sniffing position in patients with a suspected cervical spine injury can lead to further injury to the spine.

Category: Respiratory Emergencies/Obstruction

Nursing Process: Intervention

References

Andreoni, C. (2013). Pediatric considerations in emergency nursing. In B. B. Hammond & P. G. Zimmermann (Eds.), *Sheehy's manual of emergency care* (7th ed., pp. 547–570). St. Louis, MO: Elsevier Mosby.

Snow, S. K. (2012). Initial assessment. In *Emergency Nursing Pediatric Course: Provider manual* (4th ed., pp. 63–82). Des Plaines, IL: Emergency Nurses Association.

---

30. A toddler presents to the emergency department triage with their parents. The child is sitting in a tripod position, drooling with stridorous respirations, and diaphoretic. The parent states that the child was playing when they suddenly heard the child coughing. The parent denies recent illness or ill contacts, past medical history is negative for similar episodes or chronic illnesses, and immunizations are up to date. The emergency nurse recognizes that the child is most likely experiencing:

A. foreign body aspiration.
B. acute asthma exacerbation.
C. acute epiglottitis.
D. acute laryngotracheobronchitis (croup).

Rationale

A. The parent does not report any recent illness or recent ill contacts. The history of events and assessment findings are consistent with a foreign body aspiration. Patients who have ingested a foreign body will present with a variety of symptoms that include coughing, apnea, wheezing, drooling, and stridor. Airway management is the priority intervention for this patient.

B. The parent does not report any past medical history for the patient. Drooling is not an assessment finding with an asthmatic attack, and asthma symptoms would include wheezing, which is not present in this patient.

C. The parent does not report any recent illness or ill contacts. The current history of events and assessment findings are consistent with foreign body aspiration.

D. In croup, children typically experience a characteristic seal-bark cough that can be accompanied by a fever. In this case, there is no recent illness, and the child does not have a seal-bark cough.

Category (Pediatric): Respiratory Emergencies/Obstruction

Nursing Process: Analysis

Reference

O'Neal, J. (2013). Airway management. In B. B. Hammond & P. G. Zimmermann (Eds.), *Sheehy's manual of emergency care* (7th ed., pp. 77–87). St. Louis, MO: Elsevier Mosby.

---

31. A patient with end-stage renal failure is complaining of increasing shortness of breath and exercise intolerance. The emergency nurse auscultates muffled breath sounds on assessment and anticipates that the patient is at risk for developing which respiratory complication?

A. Unstable airway
B. Pulmonary embolism
C. Pleural effusion
D. Pulmonary edema

Rationale

A. Unmanaged renal failure may lead to acidosis and altered mental status. Stability of the airway should always be monitored in patients with decreasing levels of consciousness. However, muffled breath sounds indicate fluid accumulation in pleural spaces due to decreased oncotic pressure.

B. Muffled breath sounds and respiratory complications may result from an obstructing pulmonary embolism. However, a pleural effusion secondary to renal failure is more likely.

C. End-stage renal failure causes hypoalbuminemia due to reduced syntheses of albumin. Albumin is necessary in maintaining oncotic pressure, which pulls water into the circulatory system. As albumin levels decrease, so does the oncotic pressure, allowing intravascular fluid to move out of capillaries and into the pleural space.

D. Pulmonary edema is the accumulation of fluid in the extravascular spaces of the lungs. Pulmonary edema can occur in the presence of renal failure due to fluid overload and fluid shifting. However, pulmonary edema will be assessed as crackles and wheezes, as opposed to muffled breath sounds.

Category: Respiratory Emergencies/Pleural effusion

Nursing Process: Analysis

References

Rice, K. L., & Albright, M. (2012). Geriatric considerations in emergency nursing In B. B. Hammond & P. G. Zimmermann (Eds.), *Sheehy's manual of emergency care* (7th ed., pp. 571–591). St. Louis, MO: Elsevier Mosby.

Walsh, R. R. (2013). Respiratory emergencies. In B. B. Hammond & P. G. Zimmermann (Eds.), *Sheehy's manual of emergency care* (7th ed., pp. 185–199, 573). St. Louis, MO: Elsevier Mosby.

---

32. A tension pneumothorax leading to inadequate tissue perfusion is considered to be which type of shock?

A. Obstructive
B. Hypovolemic
C. Distributive
D. Cardiogenic

Rationale

A. The increasing intrathoracic pressure of a tension pneumothorax results in compression of the lungs, heart, and great vessels. Venous return decreases and cardiac output becomes inadequate, resulting in obstructive shock.

B. Hypovolemic shock is caused by an insufficient amount of circulating blood and would not be caused by a tension pneumothorax.

C. Distributive shock is caused by an abnormal distribution of intravascular volume and would not be caused by a tension pneumothorax.

D. Although a tension pneumothorax causes decreased cardiac output, it is the result of insufficient venous blood return, not the failed ability of the myocardial pump. Therefore, it would be classified as obstructive shock, not cardiogenic shock.

Category: Respiratory Emergencies/Pneumothorax

Nursing Process: Assessment

Reference

Calder, S. A. (2013). Shock. In B. B. Hammond & P. G. Zimmermann (Eds.), *Sheehy's manual of emergency care* (7th ed., pp. 213–221). St. Louis, MO: Elsevier Mosby.

---

33. A patient presents to the emergency department complaining of sudden onset of wheezing and difficulty breathing. The patient states that they sustained an acute myocardial infarction 1 month ago. On auscultation of bilateral lung fields, scattered wheezing and bibasilar crackles are heard. As the emergency nurse, which order from the provider would you question?

A. Give the patient 125 mg methylprednisolone (Solu-Medrol) intravenously
B. Place the patient on oxygen via a nonrebreather mask
C. Give the patient 2.5 mg albuterol via nebulizer
D. Give the patient 1000 mL 0.9% sodium chloride bolus over 30 minutes

Rationale

A. The administration of methylprednisolone is indicated for a patient who is wheezing and symptomatic with the complaint of dyspnea.

B. The patient has dyspnea and crackles in the bases of their lungs. Both assessment findings support the initiation of increased oxygen delivery for the patient to improve gas exchange.

C. This order is consistent with the treatment of the patient's symptoms of wheezing.

D. The patient has findings consistent with congestive heart failure or pulmonary edema; administering intravenous fluids may further impair the patient's cardiac and respiratory status and lead to further fluid overload.

Category: Respiratory Emergencies/Pulmonary edema, noncardiac

Nursing Process: Analysis

Reference

Walsh, R. (2012). Respiratory emergencies. In B. B. Hammond & P. G. Zimmermann (Eds.), *Sheehy's manual of emergency care* (7th ed., pp. 185–200). St. Louis, MO: Elsevier Mosby.

---

34. A 34-week-pregnant female arrives to triage complaining of dyspnea with exertion and right-sided chest pain since the previous evening. She admits to smoking a half-pack of cigarettes per day. Vital signs: BP 135/90 mm Hg; HR 125 beats/minute; RR 32 breaths/minute; SpO_2 85% on room air; T 37.5°C (99.5°F). The emergency nurse knows that these signs and symptoms are consistent with which of the following?

A. Pneumonia
B. HELLP syndrome
C. Pulmonary embolism
D. Asthma exacerbation

Rationale

A. The signs and symptoms of pneumonia include history of illness, fever, cough. The patient has no history of recent illness, and a mildly elevated temperature can be normal in pregnancy. The patient's current symptoms and chief complaint are not consistent with pneumonia.

B. HELLP syndrome is a severe form of preeclampsia that occurs with hemolysis, elevated liver enzymes, and low platelets. HELLP syndrome symptoms include facial edema, headache, epigastric and right upper quadrant pain, and severely elevated BP. The patient's chief complaint and current symptoms are not consistent with the presence of HELLP.

C. The signs and symptoms of a pulmonary embolism include dyspnea, hypoxia, feelings of anxiety, and chest pain. Risk factors for a pulmonary embolism include venous stasis, recent trauma, obesity, pregnancy, use of oral contraceptives, and a history of thrombosis.

D. The signs and symptoms of asthma include tachypnea, wheezing, anxiety, and dyspnea. The patient's current symptoms and chief complaint are not consistent with asthma.

Category: Respiratory Emergencies/Pulmonary embolus
Nursing Process: Analysis

Reference

Walsh, R. (2013). Respiratory emergencies. In B. B. Hammond & P. G. Zimmermann (Eds.), *Sheehy's manual of emergency care* (7th ed., pp. 185–199). St. Louis, MO: Elsevier Mosby.

---

35. Which disease process is characterized by the presence of foreign material occluding one or more pulmonary blood vessels?

A. Pulmonary embolism
B. Pulmonary edema
C. Pneumothorax
D. Pulmonary effusion

Rationale

A. Pulmonary embolism is defined as the presence of foreign material occluding one or more pulmonary blood vessels. The signs and symptoms of a pulmonary embolism include dyspnea, hypoxia, feelings of anxiety, and chest pain. Risk factors for a pulmonary embolism include venous stasis, recent trauma, obesity, pregnancy, use of oral contraceptives, and a history of thrombosis.

B. Pulmonary edema is characterized by the accumulation of fluid in the alveoli and interstitial space that inhibits the exchange of oxygen and carbon dioxide and leads to tissue hypoxia. Pulmonary embolism is defined as the presence of foreign material occluding one or more pulmonary blood vessels.

C. Pneumothorax occurs when there is an accumulation of air in the pleural space. As the air and pressure within the pleural cavity increase, a partial or complete collapse of the lung results. Pulmonary embolism is described as the presence of foreign material occluding one or more pulmonary blood vessels

D. A pleural effusion is the abnormal collection of fluid in the pleural space. Symptoms of an effusion include chest pain, dyspnea, and a dry, nonproductive cough. Pulmonary embolism is defined as the presence of foreign material occluding one or more pulmonary blood vessels.

Category: Respiratory Emergencies/Pulmonary embolus

Nursing Process: Assessment

Reference

Walsh, R. (2013). Respiratory emergencies. In B. B. Hammond & P. G. Zimmermann (Eds.), *Sheehy's manual of emergency care* (7th ed., pp. 185–199). St. Louis, MO: Elsevier Mosby.

---

36. The emergency nurse is caring for a patient with apparent ligature marks on the neck. The patient is experiencing dyspnea, hoarseness, and subcutaneous emphysema in the neck and face. The priority intervention for this patient is to:

A. prepare for laryngoscopy.
B. prepare for intubation.
C. prepare for bronchoscopy.
D. administer oxygen via mask with an oxygen reservoir (nonrebreather mask).

Rationale

A. The priority is to administer high-flow oxygen to the patient. Laryngoscopy may be indicated to identify an injury to the larynx or upper airway, but it is not the immediate priority.

B. Intubation can result in further injury or occlusion of the patient's airway. The patient should be placed on high-flow oxygen; bronchoscopy should then be considered to facilitate endotracheal tube insertion, allowing for direct visualization of the vocal cords and trachea.

C. Bronchoscopy is indicated to identify any injury to the bronchus; however, the immediate priority of care for this patient is to administer high-flow oxygen.

D. Tracheobronchial injury commonly occurs as a result of penetrating trauma but could result from blunt trauma such as a direct blow, strangulation, or clothesline-type injury. Assessment findings include dyspnea, tachypnea, hoarseness, subcutaneous emphysema in the neck, face, or upper chest, hemoptysis, and signs of airway obstruction.

Category: Respiratory Emergencies/Trauma

Nursing Process: Intervention

Reference

Day, M. W. (2014). Thoracic and neck trauma. In D. Gurney (Ed.), *Trauma Nursing Core Course: Provider manual* (7th ed., pp. 137–150). Des Plaines, IL: Emergency Nurses Association.

37. A young adult presents to triage with fever, severe headache, and stiff neck. The emergency provider diagnoses the patient with meningitis. The emergency nurse is aware that the priority for this patient is the administration of:

A. antibiotics.
B. acetaminophen (Tylenol).
C. morphine sulfate.
D. osmitrol (Mannitol).

Rationale

A. The priority medication management for a patient with meningitis, or any infection, is the prompt administration of antibiotics.

B. Acetaminophen is used for both pain and fever control; this may be an appropriate medication for this patient, but it is not the priority.

C. Pain is often associated with meningitis, but the priority is treatment of infection with the administration of antibiotics.

D. Mannitol is an osmotic diuretic and is not an appropriate medication in the treatment of meningitis. The priority for this patient is the prompt administration of antibiotics.

Category: Neurological Emergencies/Meningitis

Nursing Process: Intervention

Reference

Schuh, S., Lindner, G., Exadaktylos, K., Mühlemann, K., & Täuber, M. (2013). Determinants of timely management of acute bacterial meningitis in the ED. *American Journal of Emergency Medicine, 31*(7), 1056–1061. https://doi.org/10.1016/j.ajem.2013.03.042

---

38. A young adult presents to triage with dry mouth, blurred vision, profound fatigue, and constipation. The patient was recently diagnosed with multiple sclerosis and has begun taking a selective serotonin reuptake inhibitor (SSRI). The emergency nurse anticipates that the most likely cause of the patient's symptoms is:

A. new onset of diabetes.
B. progression of multiple sclerosis.
C. side effects related to the SSRI.
D. a hemorrhagic stroke.

Rationale

A. There is no mention of diabetes in the patient's history.

B. Although this may be possible, the most likely cause is the recent change in patient medications.

C. SSRIs have side effects such as dry mouth, constipation, urinary retention, and profound fatigue, which may indicate high serum levels of this medication and potential toxicity.

D. The patient does not demonstrate any neurological deficit that is not related to their multiple sclerosis. Therefore, the most likely cause is the recent change in patient medications.

Category: Neurological Emergencies/Chronic neurological disorders

Nursing Process: Analysis

References

Colbridge, M. (2005). Management of SSRI and related drugs overdose. *N2N: Nurse2nurse, 5*(1), 8–11.

Faguy, K. (2016). Multiple sclerosis: An update. *Radiologic Technology, 87*(5), 529–553. Retrieved from http://www.asrt.org

Oken, B., Flegal, K., Zajdel, D., Kishiyama, S., Lovera, J., Bagert, B., & Bourdette, D. (2006). Cognition and fatigue in multiple sclerosis: Potential effects of medications with central nervous system activity. *Journal of Rehabilitation Research & Development, 43*(1), 83–90. Retrieved from https://www.rehab.research.va.gov/jour/06/43/1/Oken.html

---

39. Which assessment parameter should be performed on a 26-week-pregnant female who presents with a tonic–clonic seizure?

A. Continuous electronic fetal heart monitoring
B. Measurement of abdominal girth
C. Pelvic ultrasound
D. Measurement of fundal height

Rationale

A. Continuous electronic fetal heart monitoring (EFM) provides an overall view of maternal–fetal well-being. The emergency nurse is aware that the maternal patient must maintain compensated respiratory alkalosis for the placenta to carry oxygen to the fetus. The mother may have experienced an episode of respiratory acidosis during the seizure, which could result in decreased oxygenation to the developing fetus; therefore, EFM is an important monitoring parameter in maternal–fetal well-being.

B. Measurement of abdominal girth is not an important assessment in maternal–fetal well-being.

C. Although useful, an ultrasound will not provide an up-to-date, continuous picture of maternal–fetal well-being.

D. The measurement of fundal height may be helpful to predict gestational age and viability, but it does not provide a continuous assessment of maternal–fetal well-being.

Category: Neurological Emergencies/Seizure disorders

Nursing Process: Assessment

Reference

Association of Women's Health Obstetric and Neonatal Nurses. (2009). *Fetal heart monitoring principles and practices* (5th ed.). Dubuque, IA: Kendall Hunt.

---

40. What is the least important information for the emergency nurse to obtain from a patient who has experienced a tonic–clonic seizure?

A. History of febrile seizures as a child
B. History of current medications, alcohol use, and illicit drug use
C. Pregnancy status
D. Family history of a seizure disorder

Rationale

A. The presence of febrile seizures as a child does not increase the risk for an adult to develop seizures, and most adults may not be able to recall this information.

B. Medications and substances such as benzodiazepines, narcotics, and alcohol can result in seizures.

C. This is important for a female patient who may have experienced signs and symptoms of a seizure. Seizures can result in lactic acidosis and thus impair circulation to the developing fetus.

D. A family history of seizures can contribute to the diagnosis of seizures in a relative.

Category: Neurological Emergencies/Seizure disorders

Nursing Process: Assessment

References

Chien, C., Huanga, H., Lung, F., & Lin, C. (2011). Zolpidem withdrawal delirium, seizure, and acute psychosis: Case reports and literature review. *Journal of Substance Use, 16*(4), 330–338. https://doi.org/10.3109/14659890903013067

Majlesi, N., Shih, R., Fiesseler, F. W., Hung, O., & Debellonio, R. (2010). Cocaine-associated seizures and incidence of status epilepticus. *Western Journal of Emergency Medicine, 11*(2), 157–160. Retrieved from https://www.ncbi.nlm.nih.gov/pmc/articles/PMC2908651/

Yamamoto, L., Olaes, E., & Lopez, A. (2004). Challenges in seizure management: Neurologic versus cardiac emergencies. *Topics in Emergency Medicine, 26*(3), 212–224. Retrieved from https://journals.lww.com/aenjournal/Abstract/2004/07000/Challenges_in_Seizure_Management__Neurologic.4.aspx

---

41. Assessment of a patient who was thrown from a horse 1 hour before arrival in the emergency department reveals the patient is able to move their right leg but cannot feel pain or touch. They are unable to move their left leg but can feel pain and touch. The emergency nurse is aware that this assessment finding is consistent with the following spinal cord syndrome:

A. central cord syndrome.
B. cauda equina syndrome.
C. Brown–Sequard syndrome.
D. anterior cord syndrome.

Rationale

A. Central cord syndrome results from injury to the central portion of the cord and results in motor and sensory deficits being more pronounced in the upper extremities than in the lower extremities.

B. Cauda equina syndrome results from lumbosacral nerve root compression. The patient will experience varying degrees of motor and sensory loss in the lower extremities, as well as bladder and/or bowel dysfunction.

C. Brown–Sequard syndrome is characterized by the patient experiencing ipsilateral (same side) paralysis and loss of pressure, touch, and vibration sensation, and a contralateral (opposite side) loss of pain and temperature sensation.

D. Anterior cord syndrome results from injury to the frontal portion of the cord and causes loss of motor function and pain and temperature perception below the level of the injury. The patient is still able to sense vibration, touch, pressure, and proprioception because the posterior column of the cord has remained intact.

Category: Neurological Emergencies/Spinal cord injuries
Nursing Process: Assessment

References

Crowley, M. (2014). Spinal cord and vertebral column trauma. In D. Gurney (Ed.), *Trauma Nursing Core Course: Provider manual* (7th ed., pp. 173–192). Des Plaines, IL: Emergency Nurses Association.

Wilbeck, J. (2010). Spinal trauma. In P. K. Howard & R. A. Steinmann (Eds.), *Sheehy's emergency nursing: Principles and practice* (6th ed., pp. 272–283). St. Louis, MO: Mosby Elsevier.

---

42. A patient has been receiving an intravenous infusion of norepinephrine (Levophed) for the treatment of hypotension related to the presence of spinal shock following a fracture of thoracic vertebrae 4 and accompanying spinal cord injury. Which of the following clinical signs would suggest that this intervention has had the desired effect?

A. The patient becoming less responsive
B. Capillary refill time of 4 seconds
C. A systolic blood pressure of 100
D. Urine output of 20 mL/hour and 25 mL/hour over each of the past 2 hours

Rationale

A. The patient's level of consciousness is an indication of cerebral perfusion. With the resolution of hypovolemic shock and improvement in blood pressure, the patient's level of consciousness should either remain the same or improve, but the patient should not become less responsive.

B. Prolonged capillary refill time is an indicator of tissue perfusion, but it can be affected by a variety of factors. For this reason, capillary refill is not considered a reliable indicator of shock resolution.

C. Hypotension and bradycardia are suggestive of spinal shock. Patients who have sustained a spinal cord injury resulting in sympathetic input experience no motor function, no sensation, and a loss of reflexes below the level of the spinal cord injury. A systolic BP greater than 90 mm Hg is a recognized end-point of shock resuscitation.

D. Urine output of less than 30 mL/hour is an indication of impaired renal perfusion. A urine output of greater than or equal to 30 mL/hour is considered the end-point of shock resuscitation.

Category: Neurological Emergencies/Spinal cord injuries
Nursing Process: Evaluation

Reference

Everson, F. (2013). Spinal cord and neck trauma. In B. B. Hammond & P. G. Zimmerman (Eds.), *Sheehy's manual of emergency care* (7th ed., pp. 395–405.) St. Louis, MO: Elsevier Mosby.

---

43. The emergency nurse is caring for a patient with a subdural hematoma. Which of the following assessment findings would indicate the presence of an early increase in intracranial pressure?

A. Dilated, nonreactive pupils
B. Headache
C. Bradycardia
D. Decreased respiratory effort

Rationale

A. Early assessment findings of increased intracranial pressure include headache, nausea, vomiting, amnesia, behavioral changes, and an altered level of consciousness. As pressure continues to rise, later signs and symptoms include dilated, nonreactive pupils, unresponsiveness, abnormal motor posturing, and Cushing's triad (widening pulse pressure, reflex bradycardia, and a decreased respiratory effort).

B. Early assessment findings of increased intracranial pressure include headache, nausea, vomiting, amnesia, behavioral changes, and an altered level of consciousness.

C. Early assessment findings of increased intracranial pressure include headache, nausea, vomiting, amnesia, behavioral changes, and an altered level of consciousness. As pressure continues to rise, later signs and symptoms include dilated, nonreactive pupils, unresponsiveness, abnormal motor posturing, and Cushing's triad (widening pulse pressure, reflex bradycardia, and a decreased respiratory effort).

D. Increased intracranial pressure includes predictable and chronological signs and symptoms. Early assessment findings of increased intracranial pressure include headache, nausea, vomiting, amnesia, behavioral changes, and an altered level of consciousness. As pressure continues to rise, later signs and symptoms include dilated, nonreactive pupils, unresponsiveness, abnormal motor posturing, and Cushing's triad (widening pulse pressure, reflex bradycardia, and a decreased respiratory effort).

Category: Neurological Emergencies/Increased intracranial pressure (ICP)

Nursing Process: Assessment

Reference

McLaughlin, J. C. (2014). Brain, cranial, and maxillofacial trauma. In D. Gurney (Ed.), *Trauma Nursing Core Course: Provider manual* (7th ed., pp. 105–122). Des Plaines, IL: Emergency Nurses Association.

---

44. The emergency department nurse is preparing to administer tissue plasminogen activator to a stroke patient. What percentage of the total dose should the nurse first administer to this patient as a bolus dose?

A. 1%
B. 5%
C. 10%
D. 15%

Rationale

A. 10% of the 0.9 mg/kg total dose is administered as a bolus over 1 minute. The remaining 90% of the 0.9 mg/kg dose is then administered over 60 minutes.

B. 10% of the 0.9 mg/kg total dose is administered as a bolus over 1 minute. The remaining 90% of the 0.9 mg/kg dose is then administered over 60 minutes.

C. 10% of the 0.9 mg/kg total dose is administered as a bolus over 1 minute. The remaining 90% of the 0.9 mg/kg dose is then administered over 60 minutes.

D. 10% of the 0.9 mg/kg total dose is administered as a bolus over 1 minute. The remaining 90% of the 0.9 mg/kg dose is then administered over 60 minutes.

Category: Neurological Emergencies/Stroke (ischemic or hemorrhagic)

Nursing Process: Intervention

Reference

American Stroke Association. (n.d.). *Treatment for stroke.* Retrieved from http://www.strokeassociation.org/STROKEORG/Professionals/Stroke-Resources-for-Professionals_UCM_308581_SubHomePage.jsp

---

45. Which of the following assessment findings best describes the presence of a Le Fort II fracture?

A. **A pyramidal maxillary bone fracture involving the midface**
B. A transverse maxillary bone fracture occurring above the level of the teeth
C. A complete craniofacial separation, including the maxilla, zygoma, and orbits
D. A fracture of the base of the skull resulting in cerebrospinal fluid leakage

Rationale

A. There are three types of Le Fort fractures. A Le Fort II fracture is a pyramidal maxillary bone fracture involving the midface that traverses above the bridge of the nose. A Le Fort I fracture is a transverse maxillary bone fracture occurring above the level of the teeth, causing separation of the teeth from the maxilla. A Le Fort III fracture is a complete craniofacial separation, including the maxilla, zygoma, and orbits. A fracture of the base of the skull resulting in cerebrospinal fluid leakage is a basilar skull fracture.

B. There are three types of Le Fort fractures. A Le Fort I fracture is a transverse maxillary bone fracture occurring above the level of the teeth, causing separation of the teeth from the maxilla. A Le Fort II fracture is a pyramidal maxillary bone fracture involving the midface that traverses above the bridge of the nose. A Le Fort III fracture is a complete craniofacial separation, including the maxilla, zygoma, and orbits. A fracture of the base of the skull resulting in cerebrospinal fluid leakage is a basilar skull fracture.

C. There are three types of Le Fort fractures. A Le Fort III fracture is a complete craniofacial separation, including the maxilla, zygoma, and orbits. A Le Fort I fracture is a transverse maxillary bone fracture occurring above the level of the teeth, causing separation of the teeth from the maxilla. A Le Fort II fracture is a pyramidal maxillary bone fracture involving the midface that traverses above the bridge of the nose. A fracture of the base of the skull resulting in cerebrospinal fluid leakage is a basilar skull fracture.

D. A fracture of the base of the skull resulting in cerebrospinal fluid leakage is a basilar skull fracture.

Category: Neurological Emergencies/Trauma

Nursing Process: Assessment

Reference

McLaughlin, J. C. (2014). Brain, cranial, and maxillofacial trauma. In D. Gurney (Ed.), *Trauma Nursing Core Course: Provider manual* (7th ed., pp. 105–122). Des Plaines, IL: Emergency Nurses Association.

---

46. On arrival to triage, a patient states they have experienced facial numbness and slurred speech, although the symptoms disappeared just before arrival. The patient states that they no longer wish to be seen by the emergency provider. In formulating a response to the patient's wish to leave the department, the emergency nurse should state the following to the patient:

A. "You have likely experienced a transient ischemic attack and therefore should be evaluated by the provider for appropriate care and follow-up."

B. "You should be evaluated by the provider since your symptoms will return in less than 24 hours."

C. "You are experiencing a lacunar stroke and should immediately be evaluated by the provider."

D. "A hemorrhagic stroke is the likely cause of your symptoms, and you will deteriorate rapidly."

Rationale

A. The patient's symptoms have disappeared, indicating the possible presence of a transient ischemic attack (TIA). The patient should be examined by the provider to evaluate the presence of associated risk factors and recommend appropriate follow-up care.

B. TIA is associated with an increased risk of a stroke. The patient should be evaluated and treated for risk factors to reduce the chance of a stroke in the future.

C. The risk for a subsequent TIA or stroke varies. The risk for a stroke following a TIA in less than 30 days is 13%.

D. The patient's symptoms indicate the presence of a TIA, not a lacunar stroke.

Category: Neurological Emergencies/Transient ischemic attack (TIA)

Nursing Process: Intervention

Reference

Vacca, V. (2014). Transient ischemic attack. *Nursing 2014, 44*(6), 30–36.

---

47. A patient with cerebral edema has received 1 g/kg mannitol intravenously. Which of the following clinical signs would indicate that this intervention has had the desired effect?

A. Systolic blood pressure of 80

B. Intracranial pressure reading of 60

C. A cerebral perfusion pressure decreased to 30

D. Urinary output of 500 mL in the last hour

Rationale

A. A systolic blood pressure of 80 will impair cerebral perfusion because cerebral perfusion pressure is the mean arterial pressure minus the intracranial pressure (ICP).

B. A normal ICP reading is less than 15. A reading of 60 is highly unlikely given that brain herniation would have occurred.

C. A normal cerebral perfusion pressure should be 60 or above; 30 indicates neuronal hypoxia.

D. Mannitol, an osmotic diuretic, decreases cerebral edema by pulling fluid into the vasculature for elimination by the kidneys. Increased urinary elimination means there is decreased fluid in the intracranial cavity and a potential decrease in ICP because blood, brain volume, and cerebrospinal fluid are components that contribute to ICP.

Category: Neurological Emergencies/Trauma

Nursing Process: Evaluation

Reference

Trauma.org. (2017). *Control of intracranial hypertension.* Retrieved from http://www.trauma.org/archive/neuro/icpcontrol.html

---

48. A patient arrives to the emergency department accompanied by her husband. The husband states that the patient has a history of Alzheimer's disease, and he is concerned that she has experienced a stroke. While evaluating his understanding of his wife's disease, the emergency nurse suspects he requires additional education when he states:

A. "She forgot the word for *oven* but remembered it in the car."
B. "I know she can't die from Alzheimer's disease, but I got worried that she was really having a stroke. Her mother died of a stroke."
C. "She takes her medication every day and has always been able to take care of herself."
D. "She wasn't able to make a cake today because she couldn't follow the recipe."

Rationale

A. Sometimes having trouble finding the right word is a typical age-related change.

B. Patients with Alzheimer's can develop lack of speech but do not demonstrate other stroke-like signs and symptoms.

C. Current prescribed medications do not cure Alzheimer's disease or stop it from progressing, but they may lessen the symptoms for a limited time only.

D. Alzheimer's is a progressive disease whose symptoms worsen over time. Individuals lose the ability to perform previous routine skills.

Category: Neurological Emergencies/Alzheimer's disease/dementia

Nursing Process: Evaluation

Reference

Alzheimer's Association. (2017). *10 early signs and symptoms of Alzheimer's.* Retrieved from http://www.alz.org

---

49. A young male presents to the emergency triage stating that he felt a "pop" in his head after lifting heavy weights. The patient now complains of a right-sided headache that he rates as a 10 out of 10 on the pain scale. The emergency nurse notes that the patient's right pupil is oval and sluggishly reactive to light. The emergency triage nurse will next:

A. proceed with immediate bedding.
B. place the patient in fast track.
C. place the patient in the waiting room until a room becomes available.
D. complete the medical screening exam in triage.

Rationale

A. Subarachnoid hemorrhages typically occur in younger males and may be associated with a strenuous act. Pupillary changes are typically ipsilateral in the presence of a subarachnoid hemorrhage and result from compression of cranial nerve III. This patient has a potentially life-threatening injury and should be immediately placed in an emergency bed to be seen and evaluated.

B. This patient will require an immediate computed tomography (CT) of the head and is not appropriate for fast track.

C. This patient will require an immediate CT of the head and is not appropriate for the waiting room.

D. This patient will require an immediate CT of the head, and care should not be delayed for a medical screening exam in triage.

Category: Neurological Emergencies

Nursing Process: Analysis

Reference

Hickey, J. (2013). *The clinical practice of neurological and neurosurgical nursing*. Philadelphia, PA: Lippincott.

---

50. The emergency nurse is caring for a patient with increased intracranial pressure due to a subarachnoid hemorrhage. The provider has ordered a bolus administration of intravenous mannitol. Which of the following would indicate that this medication has had the desired effect?

A. A decrease in level of consciousness
B. A partial pressure of carbon dioxide between 35 and 40 mm Hg
C. An increase in serum sodium level above 145 mEq
D. An increase in urinary output

Rationale

A. A decrease in level of consciousness would indicate a potential deterioration of the patient and may indicate an increase in intracranial pressure.

B. This is an indicator of hyperventilation. Hyperventilation can be used for short periods to reduce intracranial pressure; it is not an outcome for mannitol administration.

C. An increase in serum sodium may occur with bolus doses of hypertonic saline but does not occur with mannitol.

D. The osmotic diuretic mannitol pulls fluid from normal brain tissue, reducing intracranial pressure. This causes an increase in urine output.

Category: Neurological Emergencies/Stroke (ischemic or hemorrhagic)

Nursing Process: Evaluation

Reference

Lump, D. (2014). Managing patients with severe traumatic head injury. *Nursing 2018*, *44*(3), 30–37. https://doi.org/10.1097/01.NURSE.0000443311.50737.a8

51. Following a motor vehicle collision, an unresponsive male patient is received in the emergency department. On patient assessment, priapism is noted. Based on this finding, what intervention should the emergency nurse perform first?

A. Ensure full spinal immobilization
B. Insert a urinary drainage catheter
C. Prepare the patient for an abdominal ultrasound
D. Obtain intravenous access and begin fluid resuscitation

Rationale:

A. Priapism is a urological emergency that can occur as a result of a spinal cord injury, tumor, sickle cell disease, or the ingestion of phosphodiesterase inhibitors. The mechanism of injury in this patient, along with their inability to respond to commands, would lead the nurse to suspect a spinal cord injury.

B. The etiology of priapism is not related to urinary retention; the insertion of a urinary catheter by the nurse can result in urethral damage. The priority is to resolve the erection before penile ischemia occurs.

C. Preparing the patient for an abdominal ultrasound is not appropriate at this time. Priapism does not occur as a result of intra-abdominal injury or other pathology.

D. Obtaining IV access and beginning fluid resuscitation may be indicated for this patient, however, when a spinal cord injury is suspected, the priority is to ensure full spinal immobilization.

Category: Neurological Emergencies
Nursing Process: Intervention

Reference

Quallich, S. (2013). Genitourinary emergencies. In B. B. Hammond & P. G. Zimmermann (Eds.), *Sheehy's manual of emergency care* (7th ed., pp. 356–357). St. Louis, MO: Elsevier Mosby.

---

52. An elderly female presents to the emergency department for evaluation of headache and vomiting. The family reports that the patient sustained a fall 2 days ago, during which she struck her head. The patient's medications include lisinopril, atorvastatin, and warfarin. The emergency nurse anticipates this patient may have experienced which of the following?

A. Intraparenchymal hemorrhage
B. Epidural hematoma
C. Subdural hematoma
D. Subarachnoid hemorrhage

Rationale

A. Intraparenchymal hemorrhage usually results from a spontaneous small vessel rupture associated with uncontrolled hypertension.

B. An epidural hematoma results most commonly from injury to the middle meningeal artery. It may be caused by a blow to the side of the head, in the temporal region. Symptoms are rapid and sometimes accompanied by a brief period of lucidity, followed by a rapid deterioration in level of consciousness.

C. Subdural hematomas result from injury to the bridging veins. This injury occurs in patients on anticoagulant therapy. Symptom onset is typically slow and progressive but can also happen spontaneously if the patient receives a blow to the head or falls.

D. Most subarachnoid hemorrhages develop from rupture cerebral artery aneurysms commonly referred to as a berry aneurysm. However, the classic symptomatology is the patient's complaint of a sudden onset of "the worst headache of my life."

Category: Neurological Emergencies/Trauma

Nursing Process: Analysis

References

Broering, B. (2010). Head trauma. In P. K. Howard & R. A. Steinmann (Eds.), *Sheehy's emergency nursing: Principles and practice* (6th ed., pp. 254–271). St. Louis, MO: Mosby Elsevier.

Hickey, J. (2013). *The clinical practice of neurological and neurosurgical nursing.* Philadelphia, PA: Lippincott.

McLaughlin, J. C. (2014). Brain, cranial, and maxillofacial trauma. In D. Gurney (Ed.), *Trauma Nursing Core Course: provider manual* (7th ed., pp. 105–122). Des Plaines, IL: Emergency Nurses Association.

---

53. When assessing a patient with suspected appendicitis, the emergency nurse would expect the patient to demonstrate rebound tenderness in which area of the abdomen?

A. Right lower quadrant
B. Left lower quadrant
C. Right upper quadrant
D. Periumbilical area

Rationale

A. Rebound tenderness in the right lower quadrant is most commonly associated with appendicitis.

B. Pain in the left lower quadrant is suggestive of an ovarian cyst or diverticular disease. The appendix is located in the right lower quadrant.

C. Right upper quadrant pain is most commonly associated with inflammation or obstruction of the gallbladder.

D. An early sign of appendicitis is periumbilical pain; however, it is vague in nature, and the pain is not usually elicited with palpation over the area.

Category: Gastrointestinal, Genitourinary, Gynecology, and Obstetrical Emergencies/Gastrointestinal/Acute abdomen

Nursing Process: Assessment

References

Huether, S. E. (2009). Alterations of digestive function. In K. L. McCance & S. E. Huether., *Pathophysiology: The biologic basis for disease in adults and children* (6th ed., pp. 1452–1515). Philadelphia, PA: Elsevier.

Wolf, L., & Zimmermann, P. G. (2013). Abdominal pain and emergencies. In B. B. Hammond & P. G. Zimmermann (Eds.), *Sheehy's manual of emergency care* (7th ed., pp. 291–302). St. Louis, MO: Elsevier Mosby.

---

54. When assessing a patient who presents to the emergency department complaining of bright red rectal bleeding, what question regarding the patient's history is most important for the nurse to ask the patient?

A. "Are you diabetic?"
B. "Do you have atrial fibrillation?"
C. "Do you take nonsteroidal anti-inflammatory drugs?"
D. "Do you take iron supplements?"

Rationale

A. A history of diabetes mellitus type 1 or type 2 is not associated with an increased risk for gastrointestinal bleeding.

B. It would be important to determine if a patient with atrial fibrillation is also taking anticoagulant medications, but atrial fibrillation itself does not contribute to the patient's risk for gastrointestinal bleeding.

C. Chronic ingestion of nonsteroidal anti-inflammatory drugs is associated with an increased risk for gastrointestinal bleeding.

D. Iron supplements will cause the patient's stool to be black and tarry, and stools associated with upper gastrointestinal bleeding also appear black and tarry. However, this patient is complaining of bright red bleeding, not black and tarry stools. Therefore, the ingestion of iron supplements is not immediately relevant to the patient's assessment.

Category: Gastrointestinal, Genitourinary, Gynecology, and Obstetrical Emergencies/ Gastrointestinal/Bleeding

Nursing Process: Assessment

References

Rossoll, L. W. (2007). Abdominal emergencies. In K. S. Hoyt & J. Selfridge-Thomas (Eds.), *Emergency nursing core curriculum* (6th ed., pp. 159–186). St. Louis, MO: Saunders Elsevier.

Wolf, L., & Zimmermann, P. G. (2013). Abdominal pain and emergencies. In B. B. Hammond & P. G. Zimmermann (Eds.), *Sheehy's manual of emergency care* (7th ed., pp. 291–302). St. Louis, MO: Elsevier Mosby.

---

55. A 28-year-old female presents to the emergency department with a sudden onset of epigastric pain that radiates to the right upper quadrant. The patient is nauseated and has vomited. While obtaining the patient's medical history, the nurse also notes that the patient is 3 months postpartum. Which of the following conditions is most consistent with the patient's presenting symptoms?

A. Pancreatitis
B. Esophagitis
C. Acute gastroenteritis
D. Cholecystitis

Rationale

A. Pancreatitis usually presents as severe upper abdominal pain that radiates through to the back. The patient may also have nausea and vomiting, along with a low-grade fever.

B. Esophagitis may also present as epigastric pain with occasional vomiting. This is usually caused by the backflow of stomach acid into the esophagus. The discomfort is typically substernal and does not radiate to the abdomen.

C. Acute gastroenteritis can be bacterial or viral in origin and usually presents with nausea, vomiting, and diarrhea, occasionally to the extent of dehydration. The pain is typically described as crampy across the lower abdomen.

D. One of the most common symptoms of cholecystitis is sudden onset of epigastric pain that radiates to the right upper quadrant (especially after ingesting fried or greasy foods), and it is associated with the presence of nausea and vomiting. Pregnancy and the postpartum period predispose women to cholecystitis because of the elevation of estrogen and progesterone. These hormones cause the gallbladder to contract less and empty more slowly. The bile in the gallbladder becomes more concentrated, leading to the formation of stones.

Category: Gastrointestinal, Genitourinary, Gynecology, and Obstetrical Emergencies/Gastrointestinal/Cholecystitis

Nursing Process: Analysis

Reference

Wolf, L., & Zimmermann, P. G. (2013). Abdominal pain and emergencies In B. B. Hammond & P. G. Zimmermann (Eds.), *Sheehy's manual of emergency care* (7th ed., pp. 291–302). St. Louis, MO: Elsevier Mosby.

---

56. A patient presents to the emergency department with restlessness, severe right flank pain, nausea, and diaphoresis. The emergency nurse should anticipate preparing the patient for which diagnostic test?

A. Kidneys, ureters, and bladder radiograph
B. Intravenous pyelogram
C. Renal ultrasound
D. Helical computed tomography scan

Rationale

A. A kidneys, ureters, and bladder radiograph radiograph may visualize renal calculi, but it is not considered as sensitive an indicator as the helical computed tomography (CT) scan to make the diagnosis of renal calculi.

B. The helical CT scan has taken the place of the intravenous pyelogram as the diagnostic test of choice for renal calculi.

C. Although renal calculi may be visualized in an ultrasound, this diagnostic procedure is not considered a sensitive indicator to diagnose the presence of renal calculi.

D. This patient most likely has a renal calculus (kidney stone). The helical CT scan is the most accurate tool for the diagnosis of renal calculi.

Category: Gastrointestinal, Genitourinary, Gynecological, and Obstetrical Emergencies/Genitourinary/Renal calculi

Nursing Process: Intervention

References

Baxter, C. S. (2010). Renal and genitourinary emergencies. In P. K. Howard & R. A. Steinmann (Eds.), *Sheehy's emergency nursing: Principles and practice* (6th ed., pp. 478–489). St. Louis, MO: Mosby Elsevier.

Quallich, S. (2013). Genitourinary emergencies. In B. B. Hammond & P. G. Zimmermann (Eds.), *Sheehy's manual of emergency care* (7th ed., pp. 353–360). St. Louis, MO: Elsevier Mosby.

57. A patient is being treated in the emergency department for chronic liver disease related to cirrhosis. The emergency nurse knows that the most common cause of cirrhosis is:

A. nonalcoholic or fatty liver disease.
B. chronic hepatitis B.
C. excessive alcohol consumption.
D. end-stage cardiac disease.

Rationale

A. This form of cirrhosis is caused by fat deposits in an already inflamed liver. Risk factors include severe obesity, diabetes, and severe weight loss. As obesity rates rise, so will the incidence of fatty liver disease.

B. Hepatitis B, like hepatitis C, is due to a viral infection that causes inflammation and damage to the liver. Excessive alcohol consumption and chronic hepatitis C are common causes of cirrhosis.

C. Alcohol consumption is a common cause of cirrhosis. Alcohol is absorbed in the small intestine, and blood transports it directly to the liver, where it is then converted into a toxic chemical.

D. Patients with end-stage cardiac disease may have symptoms of chronic liver disease, but it is not a common cause of cirrhosis.

Category: Gastrointestinal, Genitourinary, Gynecology, and Obstetrical Emergencies/Gastrointestinal/Cirrhosis

Nursing Process: Assessment

References

Herrington, A. (2010). Gastrointestinal emergencies. In P. K. Howard & R. A. Steinmann (Eds.), *Sheehy's emergency nursing: Principles and practice* (6th ed., pp. 467–477). St. Louis, MO: Mosby Elsevier.

National Institute of Diabetes and Digestive and Kidney Diseases Health Information Center. (2014). *Cirrhosis.* Retrieved from https://www.niddk.nih.gov/health-information/liver-disease/cirrhosis

---

58. The emergency nurse has administered lactulose to a patient with hepatic encephalopathy. The nurse is able to determine that the medication has been effective if the patient exhibits which of the following?

A. Decreased pain
B. Increased urine output
C. Improved mental status
D. Diminished deep tendon reflexes

Rationale

A. Lactulose is a laxative and is not effective in treating a patient's pain.

B. Lactulose is a laxative and will increase the number of stools per day. It does not affect renal function, so it will not alter the patient's volume of urinary output.

C. Hepatic encephalopathy occurs as a result of the liver's inability to remove ammonia from circulation. Symptoms include personality changes, memory loss, irritability, agitation, decreased

level of consciousness, and, eventually, coma. Lactulose works to lower the pH in the colon and inhibit the diffusion of ammonia into the bloodstream, thereby lowering blood ammonia levels.

D. Chronic alcohol abuse can lead to alcoholic neuropathy; the degree of response in assessing deep tendon reflexes is not affected by the administration of lactulose.

Category: Gastrointestinal, Genitourinary, Gynecology, and Obstetrical Emergencies/Gastrointestinal/Cirrhosis

Nursing Process: Evaluation

References

Frandsen, G., & Pennington, S. S. (2014). Drug therapy for constipation and elimination problems. In *Abrams clinical drug therapy: Rationales for nursing practice* (pp. 687–699). Philadelphia, PA: Wolters Kluwer/Lippincott Williams & Wilkins.

Morton, P. G., & Fontaine, D. K. (2013). Common gastrointestinal disorders. In *Essentials of critical care nursing: A holistic approach* (10th ed., pp. 916–954). Philadelphia, PA: Walters Kluwer/Lippincott Williams & Wilkins.

---

59. A patient presents with left-sided abdominal pain and is diagnosed with diverticulitis. The emergency nurse would anticipate administering which medication to manage the patient's symptoms?

A. A proton pump inhibitor

B. An anticholinergic medication

C. An antiemetic medication

D. An antidiarrheal agent

Rationale

A. Proton pump inhibitors reduce the secretion of gastric acid and are the treatment of choice for peptic ulcer disease.

B. Anticholinergic medications reduce intestinal spasms and relieve the pain experienced by the patient with diverticulitis.

C. Fever, chills, and nausea can be symptoms associated with diverticulitis, but pain is the most common complaint. Reducing intestinal spasm with an anticholinergic medication is the recommended treatment.

D. Constipation, not diarrhea, is the most common elimination complaint associated with diverticulitis.

Category: Gastrointestinal, Genitourinary, Gynecology, and Obstetrical Emergencies/Gastrointestinal/Diverticulitis

Nursing Process: Intervention

References

Herrington, A. (2010). Gastrointestinal emergencies. In P. K. Howard & R. A. Steinmann (Eds.), *Sheehy's emergency nursing: Principles and practice* (6th ed., pp. 467–477). St. Louis, MO: Mosby Elsevier.

Rossoll, L. W. (2007). Abdominal emergencies. In K. S. Hoyt & J. Selfridge-Thomas (Eds.), *Emergency nursing core curriculum* (6th ed., pp. 159–186). St. Louis, MO: Saunders Elsevier.

---

60. Which of the following is a priority intervention for a patient with bleeding esophageal varices?
    A. Administer 2 units of whole blood
    B. Establish intravenous (IV) access with two large-caliber IV catheters
    C. Secure the patient's airway
    D. Administer high-flow oxygen via nonrebreather mask

Rationale

A. IV fluids replacement and blood administration are indicated only after the patient's airway is determined to be open and secured.

B. The patient will likely need fluid replacement, and IV access with two large-caliber catheters may be indicated. However, this can be established once the patient's airway is patent and secured.

C. Bleeding esophageal varices present an immediate threat to the patient's airway patency. The priority intervention is to determine that the airway is open, patent, and secured.

D. Oxygen administration is an important intervention, especially if the patient is showing signs of hemodynamic compromise or hypovolemic shock; however, if the patient is actively bleeding, an oxygen mask may raise the risk of aspiration.

Category: Gastrointestinal, Genitourinary, Gynecology, and Obstetrical Emergencies/Gastrointestinal/Esophageal varices

Nursing Process: Intervention

Reference

Herrington, A. (2010). Gastrointestinal emergencies. In P. K. Howard & R. A. Steinmann (Eds.), *Sheehy's emergency nursing: Principles and practice* (6th ed., pp. 467–477). St. Louis, MO: Mosby Elsevier.

---

61. A patient presents to the emergency department with a 72-hour history of vomiting and diarrhea. The patient's heart rate is elevated, skin is pale, and the patient is hard to arouse. The emergency nurse is aware that the priority management for this patient is to perform which of the following?
    A. Obtain a stool sample
    B. Establish intravenous access for administration of crystalloid fluids
    C. Administer antiemetics
    D. Maintain airway, breathing, and circulation

Rationale

A. Obtaining a stool sample to determine the cause of the gastroenteritis is important for treatment and recovery of the patient, but emergency management of the airway, breathing, and circulation should be the priority.

B. Intravenous (IV) access and administration of fluids is an important treatment because the patient is exhibiting signs of dehydration. However, priority treatment would be airway management, followed by obtaining IV access.

C. Pharmacologic management of vomiting and diarrhea will be included in the treatment, but emergency management of the airway must be considered first.

D. Because of the continued vomiting and difficulty arousing the patient, the patient's airway may become compromised. The priority would be to manage the patient's airway while establishing IV access and continuing other treatments.

Category: Gastrointestinal, Genitourinary, Gynecology, and Obstetrical Emergencies/Gastrointestinal/Gastroenteritis

Nursing Process: Intervention

Reference

Rossoll, L. W. (2007). Abdominal emergencies. In K. S. Hoyt & J. Selfridge-Thomas (Eds.), *Emergency nursing core curriculum* (6th ed., pp. 159–186). St. Louis, MO: Saunders Elsevier.

---

62. A 65-year-old patient has been diagnosed with hepatitis C. After receiving patient education regarding this diagnosis, which of the following statements made by the patient indicates their correct understanding of the disease?

A. "I'll separate my eating and drinking utensils from those used by other family members."
B. "I never used intravenous drugs or had unprotected sex with multiple partners, even when I was much younger."
C. "My partner will need to be vaccinated so they won't become infected too."
D. "I know I can be infected even though I don't have any symptoms."

Rationale

A. Hepatitis C is transmitted by contact with blood infected with the hepatitis C virus. It is not spread by sharing eating utensils or through casual contact with an infected individual.

B. Intravenous drug use and unprotected sexual contact with persons infected with the hepatitis C virus are risk factors associated with the transmission of the virus; however, persons born between 1945 and 1965 are at an additional risk to have contracted hepatitis C from medical equipment or procedures performed before the adoption of universal precautions. Blood transfusions were not screened for the hepatitis virus until 1992.

C. There is no vaccine to prevent the transmission of hepatitis C.

D. Individuals who are infected with hepatitis C may be asymptomatic for a long period of time before they develop symptoms that would lead them to seek medical care.

Category: Gastrointestinal, Genitourinary, Gynecology, and Obstetrical Emergencies/Gastrointestinal/Hepatitis

Nursing Process: Evaluation

References

Almeida, S. L. (2010). Communicable diseases. In P. K. Howard & R. A. Steinmann (Eds.), *Sheehy's emergency nursing: Principles and practice* (6th ed., pp. 513–524). St. Louis, MO: Mosby Elsevier.

Short, W. R., Kemper, M., & Jackson, J. (2013). Infectious diseases. In B. B. Hammond & P. G. Zimmermann (Eds.), *Sheehy's manual of emergency care* (7th ed., pp. 223–244). St. Louis, MO: Elsevier Mosby.

U.S. Department of Health and Human Services. (2018). *Viral hepatitis*. Retrieved from https://www.cdc.gov/hepatitis/hcv/hcvfaq.htm#section1

63. Following the insertion of a large-caliber gastric tube, which of the following nursing measures would best assist the nurse in initially determining that the gastric tube has been properly positioned in the gastrointestinal system?

A. Assessment of the pH of the gastric aspirate
B. Auscultation of instilled air over the epigastrium
C. Determination of the carbon dioxide level within the gastric tube
D. Assessing the patient for signs of respiratory distress

Rationale

A. Current research supports the validity of gastric aspirate pH measurement to lead the nurse to initially determine that the gastric tube is most likely placed in the gastrointestinal system and not the pulmonary system.

B. The instillation of air into the gastric tube, along with listening for the "whoosh" of air over the epigastrium, has been found to be an unreliable method to validate proper gastric tube placement in the stomach.

C. Early research suggests that the use of capnography may correctly determine proper placement of the gastric tube, however, further research is needed to validate this method.

D. Feeding tubes placed into the pulmonary system do not always immediately initiate signs of respiratory distress such as coughing, dyspnea, difficulty speaking, or oxygen desaturation, especially if the patient is experiencing a decreased level of consciousness.

Category: Gastrointestinal, Genitourinary, Gynecology, and Obstetrical Emergencies/Gastrointestinal/Obstructions

Nursing Process: Evaluation

References

Bourgault, A. M., Heath, J., Hooper, V., & Nesmith, E. G. (2015). Methods used by critical care nurses to verify feeding tube placement in clinical practice. *Critical Care Nurse, 35*(1). https//doi.org/10.4037/ccn2015984

Proehl, J. A., Heaton, K., Naccarato, M. K., Crowley, M. A., Storer, A., Moretz, J. D., & Li, S. (2011). Emergency nursing resource: Gastric tube placement. *Journal of Emergency Nursing, 37*(4), 357–362. https://doi.org/10.1016/j.jen.2011.04.011

---

64. A patient presents to the emergency department with complaints of upper left quadrant pain radiating to the back for the past week. The patient's serum amylase level is normal, but the serum lipase is elevated. The nurse suspects that the patient may have which of the following disease processes?

A. Peptic ulcer
B. Pyelonephritis
C. Cholecystitis
D. Pancreatitis

Rationale

A. Patients describe the pain associated with peptic ulcers as a gnawing, burning feeling located in the epigastric area. The pain often awakens patients during the night and is relieved by eating. Laboratory studies are not abnormal.

B. The serum lipase level will not be elevated in pyelonephritis.

C. The pain associated with cholecystitis is felt in the upper right quadrant and may radiate to the back. Laboratory studies may show an elevated white blood cell count, elevated bilirubin level, and elevated liver enzymes. The serum lipase level would not be elevated.

D. In acute pancreatitis, the serum amylase level will rise quickly but return to normal within 72 hours. Serum lipase will typically rise at a slower rate but remain elevated for up to 2 weeks.

Category: Gastrointestinal, Genitourinary, Gynecology, and Obstetrical Emergencies/Gastrointestinal/Pancreatitis

Nursing Process: Analysis

References

Mason, P. J. (2014). Management of patients with gastric and duodenal disorders. In J. L. Hinkle & K. H. Cheever (Eds.), *Brunner and Suddarth's textbook of medical-surgical nursing* (13th ed., pp. 1261–1284). Philadelphia, PA: Lippincott Williams & Wilkins.

Wolf, L., & Zimmermann, P. G. (2013). Abdominal pain and emergencies. In B. B. Hammond & P. G. Zimmermann (Eds.), *Sheehy's manual of emergency care* (7th ed., pp. 291–302). St. Louis, MO: Elsevier Mosby.

---

65. The emergency nurse would anticipate hospital admission for a patient newly diagnosed with renal calculi (renal stones) if the patient demonstrated which of the following?

A. Renal calculi size greater than 3 mm
B. Inability to tolerate oral fluids
C. Pain
D. Hematuria

Rationale

A. Renal calculi greater than 6 mm will be difficult to pass through the genitourinary system and may require hospitalization for stone dissolution, lithotripsy, or surgical intervention. A renal calculi less than 6 mm in size can pass through the renal system and be eliminated by the body.

B. An increased intake of oral fluids is necessary to facilitate the passage of renal calculi through the genitourinary system. Patients who are unable to tolerate oral intake will require hospital admission for intravenous fluid administration in order to facilitate the passage of the renal calculi.

C. Nonsteroidal anti-inflammatory medications and narcotic analgesics are often prescribed for patients with renal calculi. If these analgesics are not effective for pain relief, the patient should be advised to return to the emergency department, at which time hospital admission may be considered.

D. Microscopic or gross hematuria is an expected finding for a patient with renal calculi and should not necessitate hospital admission.

Category: Gastrointestinal, Genitourinary, Gynecology, and Obstetrical Emergencies/Genitourinary/Renal calculi

Nursing Process: Analysis

References

Baxter, C. S. (2010). Renal and genitourinary emergencies. In P. K. Howard & R. A. Steinmann (Eds.), *Sheehy's emergency nursing: Principles and practice* (6th ed., pp. 478–489). St. Louis, MO: Mosby Elsevier.

Jordan, K. S. (2007). Genitourinary emergencies. In K. S. Hoyt & J. Selfridge-Thomas (Eds.), *Emergency nursing core curriculum* (6th ed., pp. 387–408). St. Louis, MO: Saunders Elsevier.

Quallich, S. (2013). Genitourinary emergencies. In B. B. Hammond & P. G. Zimmermann (Eds.), *Sheehy's manual of emergency care* (7th ed., pp. 353–360). St. Louis, MO: Elsevier Mosby.

---

66. A bicyclist is brought to the emergency department after crashing into a wall and flying over the handlebars. The patient is awake and alert and is complaining of left-sided abdominal pain with nausea. Vital signs: BP 124/60 mm Hg; HR 80 beats/minute; RR 16 breaths/minute; SpO_2 98%; T 36.4°C (97.6°F). The emergency nurse would anticipate which diagnostic test to assess for possible intra-abdominal injury?

A. Diagnostic peritoneal lavage
B. Exploratory laparotomy
C. Computed tomography scan of the abdomen and pelvis with contrast
D. A focused assessment with sonography for trauma

Rationale

A. A peritoneal lavage is an invasive procedure that is indicated if the patient is hemodynamically unstable and transport to a computed tomography (CT) scanner would place the patient at risk for complications.

B. Indications for exploratory laparotomy include evidence of shock without obvious blood loss, determination of free air in the abdomen, or an alteration in level of consciousness. Vital signs are stable, and the patient does not show evidence of obvious blood loss or shock.

C. In a stable patient presenting with a potential abdominal injury, a CT scan of the abdomen and pelvis would be indicated if a FAST (focused assessment with sonography for trauma) assessment was positive for intraperitoneal fluid.

D. This patient's mechanism of injury and complaints of abdominal pain are highly suspicious for intra-abdominal injury due to blunt abdominal trauma. Because this patient is hemodynamically stable, a bedside FAST is indicated.

Category: Gastrointestinal, Genitourinary, Gynecology, and Obstetrical Emergencies/Gastrointestinal/Trauma

Nursing Process: Analysis

Reference

Harris, C. (2013). Abdominal trauma. In B. B. Hammond & P. G. Zimmermann (Eds.), *Sheehy's manual of emergency care* (7th ed., pp. 419–426). St. Louis, MO: Elsevier Mosby.

67. Following the incision and drainage of a Bartholin's gland abscess, the patient's discharge teaching instructions should include which of the following?

A. Your sexual partners will not need to be treated for this infection.
B. Take a sitz bath or soak in a bathtub with warm water several times a day.
C. You should follow up with your healthcare provider to have the drainage (Word) catheter removed in 24 hours.
D. Having an intrauterine device puts you at greater risk for developing a Bartholin's gland abscess.

Rationale

A. The most common causative organisms of the Bartholin's gland abscess are *E. coli* and *G. vaginalis.* If these organisms are the cause of the abscess, sexual partners do not require antibiotic treatment. Less commonly, *N. gonorrhea* and *C. trachomatis* have been identified by culture; in these cases, sexual partners will require antibiotic treatment.

B. The patient should be instructed to use a sitz bath or soak in a warm tub for 10–15 minutes 3–4 times per day.

C. A drainage (Word) catheter is placed in the Bartholin's gland abscess to facilitate drainage. The catheter should stay in place for several weeks.

D. The presence of an intrauterine device (IUD) places the patient at greater risk for developing pelvic inflammatory disease because of the upward migration of infectious organisms. IUDs do not increase the patient's risk for developing a Bartholin's gland abscess.

Category: Gastrointestinal, Genitourinary, Gynecology, and Obstetrical Emergencies/Gynecology/Infection

Nursing Process: Intervention

References

Jordan, K. S. (2010). Gynecologic emergencies. In P. K. Howard & R. A. Steinmann (Eds.), *Sheehy's emergency nursing: Principles and practice* (6th ed., pp. 578–589). St. Louis, MO: Mosby Elsevier.

Kelly, L. (2013). Gynecologic emergencies. In B. B. Hammond & P. G. Zimmermann (Eds.), *Sheehy's manual of emergency care* (7th ed., pp. 497–503). St. Louis, MO: Elsevier Mosby.

McNeeley, S. G. (2016). Bartholin gland cysts (Bartholin's cyst). *Merck Manual.* Retrieved from http://www.merckmanuals.com/home/women-s-health-issues/noncancerous-gynecologic-abnormalities/bartholin-gland-cysts

---

68. A female patient presents to the emergency department with complaints of right lower abdominal pain and is diagnosed as having an unruptured ectopic pregnancy in the right fallopian tube. The patient's vital signs are stable, and the ectopic pregnancy is estimated to be 3.0 cm in size. A nonsurgical treatment to terminate the ectopic pregnancy is recommended. The nurse anticipates that the patient will receive which medication?

A. Rh_o(D) immune globulin
B. Oxytocin (Pitocin)
C. Methotrexate
D. Medroxyprogesterone (Provera)

Rationale

A. If the mother is RH negative, immunization with Rho(D) immune globulin may be indicated to prevent Rh incompatibility in future pregnancies, but it will not terminate the existing ectopic pregnancy.

B. Oxytocin (Pitocin) is a uterine stimulant that is used to induce labor. Oxytocin is an effective treatment for the delivery of an intrauterine pregnancy but not an ectopic pregnancy.

C. Methotrexate is an antimetabolite that prevents further duplication of the fetal cells. It is administered intramuscularly, and the patient is then followed with quantitative serum βeta human gonadotropin (β-hCG) levels.

D. Medroxyprogesterone is a form of progesterone that helps regulate ovulation and menstrual periods. It is used to treat conditions such as absent or irregular menstrual periods; it is not indicated as a treatment for ectopic pregnancy.

Category: Gastrointestinal, Genitourinary, Gynecology, and Obstetrical Emergencies/Obstetrical/ Ectopic pregnancy

Nursing Process: Intervention

References

Jordan, K. S. (2007). Obstetric and gynecologic emergencies. In K. S. Hoyt & J. Selfridge-Thomas (Eds.), *Emergency nursing core curriculum* (6th ed., pp. 536–570). St. Louis, MO: Saunders Elsevier.

Mason, D. L. (2010). Obstetric emergencies. In P. K. Howard & R. A. Steinmann (Eds.), *Sheehy's emergency nursing: Principles and practice* (6th ed., pp. 619–629). St. Louis, MO: Mosby Elsevier.

McQueen, A. (2011). Ectopic pregnancy: Risk factors, diagnostic procedures and treatment. *Nursing Standard, 25*(37), 49–56. https://doi.org/10.7748/ns2011.05.25.37.49.c8521

---

69. While treating a patient with postpartum hemorrhage, the nurse administers 20 units of oxytocin per 1000 mL of Ringer's lactate solution. The nurse recognizes that the desired effect of this medication has occurred when:

A. the patient's blood pressure has decreased.
B. there is decreased vaginal bleeding.
C. the patient experiences a decrease in abdominal discomfort.
D. there is a softening of the uterus.

Rationale

A. Decreased blood pressure is not the desired effect of oxytocin; rather, a decrease in blood pressure may be a sign of hypovolemic shock in a postpartum patient.

B. Postpartum hemorrhage most commonly occurs as a result of uterine atony. Oxytocin is a vasoconstrictor that stimulates uterine contractions, improves uterine tone, and reduces postpartum bleeding.

C. Oxytocin will stimulate painful uterine contractions as it restores uterine tone, so abdominal discomfort is an expected effect of oxytocin administration.

D. The cause of the bleeding may likely be from uterine atony, and a soft and boggy uterus is a sign of atony. A firmer uterus is the desired effect of oxytocin administration.

Category: Gastrointestinal, Genitourinary, Gynecology, and Obstetrical Emergencies/Obstetrical/Hemorrhage

Nursing Process: Evaluation

References

Poole, J. H., & Thompson, J. E. (2013). Obstetric emergencies. In B. B. Hammond & P. G. Zimmermann (Eds.), *Sheehy's manual of emergency care* (7th ed., pp. 483–495). St. Louis, MO: Elsevier Mosby.

Adams, M., Holland, N., & Urban, C. (Eds.). (2017). Drugs for disorders and conditions of the female reproductive system. In *Pharmacology for nurses: A pathophysiologic approach* (5th ed., pp. 782–804). Boston, MA: Pearson.

---

70. A woman who is 39-weeks-pregnant presents to the emergency department. Which of the following findings would alert the emergency nurse that a vaginal delivery is imminent?

A. The patient states that her contractions are 3 minutes apart and lasting a long time.
B. The patient reports an urge to push.
C. The patient reports feeling "gush of water" 1 hour ago.
D. A pulsating umbilical cord is felt in the vagina.

Rationale

A. Contractions alone are not an indication of impending delivery. Additional findings, such as a fully dilated and effaced cervix, a bulging perineum, or a widening of the vulvovaginal area, would indicate that delivery is imminent.

B. The urge to push is associated with the second stage of labor. The mother's desire to bear down or push, or her feeling that "the baby is coming," usually indicates that delivery is imminent.

C. The rupture of membranes can occur days before a delivery, so it is not a clear indication that delivery is imminent.

D. Pressure from the baby's head can compress the umbilical cord and result in fetal hypoxia. The mother is usually repositioned to prevent the baby from compressing the cord. Delivery is not necessarily imminent; however, if the baby shows signs of fetal distress, forceps delivery may be attempted, or an emergency cesarean section may be performed.

Category: Gastrointestinal, Genitourinary, Gynecology, and Obstetrical Emergencies/Obstetrical/Emergent delivery

Nursing Process: Analysis

References

Jordan, K. S. (2007). Obstetric and gynecologic emergencies. In K. S. Hoyt & J. Selfridge-Thomas (Eds.), *Emergency nursing core curriculum* (6th ed., pp. 536–570). St. Louis, MO: Saunders Elsevier.

Mason, D. (2010). Obstetric emergencies. In P. K. Howard & R. A. Steinmann (Eds.), *Sheehy's emergency nursing: Principles and practice* (6th ed., pp. 619–629). St. Louis, MO: Mosby Elsevier.

Poole, J. H., & Thompson, J. E. (2013). Obstetric emergencies. In B. B. Hammond & P. G. Zimmermann (Eds.), *Sheehy's manual of emergency care* (7th ed., pp. 483–496). St. Louis, MO: Elsevier Mosby.

---

71. The most characteristic clinical finding in a patient with placenta previa is:

A. elevated blood pressure.
B. painless bright red vaginal bleeding.
C. vaginal discharge of blood-tinged mucus.
D. vaginal passing of tissue.

Rationale

A. A systolic blood pressure > 140 mm Hg or a diastolic blood pressure > 90 mm Hg and edema of the face, hands, and sacral area are characteristic signs of preeclampsia. Preeclampsia is a systemic disorder that does not affect the location or attachment of the placenta.

B. Painless bright red vaginal bleeding is the most characteristic clinical finding of placenta previa. In this condition, the placenta has implanted, either totally or partially, over the cervical os. As the uterus expands because of fetal growth, the implantation of the placenta is disturbed, and bleeding can occur through the cervix. The uterus is not contracting, so the bleeding is painless.

C. Blood-tinged mucus discharge, also known as a "bloody show," is a normal sign associated with impending delivery.

D. The passing of tissue, also known as the products of conception, is suggestive of a spontaneous abortion.

Category: Gastrointestinal, Genitourinary, Gynecology, and Obstetrical Emergencies/Obstetrical/Placenta previa

Nursing Process: Assessment

Reference

Benrubi, G. (2010). *Obstetric and gynecologic emergencies* (4th ed.). Philadelphia, PA: Lippincott Williams & Wilkins.

---

72. Following a precipitous delivery of a full-term infant in the emergency department, the infant is successfully intubated and adequately ventilated. The emergency nurse would begin chest compressions if the infant's heart rate is below which of the following?

A. 60–80 beats/minute
B. 90–100 beats/minute
C. 110–120 beats/minute
D. 130–150 beats/minute

Rationale

A. The American Heart Association guidelines for neonatal resuscitation recommend that chest compression be initiated if the infant's heart rate is below 60 beats/minute despite adequate ventilation.

B. The American Heart Association guidelines for neonatal resuscitation recommend that chest compression be initiated if the infant's heart rate is below 60 beats/minute despite adequate ventilation.

C. The normal heart rate for a full-term newborn is 90–170 beats/minute. Chest compressions would not be indicated for a newborn with a heart rate of 110 beats/minute.

D. This heart rate is well within the normal range for a full-term infant. Chest compressions would not be indicated.

Category (Pediatric): Gastrointestinal, Genitourinary, Gynecology, and Obstetrical Emergencies/Obstetrical/Neonatal resuscitation

Nursing Process: Assessment

Reference

Wyckoff, M. H., Aziz, K., Escobedo, M. B., Kapadia, V. S., Kattwinkel, J., Perlman, J. M., . . . Zaichkin, J. G. (2015, November 3). Neonatal resuscitation: 2015 American Heart Association guidelines update for cardiopulmonary resuscitation and emergency cardiovascular care. *Circulation, 132*, S543–S560. https://doi.org/10.1161/CIR.0000000000000267

---

73. A 25-year-old female presents to the emergency department 4 days postpartum. She has a high fever and rigors following a vaginal delivery with an episiotomy and a left sulcus laceration. On examination, the vaginal area is edematous and tender to touch, with a purpuric discoloration from the left labia that extends to the buttocks unilaterally and the presence of a "foul smelling" liquid discharge from the episiotomy site. The patient is tachycardic and tachypneic. The emergency nurse suspects this patient may have:

A. septic thrombophlebitis.
B. endometritis.
C. pelvic abscess.
D. necrotizing fasciitis.

Rationale

A. Septic thrombophlebitis is an infected thrombus, causing inflammation and bacteremia to develop in the pelvic veins. Symptoms include fever and uterine tenderness.

B. Endometritis is the most common cause of puerperal fever. However, it is most commonly the result of a caesarean section, and symptoms include abdominal pain and foul-smelling lochia. Endometritis can cause the patient to develop septic shock.

C. Pelvic abscesses may present with fever, diarrhea, dysuria, and a tender pelvic mass assessed by palpation. There is potential for the abscess to lead peritonitis, resulting in septic shock.

D. Necrotizing fasciitis is a severe wound infection involving superficial and deep fascia. It is frequently associated with episiotomy or other perineal trauma during delivery and has a high mortality rate. It can present with purpura and swelling. Without aggressive management, it can lead to sepsis, multiorgan system failure, and death.

Category: Gastrointestinal, Genitourinary, Gynecology, and Obstetrical Emergencies/Obstetrical/Postpartum infection

Nursing Process: Analysis

References

Chandraharan, E., & Arulkumaran, S. (2012). *Obstetric and intrapartum emergencies: A practical guide to management.* New York, NY: Cambridge University Press.

Macones, G. A. (2015). *Management of labor and delivery* (2nd ed.). Oxford: John Wiley & Sons.

---

74. An adolescent is being evaluated for abdominal pain. When the mother leaves the exam room to make a phone call, the patient reveals to the emergency nurse that they are being sexually fondled at school by a teacher. The priority nursing intervention for this patient is to:

A. notify the appropriate child protective services or law enforcement agency.
B. obtain consent from the mother to report the abuse to the appropriate agency.
C. report the name of the alleged abuser to law enforcement immediately.
D. discuss birth control and sexually transmitted infection prevention with the patient.

Rationale

A. Sexual abuse of children is a crime in all states. As a mandated reporter, the nurse has a legal responsibility to report alleged sexual abuse to the appropriate local agency.

B. Parental consent is not required for mandated reporting of alleged sexual abuse of a child.

C. Although child sexual assault is a crime, the investigation is the responsibility of the local child maltreatment or law enforcement agency, not the emergency nurse.

D. Discharge teaching after an appropriate examination would be done as part of the discharge process, but it is not the highest priority intervention.

Category (Pediatric): Psychosocial and Medical Emergencies/Psychosocial/Abuse and neglect
Nursing Process: Intervention

Reference

Melini, J. A. (2009.) Child sexual abuse. In D. O. Thomas & L. M. Bernardo (Eds.), *Core curriculum for pediatric emergency nursing* (2nd ed., pp. 569–579). Des Plaines, IL: Emergency Nursing Association.

---

75. When caring for a patient who has been recently diagnosed with leukemia, the emergency nurse should consider which assessment variation in this patient?

A. The sudden onset of initial symptoms is related to thrombocytosis.
B. Hepatomegaly and splenomegaly are common assessment findings in a patient with leukemia.
C. Leukemia is a nonmalignant neoplasm.
D. Early symptoms of fatigue may be related to the presence of thrombocytopenia.

Rationale

A. Thrombocytosis is not a symptom of leukemia. Thrombocytopenia, or reduced platelets, is a result of bone marrow depression and is common in patients with leukemia or those who are undergoing chemotherapy.

B. Leukemic cells may invade the liver and spleen, resulting in organ enlargement of both.

C. Leukemia is referred to as "blood cancer" and is a disease of malignant hematopoietic stem cells.

D. General malaise and fatigue are related to anemia; white blood cells proliferate in the circulatory system and result in a decreased number of mature red blood cells.

Category: Psychosocial and Medical Emergencies/Medical/Blood dyscrasias: Leukemia

Nursing Process: Assessment

Reference

Grossman, S. C., & Porth, C. M. (2014). Disorders of white blood cells and lymphoid tissues. In *Porth's pathophysiology: Concepts of altered health states* (9th ed., pp. 688–710). Philadelphia, PA: Wolters Kluwer/ Lippincott Williams & Wilkins.

---

76. A patient presents to triage, extremely tearful and visibly trembling. The patient states, "I can't take it anymore... this new medication the doctor gave me is not working! I have been taking this medication for 5 days, and I feel even more depressed than I did before!" The emergency nurse begins the patient assessment by completing the medication reconciliation and identifies that the new medication the patient has been prescribed is fluoxetine (Prozac). What intervention by the nurse would have the greatest impact for this patient?

A. Provide the patient with a benzodiazepine such as lorazepam (Ativan) to calm the patient's nerves.
B. Inform the patient that the provider will likely change the medication given that symptoms are worsening.
C. Instruct the patient to stop the medication immediately.
D. Reassure the patient that fluoxetine requires at least 1–4 weeks before a noticeable improvement in depression symptoms is evident.

Rationale

A. Antianxiety agents (benzodiazepines) should not be administered until the patient has been evaluated by their mental health provider unless otherwise instructed by the emergency provider. Selective serotonin reuptake inhibitors (SSRIs) often need a full 4 weeks to reach therapeutic effect to treat depression.

B. The nurse should never tell a patient that medication orders will be changed without first discussing the patient's symptoms with their therapist or psychiatrist.

C. SSRIs should never be stopped abruptly. Patients should be slowly weaned off the medication in conjunction with appropriate follow-up and the possibility of another medication regime being initiated.

D. SSRIs inhibit reuptake of serotonin and are used in treatment of major depressive disorders. It may take up to 4 weeks to reach therapeutic levels and see improvement. Frequent follow-up with the prescribing provider is required, and dosage may need to be adjusted if no improvement is evident within 4 weeks.

Category: Psychosocial and Medical Emergencies/Psychosocial/Depression

Nursing Process: Intervention

References

Gagnon, L. (2010). Behavioral health emergencies. In P. K. Howard & R. A. Steinmann (Eds.), *Sheehy's emergency nursing: Principles and practice* (6th ed., pp. 677–688). St. Louis, MO: Mosby Elsevier.

Manton, A. (2013). Mental health emergencies. In B. B. Hammond & P. G. Zimmermann (Eds.), *Sheehy's manual of emergency care* (7th ed., pp. 505–520). St. Louis, MO: Elsevier Mosby.

Skidmore-Roth, L. (2017). *Mosby's 2017 nursing drug reference* (30th ed.). St. Louis, MO: Elsevier.

77. A young child presents to the emergency department with signs and symptoms of diabetic ketoacidosis. The emergency nurse anticipates the need to correct the child's dehydration by administering which of the following intravenous (IV) fluids?

A. 10–20 mL/kg of 0.9% sodium chloride IV over 1–2 hours
B. 20 mL/kg of 0.9% sodium chloride rapid IV push over 15 minutes
C. 30 mL/kg bolus of 0.9% sodium chloride IV administered over 1 hour
D. 10–20 mL/kg dextrose 5% with 0.9% sodium chloride IV over 2 hours

Rationale

A. Isotonic IV fluid should be administered slowly over 1–2 hours to avoid cerebral edema.

B. Rapid infusions of large amounts of fluid may lead to cerebral edema. Isotonic IV fluid should be administered slowly over 1–2 hours to avoid cerebral edema.

C. Rapid infusions of large amounts of IV fluid may lead to fluid overload and cerebral edema; IV fluids should be administered over 1–2 hours. The recommended fluid infusion volume in the pediatric population is not 30 mL/kg; instead, the volume infused should be based on 10–20 mL/kg.

D. Dextrose should not be added to IV fluids until the child's serum blood glucose is below 250 mg/dL. The administration of dextrose 5% with 0.9% sodium chloride will not treat the acute dehydration and may cause the child's blood glucose to rise higher.

Category: Psychosocial and Medical Emergencies/Medical/Endocrine conditions: Glucose-related conditions

Nursing Process: Intervention

References

Golder, D. (2013). Childhood illness. In *Emergency Nursing Pediatric Course: Provider manual* (4th ed., pp. 147–170). Plaines, IL: Emergency Nurses Association.

Marett, B. E. (2013). Metabolic emergencies. In B. B. Hammond & P. G. Zimmermann (Eds.), *Sheehy's manual of emergency care* (7th ed., pp. 303–318). St. Louis, MO: Elsevier Mosby.

Morey, C. M. (2010). Endocrine emergencies. In P. K. Howard & R. A. Steinmann (Eds.), *Sheehy's emergency nursing: Principles and practice* (6th ed., pp. 499–512). St. Louis, MO: Mosby Elsevier.

---

78. A patient with myxedema coma is most likely to seek care in an emergency department in which season of the year?

A. Winter
B. Fall
C. Spring
D. Summer

Rationale

A. Patients with hypothyroidism have an intolerance for cooler or cold temperatures, which is related to their decreased metabolism. Myxedema coma (hypothyroid coma) is more commonly seen in the winter months because of exposure to cold temperatures or a cold environment. More than 90% of myxedema coma cases occur during the winter months, and they are more common in women over the age of 60.

B. More than 90% of myxedema coma cases occur during the winter months.

C. More than 90% of myxedema coma cases occur during the winter months.

D. More than 90% of myexedema coma cases occur during the winter months.

Category: Psychosocial and Medical Emergencies/Medical/Endocrine conditions: Thyroid
Nursing Process: Assessment

References

Marett, B. E. (2013). Metabolic emergencies. In B. B. Hammond & P. G. Zimmermann (Eds.), *Sheehy's manual of emergency care* (7th ed., pp. 303–318). St. Louis, MO: Elsevier Mosby.
Morey, C. M. (2010). Endocrine emergencies. In P. K. Howard & R. A. Steinmann (Eds.), *Sheehy's emergency nursing: Principles and practice* (6th ed., pp. 499–512). St. Louis, MO: Mosby Elsevier.

---

79. During the assessment of a young nonambulatory child, the emergency nurse identifies the presence of a possible spiral leg fracture. The parents state that the child rolled off a bed onto the floor. Based on this assessment, the emergency nurse prepares for which of the following?
A. Separate the parents and ask each what event led to the child's leg injury
B. Do not permit the parents to hold the child
C. Record all verbal interactions between the parents and emergency providers
D. Report suspicion of child maltreatment to the child protective services agency

Rationale

A. This is not the responsibility of the providers. Based on assessment and evaluation by child protective services surrounding the events leading to the child's injury, law enforcement will be responsible for determining the exact order of events.

B. There is no indication that the parents should not be allowed to hold or comfort their child. It is unknown if either parent is responsible for the injury or under which circumstances the injury occurred.

C. It is important to obtain an accurate history of the events leading to the child's injury; however, it is not necessary to record all verbal interactions between the parents and emergency personnel unless they are related to the actual events surrounding the child's injury.

D. Healthcare providers are mandated reporters and are required by law to report cases of suspected child maltreatment to the local authorities. The presence of a spiral fracture in a nonambulatory child has been associated with the presence of physical child maltreatment and is the result of an intentional twisting motion to the extremity.

Category (Pediatric): Psychosocial and Medical Emergencies/Psychosocial/Abuse and neglect
Nursing Process: Intervention

References

Black, A. (2010). Child abuse and neglect. In P. K. Howard & R. A. Steinmann (Eds.), *Sheehy's emergency nursing: Principles and practice* (6th ed., pp. 652–665). St. Louis, MO: Mosby Elsevier.
Black, A. (2012). Child maltreatment. In *Emergency Nursing Pediatric Course: Provider manual* (4th ed., pp. 343–357). Des Plaines, IL: Emergency Nurses Association.
Cohen, S. (2013). Abuse and neglect. In B. B. Hammond & P. G. Zimmermann (Eds.), *Sheehy's manual of emergency care* (7th ed., pp. 521–530). St. Louis, MO: Elsevier Mosby.

80. A patient is brought to the emergency department from an outpatient clinic following increasing agitation and the verbal and physical abuse of a staff member after being denied narcotics. The patient is speaking loudly and threatening to "blow the place up" if narcotics are not ordered to be given to him. The nurse has called for the rapid response team. Which of the following indicates an initial desired patient response to the rapid response team intervention? The patient:

A. requests removal from physical restraints.
B. follows verbal instruction.
C. requires intramuscular injection of an antianxiolytic medication.
D. tolerates being placed in seclusion.

Rationale

A. Physical restraints are not the first line of treatment interventions for an agitated patient. Yet, once applied, restraints should be removed as soon as safely possible. The patient should then be placed on constant observation.

B. According to the Emergency Nurses Association (2011), "Workplace violence (WPV) in health care is 3.8 times higher than all private industry, with the emergency department being a highly vulnerable area." Agitated, violent, and aggressive patients pose a threat to nurses and are at risk of harming themselves or those around them. Nonpharmacologic interventions, such as verbal intervention, to try to deescalate an agitated, psychotic patient should be attempted first, and an optimal response would be the patient following verbal instruction.

C. A patient requiring intramuscular injection of antianxiolytic medication is likely not able to control behavior and follow verbal instruction. This is evidence that the agitated behavior continued after the rapid response intervention.

D. Although seclusion with constant observation are a part of the treatment regimen for an agitated patient, the response of tolerating the seclusion is not sufficiently specific to indicate the expected behavioral outcome. Decreased agitation and compliance with instruction would be ideal initial responses.

Category: Psychosocial and Medical Emergencies/Psychosocial/Aggressive/violent behavior
Nursing Process: Evaluation

References

Emergency Nurses Association. (2010). *ENA workplace violence toolkit.* Retrieved from https://www.ena.org/docs/default-source/resource-library/practice-resources/toolkits/workplaceviolencetoolkit.pdf?sfvrsn=6785bc04_30

Manton, A. P. (2013). Mental health emergencies. In B. B. Hammond & P. G. Zimmermann (Eds.), *Sheehy's manual of emergency care* (7th ed., pp. 505–520). St. Louis, MO: Elsevier Mosby.

Pich, J., Hazelton, M., Sundin, D., & Kable, A. (2010). Patient-related violence against emergency department nurses. *Nursing & Health Sciences, 12*(2), 268–274. https://doi.org/10.1111/j.1442-2018.2010.00525.x

---

81. A patient was involved in a severe motor vehicle collision 2 months ago. Although the patient's injuries are healing appropriately, the patient has been treated in the emergency department 6 times for a variety of complaints since the incident. The patient reports trouble sleeping because of nightmares, fear when driving or riding in cars, and frequent thoughts of the incident. What mental health disorder should the nurse consider when assessing this patient?

A. Agoraphobia
B. Depression

C. Bipolar disorder
D. Posttraumatic stress disorder

Rationale

A. Agoraphobia (perception of an unsafe environment, feelings of being trapped, helpless, or embarrassed) may occur with posttraumatic stress disorder (PTSD) and other anxiety disorders, but these symptoms are not being reported by the patient.

B. Although stressful life events can contribute to the onset of depression, symptoms typically include depressed mood, anhedonia, difficulty concentrating, insomnia or hypersomnia, weight changes, and thoughts of suicide.

C. Symptoms of bipolar disorder include periods of depression cycling with periods of mania (including elevated, expansive, or irritable mood).

D. Patients who return often to the emergency department following a serious trauma should be questioned regarding ongoing pain, coping skills, and general well-being. Symptoms of PTSD include fear, intrusive recollections, dreams of the event, and avoidance of stimuli associated with the trauma. Early recognition of symptoms may facilitate early treatment and increase the incidence of a successful recovery.

Category: Psychosocial and Medical Emergencies/Psychosocial/Anxiety/panic

Nursing Process: Analysis

Reference

DeSelm, T. M. (2016). Mood and anxiety disorders. In J. E. Tintinalli, J. Stapczynski, O. Ma, D. M. Yealy, G. D. Meckler, & D. M. Cline (Eds.), *Tintinalli's emergency medicine: A comprehensive study guide* (8th ed.). Retrieved from http://accessemergencymedicine.mhmedical.com/content.aspx?bookid=1658&Sectionid=109448311

---

82. A patient who was diagnosed with terminal cancer 2 days previously presents to the emergency department (ED). Since receiving their diagnosis, the patient has repeatedly verbalized a desire to commit suicide, making such statements as, "I will just get my shotgun when things get bad," and "You can't stop me from driving my pickup into a tree." They are angry that their family has brought them to the ED and is continually yelling at their family members. What is the priority intervention the emergency nurse should take in this situation?

A. Explain to the family that the patient is experiencing the normal reaction of anger
B. Reassure the patient that they will be provided with resources such as hospice care
C. Recommend that the patient follow up with their primary care provider for antidepressants
D. Call for extra staff to assist

Rationale

A. Although anger is part of the stages of grief, this patient is in crisis and needs immediate psychiatric intervention.

B. The patient is too distraught to learn about end-of-life care at this time. They have likely already been provided with this information. They need immediate intervention for their current psychiatric crisis.

C. The patient is in crisis and needs immediate attention in the ED.

D. The patient has verbally expressed anger and is yelling at their family members. They are facing a very difficult situation and is not coping with it very well, making him a danger to themself, their family, and the staff. The most important priority at this time is to get the patient to a safe area so that they can receive treatment, help, and reassurance.

Category: Psychosocial and Medical Emergencies/Psychosocial/Suicidal ideation

Nursing Process: Intervention

References

Mayo Clinic. (2015). *Suicide and suicidal thoughts*. Retrieved from http://www.mayoclinic.org/diseases-conditions/suicide/basics/risk-factors/con-20033954

Smith, M., & Segal, J. (2017). Coping with grief and loss. *Helpguide.org*. Retrieved from https://www.helpguide.org/articles/grief-loss/coping-with-grief-and-loss.htm

---

83. A patient presents to the emergency department with severe swelling around their eyes and lips (angioedema). They deny any known allergies and states that they are currently taking only one medication for a recent diagnosis of hypertension. The emergency nurse recognizes that the most likely cause of the patient's angioedema is related to which of the following?

A. Midodrine (ProAmatine)
B. Losartan (Cozaar)
C. Diltiazem (Cardizem)
D. Lisinopril (Zestril)

Rationale

A. Midodrine is indicated in the treatment of orthostatic hypotension. Midodrine is an alpha-specific adrenergic agonist whose administration leads to vasoconstriction, thereby increasing the patient's vasculature tone and blood pressure. Midodrine is not indicated in the treatment of hypertension.

B. Losartan is an angiotensin II receptor blocker (ARB). ARBs are used to treat hypertension, but they are not associated with the development of angioedema as an allergic reaction to the medication. Side effects of an ARB include headache, dizziness, syncope, and weakness.

C. Diltiazem is a calcium channel blocker (CCB). CCBs are not associated with the development of angioedema as an allergic reaction to the medication. Potential side effects of CCB include dizziness, lightheadedness, headache, and fatigue. The patient is not complaining of these medication side effects.

D. Lisinopril is an angiotensin-converting enzyme inhibitor (ACE-I). Angioedema is a rare side effect attributed to the ACE-I class of antihypertensive medications. ACE-I-induced angioedema is occurring with increasing frequency because of the popularity of these medications in treating hypertension and heart failure. The incidence of angioedema is approximately 5 times greater in patients of African American descent as compared with other ethnic groups.

Category: Psychosocial and Medical Emergencies/Medical/Allergic reactions and anaphylaxis

Nursing Process: Analysis

References

Kolenc, K. M., & Dobbin, K. R. (1996). Angioedema caused by ACE inhibitor mistaken for allergic reaction. *Journal of Emergency Nursing, 22*(3), 228–231. https://doi.org/10.1016/S0099-1767(96)80116-4

Vallerand, A. H., Sanoski, C. A., & Deglin, J. H. (2015). *Davis drug guide for nurses* (14th ed.) Philadelphia, PA: F. A. Davis.

84. A patient from a skilled nursing facility is transported to the emergency department (ED) after sustaining a minor hand laceration; the bleeding has been controlled. The patient has recently been receiving high-dose chemotherapy for treatment of non-Hodgkin's lymphoma. The most appropriate area in the ED for the patient to receive treatment is in which of the following?

A. The waiting room
B. An ED room with reverse isolation precautions
C. Any available ED room
D. A quick care or rapid care minor treatment area

Rationale

A. The patient is at risk for profound neutropenia because of their chemotherapy, and every effort should be made to protect him from infection. It is not appropriate for the patient to be placed in the waiting room with other potentially infectious patients or visitors.

B. The high-dose chemotherapy used to treat Hodgkin's disease and non-Hodgkin's lymphoma results in profound neutropenia and incurs significant risk in terms of mortality and morbidity as a result of infection. Protection from infection is of vital importance, and patients should receive care in an isolation environment.

C. The patient is at risk for profound neutropenia because of their chemotherapy, and every effort should be made to protect him from infection. They should receive treatment in a room that limits their exposure to other patients and involves the fewest staff members possible.

D. The patient is at risk for profound neutropenia because of their chemotherapy, and every effort should be made to protect him from infection. A minor treatment area places the patient at risk for contracting an infectious process.

Category: Psychosocial and Medical Emergencies/Medical/Immunocompromise
Nursing Process: Analysis

Reference

Campbell, T. (1999). Feelings of oncology patients about being nursed in protective isolation as a consequence of cancer chemotherapy treatment. *Journal of Advanced Nursing, 30*(2), 439–447. https://doi.org/10.1046/j.1365-2648.1999.01099.x

---

85. Which of the following assessment findings would the emergency nurse be most concerned about in a hemophiliac patient with hemarthrosis?

A. Skin breakdown
B. Severe pain
C. Paresthesias
D. Impaired range of motion

Rationale

A. Skin breakdown is a potential finding with hemarthrosis but is not threatening to life or limb.

B. Severe pain is often noted in patients with hemarthrosis but is not limb or life threatening. Pain that is disproportionate to the injury can be associated with compartment syndrome and requires further evaluation.

C. Paresthesias can be an indicator of the presence of compartment syndrome. The collection of blood and edema can compress nerves and vasculature, reducing distal circulation and leading to tissue damage; it can be both limb and life threatening.

D. Impaired range of motion is often noted in patients with hemarthrosis but is not threatening to life or limb.

Category: Psychosocial and Medical Emergencies/Medical/Blood dyscrasias: Hemophilia

Nursing Process: Analysis

References

Bowman, S. H., & Georgopoulos, C. H. (2015). Hemophilia. In J. J. Schaider, R. M. Barkin, S. R. Hayden, R. E. Wolfe, A. Z. Barkin, P. Shayne, & P. Rosen. (Eds.), *Rosen and Barkin's 5-minute emergency medicine consult* (5th ed., pp. 502–503). Philadelphia, PA: Wolters Kluwer.

Croteau, S. E., Fleegler, E. W., & Brett-Fleegler, M. (2016). Hematologic emergencies. In K. N. Shaw & R. G. Bachur (Eds.), *Fleisher and Ludwig's textbook of pediatric emergency medicine* (7th ed., pp. 804–837). Philadelphia, PA: Wolters Kluwer.

---

86. Which of the following interventions would the emergency nurse expect to implement first in the patient who has developed signs of neuroleptic malignant syndrome?

A. Application of a cooling blanket
B. Administration of a benzodiazepine
C. Administration of a dopamine agonist
D. Insertion of a urinary catheter

Rationale

A. Application of a cooling blanket is an important intervention for treating the presence of hyperthermia in patients with neuroleptic malignant syndrome, but it is not the first treatment.

B. Patients who develop neuroleptic malignant syndrome should receive immediate intravenous benzodiazepines. Patients with neuroleptic malignant syndrome will exhibit fever, muscle rigidity, an altered level of consciousness, and dysfunction of the autonomic nervous system.

C. Administration of a dopamine agonist is an optional intervention for treating neuroleptic malignant syndrome, but it is not the first treatment.

D. Insertion of a urinary drainage catheter is an important intervention for assessing for complications of neuroleptic malignant syndrome, but it is not the first intervention to be performed.

Category: Psychosocial and Medical Emergencies/Psychosocial/Bipolar disorder

Nursing Process: Intervention

Reference

Beskind, D. L. (2015). Neuroleptic malignant syndrome. In J. J. Schaider, R. M. Barkin, S. R. Hayden, R. E. Wolfe, A. Z. Barkin, P. Shayne, & P. Rosen. (Eds.), *Rosen and Barkin's 5-minute emergency medicine consult* (5th ed., pp. 756–757). Philadelphia, PA: Wolters Kluwer.

---

87. The emergency nurse has provided discharge education to the parents of a child who experienced a febrile seizure. Which of the following statements made by the parents indicates to the emergency nurse that the teaching has been effective?

A. "Axillary temperature measurement is the preferred route for temperature measurement because it is the most accurate."
B. "Aspirin and acetaminophen (Tylenol) are the preferred medications for reducing a fever."
C. "Febrile seizures occur most often in children over the age of 2."
D. "Febrile seizures most often occur because of a rapid rise in the body's temperature."

Rationale

A. In children, a rectal temperature measurement is considered the most accurate and preferred method, especially in the very young. An axillary temperature reading is often 1–2°F lower than a rectal temperature.

B. Acetaminophen and ibuprofen are acceptable medications for fever reduction. Aspirin-containing products should be avoided in children with acute febrile illnesses because of the association with the development of Reye's syndrome.

C. The peak incidence of febrile seizures occurs in children under the age of 2, but the range is from 5 months to 5 years.

D. A rapid rise in the body's temperature, not the actual degree of the temperature, is often the cause of febrile seizures. The rapid rise irritates the immature nervous system and often causes the seizure activity.

Category (Pediatric): Psychosocial and Medical Emergencies/Medical/Fever

Nursing Process: Evaluation

References

Balamuth, F., Henretig, F. M., & Alpern, E. R. (2016). Fever. In K. N. Shaw & R. G. Bachur (Eds.), *Fleisher and Ludwig's textbook of pediatric emergency medicine* (7th ed., pp. 176–185). Philadelphia, PA: Wolters Kluwer.

Lazear, S. E., & Roberts, A. (2007). Medical emergencies. In K. S. Hoyt & J. Selfridge-Thomas (Eds.), *Emergency nursing core curriculum* (6th ed., pp. 483–509). St. Louis, MO: Saunders Elsevier.

---

88. A patient is brought to the emergency department by law enforcement after attempting to kill their brother with a knife. Presently the patient is calm, cooperative, and following directions. When performing the patient's initial assessment, which of the following would be the highest priority for the emergency nurse?

A. Offer the patient food or drink as soon as possible
B. Approach the patient early with a display of a power attitude
C. Have the patient undress completely
D. Physically restrain the patient with soft restraints

Rationale

A. It is appropriate to offer psychiatric patients food or beverage at some point, but this should not be the primary concern at the time of the initial assessment. The safety of everyone in the emergency department should be the primary concern of the emergency nurse.

B. It may be necessary to display a sense of power to the patient, either in demeanor or with a show of power through the presence of multiple security officers or other staff members in attendance. However, the show of power should only be done if it becomes absolutely necessary because of the patient's aggressive or uncooperative behavior. The highest priority is to get the patient completely undressed and all clothing searched for possible weapons.

C. It is most important that all patients who are exhibiting psychiatric emergencies be undressed completely, the patient's clothes should be checked (including pockets), and undergo a safety check for any items that could be used to harm oneself or others. Items such as guns and knives can be hidden under or inside clothing. A safe environment is one in which patients would not have access to anything that could harm themselves or others.

D. This patient is calm and cooperative, so the application of restraints is not indicated at this time.

Category: Psychosocial and Medical Emergencies/Psychosocial/Homicidal ideation

Nursing Process: Intervention

References

Citrome, L. (2015). Aggression. *Medscape*. Retrieved from http://emedicine.medscape.com/article/288689-overview#a4

Manton, A. (2013). Mental health emergencies. In B. B. Hammond & P. G. Zimmermann (Eds.), *Sheehy's manual of emergency care* (7th ed., pp. 303–318). St. Louis, MO: Elsevier Mosby.

---

89. A patient who has sustained a 4-inch laceration to the left anterior thigh arrives in the emergency department via emergency medical services. The wound had previously been bleeding profusely, however, direct pressure to the wound has reduced the blood flow. The patient is anxious and continually states, "I am a bleeder! I know I will need some factor VIII! Get it quick!" The emergency nurse is aware that this patient most likely has which of the following coagulopathies?

A. Hemophilia B
B. Hemophilia A
C. Von Willebrand disease
D. Christmas disease

Rationale

A. Hemophilia B is a sex-linked inherited disorder that results in factor IX deficiency or functionality. The hemophilia B gene is carried by the female, who passes it on to her children; however, the disease almost always manifests in males.

B. Hemophilia A is a sex-linked inherited disorder that results in factor VIII deficiency or functionality. The hemophilia A gene is carried by the female, who passes it on to her children; however, the disease is almost always found only in males.

C. Von Willebrand disease is a genetically inherited bleeding disorder. The disease is manifested in both male and female patients. Von Willebrand disease is caused by defects in the adherence of platelets, a low level of factor VIII, and decreased levels of von Willebrand factor.

D. Christmas disease is another name for hemophilia B, which is a lack of, or a decrease in the functionality of, factor IX. This disease is primarily seen in male patients.

Category: Psychosocial and Medical Emergencies/Medical/Blood dyscrasias: Hemophilia

Nursing Process: Analysis

References

Carringer, C. J., & Hammond, B. (2013). Hematologic and immunologic emergencies. In B. B. Hammond & P. G. Zimmermann (Eds.), *Sheehy's manual of emergency care* (7th ed., pp. 303–318). St. Louis, MO: Elsevier Mosby.

Smith, D. (2010). Hematologic and oncologic emergencies. In P. K. Howard & R. A. Steinmann (Eds.), *Sheehy's emergency nursing: Principles and practice* (6th ed., pp. 554–563). St. Louis, MO: Mosby Elsevier.

---

90. Which of the following statements made by a patient being treated for diabetic ketoacidosis would increase the emergency nurse's suspicion that an untoward effect was occurring during the treatment phase?

A. "I seem to have developed a pretty serious headache in the past hour."
B. "I feel like I need to urinate very badly."
C. "Can I have something for this back pain that has been getting worse?"
D. "I feel like I am aching all over."

Rationale

A. A too-rapid decrease in blood glucose level can cause the development of cerebral edema, which could be indicated by the headache. The emergency nurse should be on alert for any manifestations of increased intracranial pressure, such as dizziness, visual disturbances, nausea, vomiting, change in speech patterns, or decrease in level of consciousness.

B. This statement might be related to the patient having received several liters of fluid and actually needing to void. This is not an indicator of an untoward effect of the treatment.

C. The patient may have had to stay in bed for an extended period or may have chronic back pain issues, but back pain is not a side effect of the treatment for diabetic ketoacidosis.

D. This would not indicate a major concern related to the treatment regimen for diabetic ketoacidosis for the emergency nurse, although it is something that the nurse should discuss with the patient and the provider.

Category: Psychosocial and Medical Emergencies/Medical/Endocrine conditions: Glucose-related conditions

Nursing Process: Evaluation

References

Broering, B. (2010). Neurological emergencies. In P. K. Howard & R. A. Steinmann (Eds.), *Sheehy's emergency nursing: Principles and practice* (6th ed., pp. 457–466). St. Louis, MO: Mosby Elsevier.

Morey, C. M. (2010). Endocrine emergencies. In P. K. Howard & R. A. Steinmann (Eds.), *Sheehy's emergency nursing: Principles and practice* (6th ed., pp. 499–512). St. Louis, MO: Mosby Elsevier.

---

91. Which laboratory test would indicate that a patient's psychotic symptoms may be related to a medical condition and not a psychiatric condition?

A. A sodium level of 145 mg/dL
B. A potassium level of 4.0 mEq/L
C. A blood glucose level of 20 mg/dL
D. A calcium level of 10 mg/dL

Rationale

A. A normal sodium level 135–145 mg/dL.

B. A normal potassium level is 3.5–5.0 mEq/L.

C. A normal serum glucose level is 80–100 mg/dL. Symptoms of severe hypoglycemia include pale skin, diaphoresis, and an altered mental status, which may cause the patient to experience severe confusion and hallucinations.

D. A normal calcium level is 9.6–10.6 mg/dL.

Category: Psychosocial and Medical Emergencies/Psychosocial/Psychosis

Nursing Process: Assessment

References

Doig, A., & Huether, S. (2014). The cellular environment: Fluids and electrolytes, acids and bases. In K. McCance & S. Huether (Eds.), *Pathophysiology: The biologic basis for disease in adults and children* (pp. 103–134). St. Louis, MO: Elsevier Mosby.

Wheat, S., & Taleri, M. (2016). Psychiatric emergencies. *Primary Care: Clinics in Office Practice, 43*(2), 341–354. https://doi.org/10.1016/j.pop.2016.01.009

---

92. Which of the following laboratory trends does the emergency nurse expect to be present in a patient diagnosed with disseminated intravascular coagulation?

A. Decreased platelet count, elevated D-dimer, and prolonged prothrombin time
B. Increased platelet count, elevated D-dimer, and prolonged prothrombin time
C. Decreased platelet count, increased fibrinogen, and decreased D-dimer
D. Increased platelet count, decreased D-dimer, and prolonged prothrombin

Rationale

A. Disseminated intravascular coagulation results in a depletion of clotting factors due to diffuse microvascular clot formation. These clots are triggered by hemorrhage and dilution, often related to resuscitation after hemorrhage or the presence of a specific disease state, such as sepsis or liver disease. Platelets will decrease because of the rapid loss of blood. The D-dimer is a product of fibrin degradation.

B. The D-dimer will be elevated and the prothrombin time prolonged, but the platelet count will decrease. Platelets will decrease because of the rapid loss of blood.

C. The platelet count will decrease along with fibrinogen. Platelets will decrease because of the rapid loss of blood. Fibrinogen is rapidly depleted because of the reduction of clotting factors and formation of clots.

D. The platelet count will be decreased, and the D-dimer will be elevated. The prothrombin time will be prolonged because the clotting cascade has been disrupted, causing an interference with the blood's ability to clot.

Category: Psychosocial and Medical Emergencies/Medical/Disseminated intravascular coagulation (DIC)

Nursing Process: Assessment

References

Parker, R. (2013). Coagulopathies in the PICU: DIC and liver disease. *Critical Care Clinics, 29*(2), 319–333. https://doi.org/10.1016/j.ccc.2012.12.003

Stevenson, J. (2014). Post resuscitation care in the emergency department. In D. Gurney (Ed.), *Trauma Nursing Core Course: Provider manual* (7th ed., pp. 331–345). Des Plaines, IL: Emergency Nurses Association.

---

93. After receiving fluid resuscitation with an isotonic crystalloid solution, an emergency department patient diagnosed with septic shock remains hypotensive. Which of the following would be initiated to assist in maintaining the patient's blood pressure?

A. Transfuse hydroxyethyl starches to maintain a mean arterial pressure (MAP) of 65 mm Hg or higher
B. Addition of albumin to the current crystalloid solution to maintain a MAP of 65 mm Hg or higher
C. Transfuse packed red blood cells to maintain a MAP of 65 mm Hg or higher
D. Vasopressor to maintain a MAP of 65 mm Hg or higher

Rationale

A. The use of hydroxyethyl starches is not recommended to correct hypotension in septic shock; in some studies, it has been found to increase the risk of renal failure.

B. Currently, the use of albumin is not recommended as a solution for the treatment of hypotension during the resuscitation phase of the patient in septic shock.

C. Blood transfusions are not recommended in the management of hypotension in the presence of septic shock unless the patient's hemoglobin is 7 g/dL or lower.

D. The severe sepsis bundles recommend that if resuscitation with crystalloid does not correct the patient's hypotension, a vasopressor such as norepinephrine, epinephrine, or phenylephrine should be initiated to maintain a MAP of 65 mm Hg or higher.

Category: Psychosocial and Medical Emergencies/Medical/Sepsis and septic shock

Nursing Process: Intervention

References

Buck, K. (2014). Developing an early sepsis alert program. *Journal of Nursing Care Quarterly, 29*(20), 124–132. https://doi.org/10.1097/NCQ.0b013e3182a98182

Doble, M. (2017). Making sense of the updated sepsis definitions. *NursingCenter.* Retrieved from http://www.nursingcenter.com/ncblog/march-2016/making-sense-of-the-updated-sepsis-definitions

Keegan, J., & Wira, C. (2014). Early identification and management of patients with severe sepsis and septic shock in the emergency department. *Emergency Medicine Clinics of North America, 32*, 759–776. https://doi.org/10.1016/j.emc.2014.07.002

Miller, J. (2014). Surviving sepsis: A review of the latest guidelines. *Nursing 2017, 44*(4), 24–30. https://doi.org/10.1097/01.NURSE.0000444530.66327.de

Rhoades, C., Semonin Holleran, R., Carpenter, L., & Grissom, C. (2010). Management of the critical care patient in the emergency department. In P. K. Howard & R. A. Steinmann (Eds.), *Sheehy's emergency nursing: Principles and practice* (6th ed., pp. 211–230). St. Louis, MO: Mosby Elsevier.

Schorr, C. (2016). Nurses can help improve outcomes in severe sepsis. *American Nurse Today, 11*(3), 20–25. Retrieved from https://www.americannursetoday.com/nurses-can-help-improve-outcomes-severe-sepsis/

94. An emergency patient has been diagnosed with thrombocytopenia. The emergency nurse is aware the following laboratory value has confirmed this diagnosis:

A. White blood cell count of 8000 uL
B. Platelet count of 5000 uL
C. Platelet count of 900,000 uL
D. White blood cell count of 26,000 uL

Rationale

A. A white blood cell count (WBC) of 8000 uL is a normal value and would not define thrombocytopenia or a low platelet count.

B. Thrombocytopenia is defined as a very low platelet count. The platelet count normally ranges from 150,000 uL to 400,000 uL. A level of 5000 uL would be very low, and the patient may display bleeding tendencies. Thrombocytopenia has various causes, including failure of the bone marrow to produce platelets, and platelets being destroyed or broken down in the bloodstream, spleen, or liver.

C. This value of 900,000 uL is a markedly elevated platelet count. A normal platelet count is 150,000 uL to 400,000 uL. An elevated platelet count is referred to as thrombocytosis and can result in excessive clotting.

D. A WBC count of 26,000 uL is defined as leukocytosis and would indicate that an infectious process is present in the patient. A normal WBC count is 3600 uL to 10,400 uL.

Category: Psychosocial and Medical Emergencies/Medical/Blood dyscasias: Other coagulopathies
Nursing Process: Assessment

Reference

Lewis, S. L., Heitkemper, M. M., & Harding, M. M. (2017). Hematologic problems. In *Medical surgical nursing: Assessment and management of clinical problems* (10th ed., pp. 606–655). St. Louis, MO: Mosby.

---

95. A patient presents to the emergency department with a swollen abdomen. The patient's arms and legs are very thin, their face is round, their skin is very thin, and there is a buffalo hump between their shoulders. Pink stretch marks are noted on the abdomen. The patient has a history of long-term dexamethasone (Prednisone) use for urticaria. Vital signs include: BP 200/100 mm Hg. The emergency nurse suspects that this patient has which of the following?

A. Hashimoto disease
B. Thyrotoxicosis
C. Syndrome of inappropriate antidiuretic hormone
D. Cushing's syndrome

Rationale

A. Hashimoto disease is a condition in which the immune system attacks the thyroid gland, causing it to not function properly and decrease secretion thyroid hormones. Symptoms include fatigue, hair loss, puffy face, and increased sensitivity to cold.

B. Thyrotoxicosis is caused by severe thyroid dysfunction causing hyperthyroidism. Hyperdynamic vital signs along with central nervous system dysfunctions are common signs.

C. Syndrome of inappropriate antidiuretic hormone is caused by abnormal amounts of antidiuretic hormone being released from the pituitary gland resulting in water intoxication. This condition can be a result of head injury, infections, or certain drugs (antihypoglycemic agents, psychotropic drugs, and antineoplastic drugs). Symptoms include headache, fatigue, confusion, seizures, and weight gain.

D. Cushing's syndrome is a collection of symptoms, which can be attributed to prolonged exposure to cortisone. Classic signs and symptoms include a swelling fat pad at the base of the neck and upper spine known as a buffalo hump, hypertension, abdominal swelling, thin extremities, striations along the abdomen, and a round moon face. A tumor of the adrenal gland can also cause Cushing's syndrome.

Category: Psychosocial and Medical Emergencies/Medical/Endocrine conditions

Nursing Process: Analysis

References

Marett, B. (2013). Metabolic emergencies. In B. B. Hammond, & P. G. Zimmermann, (Eds.), *Sheehy's manual of emergency care* (7th ed., pp. 303–318). Philadelphia, PA: Mosby Elsevier.

Wall, A. (2007). Endocrine emergencies. In K. S. Hoyt & J. Selfridge-Thomas (Eds.), *Emergency nursing core curriculum* (6th ed., pp. 290–309). St. Louis, MO: Saunders Elsevier.

---

96. A patient presents to triage complaining of nausea, weakness, and fatigue. The patient appears anorexic and has hyperpigmentation to the knuckles and creases of the hands. The patient's medical history includes the presence of Addison's disease, and the provider orders a dose of hydrocortisone to be administered. The emergency nurse anticipates which of the following outcomes as a result of this medication?

A. Increase in blood pressure
B. Decrease in sodium
C. Decrease in glucose
D. Weight gain

Rationale

A. This patient is displaying symptoms of acute adrenal crisis, which can occur after abrupt cessation of methylprednisolone (Prednisone). Signs and symptoms include hypotension; tachycardia; fatigue; nausea; hyperpigmentation of the knuckles, creases in the hands, axilla, and gums; and electrolyte abnormalities: hyponatremia, hypoglycemia, hyperkalemia, and hypercalcemia. Hemodynamic stability is a high priority and is a therapeutic outcome the nurse should expect after administration of hydrocortisone.

B. Patients who present in adrenal crisis may present with hyponatremia as a result of lack of the glucocorticoid cortisol and the mineralocorticoid aldosterone. A therapeutic outcome of administration of hydrocortisone and dexamethasone is increased sodium.

C. Patients who present in adrenal crisis may present with hypoglycemia as a result of lack of the glucocorticoid cortisol. A therapeutic outcome of administration of hydrocortisone is increased glucose.

D. Patients who present in adrenal crisis will likely have recent weight loss, however, weight gain may not occur immediately with treatment. Correction of hemodynamic instability is a higher priority expected outcome.

Category: Psychosocial and Medical Emergencies/Medical/Endocrine conditions: Adrenal

Nursing Process: Evaluation

Reference

Marett, B. E. (2013). Metabolic emergencies. In B. B. Hammond & P. G. Zimmermann (Eds.), *Sheehy's manual of emergency care* (7th ed., pp. 303–318). St. Louis, MO: Elsevier Mosby.

---

97. The emergency nurse is assessing a patient with a history of sickle cell disease (SCD). The patient tells the nurse that he is experiencing wheezing, fever, and shortness of breath. Which high-morbidity complication of SCD would the emergency nurse suspect this patient is experiencing?

A. Priapism
B. Acute chest syndrome
C. Cholecystitis
D. Splenic sequestration

Rationale

A. Priapism is a painful erection and a genitourinary emergency in which red blood cells sickle and become lodged in the microvasculature, which leads to entrapment of blood in the penis. Symptoms do not typically include fever, wheezing, or dyspnea. Priapism is not associated with high mortality rates in patients with SCD.

B. Acute chest syndrome occurs when sickle-shaped red blood cells attach to the lung endothelium that is already inflamed, and the failure of the lung tissue to be reoxygenated leads to additional inflammation and lung infarction. Acute chest syndrome is the cause of death in approximately 25% of all deaths in people with SCD. Symptoms include chest pain, dyspnea, fever, cough, wheezing, hypoxemia, and pulmonary infiltrates.

C. While patients with SCD may be at higher risk for cholecystitis, presenting symptoms typically include right upper quadrant abdominal pain, nausea, vomiting, and diarrhea. Cholecystitis is not associated with high mortality rates in patients with SCD.

D. Patients with SCD are at high risk for splenic issues, this complication occurs primarily in children. Splenic sequestration occurs when large amounts of blood become pooled in the spleen; because the spleen can hold one-fifth of the bodies blood supply, there are high mortality rates associated with splenic sequestration resulting in cardiovascular collapse. Symptoms would be abdominal pain and signs of hypovolemic shock, weakness, pallor, tachycardia, and hypotension.

Category: Psychosocial and Medical Emergencies/Medical/Blood dyscrasias: Sickle cell crisis

Nursing Process: Analysis

References

Kline, N. E. (2013). Alterations of hematologic function in children. In K. L. McCance, S. E. Huether, V. L. Brashers, & N. S. Rote (Eds.), *Pathophysiology: The biologic basis for disease in adults and children* (7th ed., pp. 1055–1082). St. Louis, MO: Mosby.

Smith, D. A. (2010). Hematologic and oncologic emergencies. In P. K. Howard & R. A. Steinmann (Eds.), *Sheehy's emergency nursing: Principles and practice* (6th ed., pp. 554–563). St. Louis, MO: Elsevier.

98. Which of the following conditions is a rare, life-threatening, and serious complication of hypothyroidism?

A. Adrenal crisis
B. Myxedema coma
C. Thyroid storm
D. Cushing's syndrome

Rationale

A. Adrenal crisis, also known as acute adrenal insufficiency, is a life-threatening condition caused by a decrease in cortisol and aldosterone levels. This results in sodium and water loss from both the kidneys and gastrointestinal tract, causing the patient to become hypotensive and hypovolemic. As the body loses sodium, there is an increase in potassium, leading to hyperkalemia and the development of fatal dysrhythmias. Treatment includes fluid replacement, correction of hyperkalemia, and hydrocortisone administration.

B. Myxedema coma is a rare, life-threatening, and serious complication of hypothyroidism that affects older patients with pulmonary or vascular disease. Patients complain of fatigue, shortness of breath, and weight gain, and may experience tongue swelling. Treatment includes support of the patient's airway, breathing, and circulation (ABCs), as well as thyroid hormone replacement.

C. Thyroid storm, also known as thyrotoxic crisis, is a rare, life-threatening, and serious complication of hyperthyroidism. Patients present with agitation, tachydysrhythmias, tachypnea, and fever. Treatment includes support of the patient's ABCs, fever control, propylthiouracil, and iodine.

D. Cushing's syndrome is the result of prolonged exposure to glucocorticoids (either endogenous or exogenous) that causes the patient to develop a cushingoid appearance. There is an increased amount of adipose tissue to the face, upper back, and base of the neck.

Category: Psychosocial and Medical Emergencies/Medical/Endocrine conditions

Nursing Process: Assessment

References

Marrett, B. (2013). Metabolic emergencies. In B. B. Hammond & P. G. Zimmermann (Eds.), *Sheehy's manual of emergency care* (7th ed., pp. 303–317). St. Louis, MO: Elsevier Mosby.

Morey, C. (2010). Endocrine emergencies. In P. K. Howard & R. A. Steinmann (Eds.), *Sheehy's emergency nursing: Principles and practice* (6th ed., pp. 499–511). St. Louis, MO: Mosby Elsevier

Wall, S. W. (2007). Endocrine emergencies. In K. S. Hoyt & J. Selfridge-Thomas (Eds.), *Emergency nursing core curriculum* (6th ed., pp. 290–309). St. Louis, MO: Saunders Elsevier.

---

99. Parents arrive to triage with their toddler, whose hand was caught in the car door, resulting in amputation of the index finger. The amputated part has been wrapped in gauze, which is presented to the triage nurse. The emergency nurse is aware that the proper way to care for the amputated part is to:

A. wrap the amputated part with sterile gauze soaked in tap water, place in a sealed bag, place the sealed bag in another bag, and place in tepid water.
B. wrap the amputated part in sterile gauze soaked with hibiclens and saline, place the part in a sealed bag, place the sealed bag in another bag, and place in ice water.

C. wrap the amputated part with dry sterile gauze, place in a sealed bag, place the sealed bag in another bag, and place in tepid water.
D. wrap the amputated part in sterile gauze moistened by saline, place the part in a sealed bag, place the sealed bag in another bag, and place in ice water.

Rationale

A. The amputated part should not be wrapped with gauze in tap water, and it should be placed in an ice bath, not tepid water. There are numerous organisms in tap water that can lead to infection and prevent successful reimplantation of the amputated part.

B. Hibiclens-soaked gauze may actually cause more damage to the soft tissue of the amputated part. Hibiclens is an antimicrobial soap that can damage the tissue of the amputated part and prevent reimplantation. For best results, the part needs to be placed in sterile gauze moistened with saline.

C. The amputated part should not be allowed to dry out because this can prevent successful reimplantation. The amputated part should be wrapped in sterile gauze that has been soaked in sterile saline and placed in an ice water bath.

D. For best results regarding successful reimplantation of an amputated part, it is best to keep the amputated part wrapped in sterile gauze that has been gently moistened with sterile saline and place it in a plastic bag. Next, place this bag into a second plastic bag containing ice. The double-wrapped amputated part is then placed in a container with saline. Double-bagging the amputated part prevents it from coming in direct contact with the iced saline solution. The amputated part should not be allowed to freeze or be submerged in water.

Category: Maxillofacial, Ocular, Orthopedic, and Wound Emergencies/Orthopedic/Amputation
Nursing Process: Intervention

Reference

Bratcher, C. M. (2014). Musculoskeletal trauma. In D. Gurney (Ed.), *Trauma Nursing Core Course: Provider manual* (7th ed., pp. 193–204). Des Plaines, IL: Emergency Nurses Association.

---

100. When caring for a variety of patients, the emergency nurse is knowledgeable that the patient with the least risk for developing compartment syndrome would be a patient with which of the following injuries?

A. A patient with a venomous snake bite to the forearm
B. A crush injury to the shaft of the femur
C. A patient with a circumferential full thickness burn to the calf
D. A nondisplaced fracture to the medial malleolus

Rationale

A. Snake bites are soft tissue injuries that can lead to edema in the compartment, making the patient more at risk for developing compartment syndrome.

B. Crush injuries tend to be associated with compartment syndrome because they cause swelling of the soft tissues, which can increase the intracompartmental pressure. In addition, pressure from an outside force, such as when a heavy object falls on a patient, can increase the risk of developing compartment syndrome.

C. Circumferential burn injuries are associated with increased risk for compartment syndrome. Soft tissue injuries and burns are associated with edema, which causes an increase in intracompartmental pressure. This type of injury may require a fasciotomy or escharotomy to relieve the compartment pressure.

D. Most malleolus fractures are associated with inversion or eversion injuries related to ankle sprains. This fracture is nondisplaced, and the patient most likely will need only to be splinted or have a cast applied to the ankle area. The risk for compartment syndrome with this type of fracture is generally low.

Category: Maxillofacial, Ocular, Orthopedic, and Wound Emergencies/Orthopedic/Compartment syndrome

Nursing Process: Analysis

Reference

Halpren, J. (2013). Musculoskeletal trauma. In B. B. Hammond & P. G. Zimmerman (Eds.), *Sheehy's manual of emergency care* (7th ed., pp. 427–437). St. Louis, MO: Elsevier Mosby.

---

101. The emergency nurse is discharging a patient who developed back pain 1 week ago after bending over to pick up a young child. The emergency nurse determines that patient teaching has been effective when the patient states which of the following?

A. "Nonsteroidal anti-inflammatory drugs and acetaminophen (Tylenol) are not effective in relieving my back pain."
B. "I need to limit my activity and rest my back as much as possible."
C. "It is important that I stop smoking so that I will heal faster."
D. "I should only use ice and heat during the first 24 hours of my back pain."

Rationale

A. Anti-inflammatories and acetaminophen are good options for pain relief and are very effective pain relievers.

B. It is important and can actually help back pain to stay active with activities that don't strain the back, such as walking. The emergency nurse should teach proper body mechanics, especially when it comes to lifting, and instruct the patient to avoid movements that may cause strain to the back.

C. Smoking is associated with delayed healing for low back pain. Encouraging smoking cessation is very important for most health conditions and can assist with healing for low back pain.

D. Ice and heat are good options for back pain relief and should not be limited to the first day.

Category: Maxillofacial, Ocular, Orthopedic, and Wound Emergencies/Orthopedic/Low back pain

Nursing Process: Evaluation

References

Cerepani, M. J., & Ramponi, D. R. (2007). Orthopedic emergencies. In K. S. Hoyt & J. Selfridge-Thomas (Eds.), *Emergency nursing core curriculum* (6th ed., pp. 585–603). St. Louis, MO: Saunders Elsevier.

Rouzier, P. (2010). *The sports medicine patient advisor* (3rd ed.). Amherst, MA: SportsMedPress.

102. A patient presents to the emergency department by emergency medical services (EMS) in complete cervical spine immobilization. The patient is intoxicated, and EMS reports that the patient had been drinking and jumped off the second floor of a parking garage and landed on their heels. The patient is found to have bilateral calcaneal fractures. The emergency nurse also anticipates the patient may have experienced which of the following injuries?

A. Spinous process fracture of thoracic vertebrae 6 (T6)
B. Spiral fracture of the femur
C. Bilateral bipartite patella
D. Burst fracture of lumbar vertebrae 1 (L1)

Rationale

A. Axial loading injuries are associated with burst fractures of the spine, which is the correct answer to this question. Spinous process fractures are more commonly associated with direct blows to the back, motor vehicle collisions, falls, or sudden twisting motions.

B. There may be other fractures associated with axial loading injuries, but the mechanism of the calcaneal fracture would not result in a spiral fracture of the femur.

C. Bipartite patella is a type of congenital abnormality of the patella and is not associated with trauma.

D. Calcaneal fractures, especially in injuries that involve the patient landing on their feet, is a type of axial loading injury where other injuries must be considered. Injuries associated with calcaneal fractures include burst fracture of the spine, tibial plateau fracture, and internal organ injuries.

Category: Maxillofacial, Ocular, Orthopedic, and Wound Emergencies/Orthopedic/Trauma
Nursing Process: Analysis

Reference

Crowley, M. (2014). Spinal cord and vertebral column trauma. In D. Gurney (Ed.), *Trauma Nursing Core Course: Provider manual* (7th ed., pp. 173–192). Des Plaines, IL: Emergency Nurses Association.

---

103. A patient is being discharged from the emergency department with a lower leg cast. The patient is concerned about how they will be able to walk up and down the steps with crutches at home. The emergency nurse will instruct the patient that the proper technique to go up and down stairs is:

A. up with the "bad" leg and down with the "good" leg.
B. up with the "bad" leg and down with the "bad" leg.
C. up with the "good" leg and down with the "bad" leg.
D. up with the "good" leg and down with the "good" leg.

Rationale

A. Going up stairs, the uninjured (good) leg goes up on the first step, followed by the injured (bad) leg and crutches. Going down stairs, place crutches down one step, step down with the injured (bad) leg, and follow with the uninjured (good) leg.

B. Going up stairs, the uninjured (good) leg goes up on the first step, followed by the injured (bad) leg and crutches. Going down stairs, place crutches down one step, step down with the injured (bad) leg, and follow with the uninjured (good) leg.

C. Going up stairs, the uninjured (good) leg goes up on the first step, followed by the injured (bad) leg and crutches. Going down stairs, place crutches down one step, step down with the injured (bad) leg, and follow with the uninjured (good) leg.

D. Going up stairs, the uninjured (good) leg goes up on the first step, followed by the injured (bad) leg and crutches. Going down stairs, place crutches down one step, step down with the injured (bad) leg, and follow with the uninjured (good) leg.

Category: Maxillofacial, Ocular, Orthopedic, and Wound Emergencies/Orthopedic/Fracture/dislocation
Nursing Process: Evaluation

Reference

Ramponi, D., & Cerepani, M. J. (2007). Orthopedic trauma. In K. S. Hoyt & J. Selfridge-Thomas (Eds.), *Emergency nursing core curriculum* (6th ed., pp. 891–928). St. Louis, MO: Saunders Elsevier.

---

104. The emergency nurse is caring for a patient with a pelvic fracture. At the beginning of the assessment, the nurse notes the presence of distal pulses with good motor and sensory function of the lower extremities. However, during ongoing assessments, the nurse is no longer able to palpate distal pulses, and the patient has an altered mental status. Which of the following could be responsible for this change in the patient's status?

A. Fat embolism
B. Hemorrhage
C. Compartment syndrome
D. Neurogenic shock

Rationale

A. Most instances of fat embolism are asymptomatic, but in symptomatic patients, there is a classic triad presentation of decreased mental status, starting with restlessness and agitation; respiratory distress, including dyspnea and hypoxia; and petechial rash on the head, neck, anterior thorax, conjunctivae, buccal mucous membranes, and axillae.

B. Signs and symptoms of decompensated or progressive shock include an altered level of consciousness, the presence of weak, thready pulses, and cool, clammy, cyanotic skin as the blood shunts to vital organs.

C. The six Ps associated with compartment syndrome are pain, pressure, pallor, pulses, paresthesia, and paralysis. Compartment syndrome does not directly result in an altered mental status change.

D. Neurogenic shock is a type of distributive shock that occurs as a result of maldistribution of an adequate circulating blood volume. It usually occurs with spinal cord injury, resulting in the loss of sympathetic nervous system control of vascular tone, which produces venous and arterial vasodilation.

Category: Maxillofacial, Ocular, Orthopedic, and Wound Emergencies/Orthopedic
Nursing Process: Analysis

References

Bratcher, C. M. (2014) Musculoskeletal trauma. In D. Gurney (Ed.), *Trauma Nursing Core Course: Provider manual* (7th ed., pp. 193–204, Des Plaines, IL: Emergency Nursing Association.
Pentecost, D. A., & Smith, S. G. (2014). Shock. In D. Gurney (Ed.), *Trauma Nursing Core Course: Provider manual* (7th ed., pp. 73–90). Des Plaines, IL: Emergency Nursing Association.
Stevenson, J. (2014). Post resuscitation care in the emergency department. In D. Gurney (Ed.), *Trauma Nursing Core Course: Provider manual* (7th ed., pp. 331–344). Des Plaines, IL: Emergency Nursing Association.

---

105. The emergency nurse is aware that patients with gout will experience periodic exacerbation of painful joint inflammation, resulting in acute painful episodes to be treated with the following medication:

A. allopurinol.
B. antibiotics.
C. nonsteroidal anti-inflammatory medications.
D. bisphosphonates.

Rationale

A. Allopurinol impairs conversion of xanthine to uric acid, thus inhibiting urate synthesis. This medication is used for chronic gout, not for acute episodic flare-ups of gout.

B. Gout is a disorder of purine metabolism characterized by monosodium urate crystal deposits in specific periarticular and subcutaneous tissues that lead to acute attacks of inflammatory arthritis. Antibiotics are not helpful in the treatment of gout.

C. Although indomethacin (Indocin) often is preferred, almost any nonsteroidal anti-inflammatory medications is effective in treating acute gout if prescribed in anti-inflammatory doses. Colchicine, a traditional therapy for gout, can be dramatically effective if initiated shortly after onset of acute symptoms.

D. Bisphosphonates are antiresorptive agents used to slow bone resorption and maintain bone mineral density. They help to prevent fractures and bone loss but are not indicated in the treatment of gout.

Category: Maxillofacial, Ocular, Orthopedic, and Wound Emergencies/Orthopedic/Inflammatory conditions

Nursing Process: Intervention

Reference

National Association of Orthopaedic Nurses. (2013). Arthritis & connective tissue disorders. In *Core curriculum for orthopaedic nursing* (7th ed., pp. 335–376). Chicago, IL: Author.

---

106. A patient arrives by emergency medical services (EMS) to the emergency department. EMS reports that the patient jumped from a third-story balcony when the support structure gave way. The patient landed on both feet and has been found to have a compression fracture of the lumbar spine with significant pain. Neurological assessment indicates the spine is intact, and the patient has no other complaints of pain. Glasgow Coma Scale score is 15, with no reported loss of consciousness. In addition to the compression fracture of the lumbar spine, this patient should also be evaluated for the presence of a:

A. hidden foreign body impalement.
B. femur fracture.
C. subdural hematoma.
D. calcaneus fracture.

Rationale

A. Impalement of a hidden foreign body results from penetrating trauma. This results in an open wound from the foreign object that may or may not be present.

B. Femur fractures result from high-energy transfer. Femur fractures can occur in conjunction with knee trauma or result from a direct blow to the femur. Signs and symptoms include pain radiating to the groin, swollen thigh, and limited range of motion. Femur fractures may result in significant blood loss into the surrounding tissue.

C. Subdural hematoma occurs because of hemorrhage in the subdural space and may be either acute (after severe trauma) or chronic (over a period of days or weeks). Risk increases in those who use anticoagulants; alcoholics; and the elderly (cerebral atrophy).

D. Calcaneus fractures can occur in jumps or falls when the patient lands directly on their feet. The energy load of landing feet first can result in calcaneus fractures as well as vertebral body fractures.

Category: Maxillofacial, Ocular, Orthopedic, and Wound Emergencies/Orthopedic/Fractures/dislocations

Nursing Process: Analysis

Reference

Solheim, J. (2013). Assessment and stabilization of the trauma patient. In B. B. Hammond & P. G. Zimmermann (Eds.), *Sheehy's manual of emergency care* (7th ed., pp. 369–378). St. Louis, MO: Elsevier Mosby.

---

107. A young patient presents to triage with complaints of left ankle pain. The patient reports that while playing basketball, they lost their balance and landed hard on their left foot; a "popping" sound in the ankle followed. The ankle is swollen and painful, and the patient is unable to bear weight on the left foot. The patient is exhibiting signs and symptoms of what type of ankle injury?

A. Avulsion fracture
B. Sprain
C. Dislocation
D. Strain

Rationale

A. An avulsion fracture occurs when a muscle mass contracts forcefully, causing a bone fragment to tear off at the muscle insertion site. Ligaments can also tear fragments from bone.

B. A sprain is the result of injury to the ankle ligaments that have been stretched or torn by excessive force. Ankle sprains are often associated with sports activities. They are graded according to degree of damage and the amount of instability present.

C. Dislocation requires a large amount of force to the affected joint. The ankle is plantar flexed with the foot inverted or even diverted under stress and occurs more frequently in children and adolescents. Presence of neurovascular compromise is possible with a dislocation.

D. A strain is the stretching or tearing of a muscle or tendon from bone as the result of excessive force. Strains are graded according to severity in a similar manner to sprains.

Category (Pediatric): Maxillofacial, Ocular, Orthopedic, and Wound Emergencies/Orthopedic/Strains/sprains

Nursing Process: Assessment

Reference

Halpern, J. S. (2013). Musculoskeletal trauma. In B. B. Hammond & P. G. Zimmermann (Eds.), *Sheehy's manual of emergency care* (7th ed., pp. 427–438). St. Louis, MO: Elsevier Mosby.

---

108. A patient with a laceration to the middle phalanx of the palmar side of the index finger from a kitchen knife presents to triage. Bleeding has been controlled. After examining the patient for possible tendon injury, the emergency nurse anticipates preparing the patient for wound closure by first:

A. cleansing the wound.
B. administering antibiotics.
C. providing anesthesia with lidocaine and epinephrine into the affected finger.
D. administering an opioid analgesia.

Rationale

A. Remove visible contamination and dried blood by using a 4 x 4 sponge and cleansing agent.

B. Prophylactic use of antibiotics is controversial unless the wound is considered a high-risk contaminated wound.

C. 0.5–2.0% lidocaine is often used because of a rapid onset (1–2 minutes) of action. Epinephrine, however, is contraindicated for distal areas (e.g., fingers, toes, nose, and earlobes) because of vasoconstrictive effects of the epinephrine.

D. Use of opioid analgesia is not indicated for pain associated with minor lacerations.

Category: Maxillofacial, Ocular, Orthopedic, and Wound Emergencies/Wound/Lacerations
Nursing Process: Intervention

Reference

Bratcher, C. M. (2014). Musculoskeletal trauma. In D. Gurney (Ed.), *Trauma Nursing Core Course: Provider manual* (7th ed., pp. 193–204). Des Plaines, IL: Emergency Nurses Association.

---

109. A patient presents to the emergency department with a shortened, deformed, and outwardly rotated right leg. The patient requires the application of a traction splint. The splint has been appropriately applied when:

A. the affected limb begins to swell.
B. the patient reports an increase in pain.
C. the dorsalis pedis pulse is faint.
D. the patient reports a decrease in pain.

Rationale

A. Proper stabilization of the limb will decrease pain and correct circulatory compromise. Swelling would be an indicator of internal bleeding and improper placement of the splint.

B. Splinting and stabilization of the limb will decrease the patient's pain. Loss of a previously present palpable pulse, change in temperature, or an increase in pain are indications that the splint should be removed.

C. Proper stabilization will decrease pain and correct circulatory compromise to the limb. Loss of a previously present palpable pulse, change in temperature, or an increase in pain are indications that the splint should be removed.

D. Splinting is performed when there is a deformity, pain, crepitus, edema, and/or circulatory compromise to the limb. Stabilization of the limb will decrease pain.

Category: Maxillofacial, Ocular, Orthopedic, and Wound Emergencies/Orthopedic/Fractures/dislocations

Nursing Process: Evaluation

References

Bratcher, C. A. (2014). Musculoskeletal trauma. In D. Gurney (Ed.), *Trauma Nursing Core Course: Provider manual* (7th ed., pp. 193–204). Des Plaines, IL: Emergency Nurses Association.

Cerepani, M. J. (2010). Orthopedic and neurovascular trauma. In P. K. Howard & R. A. Steinmann (Eds.), *Sheehy's emergency nursing principles and practice* (6th ed., pp. 313–339). St. Louis, MO: Mosby Elsevier.

---

110. A college student presents to triage complaining of a constant buzzing sound in their ear. On examination, an insect is seen in the ear canal. The physician has instilled viscous lidocaine in the ear of the patient. The emergency nurse identifies that this treatment has been effective when the patient states which of the following?

A. "My ear feels numb."
B. "I no longer hear the buzzing sound in my ear, I don't think the insect is moving."
C. "My ear no longer hurts."
D. "My hearing has improved in that ear now."

Rationale

A. The instillation is to immobilize the insect, not numb the ear canal.

B. Live insects in the ear canal should be immobilized before removal is attempted. The administration of viscous lidocaine will immobilize the insect and stop the buzzing sound the patient has been experiencing. Mineral oil, microscope oil, and viscous lidocaine have all been used successfully for this purpose.

C. The instillation is to immobilize the insect to decrease the likelihood of fragmentation during removal.

D. The placement of viscous lidocaine will decrease sound conduction and should not improve the patient's ability to hear.

Category: Maxillofacial, Ocular, Orthopedic, and Wound Emergencies/Maxillofacial/Foreign bodies

Nursing Process: Evaluation

References

Kwong, A. (2017). Ear foreign body removal procedures. *Medscape.* Retrieved from http://emedicine.medscape.com/article/80507-overview

Nolan, E. G. (2010). Dental, ear, nose, throat and facial emergencies. In P. K. Howard & R. A. Steinmann (Eds.), *Sheehy's emergency nursing: Principles and practice* (6th ed., pp. 590–601). St. Louis, MO: Mosby Elsevier.

---

111. A patient presents to the emergency department complaining of decreased vision, an intense headache, and the appearance of halos around lights with photophobia. The emergency nurse identifies these symptoms as being consistent with the development of which of the following?

A. Central retinal artery occlusion
B. Glaucoma
C. Corneal abrasion
D. Iritis

Rationale

A. Central retinal artery occlusion is associated with the sudden of loss of vision in the affected eye. It is considered an ophthalmology emergency and requires immediate intervention to prevent permanent loss of vision in the affected eye.

B. The patient's presenting signs and symptoms are consistent with the presence of glaucoma.

C. A patient with corneal abrasion would experience photophobia with the development of excessive tearing and pain in the affected eye.

D. Iritis is associated with the development of intense unilateral pain, irritated conjunctiva, edema, and excessive tearing with photophobia.

Category: Maxillofacial, Ocular, Orthopedic, and Wound Emergencies/Ocular/Glaucoma
Nursing Process: Assessment

Reference

Gerhart, A. E. (2007). Ocular emergencies. In K. S. Hoyt & J. Selfridge-Thomas (Eds.), *Emergency nursing core curriculum* (6th ed., pp. 571–584). St. Louis, MO: Saunders Elsevier.

---

112. The emergency nurse is preparing to dress a stage 2 pressure injury on the shoulder of a patient. Which solution would be most appropriate to cleanse the wound bed with?

A. Ringer's lactate solution
B. Povidone iodine (Betadine)
C. Hydrogen peroxide
D. Tap water

Rationale

A. Ringer's lactate solution is not an appropriate choice for wound bed cleansing. Normal saline would be a more appropriate choice.

B. Povidone iodine is an inappropriate solution to use for wound bed cleansing because it can result in a reduction of defenses and lead to increased bacterial growth.

C. Hydrogen peroxide is inappropriate for wound bed cleansing because it can lead to the damage of healthy tissue.

D. Potable water (water that is suitable for drinking) or normal saline is appropriate for cleansing of the wound bed.

Category: Maxillofacial, Ocular, Orthopedic, and Wound Emergencies/Wound/Pressure ulcers

Nursing Process: Intervention

Reference

National Pressure Ulcer Advisory Panel, European Pressure Ulcer Advisory Panel, and Pan Pacific Pressure Injury Alliance. (2014). *Prevention and treatment of pressure ulcers: Quick reference guide.* E. Haesler (Ed.). Osborne Park, Australia: Cambridge Media. Retrieved from http://www.npuap.org/wp-content/uploads/2014/08/Updated-10-16-14-Quick-Reference-Guide-DIGITAL-NPUAP-EPUAP-PPPIA-16Oct2014.pdf

---

113. Which patient would be least likely to require a tetanus booster shot?

A. The 70-year-old patient with burns on the leg
B. The 13-year-old patient with a facial laceration
C. The 24-year-old patient who stepped on a nail
D. The 35-year-old pregnant female who sustained a laceration to the hand

Rationale

A. Burns are a break in skin integrity, so the patient must have current tetanus immunization.

B. An adolescent patient does not require a tetanus booster if up to date on vaccinations. The current vaccination schedule requires children to receive a tetanus booster between 11 and 12 years of age.

C. Puncture wounds are typically deep and would require the patient to have current tetanus immunization.

D. Pregnancy is not a contraindication to receiving tetanus immunization; therefore, it is important to determine that this patient is current in her tetanus immunization.

Category: Maxillofacial, Ocular, Orthopedic, and Wound Emergencies/Wound/Trauma

Nursing Process: Assessment

References

Centers for Disease Control and Prevention. (2018). *Recommended immunization schedule for persons aged 0 through 18 years, 2018.* Retrieved from http://www.cdc.gov/vaccines/schedules/hcp/imz/child-adolescent.html

Denke, N. (2010). Wound management. In P. K. Howard & R. A. Steinmann (Eds.), *Sheehy's emergency nursing: Principles and practice* (6th ed., pp. 119–126). St. Louis, MO: Mosby Elsevier.

---

114. A patient presents with complaints of generalized muscle spasms, pain, and headache. The patient reports stepping on a nail 2 days ago. Which bacterial organism does the emergency nurse anticipate to be the cause of the patient's symptoms?

A. Group A streptococcus
B. *Clostridium tetani*
C. *Staphylococcus aureus*
D. *Clostridium perfringens*

Rationale

A. Group A streptococcus is found in the tissues of the throat and skin. The initial presentation of a streptococcus infection includes fever, erythema, purulent discharge, or an abscess and may progress to necrotizing fasciitis. Infections from group A streptococcus do not cause generalized muscle spasms.

B. Puncture wounds place the patient at risk for developing tetanus from the *Clostridium tetani* organism. Restlessness, muscle spasms, pain, and headache are initial symptoms of tetanus.

C. *Staphylococcus aureus* is a causative agent for skin infections. The infection first appears as a localized abscess of the superficial subcutaneous tissues; the infection may also spread systemically.

D. *Clostridium perfringens* is also referred to as gas gangrene, a tightening edema that results in hypoxia and crepitus of the soft tissues. Crepitus is the result of hydrogen sulfide and carbon dioxide within the tissue. A radiograph (X-ray) of the infected area will demonstrate the presence of gas bubbles within the tissue.

Category: Maxillofacial, Ocular, Orthopedic, and Wound Emergencies/Wound/Puncture wounds
Nursing Process: Analysis

Reference

Ramirez, E. G. (2007). Wounds and wound management. In K. S. Hoyt & J. Selfridge-Thomas (Eds.), *Emergency nursing core curriculum* (6th ed., pp. 738–759). St. Louis, MO: Saunders Elsevier.

---

115. A patient arrives to the emergency department complaining of sudden onset of severe jaw pain that radiates to their ear. The patient states that they are having difficulty speaking because of the excessive pain. The pain started as they were biting into a large sandwich. The emergency nurse anticipates that this patient has which of the following?

A. Angina
B. Trigeminal neuralgia
C. Dental pain
D. Temporomandibular joint syndrome

Rationale

A. The pain from myocardial ischemia can often be referred to the neck and jaw. The nurse should keep an index of suspicion for angina as the cause of the patient's jaw pain until a detailed history has been obtained.

B. Trigeminal neuralgia is usually a sharp, severe stabbing recurrent pain that is paroxysmal and lasts from seconds to minutes. The recurrent pain is usually unilateral and occurs in one or more branches of the trigeminal nerve.

C. Dental pain is generally constant and throbbing in nature.

D. Temporomandibular joint (TMJ) syndrome is also referred to as myofascial pain dysfunction (MPD). It has several causes, including stress, malocclusion, dental disease, disease of the TMJ tissues, and poorly fitting dentures. Symptoms range from a mild ache to severe, sharp pain. The patient usually experiences pain with movement of the joint, particularly with chewing. The pain is often referred to the ear on the affected side.

Category: Maxillofacial, Ocular, Orthopedic, and Wound Emergencies/Maxillofacial/Temporomandibular joint (TMJ) dislocation

Nursing Process: Assessment

References

Egging, D. (2013). Facial, ENT, and dental emergencies. In B. B. Hammond & P. G. Zimmermann (Eds.), *Sheehy's manual of emergency care* (7th ed., pp. 275–284). St. Louis, MO: Elsevier Mosby.

Grubbs, L. (2015). Head, face, and neck. In *Advanced assessment* (3rd ed., pp. 76–95). Philadelphia, PA: F. A. Davis.

---

116. A patient presents to triage with the complaint of a foreign body sensation and excessive pain to their left eye but denies any recent change to their vision. The patient states they were treated earlier in the week for conjunctivitis. The emergency nurse anticipates that this patient is experiencing which of the following conditions?

A. Uveitis
B. Subconjunctival hemorrhage
C. Keratitis
D. Episcleritis

Rationale

A. Uveitis or iritis is the inflammation of the uveal tract, including the iris, ciliary body, and choroid. Uveitis can be caused by inflammation, infection, or trauma. The patient frequently complains of decreased vision, photophobia, excessive tearing, and eye pain. Constriction of the pupil is usually present with uveitis.

B. Subconjunctival hemorrhage of the eye is most frequently caused by the rupture of small capillaries from trauma, coughing, sneezing, or rubbing of the eye. Although striking to look at, it is usually a benign and self-limiting condition and is not associated with vision loss, photophobia, or pain. However, patients should be instructed to avoid aspirin-containing products and nonsteroidal anti-inflammatory agents until the appearance of blood has disappeared from the conjunctiva.

C. Keratitis is the inflammation of the cornea. Symptoms may include pain, photophobia, purulent discharge, and decreased vision. Keratitis may occur secondary to preexisting or recent history of conjunctivitis and can result in cornea ulcerations, opacities, and blindness if untreated.

D. Episcleritis is an inflammatory condition affecting the episcleritis, located between the conjunctiva and the sclera. Episcleritis usually does not affect vision, is self-limiting, and is generally painless. Episcleritis can be associated with localized engorged vessels and nodular changes.

Category: Maxillofacial, Ocular, Orthopedic, and Wound Emergencies/Ocular/Infections

Nursing Process: Assessment

References

Egging, D. (2010). Ocular emergencies. In P. K. Howard & R. A. Steinmann (Eds.), *Sheehy's emergency nursing principles and practice* (6th ed., pp. 601–618). St. Louis, MO: Elsevier Mosby.

Goolsby, M. (2015). The eye. In M. Goolsby & L. Grubbs (Eds.), *Advanced assessment* (3rd ed., pp. 96–122). Philadelphia, PA: F. A. Davis.

Solheim, J. (2013). Facial, ocular, ENT and dental trauma. In B. B. Hammond & P. G. Zimmermann (Eds.), *Sheehy's manual of emergency care* (7th ed., pp. 439–452). St. Louis, MO: Elsevier Mosby.

117. A patient rushes into triage and stating that there is something in their eye. A large sliver of wood is noted to be impaled in the patient's right eye. Following completion of the visual acuity (Snellen) exam, what is the next intervention that the emergency nurse should perform for this patient?

A. Instill a topical ophthalmic anesthetic
B. Irrigate the eye as soon as possible
C. Apply a cotton patch to the unaffected eye
D. Place a rigid eye shield over the affected orbit

Rationale

A. There is no indication that this patient has any pain. Nothing should be put in the eye that might increase the pressure.

B. Irrigation with any type of fluid would cause a wood splinter to "swell." No pressure or any form of manipulation should be applied to the eye or the wooden splinter.

C. Applying a patch to the unaffected eye will act to limit concomitant movement of the unaffected eye.

D. It is important to immobilize the penetrating object to avoid increasing the extent of damage and to prevent further disruption of the orbit.

Category: Maxillofacial, Ocular, Orthopedic, and Wound Emergencies/Ocular/Foreign bodies
Nursing Process: Intervention

References

Egging, D. (2010). Ocular emergencies. In P. K. Howard & R. A. Steinmann (Eds.), *Sheehy's emergency nursing: Principles and practice* (6th ed., pp. 602–618). St. Louis, MO: Mosby Elsevier.

Egging, D. (2014). Ocular trauma. In D. Gurney (Ed.), *Trauma Nursing Core Course: Provider manual* (7th ed., pp. 123–136). Des Plaines, IL: Emergency Nurses Association.

---

118. A patient presents to the emergency department with a history of blunt force trauma to their face. The patient relates falling down and striking their face on the floor. There is periorbital bruising and edema around the left eye, and the patient is complaining of diplopia. Which of the following assessment findings would confirm a diagnosis of an orbital rim fracture with entrapment of extraocular muscles?

A. Decreased ability to look upward
B. Teardrop shape of their left pupil
C. Presence of blood in the anterior chamber
D. Complaint of halos around lights

Rationale

A. The decreased ability to look upward is the result of entrapment of extraocular muscles within the fracture site.

B. The presence of a teardrop-shaped pupil is a definitive sign of a ruptured globe. Patients with a ruptured globe will have a shallow-appearing anterior chamber, diminished or absent vision in the affected eye, severe ocular pain, and the leakage of vitreous humor from the eye.

C. Blood in the anterior chamber of the eye is a definitive sign for the presence of hyphema.

D. The complaint or presence of halos seen around lights is characteristic for the presence of glaucoma.

Category: Maxillofacial, Ocular, Orthopedic, and Wound Emergencies/Maxillofacial/Trauma
Nursing Process: Assessment

Reference

Solheim, J. (2013). Facial, ocular, ENT, and dental trauma. In B. B. Hammond & P. G. Zimmermann (Eds.), *Sheehy's manual of emergency care* (7th ed., pp. 439–452). St. Louis, MO: Elsevier Mosby.

---

119. While at triage, the emergency nurse assesses a patient who presents with a complaint of increasing difficulty speaking. The patient's voice is muffled, they are drooling, and the left side of their face is markedly swollen. The patient's tongue is protruding slightly through their lips. The patient indicates that they were recently assaulted. The emergency nurse anticipates that this patient has which of the following?

A. Pharyngitis
B. Peritonsillar abscess
C. Ludwig's angina
D. Tonsillitis

Rationale

A. Pharyngitis is the inflammation of the pharynx, often occurring in conjunction with the common cold. The patient will experience a reddened throat, swollen tonsils, and the presence of exudate on the tonsils.

B. Peritonsillar abscess is a purulent collection around the tonsils that can develop into a deeper tissue infection. It is often associated with a recent episode of pharyngitis or tonsillitis. If left untreated, the abscess can cause airway compromise.

C. Ludwig's angina is a potentially fatal cellulitis that involves the floor of the mouth and the neck. The patient may have a history of a recent dental abscess that is unresponsive to therapy, or they may have experienced recent dental trauma. Signs and symptoms include swelling of the submandibular and sublingual spaces, dysphagia, drooling, and a muffled voice.

D. Tonsillitis is swelling or inflammation of the tonsils. Symptoms are similar to pharyngitis and may result in a feeling of fullness in the throat, in conjunction with ear pain and generalized malaise.

Category: Maxillofacial, Ocular, Orthopedic, and Wound Emergencies/Maxillofacial/Infections
Nursing Process: Analysis

References

Egging, D. (2013). Facial, ENT, and dental emergencies. In B. B. Hammond & P. G. Zimmermann (Eds.), *Sheehy's manual of emergency care* (7th ed., pp. 275–284). St. Louis, MO: Elsevier Mosby.
Nolan, E. G. (2010). Dental, ear, nose, throat and facial emergencies. In P. K. Howard & R. A. Steinmann (Eds.), *Sheehy's emergency nursing: Principles and practice* (6th ed., pp. 590–601). St. Louis, MO: Mosby Elsevier.

---

120. A patient with burns to their anterior trunk and both arms from a camp fire presents to the emergency department. Based on the "rule of nines," the patient's estimated total body surface area burned is:

A. 36%.
B. 18%.
C. 45%.
D. 40%.

Rationale

A. The rule of nines is a method that divides areas of the body into multiples of 9. The perineum is 1%; each arm is 9%; the anterior trunk is 18%; the posterior trunk is 18%; the head is 9%; and each leg is 18%. This case involves both arms (9% + 9%) and the anterior trunk (18%), for a total body surface area (TBSA) of 36%.

B. This percentage would underestimate the percentage of body burned and result in inadequate fluid resuscitation for the patient.

C. This percentage is an overestimation of the total burn area and may result in excessive fluid resuscitation, leading to fluid overload.

D. Based on the rule of nines, it would not be possible to calculate this percentage of TBSA.

Category: Environment and Toxicology Emergencies, and Communicable Diseases/Environment/Burns
Nursing Process: Assessment

Reference

Provins-Churbock, C. (2014). Surface and burn trauma. In D. Gurney (Ed.), *Trauma Nursing Core Course: Provider manual* (7th ed., pp. 205–222). Des Plaines, IL: Emergency Nurses Association.

---

121. A patient was brought into the emergency department following a house fire that was believed to have started as a result of a gas leak. The patient's skin is flushed, they are not oriented to time, place, or person, and they are complaining of nausea associated with a severe headache. What should be performed first to properly care for this patient?

A. Obtain a carboxyhemoglobin level
B. Provide continuous pulse oximetry
C. Obtain an arterial blood gas test
D. Provide continuous capnography

Rationale

A. The patient is at high risk for carbon monoxide poisoning. To adequately determine the patient's level of carbon monoxide poisoning, a carboxyhemoglobin level must be obtained. The patient is exhibiting signs of elevated carboxyhemoglobin levels, which include headache, disorientation, nausea, dizziness, tachycardia, and flushing. In later stages, if the levels of carboxyhemoglobin are allowed to rise, coma, seizures, and death could result.

B. Pulse oximetry measures saturation of oxygen. The pulse oximeter cannot differentiate between hemoglobin saturated with carbon monoxide and hemoglobin saturated with oxygen, and it can provide a false reading of oxygen saturation. The carbon monoxide binds to the hemoglobin, displacing oxygen. The oxygen saturation level could therefore display normal values in error.

C. The oxygen dissolved in the blood plasma (PaO_2) is usually unaffected by carbon monoxide poisoning. An arterial blood gas test will not provide the information required to evaluate the patient's level of carbon monoxide poisoning.

D. Capnography is the measurement of expired carbon dioxide levels in the airway and is not a measurement of carboxyhemoglobin.

Category: Environment and Toxicology Emergencies, and Communicable Diseases/Environment/Burns

Nursing Process: Intervention

Reference

Ribbins, K. M., & DeVries, M. (2013). Burns. In B. B. Hammond & P. G. Zimmermann (Eds.), *Sheehy's manual of emergency care* (7th ed., pp. 453–462). St. Louis, MO: Elsevier Mosby.

---

122. After unintentionally being sprayed by a crop duster, a patient presents to the emergency department with excessive tearing, salivation, nausea, vomiting, and bradycardia. The emergency nurse should anticipate the administration of which intravenous medication to this patient?

A. Naloxone (Narcan)
B. Atropine (atropine sulfate)
C. Sodium nitrite
D. Flumazenil (Romazicon)

Rationale

A. Naloxone is used to treat opiate ingestion or an opiate intravenous (IV) overdose; it is not indicated in the treatment of organophosphate poisoning.

B. An immediate treatment for organophosphate poisoning is the administration of IV atropine.

C. Sodium nitrite is the antidote for cyanide poisoning; it is not used in the treatment of organophosphate poisoning.

D. Flumazenil is used in the treatment of benzodiazepine overdoses; it is not indicated in the treatment of organophosphate poisoning.

Category: Environment and Toxicology Emergencies, and Communicable Diseases/Environment/ Chemical exposure

Nursing Process: Intervention

References

Badillo, R. B., Hovseth, K., & Schaffer, S. (2013). Toxicologic emergencies. In B. B. Hammond & P. G. Zimmermann (Eds.), *Sheehy's manual of emergency care* (7th ed., pp. 319–331). St. Louis, MO: Elsevier Mosby.
Sturr, P. (2010). Toxicologic emergencies. In P. K. Howard & R. A. Steinmann (Eds.), *Sheehy's emergency nursing: Principles and practice* (6th ed., pp. 564–577). St. Louis, MO: Mosby Elsevier.

---

123. The most important factor in the survival of a drowning victim is:

A. **immediate cardiopulmonary resuscitation.**
B. the speed of rewarming the victim while in the emergency department.
C. the type of water (saltwater or freshwater) that the victim was found in.
D. an initial Glasgow Coma Score of 3 or greater.

Rationale

A. Field resuscitation of the near-drowning victim is crucial for survival. Performing an immediate basic life support procedure on the victim after removal from the water has been cited as a significant factor in the victim's survival.

B. Rewarming efforts should be aggressive if the victim's core temperature is below 30°C (86°F) but does not outweigh early cardiopulmonary resuscitation in survivability.

C. Although saltwater and freshwater differ significantly in composition, these differences do not affect survival in near-drowning incidents. Immediate basic life support for the drowning victim is a significant factor in survival.

D. A patient's initial Glasgow Coma Scale score has not been shown to increase survival in drowning incidents.

Category: Environment and Toxicology Emergencies, and Communicable Diseases/Environment/ Submersion injury

Nursing Process: Analysis

Reference

Sedlak, K. (2013). Environmental emergencies. In B. B. Hammond & P. G. Zimmermann (Eds.), *Sheehy's manual of emergency care* (7th ed., pp. 333–344). St. Louis, MO: Elsevier Mosby.

---

124. A patient arrives at the emergency department after a sudden onset of severe pain to the left calf area while playing tennis. The provider performs a Thompson test on the patient's left calf, which is positive and indicates an Achilles tendon injury. The patient reports that they were recently taking an antibiotic. The emergency nurse is aware that the following antibiotic is associated with the development of an Achilles tendon injury:

A. **ciprofloxacin (Cipro).**
B. cephalexin (Keflex).
C. azithromycin (Zithromax).
D. amoxicillin (Amoxil).

Rationale

A. An FDA safety review has shown that the systemic use of fluoroquinolones (i.e., tablets, capsules, and injectable) is associated with disabling and potentially permanent serious side effects that can involve the tendons, muscles, joints, nerves, and the central nervous system.

B. Cephalexin is not associated with Achilles tendon injuries.

C. Azithromycin is not associated with Achilles tendon injuries.

D. Amoxicillin is not associated with Achilles tendon injuries.

Category: Environment and Toxicology Emergencies, and Communicable Diseases/Toxicology/Drug interactions

Nursing Process: Analysis

Reference

U.S. Food and Drug Administration. (2016, May 12). *FDA Drug Safety Communication: FDA updates warnings for oral and injectable fluoroquinolone antibiotics due to disabling side effects*. Retrieved from http://www.fda.gov/Drugs/DrugSafety/ucm511530.htm

---

125. The emergency nurse is caring for a child who presents with a red ring-shaped rash to the right leg. The nurse anticipates that the provider will prescribe which of the following treatments?

A. Oral antifungal medication
B. Topical antibiotic medication
C. Oral antibiotic medication
D. Topical antifungal medication

Rationale

A. Ringworm of the skin is usually responsive to topical antifungal medications.

B. Ringworm is a fungal infection and requires treatment with an antifungal medication. Topical antibiotic medication is not appropriate and will not eliminate the tinea infestation.

C. Ringworm is a fungal infection and requires treatment with an antifungal medication.

D. The patient is presenting with classic signs of tinea, or ringworm. Tinea on the skin should be treated with a topical antifungal medication.

Category (Pediatric): Environment and Toxicology Emergencies, and Communicable Diseases/Environment/Parasite and fungal infestations

Nursing Process: Intervention

Reference

Centers for Disease Control and Prevention. (2015). *Ringworm*. Retrieved from http://www.cdc.gov/fungal/diseases/ringworm/index.html

---

126. An adult patient who has been diagnosed with Lyme disease presents to the emergency department with a complaint of left-sided facial weakness for 2 days. On assessment, the nurse notes unilateral facial drooping on the left side, and drooling. The patient is alert and oriented. Gait is normal, and strength is equal in both arms and legs. Vital signs: BP 140/78 mm Hg; HR 92 beats/minute; RR 20 breaths/minute; SpO_2 99%; T 36.8°C (98.2°F). Which of the following is the most likely cause of this patient's signs and symptoms?

A. Bell's palsy
B. Transient ischemic attack
C. Allergic reaction
D. Ischemic stroke

Rationale

A. Bell's palsy is a common manifestation in the later stages of Lyme disease. The lack of unilateral weakness in the extremities makes stroke a less probable diagnosis.

B. A transient ischemic attack is usually a brief neurologic event. This patient has had facial weakness for 2 days, which makes this diagnosis unlikely.

C. Unilateral facial weakness is not a common symptom of an allergic reaction.

D. If the patient was having an ischemic stroke, the nurse would expect to see unilateral extremity weakness on the same side as the facial weakness. Speech and gait may be affected. It is possible that the patient in this scenario is having a stroke; however, it is not the most likely diagnosis.

Category: Environment and Toxicology Emergencies, and Communicable Diseases/Environment/ Vector-borne illnesses

Nursing Process: Assessment

References

Centers for Disease Control and Prevention. (2016). *Ticks*. Retrieved from http://www.cdc.gov/ticks/index.html

Sedlak, S. K. (2013). Bite and sting emergencies. In B. B. Hammond & P. G. Zimmermann (Eds.), *Sheehy's manual of emergency care* (7th ed., pp. 232–243). St. Louis, MO: Elsevier Mosby.

---

127. The emergency nurse is caring for a child who has been diagnosed with rubeola (measles). The nurse anticipates that the patient will require which of the following interventions?

A. **Measles, mumps, rubella vaccination**
B. Intravenous antibiotics
C. Isolation with standard and droplet precautions
D. Vitamin K injection

Rationale

A. Patients with rubeola who have not been previously vaccinated should be offered vaccination as postexposure prophylaxis.

B. Rubeola is caused by a virus. Antibiotics would only be appropriate if the patient has a concurrent bacterial infection.

C. Patients with rubeola should be placed in isolation with standard and airborne precautions to prevent the spread of infection. Droplet precautions are not indicated for this patient.

D. Some patients with severe cases of rubeola may require vitamin A if they have a deficiency; however, vitamin K is not indicated for treatment of rubeola.

Category (Pediatric): Environment and Toxicology Emergencies, and Communicable Diseases/ Communicable Diseases/Childhood diseases

Nursing Process: Intervention

Reference

Centers for Disease Control and Prevention. (2016). *About measles*. Retrieved from http://www.cdc.gov/measles/about/

128. A patient is brought to the emergency department after cleaning solution is unintentionally splashed over the patient's face and eyes. Irrigation is currently in progress. Which of the following would indicate to the emergency nurse that effective eye irrigation has occurred?

A. 1.0 L of dextrose and water has been used for irrigation
B. Eye pH of 7.25 after irrigation
C. Clear sclera after irrigation
D. Visual acuity of 20/20 after irrigation

Rationale

A. Irrigation may need to continue for up to 60 minutes or longer and is not limited to 1.0 L. Irrigation fluids should be normal saline or Ringer's lactate solution, not dextrose-containing fluids.

B. If possible, a pH value of the eye should be obtained before starting irrigation and repeated after copious eye irrigation has been completed. The irrigation should be continued until the eye pH is between 7.0 and 7.5. Cleaning fluids are generally alkalotic, causing an elevated pH level.

C. The sclera may appear injected or reddened because of irritation from the irrigation or chemical injury and should not be a determinant to discontinue irrigation. Eye pH should be the guide when to discontinue the irrigation.

D. Although a visual acuity of 20/20 is normal, it would not be an indicator that eye irrigation should be discontinued. The eye pH should be measured and irrigation continued until a pH of 7.0–7.5 is maintained.

Category: Environment and Toxicology Emergencies, and Communicable Diseases/Toxicology/Acid and alkali
Nursing Process: Evaluation

Reference

Egging, D. (2013). Ocular emergencies. In B. B. Hammond & P. G. Zimmermann (Eds.), *Sheehy's manual of emergency care* (7th ed., pp. 285–290). St. Louis, MO: Elsevier Mosby.

---

129. The emergency nurse is aware that the cyanide antidote kit contains:

A. acetylcysteine.
B. dimercaprol.
C. amyl nitrite.
D. sodium polystyrene sulfonate.

Rationale

A. Acetylcysteine increases liver stores of glutathione for acetaminophen toxicity.

B. Dimercaprol is used for chelation therapy in acute lead encephalopathy.

C. Amyl nitrite is a focused therapy for cyanide poisoning.

D. Sodium polystyrene sulfonate or kayexalate is indicated for hyperkalemia.

Category: Environment and Toxicology Emergencies, and Communicable Diseases/Toxicology/Cyanide

Nursing Process: Assessment

References

Badillo, R., Hovseth, K., & Schaffer, S. (2013). Toxicologic emergencies. In B. B. Hammond & P. G. Zimmermann (Eds.), *Sheehy's manual of emergency care* (7th ed., pp. 319–332). St. Louis, MO: Elsevier Mosby.

Philips, M. (2007). Toxicologic emergences. In K. S. Hoyt & J. Selfridge-Thomas (Eds.), *Emergency nursing core curriculum* (6th ed., pp. 604–658). St. Louis, MO: Saunders Elsevier.

Rader, J., Terry, D., & Trujillo, L. A. (Eds.). (2017). *Nursing 2017 drug handbook* (37th ed.). Philadelphia, PA: Wolters Kluwer.

130. A patient presents to the emergency department after taking an overdose of beta blocker medication. Which of the following signs and/or symptoms indicate that the treatment has been effective?

A. Increasing glucose level
B. Lowering blood pressure
C. Decreasing heart rate
D. Decreasing level of consciousness

Rationale

A. Hypoglycemia can occur with beta blocker overdoses, so an increasing blood glucose level would indicate that treatment is effective.

B. Beta blocker overdose blocks the beta receptors of the heart, which results in hypotension. The goal of treatment for a beta blocker overdose would be to increase blood pressure.

C. A treatment goal for beta blocker overdose would be to increase the patient's heart rate because bradycardia can occur.

D. Altered mental status can occur, so a treatment goal would be to increase the patient's level of consciousness.

Category: Environment and Toxicology Emergencies, and Communicable Diseases/Toxicology/Overdose and ingestions

Nursing Process: Evaluation

Reference

Badillo, R., Hovseth, K., & Schaffer, S. (2013). Toxicologic emergencies. In B. B. Hammond & P. G. Zimmermann (Eds.), *Sheehy's manual of emergency care* (7th ed., pp. 319–332). St. Louis, MO: Elsevier Mosby.

---

131. A patient arrives to emergency department following recent ingestion of cocaine. Which of the following symptoms being exhibited by the patient would cause the nurse the greatest concern?

A. Auditory hallucinations
B. Fever
C. Poor appetite
D. Abdominal pain

Rationale

A. Auditory hallucinations may result from cocaine use.

B. A patient who presents with fever and reporting recent cocaine use is at increased risk of complications. Although cocaine effects may display hyperthermia, other complications may also present with elevations in temperature, such as aspiration or wound infections.

C. Chronic use of cocaine can result in poor appetite and malnourishment.

D. Patients may report abdominal pain with cocaine use.

Category: Environment and Toxicology Emergencies, and Communicable Diseases/Toxicology/Substance abuse

Nursing Process: Analysis

Reference

Badillo, R. B., Hovseth, K., & Schaffer, S. (2013). Toxicologic emergencies. In B. B. Hammond & P. G. Zimmermann, (Eds.), *Sheehy's manual of emergency care* (7th ed., pp. 319–332). St. Louis, MO: Elsevier Mosby.

---

132. A patient presents to the emergency department in acute alcohol withdrawal. The alcohol withdrawal treatment protocol is initiated for this patient. Which change in the patient's condition would indicate to the nurse that the treatment is having its intended effect?

A. Increased blood pressure
B. Decreased heart rate
C. Increased temperature
D. Increased motor activity

Rationale

A. Hypertension can occur with alcohol withdrawal. A desired outcome would be to decrease the patient's blood pressure.

B. In alcohol withdrawal, tachycardia can occur. A decreased heart rate is a positive effect from the initiation of treatment for alcohol withdrawal.

C. A low-grade fever may accompany alcohol withdrawal. An intended effect of treatment would be to decrease the patient's temperature.

D. Tremulousness and motor hyperactivity can occur in alcohol withdrawal. The goal would be to decrease motor activity and the presence of tremors.

Category: Environment and Toxicology Emergencies, and Communicable Diseases/Toxicology/Withdrawal syndrome

Nursing Process: Evaluation

Reference

Badillo, R. B., Hovseth, K., & Schaffer, S. (2013). Toxicologic emergencies. In B. B. Hammond & P. G. Zimmermann (Eds.), *Sheehy's manual of emergency care* (7th ed., pp. 319–332). St. Louis, MO: Elsevier Mosby.

---

133. You are caring for a patient who has presented directly from their primary care provider for hydration therapy secondary to 2 days of watery diarrhea and the presence of blood in their stool. Which of the following statements by the patient would be concerning for a *Clostridium difficile* infection?

A. "I work at a daycare with toddlers all day."
B. "I've been taking penicillin for this infection in my leg for several weeks."
C. "I work on a farm around cattle and livestock every day."
D. "I just returned from traveling in Africa for 2 weeks."

Rationale

A. Working in and around young children would not be a risk factor for contracting a *Clostridium difficile* (*C. difficle*) infection.

B. Risk factors for contracting *Clostridium difficile* include antibiotic exposure, proton pump inhibitor use, gastrointestinal surgery/manipulation, long length of stay in a healthcare setting, serious underlying illness, immunocompromising conditions, and advanced age.

C. Working in and around livestock is not a risk factor for a contracting a *C. difficile* infection.

D. International travel is not a risk factor for contracting a *C. difficile* infection.

Category: Environment and Toxicology Emergencies, and Communicable Diseases/Communicable Disease/*C. difficile*

Nursing Process: Analysis

Reference

Centers for Disease Control and Prevention. (2012). *Frequently asked questions about Clostridium difficile for health-care providers*. Retrieved from http://www.cdc.gov/HAI/organisms/cdiff/Cdiff_faqs_HCP.html

---

134. The nurse is caring for a patient who presents with a fracture of the radius. The patient provides a history of having human immunodeficiency virus and is taking multiple medications for tuberculosis. Which physical finding should the nurse assess for that is related to potential complications from the tuberculosis medications?

A. Urine is orange colored.
B. Skin has a yellow tinge.
C. Patient reports having diarrhea.
D. Patient reports presence of tinnitus.

Rationale

A. Rifabutin (Mycobutin) is a medication used for tuberculosis and has a side effect of causing discoloration of all body fluids (urine, sputum, tears, sweat). Other classic medications include isoniazid, which can cause peripheral neuropathy (so B_6 is given concurrently), and ethambutol (Myambutol), which can cause ocular toxicity.

B. The medications used for tuberculosis are hepatotoxic, and the risk is increased if the client drinks alcohol. Liver function tests will need to be performed. Immunosuppressed clients, such as those who are human immunodeficiency virus positive are at risk for contracting tuberculosis.

C. Diarrhea is not a common complication of the medications typically used as part of the multidrug regime for tuberculosis.

D. Tinnitus (ringing in the ears) is not a common complication of the medications typically used as part of the multidrug regime for tuberculosis. It is a side effect of high doses of nonsteroidal anti-inflammatories.

Category: Environment and Toxicology Emergencies, and Communicable Diseases/Communicable Diseases/Tuberculosis

Nursing Process: Assessment

Reference

Lewis, S. L., Bucher, L., Heitkemper, M. M., & Harding, M. M. (2017). Lower respiratory problems. In *Medical-surgical nursing* (10th ed., pp. 499–537). St. Louis, MO: Elsevier.

---

135. Following introduction of the participants, which of the following statements would be used at the beginning of a critical incident stress debriefing?

A. "Can you tell me what you think should have been done differently?"
B. "Can you provide me with a brief description of what happened during the situation from your viewpoint?"
C. "Can you tell us what you perceive to be the positive outcomes of this event?"
D. "Can you describe how you are feeling after going through this event?"

Rationale

A. A debriefing is not a critique of the event, but a systematic review of the events that allows peers to discuss their thoughts and feelings in a safe environment.

B. This question will get the conversation started; it is easier to describe what happened before discussing the impact of the event.

C. A debriefing is not a critique of the event. Opening the conversation with what happened will help get the conversation started.

D. It is often difficult to express feelings initially because many participants have not processed the impact of this event at this stage of the debriefing. Beginning with the facts of the event can better start the conversation.

Category: Professional Issues/Nurse/Critical Incident Stress Management

Cognitive Level: Application

References

Davies, J. (2013). Critical incident stress debriefing from a traumatic event. *Psychology Today*. Retrieved from https://www.psychologytoday.com/blog/crimes-and-misdemeanors/201302/critical-incident-stress-debriefing-traumatic-event

Healy, M. M., & Gurney, D. (2014). Psychosocial aspects of trauma care. In D. Gurney (Ed.), *Trauma Nursing Core Course: Provider manual* (7th ed., pp. 295–309). Des Plaines, IL: Emergency Nurses Association.

136. A patient with a known history of alcohol abuse was found lying on the sidewalk and brought to the emergency department by emergency medical services. The patient is confused, speech is slurred, and there is a strong smell of alcohol on the patient's breath. After placing the patient in a treatment area, what is the next action performed by the emergency nurse?

A. **Request an evaluation by the physician**
B. Request a blood alcohol level to be drawn
C. Initiate intravenous (IV) access and begin an infusion of a thiamine-containing IV fluid
D. Begin the process for referral to a detoxification unit

Rationale

A. The patient's altered mental status must be a factor in determining the patient's immediate need for care. Possible etiologies of an altered level of consciousness for this patient might include head trauma, seizure disorder, hyperglycemia, or stroke. Emergency nurses are ethically and legally bound to provide the same standard of care to patients regardless of the known or presumed mechanism of injury and should prioritize care according the patient's current status and the likelihood of life-threatening conditions should there be a delay in care. Patients who frequently visit the emergency department may eventually have a health emergency and are entitled to the same level of care as a patient not frequently seen.

B. The patient's altered mental status must drive the triage decision. Although a blood alcohol level test may be indicated, the patient should first be assessed to determine other possible, more serious etiologies for a confused mental state.

C. A lack of thiamine (vitamin B_1) is common in patients with alcoholism. The deficiency can result in encephalopathy and damage to the areas of the brain that control memory. The etiology of the patient's change in mental status must be determined before any treatment decisions are made. If it is decided that the patient's confusion is due to alcohol abuse, then an IV containing thiamine would be appropriate.

D. The priority of care for this patient is understanding the etiology of the altered mental status change. A referral to a detoxification unit may be indicated if alcohol abuse is found to be the basis of the patient's confusion, but that cannot be determined until more serious etiologies, such as head trauma, stroke, hyperglycemia, or seizure disorder, have been ruled out.

Category: Professional Issues/Nurse/Ethical dilemmas

Cognitive Level: Application

References

Center for Medicare Services. (2015). *The CMS hospital conditions of participation and interpretive guidelines.* Brentwood, TN: HCPro.

Dimeo, P., & Ballard, D. (2011). *Law for nurse leaders.* New York, NY: Springer.

Williamson, D. M. (2013). Alcohol abuse. In B. B. Hammond & P. G. Zimmermann (Eds.), *Sheehy's manual of emergency care* (7th ed., pp. 137–146). St. Louis, MO: Elsevier Mosby.

---

137. When caring for a patient who has experienced an act of interpersonal violence, it is important the emergency nurse perform which of the following?

A. Use only fluorescent lights when photographing injuries
B. Document patient statements using proper medical terminology

C. Label bullet wounds as "entrance" and "exit"
D. Recognize items that may have forensic value

Rationale

A. Fluorescent lights may give bruises a yellow or green tint when photographed. The nurse should photograph these injuries using several different light sources.

B. When documenting the patient's report of the events, best practice is to directly quote the patient using the patient's words, placed within quotation marks, rather than proper medical terminology. This supports the documentation as an accurate and unbiased report of the patient's statements.

C. Differentiating between entrance and exit wounds of a projectile is beyond the education and training of the emergency nurse. Wounds should be identified by their anatomical location.

D. Stabilization of the patient's physical condition is always the nurse's priority, but because the nurse may have contact with the patient before law enforcement is involved, it becomes the nurse's responsibility to recognize, properly collect, and store evidence with potential forensic value.

Category: Professional Issues/Patient/Forensic evidence collection

Cognitive Level: Recall

Reference

Sheridan, D. J., Nash, K. R., & Bresee, H. (2010). Forensic nursing in the emergency department. In P. K. Howard & R. A. Steinmann (Eds.), *Sheehy's emergency nursing: Principles and practice* (6th ed., pp. 174–186). St. Louis, MO: Mosby Elsevier.

---

138. Nursing staff in the emergency department voice a concern that blood culture contamination rates are high. What is the initial step the nurses should complete to develop a new, evidence-based blood-drawing protocol?

A. Collect the evidence
B. Develop the clinical question
C. Evaluate the hierarchy of evidence
D. Identify patient preferences and values

Rationale

A. Collecting the evidence is accomplished through a review of the literature. This review provides the foundation of the best evidence available to address the clinical question; therefore, the initial step is to define the problem.

B. Defining the problem in the form of a clinical question provides direction for the remainder of the research and protocol development process.

C. Evidence must be evaluated to determine if it is valid, reliable, and applicable to the nurses' hospital setting and emergency department population.

D. Once the evidence has been collected and evaluated, personal clinical expertise and patient preferences and values are incorporated into the development of the new, evidence-based protocol.

Category: Professional Issues/Nurse/Evidence-based practice

Cognitive Level: Application

Reference

Howard, P. K. (2007). Research and evidence-based practice. In K. S. Hoyt & J. Selfridge-Thomas (Eds.), *Emergency nursing core curriculum* (6th ed., pp. 1057–1071). St. Louis, MO: Saunders Elsevier.

---

139. The emergency nurse is caring for a 10-year-old trauma patient who is unresponsive and hemodynamically unstable because of severe internal hemorrhage. The trauma surgeon has ordered that the massive transfusion protocol (MTP) be initiated for this patient. The family is refusing the blood transfusion because of their religious beliefs. Although the patient's family is refusing to consent to the MTP treatment, the nurse should plan to:

A. initiate the transfusion protocol.
B. provide comfort measures only.
C. ask the family to sign a Do Not Resuscitate form.
D. complete an incident report for not initiating the transfusion protocol.

Rationale

A. In the event that a child presents and the family refuses essential medical care, protective custody of the child is indicated to allow necessary treatment to be initiated. Adults have autonomous rights, but they cannot be imposed on a child.

B. In the event that a child presents and the family refuses essential medical care, protective custody of the child is indicated to allow necessary treatment to be initiated. Adults have autonomous rights, but they cannot be imposed on a child.

C. In the event that a child presents and the family refuses essential medical care, protective custody of the child is indicated to allow necessary treatment. Adults have autonomous rights, but they cannot be imposed on a child

D. In the event that a severely injured or ill child presents and the family refuses essential medical care, protective custody of the child is indicated to allow the necessary treatment to be initiated. Adults have autonomous rights, but they cannot be imposed on a child.

Category (Pediatric): Professional Issues/Patient/Cultural considerations

Cognitive Level: Application

Reference

Heilicser, B. (2013). Ethical dilemmas in emergency nursing. In B. B. Hammond & P. G. Zimmermann (Eds.), *Sheehy's manual of emergency care* (7th ed., pp. 43–48). St. Louis, MO: Elsevier Mosby.

---

140. Which of the following is the most effective method for an emergency nurse to reinforce a patient's understanding of their discharge instructions?

A. Assist the patient in scheduling a follow-up appointment with their primary care provider
B. Provide written discharge instructions

C. Arrange for a follow-up phone call
D. Demonstrate all procedures before discharge

Rationale

A. Assisting the patient in making a follow-up appointment is important, however, it will not reinforce instructions at the time of discharge.

B. Written discharge instructions are an effective means of reinforcing a patient's understanding.

C. Follow-up phone calls are an important tool for the nurse to evaluate the effectiveness of patient teaching, but these calls are not an effective reinforcement of instructions at the time of discharge.

D. A return demonstration by the patient will identify the need for reinforcement of instruction or additional teaching, but it is not the most effective method to reinforce a patient's understanding of their discharge instructions.

Category: Professional Issues/Patient/Discharge planning

Cognitive Level: Analysis

Reference

Powell, K. K., & Daniels, J. H. (2007). Education: Professional, patient, and community. In K. S. Hoyt & J. Selfridge-Thomas (Eds.), *Emergency nursing core curriculum* (6th ed., pp. 997–1009). St. Louis, MO: Saunders Elsevier.

---

141. Hospital staff who access the medical record of a patient whom they have no responsibility to care for would be in violation of which federal regulation?

A. Reportable conditions
B. Emergency Medical Treatment and Active Labor Act
C. Health Insurance Portability and Accountability Act
D. Advance directives

Rationale

A. Reportable conditions include errors in assessment or implementation of patient conditions; failure to act as a patient advocate; falls; medication errors; or unsafe or malfunctioning equipment. Reportable conditions are governed by state laws and require breach of patient confidentiality for the reporting of these types of events.

B. Emergency Medical Treatment and Active Labor Act regulations are enforced to ensure that any patient asking for treatment is given a medical screening and any life-stabilizing treatment regardless of their ability to pay.

C. The Health Insurance Portability and Accountability Act's privacy regulations protect personal health information and require that the information only be accessed by authorized entities, such as healthcare providers, who are involved in the planning and care of the patient.

D. Advance directives involve a federal law that requires hospitalized patients to be provided with information regarding written statements to healthcare providers about treatment choices if a terminal or irreversible illness occurs.

Category: Professional Issues/System/Federal regulations

Cognitive Level: Application

References

Brous, E. A. (2010). Legal and regulatory constructs. In P. K. Howard & R. A. Steinmann (Eds.), *Sheehy's emergency nursing: Principles and practice* (6th ed., pp. 16–25). St. Louis, MO: Mosby Elsevier.

Hammond B. B., & Zimmermann, P. G. (Eds.). (2013). Legal issues for emergency nurses. In *Sheehy's manual of emergency care* (7th ed., pp. 3–9). St. Louis, MO: Elsevier Mosby.

---

142. Following the death of a patient in the emergency department, who determines if the patient's organs and tissues are suitable for donation?

A. The local medical examiner
B. The emergency physician
C. A representative of the organ procurement organization
D. The patient's legal next-of-kin

Rationale

A. In compliance with state and local regulations, the medical examiner must be notified of any death that occurs in the emergency department. In some cases, law enforcement protocols must be followed, but the representative of the organ procurement organization, not the medical examiner, determines the patient's suitability for organ donation.

B. A representative from the organ procurement organization is responsible for determining if the patient's organs are suitable for donation; the emergency department physician cannot make this determination.

C. In 1998, the U.S. Department of Health and Human Services ruled that hospitals must notify their organ procurement organization of any patient who dies in their hospital or whose death is imminent.

D. The patient's legal next-of-kin must provide consent for donation, but it is the responsibility of the representative from the hospital's designated organ procurement organization to determine if the organs and tissues are suitable for donation.

Category: Professional Issues/Patient/End-of-life issues: Organ and tissue donation

Cognitive Level: Recall

References

Bonalumi, N. (2010). Organ and tissue donation. In P. K. Howard & R. A. Steinmann (Eds.), *Sheehy's emergency nursing: Principles and practice* (6th ed., pp. 155–160). St. Louis, MO: Mosby Elsevier.

Cronin, T. D. (2013). End-of-life issues for emergency nurses. In B. B. Hammond & P. G. Zimmermann (Eds.), *Sheehy's manual of emergency care* (7th ed., pp. 179–182). St. Louis, MO: Elsevier Mosby.

---

143. The emergency department is notified that a patient will soon be arriving via emergency medical services. The patient was involved in a possible shooting, and the police are requesting that the patient's hands be "bagged." The emergency nurse is aware that the police are requesting that which of the following actions be performed when the patient arrives?

A. Place a sterile drape over each hand and secure at the wrist.
B. Place a clear plastic bag over each hand and secure at the wrist.
C. Place a paper bag over each hand and secure at the wrist.
D. Wrap each hand in a towel and secure at the wrist.

Rationale

A. A sterile drape is not required; each hand should be bagged with an individual paper bag and sealed at the wrist until police can arrive to assess the hands for evidence.

B. Plastic bags can harbor moisture and may alter the evidence. Each hand should be bagged with an individual paper bag and sealed at the wrist until police can arrive to assess the hands for evidence.

C. Place a paper bag over each hand and seal at the wrist with tape. Police will need to assess the hands for gunpowder residue testing and for evidence under the nails or on the hands.

D. Towels can harbor moisture, and key evidence could be removed by the towel, especially if the hand has open wounds. Each hand should be bagged with an individual paper bag and sealed at the wrist until police can arrive to assess the hands for evidence.

Category: Professional Issues/Patient/Forensic evidence collection
Cognitive Level: Application

References

Eckes-Roper, J. (2013). Forensics. In B. B. Hammond & P. G. Zimmermann (Eds.), *Sheehy's manual of emergency care* (7th ed., pp. 49–58). St. Louis, MO: Elsevier Mosby.
Sheridan, D., Nash, K., & Bresee, H. (2010). Forensic nursing in the emergency department. In P. K. Howard & R. A. Steinmann (Eds.), *Sheehy's emergency nursing: Principles and practice* (6th ed., pp. 174–186). St. Louis, MO: Mosby Elsevier.

---

144. The emergency nurse is preparing a treatment room for procedural sedation. Review of the preprocedure checklist identifies that the patient's ASA (American Society of Anesthesiologists) physical status classification is a level 3. The nurse should perform which of the following actions?

A. Refuse to do the procedure and call the nursing supervisor.
B. Continue to set up the treatment room for the procedure as indicated and ensure that end-tidal CO_2 capnography is readily available.
C. Discuss with the patient's physician that an ASA class 3 indicates that the patient has a history of severe systemic disease and therefore may require an anesthesia consult, or the procedure may be performed more safely in the operating room.
D. Request that the emergency department charge nurse immediately notify the on-call anesthesiologist of the procedure.

Rationale

A. The nurse should discuss with the emergency department physician that according to hospital policy, an ASA class 3 patient should have the procedure performed with readily available anesthesia support or in the operating room.

B. End-tidal CO_2 is considered the gold standard for early recognition of potential airway compromise during sedation and monitoring of the patient during sedation procedures. An ASA class 3 patient has two or more comorbidities and possibly should have the procedure performed with readily available anesthesia support or in the operating room. The emergency room nurse should be aware of ASA classifications to identify those patients who may experience complications when receiving anesthesia agents.

C. Patients who are an ASA class 3 or higher are considered to be at increased risk for complications as compared with patients with a lower ASA score. An ASA class 3 patient has two or more comorbidities and possibly should have the procedure performed with readily available anesthesia support or in the operating room. The emergency department nurse is aware that ASA classifications provide criteria to identify patients who may experience complications when receiving anesthesia agents.

D. The emergency department nurse should discuss the ASA classification and review the institutional policies with the emergency department physician who designed the ASA classification before notifying the on-call anesthesiologist.

Category: Professional Issues/Patient/Pain management and procedural sedation

Cognitive Level: Application

Reference

McCauley, L. W. (2013). Procedural sedation. In B. B. Hammond & P. G. Zimmermann (Eds.), *Sheehy's manual of emergency care* (7th ed., pp. 161–166). St. Louis, MO: Elsevier Mosby.

---

145. A nationwide initiative being used in emergency departments to increase patient safety during nurses' change-of-shift report is to perform a:

A. uninterrupted report.
B. bedside report.
C. designated timed report.
D. taped report.

Rationale

A. Nurses should be uninterrupted in medication administration to reduce errors, however, interactive change-of-shift report at the bedside has been proved to increase patient safety.

B. Having nurses conduct the change-of-shift report directly at the patient's bedside has been proven to enhance patient safety and satisfaction.

C. Report during shift change is variable depending on the number of patients and the acuity of the patient assignment. Conducting the change-of-shift report at the bedside has been proved to improve patient safety and satisfaction.

D. Performing a taped report does not allow for direct interaction between the nursing staff. Conducting nurses' change-of-shift report directly at the patient's bedside has been proved to improve patient safety and satisfaction.

Category: Professional Issues/Patient/Patient safety

Cognitive Level: Analysis

Reference

Baker, S. (2009). *Excellence in the emergency department: How to get results.* Gulf Breeze, FL: Fire Starter.

---

146. There are five mission areas of emergency response according to the Federal Emergency Management Agency. The five phases are prevention, protection, response, recovery, and:

A. education.
B. management.
C. evacuation.
D. mitigation.

Rationale

A. Education is an important part of disaster management and includes educating personnel, administration, and the public for everyone's safety. However, education is performed throughout all four phases of disaster management: mitigation, preparedness, response, and recovery.

B. Managing the situation is the responsibility of leaders before, during, and after a mass casualty or disaster event. This is done throughout the five phases of emergency management, mitigation, preparedness, response, and recovery.

C. Evacuation is removing people and animals from an incident to protect them from danger. This is done during a mass casualty or disaster event and is part of the response phase of disaster management.

D. Mitigation is preventing future emergencies or minimizing their effects. According to the Federal Emergency Management Agency, this is an important step in emergency management. Mitigation happens both before and after a disaster. Buying flood and fire insurance for your home is an example of mitigation.

Category: Professional Issues/System/Disaster management

Cognitive Level: Analysis

Reference

Federal Emergency Management Agency. (2016). *Fundamentals of emergency management: Lesson 1: Emergency management overview.* Retrieved from https://emilms.fema.gov/IS230c/FEMsummary.htm

---

147. An emergency department guideline being used to improve patient safety is to weigh all children in:

A. grains.
B. pounds.
C. ounces.
D. kilograms.

Rationale

A. Weights in kilograms are safer in pediatric nursing because medications for children are ordered in calculations by kilograms. This will reduce the incidence of both mathematical errors and medication errors.

B. A scale that measures only in kilograms is best practice for pediatric care in the emergency department. Medication doses for children are calculated by the patient's weight in kilograms; therefore, the child should be weighed in kilograms.

C. Weights in kilograms are safer in pediatric nursing because medications for children are ordered in calculations by kilograms. This will reduce the incidence of both mathematical errors and medication errors

D. Medication dosages for children are based on the patient's kilogram weight, and dosages are subsequently ordered in milligrams per kilogram. Weighing all children in kilograms will reduce the incidence of both mathematical errors and medication errors.

Category (Pediatric): Professional Issues/System/Risk management

Cognitive Level: Recall

Reference

Binder, R. C. (2012). Medication administration. *Emergency Nursing Pediatric Course: Provider manual* (4th ed., pp. 115–122). Des Plaines, IL: Emergency Nurses Association.

---

148. A patient arrives by ambulance to the emergency department demonstrating delusions, hallucinations, and suicidal ideation. The patient refuses all medical treatment. The emergency nurse is aware that the healthcare team can legally treat the patient based on which type of consent?

A. Express consent
B. Involuntary consent
C. Implied consent
D. Informed consent

Rationale

A. Express consent is given voluntarily when an individual seeks medical treatment; this type of consent is predicated on the patient's mental capacity.

B. When an individual refuses to consent to needed medical treatment and is deemed gravely disabled or a danger to self or others, then a physician, peace officer, or licensed mental health professional (e.g., psychiatrist, psychologist, licensed clinical professional counselor, licensed clinical social worker) can complete a certificate and petition for involuntary treatment of the patient. Documentation must include a psychiatric evaluation.

C. Implied consent is used when an individual is in a life- or limb-threatening situation and is unable to provide express consent.

D. Before a procedure, a physician describes the procedure to be performed, alternatives to the procedure, risks and benefits of the procedure, and the patient's understanding of the procedure and its alternatives, risks, and benefits.

Category: Professional Issues/System/Patient consent for treatment

Cognitive Level: Application

Reference

Jagmin, M. (2007). Legal and regulatory issues. In K. S. Hoyt & J. Selfridge-Thomas (Eds.), *Emergency nursing core curriculum* (6th ed., pp. 1033–1045). St. Louis, MO: Saunders Elsevier.

---

149. Which of the following is a mandatory reportable disease to the Centers for Disease Control and Prevention?

A. Urinary tract infections
B. Pneumonia
C. Hand, foot, and mouth disease
D. Measles (rubeola)

Rationale

A. UTIs are typically bacterial in nature and are not contagious. UTIs do not need to be reported to the Centers for Disease Control and Prevention.

B. Pneumonia can be either bacterial or viral but does not need to be reported to the CDC. The total number of cases may be reported within a given region, but it is not a mandatory disease to report.

C. Hand, foot, and mouth disease is highly contagious viral illness that causes sores to the hands, feet, and mouth. It is not a reportable disease to the CDC, but it should be reported to anyone who may have come into contact with the virus.

D. Measles (rubeola) is an acute and highly contagious viral illness caused by the rubeola virus. It must be reported by phone to the CDC by the patient's provider.

Category: Professional Issues/System/Symptom surveillance: Mandatory reporting of disease

Nursing Process: Recall

Reference

Jagmin, M. (2007). Legal and regulatory issues. In K. S. Hoyt & J. Selfridge-Thomas (Eds.), *Emergency nursing core curriculum* (6th ed., pp. 1033–1045). St. Louis, MO: Saunders.

---

150. While working in triage, the emergency nurse is speaking on the phone to an individual who is seeking medical advice for abdominal pain. What is the appropriate response for the emergency triage nurse to give to this patient?

A. "It sounds like you have a viral infection. Be sure to increase your fluids and avoid dairy products."
B. "I will call you back after I speak to the emergency provider. Can you tell me more about the pain that you are experiencing?"
C. "It is very busy here right now; I think you should just wait and be seen by your physician tomorrow."
D. "I cannot answer your question over the phone; the emergency department is open 24 hours a day, and we can evaluate you here in person if you wish to be seen."

Rationale

A. The emergency nurse should not provide any medical advice over the phone unless the facility has a designated telephone triage program and the nurse has completed the appropriate education for this program.

B. It is inappropriate for the nurse to provide any medical advice over the phone to a potential patient; this would not be an appropriate answer.

C. The nurse does not have the knowledge to provide this type of advice over the phone; the patient should be advised to come to the emergency department for an evaluation.

D. Unless a hospital is equipped for a formal telephone triage system, the Emergency Nurses Association does not support a nurse providing medical advice over the phone. Patients should be advised that they can come to the emergency department to be properly evaluated.

Category: Professional Issues/System/Triage

Cognitive Level: Application

Reference

Gilboy, N. (2013). Triage. In B. B. Hammond & P. G. Zimmermann (Eds.), *Sheehy's manual of emergency care* (7th ed., pp. 61–75). St. Louis, MO: Elsevier Mosby.

SELF-DIAGNOSTIC PROFILE

How to Use the Self-Assessment Worksheet

1. Indicate on your answer sheet whether your answers are correct or incorrect.
2. Note the items you answered incorrectly.
3. Count the total number of items you answered incorrectly in each category.
4. Compare the total number of items you answered incorrectly in each category with the total number of items per category. This information will give you an idea of where you will need to focus your continued study.

Content Category	Questions Answered Incorrectly	Total Number of Questions Answered Incorrectly in Each Category	Total Number of Questions in Each CEN Content Category
Cardiovascular Emergencies			20
Respiratory Emergencies			16
Neurological Emergencies			16
Gastrointestinal, Genitourinary, Gynecology, and Obstetrical Emergencies			21
Psychosocial and Medical Emergencies			25
Maxillofacial, Ocular, Orthopedic, and Wound Emergencies			21
Environment and Toxicology Emergencies, and Communicable Diseases			15
Professional Issues			16

Answer Sheets for Practice Examinations

Practice Examination Answer Sheet

1. ○ A ○ B ○ C ○ D	31. ○ A ○ B ○ C ○ D	61. ○ A ○ B ○ C ○ D	91. ○ A ○ B ○ C ○ D	121. ○ A ○ B ○ C ○ D
2. ○ A ○ B ○ C ○ D	32. ○ A ○ B ○ C ○ D	62. ○ A ○ B ○ C ○ D	92. ○ A ○ B ○ C ○ D	122. ○ A ○ B ○ C ○ D
3. ○ A ○ B ○ C ○ D	33. ○ A ○ B ○ C ○ D	63. ○ A ○ B ○ C ○ D	93. ○ A ○ B ○ C ○ D	123. ○ A ○ B ○ C ○ D
4. ○ A ○ B ○ C ○ D	34. ○ A ○ B ○ C ○ D	64. ○ A ○ B ○ C ○ D	94. ○ A ○ B ○ C ○ D	124. ○ A ○ B ○ C ○ D
5. ○ A ○ B ○ C ○ D	35. ○ A ○ B ○ C ○ D	65. ○ A ○ B ○ C ○ D	95. ○ A ○ B ○ C ○ D	125. ○ A ○ B ○ C ○ D
6. ○ A ○ B ○ C ○ D	36. ○ A ○ B ○ C ○ D	66. ○ A ○ B ○ C ○ D	96. ○ A ○ B ○ C ○ D	126. ○ A ○ B ○ C ○ D
7. ○ A ○ B ○ C ○ D	37. ○ A ○ B ○ C ○ D	67. ○ A ○ B ○ C ○ D	97. ○ A ○ B ○ C ○ D	127. ○ A ○ B ○ C ○ D
8. ○ A ○ B ○ C ○ D	38. ○ A ○ B ○ C ○ D	68. ○ A ○ B ○ C ○ D	98. ○ A ○ B ○ C ○ D	128. ○ A ○ B ○ C ○ D
9. ○ A ○ B ○ C ○ D	39. ○ A ○ B ○ C ○ D	69. ○ A ○ B ○ C ○ D	99. ○ A ○ B ○ C ○ D	129. ○ A ○ B ○ C ○ D
10. ○ A ○ B ○ C ○ D	40. ○ A ○ B ○ C ○ D	70. ○ A ○ B ○ C ○ D	100. ○ A ○ B ○ C ○ D	130. ○ A ○ B ○ C ○ D
11. ○ A ○ B ○ C ○ D	41. ○ A ○ B ○ C ○ D	71. ○ A ○ B ○ C ○ D	101. ○ A ○ B ○ C ○ D	131. ○ A ○ B ○ C ○ D
12. ○ A ○ B ○ C ○ D	42. ○ A ○ B ○ C ○ D	72. ○ A ○ B ○ C ○ D	102. ○ A ○ B ○ C ○ D	132. ○ A ○ B ○ C ○ D
13. ○ A ○ B ○ C ○ D	43. ○ A ○ B ○ C ○ D	73. ○ A ○ B ○ C ○ D	103. ○ A ○ B ○ C ○ D	133. ○ A ○ B ○ C ○ D
14. ○ A ○ B ○ C ○ D	44. ○ A ○ B ○ C ○ D	74. ○ A ○ B ○ C ○ D	104. ○ A ○ B ○ C ○ D	134. ○ A ○ B ○ C ○ D
15. ○ A ○ B ○ C ○ D	45. ○ A ○ B ○ C ○ D	75. ○ A ○ B ○ C ○ D	105. ○ A ○ B ○ C ○ D	135. ○ A ○ B ○ C ○ D
16. ○ A ○ B ○ C ○ D	46. ○ A ○ B ○ C ○ D	76. ○ A ○ B ○ C ○ D	106. ○ A ○ B ○ C ○ D	136. ○ A ○ B ○ C ○ D
17. ○ A ○ B ○ C ○ D	47. ○ A ○ B ○ C ○ D	77. ○ A ○ B ○ C ○ D	107. ○ A ○ B ○ C ○ D	137. ○ A ○ B ○ C ○ D
18. ○ A ○ B ○ C ○ D	48. ○ A ○ B ○ C ○ D	78. ○ A ○ B ○ C ○ D	108. ○ A ○ B ○ C ○ D	138. ○ A ○ B ○ C ○ D
19. ○ A ○ B ○ C ○ D	49. ○ A ○ B ○ C ○ D	79. ○ A ○ B ○ C ○ D	109. ○ A ○ B ○ C ○ D	139. ○ A ○ B ○ C ○ D
20. ○ A ○ B ○ C ○ D	50. ○ A ○ B ○ C ○ D	80. ○ A ○ B ○ C ○ D	110. ○ A ○ B ○ C ○ D	140. ○ A ○ B ○ C ○ D
21. ○ A ○ B ○ C ○ D	51. ○ A ○ B ○ C ○ D	81. ○ A ○ B ○ C ○ D	111. ○ A ○ B ○ C ○ D	141. ○ A ○ B ○ C ○ D
22. ○ A ○ B ○ C ○ D	52. ○ A ○ B ○ C ○ D	82. ○ A ○ B ○ C ○ D	112. ○ A ○ B ○ C ○ D	142. ○ A ○ B ○ C ○ D
23. ○ A ○ B ○ C ○ D	53. ○ A ○ B ○ C ○ D	83. ○ A ○ B ○ C ○ D	113. ○ A ○ B ○ C ○ D	143. ○ A ○ B ○ C ○ D
24. ○ A ○ B ○ C ○ D	54. ○ A ○ B ○ C ○ D	84. ○ A ○ B ○ C ○ D	114. ○ A ○ B ○ C ○ D	144. ○ A ○ B ○ C ○ D
25. ○ A ○ B ○ C ○ D	55. ○ A ○ B ○ C ○ D	85. ○ A ○ B ○ C ○ D	115. ○ A ○ B ○ C ○ D	145. ○ A ○ B ○ C ○ D
26. ○ A ○ B ○ C ○ D	56. ○ A ○ B ○ C ○ D	86. ○ A ○ B ○ C ○ D	116. ○ A ○ B ○ C ○ D	146. ○ A ○ B ○ C ○ D
27. ○ A ○ B ○ C ○ D	57. ○ A ○ B ○ C ○ D	87. ○ A ○ B ○ C ○ D	117. ○ A ○ B ○ C ○ D	147. ○ A ○ B ○ C ○ D
28. ○ A ○ B ○ C ○ D	58. ○ A ○ B ○ C ○ D	88. ○ A ○ B ○ C ○ D	118. ○ A ○ B ○ C ○ D	148. ○ A ○ B ○ C ○ D
29. ○ A ○ B ○ C ○ D	59. ○ A ○ B ○ C ○ D	89. ○ A ○ B ○ C ○ D	119. ○ A ○ B ○ C ○ D	149. ○ A ○ B ○ C ○ D
30. ○ A ○ B ○ C ○ D	60. ○ A ○ B ○ C ○ D	90. ○ A ○ B ○ C ○ D	120. ○ A ○ B ○ C ○ D	150. ○ A ○ B ○ C ○ D

Self-Diagnostic Profile

How to Use the Self-Assessment Worksheet

1. Indicate on your answer sheet whether your answers are correct or incorrect.
2. Note the items you answered incorrectly.
3. Count the total number of items you answered incorrectly in each category.
4. Compare the total number of items you answered incorrectly in each category with the total number of items per category. This information will give you an idea of where you will need to focus your continued study.

Content Category	Questions Answered Incorrectly	Total Number of Questions Answered Incorrectly in Each Category	Total Number of Questions in Each CEN Content Category
Cardiovascular Emergencies			20
Respiratory Emergencies			16
Neurological Emergencies			16
Gastrointestinal, Genitourinary, Gynecology, and Obstetrical Emergencies			21
Psychosocial and Medical Emergencies			25
Maxillofacial, Ocular, Orthopedic, and Wound Emergencies			21
Environment and Toxicology Emergencies, and Communicable Diseases			15
Professional Issues			16

Practice Examination Answer Sheet

1. ○A ○B ○C ○D	31. ○A ○B ○C ○D	61. ○A ○B ○C ○D	91. ○A ○B ○C ○D	121. ○A ○B ○C ○D
2. ○A ○B ○C ○D	32. ○A ○B ○C ○D	62. ○A ○B ○C ○D	92. ○A ○B ○C ○D	122. ○A ○B ○C ○D
3. ○A ○B ○C ○D	33. ○A ○B ○C ○D	63. ○A ○B ○C ○D	93. ○A ○B ○C ○D	123. ○A ○B ○C ○D
4. ○A ○B ○C ○D	34. ○A ○B ○C ○D	64. ○A ○B ○C ○D	94. ○A ○B ○C ○D	124. ○A ○B ○C ○D
5. ○A ○B ○C ○D	35. ○A ○B ○C ○D	65. ○A ○B ○C ○D	95. ○A ○B ○C ○D	125. ○A ○B ○C ○D
6. ○A ○B ○C ○D	36. ○A ○B ○C ○D	66. ○A ○B ○C ○D	96. ○A ○B ○C ○D	126. ○A ○B ○C ○D
7. ○A ○B ○C ○D	37. ○A ○B ○C ○D	67. ○A ○B ○C ○D	97. ○A ○B ○C ○D	127. ○A ○B ○C ○D
8. ○A ○B ○C ○D	38. ○A ○B ○C ○D	68. ○A ○B ○C ○D	98. ○A ○B ○C ○D	128. ○A ○B ○C ○D
9. ○A ○B ○C ○D	39. ○A ○B ○C ○D	69. ○A ○B ○C ○D	99. ○A ○B ○C ○D	129. ○A ○B ○C ○D
10. ○A ○B ○C ○D	40. ○A ○B ○C ○D	70. ○A ○B ○C ○D	100. ○A ○B ○C ○D	130. ○A ○B ○C ○D
11. ○A ○B ○C ○D	41. ○A ○B ○C ○D	71. ○A ○B ○C ○D	101. ○A ○B ○C ○D	131. ○A ○B ○C ○D
12. ○A ○B ○C ○D	42. ○A ○B ○C ○D	72. ○A ○B ○C ○D	102. ○A ○B ○C ○D	132. ○A ○B ○C ○D
13. ○A ○B ○C ○D	43. ○A ○B ○C ○D	73. ○A ○B ○C ○D	103. ○A ○B ○C ○D	133. ○A ○B ○C ○D
14. ○A ○B ○C ○D	44. ○A ○B ○C ○D	74. ○A ○B ○C ○D	104. ○A ○B ○C ○D	134. ○A ○B ○C ○D
15. ○A ○B ○C ○D	45. ○A ○B ○C ○D	75. ○A ○B ○C ○D	105. ○A ○B ○C ○D	135. ○A ○B ○C ○D
16. ○A ○B ○C ○D	46. ○A ○B ○C ○D	76. ○A ○B ○C ○D	106. ○A ○B ○C ○D	136. ○A ○B ○C ○D
17. ○A ○B ○C ○D	47. ○A ○B ○C ○D	77. ○A ○B ○C ○D	107. ○A ○B ○C ○D	137. ○A ○B ○C ○D
18. ○A ○B ○C ○D	48. ○A ○B ○C ○D	78. ○A ○B ○C ○D	108. ○A ○B ○C ○D	138. ○A ○B ○C ○D
19. ○A ○B ○C ○D	49. ○A ○B ○C ○D	79. ○A ○B ○C ○D	109. ○A ○B ○C ○D	139. ○A ○B ○C ○D
20. ○A ○B ○C ○D	50. ○A ○B ○C ○D	80. ○A ○B ○C ○D	110. ○A ○B ○C ○D	140. ○A ○B ○C ○D
21. ○A ○B ○C ○D	51. ○A ○B ○C ○D	81. ○A ○B ○C ○D	111. ○A ○B ○C ○D	141. ○A ○B ○C ○D
22. ○A ○B ○C ○D	52. ○A ○B ○C ○D	82. ○A ○B ○C ○D	112. ○A ○B ○C ○D	142. ○A ○B ○C ○D
23. ○A ○B ○C ○D	53. ○A ○B ○C ○D	83. ○A ○B ○C ○D	113. ○A ○B ○C ○D	143. ○A ○B ○C ○D
24. ○A ○B ○C ○D	54. ○A ○B ○C ○D	84. ○A ○B ○C ○D	114. ○A ○B ○C ○D	144. ○A ○B ○C ○D
25. ○A ○B ○C ○D	55. ○A ○B ○C ○D	85. ○A ○B ○C ○D	115. ○A ○B ○C ○D	145. ○A ○B ○C ○D
26. ○A ○B ○C ○D	56. ○A ○B ○C ○D	86. ○A ○B ○C ○D	116. ○A ○B ○C ○D	146. ○A ○B ○C ○D
27. ○A ○B ○C ○D	57. ○A ○B ○C ○D	87. ○A ○B ○C ○D	117. ○A ○B ○C ○D	147. ○A ○B ○C ○D
28. ○A ○B ○C ○D	58. ○A ○B ○C ○D	88. ○A ○B ○C ○D	118. ○A ○B ○C ○D	148. ○A ○B ○C ○D
29. ○A ○B ○C ○D	59. ○A ○B ○C ○D	89. ○A ○B ○C ○D	119. ○A ○B ○C ○D	149. ○A ○B ○C ○D
30. ○A ○B ○C ○D	60. ○A ○B ○C ○D	90. ○A ○B ○C ○D	120. ○A ○B ○C ○D	150. ○A ○B ○C ○D

Self-Diagnostic Profile

How to Use the Self-Assessment Worksheet

1. Indicate on your answer sheet whether your answers are correct or incorrect.
2. Note the items you answered incorrectly.
3. Count the total number of items you answered incorrectly in each category.
4. Compare the total number of items you answered incorrectly in each category with the total number of items per category. This information will give you an idea of where you will need to focus your continued study.

Content Category	Questions Answered Incorrectly	Total Number of Questions Answered Incorrectly in Each Category	Total Number of Questions in Each CEN Content Category
Cardiovascular Emergencies			20
Respiratory Emergencies			16
Neurological Emergencies			16
Gastrointestinal, Genitourinary, Gynecology, and Obstetrical Emergencies			21
Psychosocial and Medical Emergencies			25
Maxillofacial, Ocular, Orthopedic, and Wound Emergencies			21
Environment and Toxicology Emergencies, and Communicable Diseases			15
Professional Issues			16

Practice Examination Answer Sheet

1. ○A ○B ○C ○D	31. ○A ○B ○C ○D	61. ○A ○B ○C ○D	91. ○A ○B ○C ○D	121. ○A ○B ○C ○D
2. ○A ○B ○C ○D	32. ○A ○B ○C ○D	62. ○A ○B ○C ○D	92. ○A ○B ○C ○D	122. ○A ○B ○C ○D
3. ○A ○B ○C ○D	33. ○A ○B ○C ○D	63. ○A ○B ○C ○D	93. ○A ○B ○C ○D	123. ○A ○B ○C ○D
4. ○A ○B ○C ○D	34. ○A ○B ○C ○D	64. ○A ○B ○C ○D	94. ○A ○B ○C ○D	124. ○A ○B ○C ○D
5. ○A ○B ○C ○D	35. ○A ○B ○C ○D	65. ○A ○B ○C ○D	95. ○A ○B ○C ○D	125. ○A ○B ○C ○D
6. ○A ○B ○C ○D	36. ○A ○B ○C ○D	66. ○A ○B ○C ○D	96. ○A ○B ○C ○D	126. ○A ○B ○C ○D
7. ○A ○B ○C ○D	37. ○A ○B ○C ○D	67. ○A ○B ○C ○D	97. ○A ○B ○C ○D	127. ○A ○B ○C ○D
8. ○A ○B ○C ○D	38. ○A ○B ○C ○D	68. ○A ○B ○C ○D	98. ○A ○B ○C ○D	128. ○A ○B ○C ○D
9. ○A ○B ○C ○D	39. ○A ○B ○C ○D	69. ○A ○B ○C ○D	99. ○A ○B ○C ○D	129. ○A ○B ○C ○D
10. ○A ○B ○C ○D	40. ○A ○B ○C ○D	70. ○A ○B ○C ○D	100. ○A ○B ○C ○D	130. ○A ○B ○C ○D
11. ○A ○B ○C ○D	41. ○A ○B ○C ○D	71. ○A ○B ○C ○D	101. ○A ○B ○C ○D	131. ○A ○B ○C ○D
12. ○A ○B ○C ○D	42. ○A ○B ○C ○D	72. ○A ○B ○C ○D	102. ○A ○B ○C ○D	132. ○A ○B ○C ○D
13. ○A ○B ○C ○D	43. ○A ○B ○C ○D	73. ○A ○B ○C ○D	103. ○A ○B ○C ○D	133. ○A ○B ○C ○D
14. ○A ○B ○C ○D	44. ○A ○B ○C ○D	74. ○A ○B ○C ○D	104. ○A ○B ○C ○D	134. ○A ○B ○C ○D
15. ○A ○B ○C ○D	45. ○A ○B ○C ○D	75. ○A ○B ○C ○D	105. ○A ○B ○C ○D	135. ○A ○B ○C ○D
16. ○A ○B ○C ○D	46. ○A ○B ○C ○D	76. ○A ○B ○C ○D	106. ○A ○B ○C ○D	136. ○A ○B ○C ○D
17. ○A ○B ○C ○D	47. ○A ○B ○C ○D	77. ○A ○B ○C ○D	107. ○A ○B ○C ○D	137. ○A ○B ○C ○D
18. ○A ○B ○C ○D	48. ○A ○B ○C ○D	78. ○A ○B ○C ○D	108. ○A ○B ○C ○D	138. ○A ○B ○C ○D
19. ○A ○B ○C ○D	49. ○A ○B ○C ○D	79. ○A ○B ○C ○D	109. ○A ○B ○C ○D	139. ○A ○B ○C ○D
20. ○A ○B ○C ○D	50. ○A ○B ○C ○D	80. ○A ○B ○C ○D	110. ○A ○B ○C ○D	140. ○A ○B ○C ○D
21. ○A ○B ○C ○D	51. ○A ○B ○C ○D	81. ○A ○B ○C ○D	111. ○A ○B ○C ○D	141. ○A ○B ○C ○D
22. ○A ○B ○C ○D	52. ○A ○B ○C ○D	82. ○A ○B ○C ○D	112. ○A ○B ○C ○D	142. ○A ○B ○C ○D
23. ○A ○B ○C ○D	53. ○A ○B ○C ○D	83. ○A ○B ○C ○D	113. ○A ○B ○C ○D	143. ○A ○B ○C ○D
24. ○A ○B ○C ○D	54. ○A ○B ○C ○D	84. ○A ○B ○C ○D	114. ○A ○B ○C ○D	144. ○A ○B ○C ○D
25. ○A ○B ○C ○D	55. ○A ○B ○C ○D	85. ○A ○B ○C ○D	115. ○A ○B ○C ○D	145. ○A ○B ○C ○D
26. ○A ○B ○C ○D	56. ○A ○B ○C ○D	86. ○A ○B ○C ○D	116. ○A ○B ○C ○D	146. ○A ○B ○C ○D
27. ○A ○B ○C ○D	57. ○A ○B ○C ○D	87. ○A ○B ○C ○D	117. ○A ○B ○C ○D	147. ○A ○B ○C ○D
28. ○A ○B ○C ○D	58. ○A ○B ○C ○D	88. ○A ○B ○C ○D	118. ○A ○B ○C ○D	148. ○A ○B ○C ○D
29. ○A ○B ○C ○D	59. ○A ○B ○C ○D	89. ○A ○B ○C ○D	119. ○A ○B ○C ○D	149. ○A ○B ○C ○D
30. ○A ○B ○C ○D	60. ○A ○B ○C ○D	90. ○A ○B ○C ○D	120. ○A ○B ○C ○D	150. ○A ○B ○C ○D

Self-Diagnostic Profile

How to Use the Self-Assessment Worksheet

1. Indicate on your answer sheet whether your answers are correct or incorrect.
2. Note the items you answered incorrectly.
3. Count the total number of items you answered incorrectly in each category.
4. Compare the total number of items you answered incorrectly in each category with the total number of items per category. This information will give you an idea of where you will need to focus your continued study.

Content Category	Questions Answered Incorrectly	Total Number of Questions Answered Incorrectly in Each Category	Total Number of Questions in Each CEN Content Category
Cardiovascular Emergencies			20
Respiratory Emergencies			16
Neurological Emergencies			16
Gastrointestinal, Genitourinary, Gynecology, and Obstetrical Emergencies			21
Psychosocial and Medical Emergencies			25
Maxillofacial, Ocular, Orthopedic, and Wound Emergencies			21
Environment and Toxicology Emergencies, and Communicable Diseases			15
Professional Issues			16

Practice Examination Answer Sheet

1. ○ A ○ B ○ C ○ D	31. ○ A ○ B ○ C ○ D	61. ○ A ○ B ○ C ○ D	91. ○ A ○ B ○ C ○ D	121. ○ A ○ B ○ C ○ D
2. ○ A ○ B ○ C ○ D	32. ○ A ○ B ○ C ○ D	62. ○ A ○ B ○ C ○ D	92. ○ A ○ B ○ C ○ D	122. ○ A ○ B ○ C ○ D
3. ○ A ○ B ○ C ○ D	33. ○ A ○ B ○ C ○ D	63. ○ A ○ B ○ C ○ D	93. ○ A ○ B ○ C ○ D	123. ○ A ○ B ○ C ○ D
4. ○ A ○ B ○ C ○ D	34. ○ A ○ B ○ C ○ D	64. ○ A ○ B ○ C ○ D	94. ○ A ○ B ○ C ○ D	124. ○ A ○ B ○ C ○ D
5. ○ A ○ B ○ C ○ D	35. ○ A ○ B ○ C ○ D	65. ○ A ○ B ○ C ○ D	95. ○ A ○ B ○ C ○ D	125. ○ A ○ B ○ C ○ D
6. ○ A ○ B ○ C ○ D	36. ○ A ○ B ○ C ○ D	66. ○ A ○ B ○ C ○ D	96. ○ A ○ B ○ C ○ D	126. ○ A ○ B ○ C ○ D
7. ○ A ○ B ○ C ○ D	37. ○ A ○ B ○ C ○ D	67. ○ A ○ B ○ C ○ D	97. ○ A ○ B ○ C ○ D	127. ○ A ○ B ○ C ○ D
8. ○ A ○ B ○ C ○ D	38. ○ A ○ B ○ C ○ D	68. ○ A ○ B ○ C ○ D	98. ○ A ○ B ○ C ○ D	128. ○ A ○ B ○ C ○ D
9. ○ A ○ B ○ C ○ D	39. ○ A ○ B ○ C ○ D	69. ○ A ○ B ○ C ○ D	99. ○ A ○ B ○ C ○ D	129. ○ A ○ B ○ C ○ D
10. ○ A ○ B ○ C ○ D	40. ○ A ○ B ○ C ○ D	70. ○ A ○ B ○ C ○ D	100. ○ A ○ B ○ C ○ D	130. ○ A ○ B ○ C ○ D
11. ○ A ○ B ○ C ○ D	41. ○ A ○ B ○ C ○ D	71. ○ A ○ B ○ C ○ D	101. ○ A ○ B ○ C ○ D	131. ○ A ○ B ○ C ○ D
12. ○ A ○ B ○ C ○ D	42. ○ A ○ B ○ C ○ D	72. ○ A ○ B ○ C ○ D	102. ○ A ○ B ○ C ○ D	132. ○ A ○ B ○ C ○ D
13. ○ A ○ B ○ C ○ D	43. ○ A ○ B ○ C ○ D	73. ○ A ○ B ○ C ○ D	103. ○ A ○ B ○ C ○ D	133. ○ A ○ B ○ C ○ D
14. ○ A ○ B ○ C ○ D	44. ○ A ○ B ○ C ○ D	74. ○ A ○ B ○ C ○ D	104. ○ A ○ B ○ C ○ D	134. ○ A ○ B ○ C ○ D
15. ○ A ○ B ○ C ○ D	45. ○ A ○ B ○ C ○ D	75. ○ A ○ B ○ C ○ D	105. ○ A ○ B ○ C ○ D	135. ○ A ○ B ○ C ○ D
16. ○ A ○ B ○ C ○ D	46. ○ A ○ B ○ C ○ D	76. ○ A ○ B ○ C ○ D	106. ○ A ○ B ○ C ○ D	136. ○ A ○ B ○ C ○ D
17. ○ A ○ B ○ C ○ D	47. ○ A ○ B ○ C ○ D	77. ○ A ○ B ○ C ○ D	107. ○ A ○ B ○ C ○ D	137. ○ A ○ B ○ C ○ D
18. ○ A ○ B ○ C ○ D	48. ○ A ○ B ○ C ○ D	78. ○ A ○ B ○ C ○ D	108. ○ A ○ B ○ C ○ D	138. ○ A ○ B ○ C ○ D
19. ○ A ○ B ○ C ○ D	49. ○ A ○ B ○ C ○ D	79. ○ A ○ B ○ C ○ D	109. ○ A ○ B ○ C ○ D	139. ○ A ○ B ○ C ○ D
20. ○ A ○ B ○ C ○ D	50. ○ A ○ B ○ C ○ D	80. ○ A ○ B ○ C ○ D	110. ○ A ○ B ○ C ○ D	140. ○ A ○ B ○ C ○ D
21. ○ A ○ B ○ C ○ D	51. ○ A ○ B ○ C ○ D	81. ○ A ○ B ○ C ○ D	111. ○ A ○ B ○ C ○ D	141. ○ A ○ B ○ C ○ D
22. ○ A ○ B ○ C ○ D	52. ○ A ○ B ○ C ○ D	82. ○ A ○ B ○ C ○ D	112. ○ A ○ B ○ C ○ D	142. ○ A ○ B ○ C ○ D
23. ○ A ○ B ○ C ○ D	53. ○ A ○ B ○ C ○ D	83. ○ A ○ B ○ C ○ D	113. ○ A ○ B ○ C ○ D	143. ○ A ○ B ○ C ○ D
24. ○ A ○ B ○ C ○ D	54. ○ A ○ B ○ C ○ D	84. ○ A ○ B ○ C ○ D	114. ○ A ○ B ○ C ○ D	144. ○ A ○ B ○ C ○ D
25. ○ A ○ B ○ C ○ D	55. ○ A ○ B ○ C ○ D	85. ○ A ○ B ○ C ○ D	115. ○ A ○ B ○ C ○ D	145. ○ A ○ B ○ C ○ D
26. ○ A ○ B ○ C ○ D	56. ○ A ○ B ○ C ○ D	86. ○ A ○ B ○ C ○ D	116. ○ A ○ B ○ C ○ D	146. ○ A ○ B ○ C ○ D
27. ○ A ○ B ○ C ○ D	57. ○ A ○ B ○ C ○ D	87. ○ A ○ B ○ C ○ D	117. ○ A ○ B ○ C ○ D	147. ○ A ○ B ○ C ○ D
28. ○ A ○ B ○ C ○ D	58. ○ A ○ B ○ C ○ D	88. ○ A ○ B ○ C ○ D	118. ○ A ○ B ○ C ○ D	148. ○ A ○ B ○ C ○ D
29. ○ A ○ B ○ C ○ D	59. ○ A ○ B ○ C ○ D	89. ○ A ○ B ○ C ○ D	119. ○ A ○ B ○ C ○ D	149. ○ A ○ B ○ C ○ D
30. ○ A ○ B ○ C ○ D	60. ○ A ○ B ○ C ○ D	90. ○ A ○ B ○ C ○ D	120. ○ A ○ B ○ C ○ D	150. ○ A ○ B ○ C ○ D

Self-Diagnostic Profile

How to Use the Self-Assessment Worksheet

1. Indicate on your answer sheet whether your answers are correct or incorrect.
2. Note the items you answered incorrectly.
3. Count the total number of items you answered incorrectly in each category.
4. Compare the total number of items you answered incorrectly in each category with the total number of items per category. This information will give you an idea of where you will need to focus your continued study.

Content Category	Questions Answered Incorrectly	Total Number of Questions Answered Incorrectly in Each Category	Total Number of Questions in Each CEN Content Category
Cardiovascular Emergencies			20
Respiratory Emergencies			16
Neurological Emergencies			16
Gastrointestinal, Genitourinary, Gynecology, and Obstetrical Emergencies			21
Psychosocial and Medical Emergencies			25
Maxillofacial, Ocular, Orthopedic, and Wound Emergencies			21
Environment and Toxicology Emergencies, and Communicable Diseases			15
Professional Issues			16

Practice Examination Answer Sheet

1. ○ A ○ B ○ C ○ D	31. ○ A ○ B ○ C ○ D	61. ○ A ○ B ○ C ○ D	91. ○ A ○ B ○ C ○ D	121. ○ A ○ B ○ C ○ D
2. ○ A ○ B ○ C ○ D	32. ○ A ○ B ○ C ○ D	62. ○ A ○ B ○ C ○ D	92. ○ A ○ B ○ C ○ D	122. ○ A ○ B ○ C ○ D
3. ○ A ○ B ○ C ○ D	33. ○ A ○ B ○ C ○ D	63. ○ A ○ B ○ C ○ D	93. ○ A ○ B ○ C ○ D	123. ○ A ○ B ○ C ○ D
4. ○ A ○ B ○ C ○ D	34. ○ A ○ B ○ C ○ D	64. ○ A ○ B ○ C ○ D	94. ○ A ○ B ○ C ○ D	124. ○ A ○ B ○ C ○ D
5. ○ A ○ B ○ C ○ D	35. ○ A ○ B ○ C ○ D	65. ○ A ○ B ○ C ○ D	95. ○ A ○ B ○ C ○ D	125. ○ A ○ B ○ C ○ D
6. ○ A ○ B ○ C ○ D	36. ○ A ○ B ○ C ○ D	66. ○ A ○ B ○ C ○ D	96. ○ A ○ B ○ C ○ D	126. ○ A ○ B ○ C ○ D
7. ○ A ○ B ○ C ○ D	37. ○ A ○ B ○ C ○ D	67. ○ A ○ B ○ C ○ D	97. ○ A ○ B ○ C ○ D	127. ○ A ○ B ○ C ○ D
8. ○ A ○ B ○ C ○ D	38. ○ A ○ B ○ C ○ D	68. ○ A ○ B ○ C ○ D	98. ○ A ○ B ○ C ○ D	128. ○ A ○ B ○ C ○ D
9. ○ A ○ B ○ C ○ D	39. ○ A ○ B ○ C ○ D	69. ○ A ○ B ○ C ○ D	99. ○ A ○ B ○ C ○ D	129. ○ A ○ B ○ C ○ D
10. ○ A ○ B ○ C ○ D	40. ○ A ○ B ○ C ○ D	70. ○ A ○ B ○ C ○ D	100. ○ A ○ B ○ C ○ D	130. ○ A ○ B ○ C ○ D
11. ○ A ○ B ○ C ○ D	41. ○ A ○ B ○ C ○ D	71. ○ A ○ B ○ C ○ D	101. ○ A ○ B ○ C ○ D	131. ○ A ○ B ○ C ○ D
12. ○ A ○ B ○ C ○ D	42. ○ A ○ B ○ C ○ D	72. ○ A ○ B ○ C ○ D	102. ○ A ○ B ○ C ○ D	132. ○ A ○ B ○ C ○ D
13. ○ A ○ B ○ C ○ D	43. ○ A ○ B ○ C ○ D	73. ○ A ○ B ○ C ○ D	103. ○ A ○ B ○ C ○ D	133. ○ A ○ B ○ C ○ D
14. ○ A ○ B ○ C ○ D	44. ○ A ○ B ○ C ○ D	74. ○ A ○ B ○ C ○ D	104. ○ A ○ B ○ C ○ D	134. ○ A ○ B ○ C ○ D
15. ○ A ○ B ○ C ○ D	45. ○ A ○ B ○ C ○ D	75. ○ A ○ B ○ C ○ D	105. ○ A ○ B ○ C ○ D	135. ○ A ○ B ○ C ○ D
16. ○ A ○ B ○ C ○ D	46. ○ A ○ B ○ C ○ D	76. ○ A ○ B ○ C ○ D	106. ○ A ○ B ○ C ○ D	136. ○ A ○ B ○ C ○ D
17. ○ A ○ B ○ C ○ D	47. ○ A ○ B ○ C ○ D	77. ○ A ○ B ○ C ○ D	107. ○ A ○ B ○ C ○ D	137. ○ A ○ B ○ C ○ D
18. ○ A ○ B ○ C ○ D	48. ○ A ○ B ○ C ○ D	78. ○ A ○ B ○ C ○ D	108. ○ A ○ B ○ C ○ D	138. ○ A ○ B ○ C ○ D
19. ○ A ○ B ○ C ○ D	49. ○ A ○ B ○ C ○ D	79. ○ A ○ B ○ C ○ D	109. ○ A ○ B ○ C ○ D	139. ○ A ○ B ○ C ○ D
20. ○ A ○ B ○ C ○ D	50. ○ A ○ B ○ C ○ D	80. ○ A ○ B ○ C ○ D	110. ○ A ○ B ○ C ○ D	140. ○ A ○ B ○ C ○ D
21. ○ A ○ B ○ C ○ D	51. ○ A ○ B ○ C ○ D	81. ○ A ○ B ○ C ○ D	111. ○ A ○ B ○ C ○ D	141. ○ A ○ B ○ C ○ D
22. ○ A ○ B ○ C ○ D	52. ○ A ○ B ○ C ○ D	82. ○ A ○ B ○ C ○ D	112. ○ A ○ B ○ C ○ D	142. ○ A ○ B ○ C ○ D
23. ○ A ○ B ○ C ○ D	53. ○ A ○ B ○ C ○ D	83. ○ A ○ B ○ C ○ D	113. ○ A ○ B ○ C ○ D	143. ○ A ○ B ○ C ○ D
24. ○ A ○ B ○ C ○ D	54. ○ A ○ B ○ C ○ D	84. ○ A ○ B ○ C ○ D	114. ○ A ○ B ○ C ○ D	144. ○ A ○ B ○ C ○ D
25. ○ A ○ B ○ C ○ D	55. ○ A ○ B ○ C ○ D	85. ○ A ○ B ○ C ○ D	115. ○ A ○ B ○ C ○ D	145. ○ A ○ B ○ C ○ D
26. ○ A ○ B ○ C ○ D	56. ○ A ○ B ○ C ○ D	86. ○ A ○ B ○ C ○ D	116. ○ A ○ B ○ C ○ D	146. ○ A ○ B ○ C ○ D
27. ○ A ○ B ○ C ○ D	57. ○ A ○ B ○ C ○ D	87. ○ A ○ B ○ C ○ D	117. ○ A ○ B ○ C ○ D	147. ○ A ○ B ○ C ○ D
28. ○ A ○ B ○ C ○ D	58. ○ A ○ B ○ C ○ D	88. ○ A ○ B ○ C ○ D	118. ○ A ○ B ○ C ○ D	148. ○ A ○ B ○ C ○ D
29. ○ A ○ B ○ C ○ D	59. ○ A ○ B ○ C ○ D	89. ○ A ○ B ○ C ○ D	119. ○ A ○ B ○ C ○ D	149. ○ A ○ B ○ C ○ D
30. ○ A ○ B ○ C ○ D	60. ○ A ○ B ○ C ○ D	90. ○ A ○ B ○ C ○ D	120. ○ A ○ B ○ C ○ D	150. ○ A ○ B ○ C ○ D

Self-Diagnostic Profile

How to Use the Self-Assessment Worksheet

1. Indicate on your answer sheet whether your answers are correct or incorrect.
2. Note the items you answered incorrectly.
3. Count the total number of items you answered incorrectly in each category.
4. Compare the total number of items you answered incorrectly in each category with the total number of items per category. This information will give you an idea of where you will need to focus your continued study.

Content Category	Questions Answered Incorrectly	Total Number of Questions Answered Incorrectly in Each Category	Total Number of Questions in Each CEN Content Category
Cardiovascular Emergencies			20
Respiratory Emergencies			16
Neurological Emergencies			16
Gastrointestinal, Genitourinary, Gynecology, and Obstetrical Emergencies			21
Psychosocial and Medical Emergencies			25
Maxillofacial, Ocular, Orthopedic, and Wound Emergencies			21
Environment and Toxicology Emergencies, and Communicable Diseases			15
Professional Issues			16

Practice Examination Answer Sheet

1. ○ A ○ B ○ C ○ D	31. ○ A ○ B ○ C ○ D	61. ○ A ○ B ○ C ○ D	91. ○ A ○ B ○ C ○ D	121. ○ A ○ B ○ C ○ D
2. ○ A ○ B ○ C ○ D	32. ○ A ○ B ○ C ○ D	62. ○ A ○ B ○ C ○ D	92. ○ A ○ B ○ C ○ D	122. ○ A ○ B ○ C ○ D
3. ○ A ○ B ○ C ○ D	33. ○ A ○ B ○ C ○ D	63. ○ A ○ B ○ C ○ D	93. ○ A ○ B ○ C ○ D	123. ○ A ○ B ○ C ○ D
4. ○ A ○ B ○ C ○ D	34. ○ A ○ B ○ C ○ D	64. ○ A ○ B ○ C ○ D	94. ○ A ○ B ○ C ○ D	124. ○ A ○ B ○ C ○ D
5. ○ A ○ B ○ C ○ D	35. ○ A ○ B ○ C ○ D	65. ○ A ○ B ○ C ○ D	95. ○ A ○ B ○ C ○ D	125. ○ A ○ B ○ C ○ D
6. ○ A ○ B ○ C ○ D	36. ○ A ○ B ○ C ○ D	66. ○ A ○ B ○ C ○ D	96. ○ A ○ B ○ C ○ D	126. ○ A ○ B ○ C ○ D
7. ○ A ○ B ○ C ○ D	37. ○ A ○ B ○ C ○ D	67. ○ A ○ B ○ C ○ D	97. ○ A ○ B ○ C ○ D	127. ○ A ○ B ○ C ○ D
8. ○ A ○ B ○ C ○ D	38. ○ A ○ B ○ C ○ D	68. ○ A ○ B ○ C ○ D	98. ○ A ○ B ○ C ○ D	128. ○ A ○ B ○ C ○ D
9. ○ A ○ B ○ C ○ D	39. ○ A ○ B ○ C ○ D	69. ○ A ○ B ○ C ○ D	99. ○ A ○ B ○ C ○ D	129. ○ A ○ B ○ C ○ D
10. ○ A ○ B ○ C ○ D	40. ○ A ○ B ○ C ○ D	70. ○ A ○ B ○ C ○ D	100. ○ A ○ B ○ C ○ D	130. ○ A ○ B ○ C ○ D
11. ○ A ○ B ○ C ○ D	41. ○ A ○ B ○ C ○ D	71. ○ A ○ B ○ C ○ D	101. ○ A ○ B ○ C ○ D	131. ○ A ○ B ○ C ○ D
12. ○ A ○ B ○ C ○ D	42. ○ A ○ B ○ C ○ D	72. ○ A ○ B ○ C ○ D	102. ○ A ○ B ○ C ○ D	132. ○ A ○ B ○ C ○ D
13. ○ A ○ B ○ C ○ D	43. ○ A ○ B ○ C ○ D	73. ○ A ○ B ○ C ○ D	103. ○ A ○ B ○ C ○ D	133. ○ A ○ B ○ C ○ D
14. ○ A ○ B ○ C ○ D	44. ○ A ○ B ○ C ○ D	74. ○ A ○ B ○ C ○ D	104. ○ A ○ B ○ C ○ D	134. ○ A ○ B ○ C ○ D
15. ○ A ○ B ○ C ○ D	45. ○ A ○ B ○ C ○ D	75. ○ A ○ B ○ C ○ D	105. ○ A ○ B ○ C ○ D	135. ○ A ○ B ○ C ○ D
16. ○ A ○ B ○ C ○ D	46. ○ A ○ B ○ C ○ D	76. ○ A ○ B ○ C ○ D	106. ○ A ○ B ○ C ○ D	136. ○ A ○ B ○ C ○ D
17. ○ A ○ B ○ C ○ D	47. ○ A ○ B ○ C ○ D	77. ○ A ○ B ○ C ○ D	107. ○ A ○ B ○ C ○ D	137. ○ A ○ B ○ C ○ D
18. ○ A ○ B ○ C ○ D	48. ○ A ○ B ○ C ○ D	78. ○ A ○ B ○ C ○ D	108. ○ A ○ B ○ C ○ D	138. ○ A ○ B ○ C ○ D
19. ○ A ○ B ○ C ○ D	49. ○ A ○ B ○ C ○ D	79. ○ A ○ B ○ C ○ D	109. ○ A ○ B ○ C ○ D	139. ○ A ○ B ○ C ○ D
20. ○ A ○ B ○ C ○ D	50. ○ A ○ B ○ C ○ D	80. ○ A ○ B ○ C ○ D	110. ○ A ○ B ○ C ○ D	140. ○ A ○ B ○ C ○ D
21. ○ A ○ B ○ C ○ D	51. ○ A ○ B ○ C ○ D	81. ○ A ○ B ○ C ○ D	111. ○ A ○ B ○ C ○ D	141. ○ A ○ B ○ C ○ D
22. ○ A ○ B ○ C ○ D	52. ○ A ○ B ○ C ○ D	82. ○ A ○ B ○ C ○ D	112. ○ A ○ B ○ C ○ D	142. ○ A ○ B ○ C ○ D
23. ○ A ○ B ○ C ○ D	53. ○ A ○ B ○ C ○ D	83. ○ A ○ B ○ C ○ D	113. ○ A ○ B ○ C ○ D	143. ○ A ○ B ○ C ○ D
24. ○ A ○ B ○ C ○ D	54. ○ A ○ B ○ C ○ D	84. ○ A ○ B ○ C ○ D	114. ○ A ○ B ○ C ○ D	144. ○ A ○ B ○ C ○ D
25. ○ A ○ B ○ C ○ D	55. ○ A ○ B ○ C ○ D	85. ○ A ○ B ○ C ○ D	115. ○ A ○ B ○ C ○ D	145. ○ A ○ B ○ C ○ D
26. ○ A ○ B ○ C ○ D	56. ○ A ○ B ○ C ○ D	86. ○ A ○ B ○ C ○ D	116. ○ A ○ B ○ C ○ D	146. ○ A ○ B ○ C ○ D
27. ○ A ○ B ○ C ○ D	57. ○ A ○ B ○ C ○ D	87. ○ A ○ B ○ C ○ D	117. ○ A ○ B ○ C ○ D	147. ○ A ○ B ○ C ○ D
28. ○ A ○ B ○ C ○ D	58. ○ A ○ B ○ C ○ D	88. ○ A ○ B ○ C ○ D	118. ○ A ○ B ○ C ○ D	148. ○ A ○ B ○ C ○ D
29. ○ A ○ B ○ C ○ D	59. ○ A ○ B ○ C ○ D	89. ○ A ○ B ○ C ○ D	119. ○ A ○ B ○ C ○ D	149. ○ A ○ B ○ C ○ D
30. ○ A ○ B ○ C ○ D	60. ○ A ○ B ○ C ○ D	90. ○ A ○ B ○ C ○ D	120. ○ A ○ B ○ C ○ D	150. ○ A ○ B ○ C ○ D

Self-Diagnostic Profile

How to Use the Self-Assessment Worksheet

1. Indicate on your answer sheet whether your answers are correct or incorrect.
2. Note the items you answered incorrectly.
3. Count the total number of items you answered incorrectly in each category.
4. Compare the total number of items you answered incorrectly in each category with the total number of items per category. This information will give you an idea of where you will need to focus your continued study.

Content Category	Questions Answered Incorrectly	Total Number of Questions Answered Incorrectly in Each Category	Total Number of Questions in Each CEN Content Category
Cardiovascular Emergencies			20
Respiratory Emergencies			16
Neurological Emergencies			16
Gastrointestinal, Genitourinary, Gynecology, and Obstetrical Emergencies			21
Psychosocial and Medical Emergencies			25
Maxillofacial, Ocular, Orthopedic, and Wound Emergencies			21
Environment and Toxicology Emergencies, and Communicable Diseases			15
Professional Issues			16

Practice Examination Answer Sheet

1. ○ A ○ B ○ C ○ D	31. ○ A ○ B ○ C ○ D	61. ○ A ○ B ○ C ○ D	91. ○ A ○ B ○ C ○ D	121. ○ A ○ B ○ C ○ D
2. ○ A ○ B ○ C ○ D	32. ○ A ○ B ○ C ○ D	62. ○ A ○ B ○ C ○ D	92. ○ A ○ B ○ C ○ D	122. ○ A ○ B ○ C ○ D
3. ○ A ○ B ○ C ○ D	33. ○ A ○ B ○ C ○ D	63. ○ A ○ B ○ C ○ D	93. ○ A ○ B ○ C ○ D	123. ○ A ○ B ○ C ○ D
4. ○ A ○ B ○ C ○ D	34. ○ A ○ B ○ C ○ D	64. ○ A ○ B ○ C ○ D	94. ○ A ○ B ○ C ○ D	124. ○ A ○ B ○ C ○ D
5. ○ A ○ B ○ C ○ D	35. ○ A ○ B ○ C ○ D	65. ○ A ○ B ○ C ○ D	95. ○ A ○ B ○ C ○ D	125. ○ A ○ B ○ C ○ D
6. ○ A ○ B ○ C ○ D	36. ○ A ○ B ○ C ○ D	66. ○ A ○ B ○ C ○ D	96. ○ A ○ B ○ C ○ D	126. ○ A ○ B ○ C ○ D
7. ○ A ○ B ○ C ○ D	37. ○ A ○ B ○ C ○ D	67. ○ A ○ B ○ C ○ D	97. ○ A ○ B ○ C ○ D	127. ○ A ○ B ○ C ○ D
8. ○ A ○ B ○ C ○ D	38. ○ A ○ B ○ C ○ D	68. ○ A ○ B ○ C ○ D	98. ○ A ○ B ○ C ○ D	128. ○ A ○ B ○ C ○ D
9. ○ A ○ B ○ C ○ D	39. ○ A ○ B ○ C ○ D	69. ○ A ○ B ○ C ○ D	99. ○ A ○ B ○ C ○ D	129. ○ A ○ B ○ C ○ D
10. ○ A ○ B ○ C ○ D	40. ○ A ○ B ○ C ○ D	70. ○ A ○ B ○ C ○ D	100. ○ A ○ B ○ C ○ D	130. ○ A ○ B ○ C ○ D
11. ○ A ○ B ○ C ○ D	41. ○ A ○ B ○ C ○ D	71. ○ A ○ B ○ C ○ D	101. ○ A ○ B ○ C ○ D	131. ○ A ○ B ○ C ○ D
12. ○ A ○ B ○ C ○ D	42. ○ A ○ B ○ C ○ D	72. ○ A ○ B ○ C ○ D	102. ○ A ○ B ○ C ○ D	132. ○ A ○ B ○ C ○ D
13. ○ A ○ B ○ C ○ D	43. ○ A ○ B ○ C ○ D	73. ○ A ○ B ○ C ○ D	103. ○ A ○ B ○ C ○ D	133. ○ A ○ B ○ C ○ D
14. ○ A ○ B ○ C ○ D	44. ○ A ○ B ○ C ○ D	74. ○ A ○ B ○ C ○ D	104. ○ A ○ B ○ C ○ D	134. ○ A ○ B ○ C ○ D
15. ○ A ○ B ○ C ○ D	45. ○ A ○ B ○ C ○ D	75. ○ A ○ B ○ C ○ D	105. ○ A ○ B ○ C ○ D	135. ○ A ○ B ○ C ○ D
16. ○ A ○ B ○ C ○ D	46. ○ A ○ B ○ C ○ D	76. ○ A ○ B ○ C ○ D	106. ○ A ○ B ○ C ○ D	136. ○ A ○ B ○ C ○ D
17. ○ A ○ B ○ C ○ D	47. ○ A ○ B ○ C ○ D	77. ○ A ○ B ○ C ○ D	107. ○ A ○ B ○ C ○ D	137. ○ A ○ B ○ C ○ D
18. ○ A ○ B ○ C ○ D	48. ○ A ○ B ○ C ○ D	78. ○ A ○ B ○ C ○ D	108. ○ A ○ B ○ C ○ D	138. ○ A ○ B ○ C ○ D
19. ○ A ○ B ○ C ○ D	49. ○ A ○ B ○ C ○ D	79. ○ A ○ B ○ C ○ D	109. ○ A ○ B ○ C ○ D	139. ○ A ○ B ○ C ○ D
20. ○ A ○ B ○ C ○ D	50. ○ A ○ B ○ C ○ D	80. ○ A ○ B ○ C ○ D	110. ○ A ○ B ○ C ○ D	140. ○ A ○ B ○ C ○ D
21. ○ A ○ B ○ C ○ D	51. ○ A ○ B ○ C ○ D	81. ○ A ○ B ○ C ○ D	111. ○ A ○ B ○ C ○ D	141. ○ A ○ B ○ C ○ D
22. ○ A ○ B ○ C ○ D	52. ○ A ○ B ○ C ○ D	82. ○ A ○ B ○ C ○ D	112. ○ A ○ B ○ C ○ D	142. ○ A ○ B ○ C ○ D
23. ○ A ○ B ○ C ○ D	53. ○ A ○ B ○ C ○ D	83. ○ A ○ B ○ C ○ D	113. ○ A ○ B ○ C ○ D	143. ○ A ○ B ○ C ○ D
24. ○ A ○ B ○ C ○ D	54. ○ A ○ B ○ C ○ D	84. ○ A ○ B ○ C ○ D	114. ○ A ○ B ○ C ○ D	144. ○ A ○ B ○ C ○ D
25. ○ A ○ B ○ C ○ D	55. ○ A ○ B ○ C ○ D	85. ○ A ○ B ○ C ○ D	115. ○ A ○ B ○ C ○ D	145. ○ A ○ B ○ C ○ D
26. ○ A ○ B ○ C ○ D	56. ○ A ○ B ○ C ○ D	86. ○ A ○ B ○ C ○ D	116. ○ A ○ B ○ C ○ D	146. ○ A ○ B ○ C ○ D
27. ○ A ○ B ○ C ○ D	57. ○ A ○ B ○ C ○ D	87. ○ A ○ B ○ C ○ D	117. ○ A ○ B ○ C ○ D	147. ○ A ○ B ○ C ○ D
28. ○ A ○ B ○ C ○ D	58. ○ A ○ B ○ C ○ D	88. ○ A ○ B ○ C ○ D	118. ○ A ○ B ○ C ○ D	148. ○ A ○ B ○ C ○ D
29. ○ A ○ B ○ C ○ D	59. ○ A ○ B ○ C ○ D	89. ○ A ○ B ○ C ○ D	119. ○ A ○ B ○ C ○ D	149. ○ A ○ B ○ C ○ D
30. ○ A ○ B ○ C ○ D	60. ○ A ○ B ○ C ○ D	90. ○ A ○ B ○ C ○ D	120. ○ A ○ B ○ C ○ D	150. ○ A ○ B ○ C ○ D

Self-Diagnostic Profile

How to Use the Self-Assessment Worksheet

1. Indicate on your answer sheet whether your answers are correct or incorrect.
2. Note the items you answered incorrectly.
3. Count the total number of items you answered incorrectly in each category.
4. Compare the total number of items you answered incorrectly in each category with the total number of items per category. This information will give you an idea of where you will need to focus your continued study.

Content Category	Questions Answered Incorrectly	Total Number of Questions Answered Incorrectly in Each Category	Total Number of Questions in Each CEN Content Category
Cardiovascular Emergencies			20
Respiratory Emergencies			16
Neurological Emergencies			16
Gastrointestinal, Genitourinary, Gynecology, and Obstetrical Emergencies			21
Psychosocial and Medical Emergencies			25
Maxillofacial, Ocular, Orthopedic, and Wound Emergencies			21
Environment and Toxicology Emergencies, and Communicable Diseases			15
Professional Issues			16

Practice Examination Answer Sheet

1. ○A ○B ○C ○D	31. ○A ○B ○C ○D	61. ○A ○B ○C ○D	91. ○A ○B ○C ○D	121. ○A ○B ○C ○D
2. ○A ○B ○C ○D	32. ○A ○B ○C ○D	62. ○A ○B ○C ○D	92. ○A ○B ○C ○D	122. ○A ○B ○C ○D
3. ○A ○B ○C ○D	33. ○A ○B ○C ○D	63. ○A ○B ○C ○D	93. ○A ○B ○C ○D	123. ○A ○B ○C ○D
4. ○A ○B ○C ○D	34. ○A ○B ○C ○D	64. ○A ○B ○C ○D	94. ○A ○B ○C ○D	124. ○A ○B ○C ○D
5. ○A ○B ○C ○D	35. ○A ○B ○C ○D	65. ○A ○B ○C ○D	95. ○A ○B ○C ○D	125. ○A ○B ○C ○D
6. ○A ○B ○C ○D	36. ○A ○B ○C ○D	66. ○A ○B ○C ○D	96. ○A ○B ○C ○D	126. ○A ○B ○C ○D
7. ○A ○B ○C ○D	37. ○A ○B ○C ○D	67. ○A ○B ○C ○D	97. ○A ○B ○C ○D	127. ○A ○B ○C ○D
8. ○A ○B ○C ○D	38. ○A ○B ○C ○D	68. ○A ○B ○C ○D	98. ○A ○B ○C ○D	128. ○A ○B ○C ○D
9. ○A ○B ○C ○D	39. ○A ○B ○C ○D	69. ○A ○B ○C ○D	99. ○A ○B ○C ○D	129. ○A ○B ○C ○D
10. ○A ○B ○C ○D	40. ○A ○B ○C ○D	70. ○A ○B ○C ○D	100. ○A ○B ○C ○D	130. ○A ○B ○C ○D
11. ○A ○B ○C ○D	41. ○A ○B ○C ○D	71. ○A ○B ○C ○D	101. ○A ○B ○C ○D	131. ○A ○B ○C ○D
12. ○A ○B ○C ○D	42. ○A ○B ○C ○D	72. ○A ○B ○C ○D	102. ○A ○B ○C ○D	132. ○A ○B ○C ○D
13. ○A ○B ○C ○D	43. ○A ○B ○C ○D	73. ○A ○B ○C ○D	103. ○A ○B ○C ○D	133. ○A ○B ○C ○D
14. ○A ○B ○C ○D	44. ○A ○B ○C ○D	74. ○A ○B ○C ○D	104. ○A ○B ○C ○D	134. ○A ○B ○C ○D
15. ○A ○B ○C ○D	45. ○A ○B ○C ○D	75. ○A ○B ○C ○D	105. ○A ○B ○C ○D	135. ○A ○B ○C ○D
16. ○A ○B ○C ○D	46. ○A ○B ○C ○D	76. ○A ○B ○C ○D	106. ○A ○B ○C ○D	136. ○A ○B ○C ○D
17. ○A ○B ○C ○D	47. ○A ○B ○C ○D	77. ○A ○B ○C ○D	107. ○A ○B ○C ○D	137. ○A ○B ○C ○D
18. ○A ○B ○C ○D	48. ○A ○B ○C ○D	78. ○A ○B ○C ○D	108. ○A ○B ○C ○D	138. ○A ○B ○C ○D
19. ○A ○B ○C ○D	49. ○A ○B ○C ○D	79. ○A ○B ○C ○D	109. ○A ○B ○C ○D	139. ○A ○B ○C ○D
20. ○A ○B ○C ○D	50. ○A ○B ○C ○D	80. ○A ○B ○C ○D	110. ○A ○B ○C ○D	140. ○A ○B ○C ○D
21. ○A ○B ○C ○D	51. ○A ○B ○C ○D	81. ○A ○B ○C ○D	111. ○A ○B ○C ○D	141. ○A ○B ○C ○D
22. ○A ○B ○C ○D	52. ○A ○B ○C ○D	82. ○A ○B ○C ○D	112. ○A ○B ○C ○D	142. ○A ○B ○C ○D
23. ○A ○B ○C ○D	53. ○A ○B ○C ○D	83. ○A ○B ○C ○D	113. ○A ○B ○C ○D	143. ○A ○B ○C ○D
24. ○A ○B ○C ○D	54. ○A ○B ○C ○D	84. ○A ○B ○C ○D	114. ○A ○B ○C ○D	144. ○A ○B ○C ○D
25. ○A ○B ○C ○D	55. ○A ○B ○C ○D	85. ○A ○B ○C ○D	115. ○A ○B ○C ○D	145. ○A ○B ○C ○D
26. ○A ○B ○C ○D	56. ○A ○B ○C ○D	86. ○A ○B ○C ○D	116. ○A ○B ○C ○D	146. ○A ○B ○C ○D
27. ○A ○B ○C ○D	57. ○A ○B ○C ○D	87. ○A ○B ○C ○D	117. ○A ○B ○C ○D	147. ○A ○B ○C ○D
28. ○A ○B ○C ○D	58. ○A ○B ○C ○D	88. ○A ○B ○C ○D	118. ○A ○B ○C ○D	148. ○A ○B ○C ○D
29. ○A ○B ○C ○D	59. ○A ○B ○C ○D	89. ○A ○B ○C ○D	119. ○A ○B ○C ○D	149. ○A ○B ○C ○D
30. ○A ○B ○C ○D	60. ○A ○B ○C ○D	90. ○A ○B ○C ○D	120. ○A ○B ○C ○D	150. ○A ○B ○C ○D

Self-Diagnostic Profile

How to Use the Self-Assessment Worksheet

1. Indicate on your answer sheet whether your answers are correct or incorrect.
2. Note the items you answered incorrectly.
3. Count the total number of items you answered incorrectly in each category.
4. Compare the total number of items you answered incorrectly in each category with the total number of items per category. This information will give you an idea of where you will need to focus your continued study.

Content Category	Questions Answered Incorrectly	Total Number of Questions Answered Incorrectly in Each Category	Total Number of Questions in Each CEN Content Category
Cardiovascular Emergencies			20
Respiratory Emergencies			16
Neurological Emergencies			16
Gastrointestinal, Genitourinary, Gynecology, and Obstetrical Emergencies			21
Psychosocial and Medical Emergencies			25
Maxillofacial, Ocular, Orthopedic, and Wound Emergencies			21
Environment and Toxicology Emergencies, and Communicable Diseases			15
Professional Issues			16

Practice Examination Answer Sheet

1. ○ A ○ B ○ C ○ D	31. ○ A ○ B ○ C ○ D	61. ○ A ○ B ○ C ○ D	91. ○ A ○ B ○ C ○ D	121. ○ A ○ B ○ C ○ D
2. ○ A ○ B ○ C ○ D	32. ○ A ○ B ○ C ○ D	62. ○ A ○ B ○ C ○ D	92. ○ A ○ B ○ C ○ D	122. ○ A ○ B ○ C ○ D
3. ○ A ○ B ○ C ○ D	33. ○ A ○ B ○ C ○ D	63. ○ A ○ B ○ C ○ D	93. ○ A ○ B ○ C ○ D	123. ○ A ○ B ○ C ○ D
4. ○ A ○ B ○ C ○ D	34. ○ A ○ B ○ C ○ D	64. ○ A ○ B ○ C ○ D	94. ○ A ○ B ○ C ○ D	124. ○ A ○ B ○ C ○ D
5. ○ A ○ B ○ C ○ D	35. ○ A ○ B ○ C ○ D	65. ○ A ○ B ○ C ○ D	95. ○ A ○ B ○ C ○ D	125. ○ A ○ B ○ C ○ D
6. ○ A ○ B ○ C ○ D	36. ○ A ○ B ○ C ○ D	66. ○ A ○ B ○ C ○ D	96. ○ A ○ B ○ C ○ D	126. ○ A ○ B ○ C ○ D
7. ○ A ○ B ○ C ○ D	37. ○ A ○ B ○ C ○ D	67. ○ A ○ B ○ C ○ D	97. ○ A ○ B ○ C ○ D	127. ○ A ○ B ○ C ○ D
8. ○ A ○ B ○ C ○ D	38. ○ A ○ B ○ C ○ D	68. ○ A ○ B ○ C ○ D	98. ○ A ○ B ○ C ○ D	128. ○ A ○ B ○ C ○ D
9. ○ A ○ B ○ C ○ D	39. ○ A ○ B ○ C ○ D	69. ○ A ○ B ○ C ○ D	99. ○ A ○ B ○ C ○ D	129. ○ A ○ B ○ C ○ D
10. ○ A ○ B ○ C ○ D	40. ○ A ○ B ○ C ○ D	70. ○ A ○ B ○ C ○ D	100. ○ A ○ B ○ C ○ D	130. ○ A ○ B ○ C ○ D
11. ○ A ○ B ○ C ○ D	41. ○ A ○ B ○ C ○ D	71. ○ A ○ B ○ C ○ D	101. ○ A ○ B ○ C ○ D	131. ○ A ○ B ○ C ○ D
12. ○ A ○ B ○ C ○ D	42. ○ A ○ B ○ C ○ D	72. ○ A ○ B ○ C ○ D	102. ○ A ○ B ○ C ○ D	132. ○ A ○ B ○ C ○ D
13. ○ A ○ B ○ C ○ D	43. ○ A ○ B ○ C ○ D	73. ○ A ○ B ○ C ○ D	103. ○ A ○ B ○ C ○ D	133. ○ A ○ B ○ C ○ D
14. ○ A ○ B ○ C ○ D	44. ○ A ○ B ○ C ○ D	74. ○ A ○ B ○ C ○ D	104. ○ A ○ B ○ C ○ D	134. ○ A ○ B ○ C ○ D
15. ○ A ○ B ○ C ○ D	45. ○ A ○ B ○ C ○ D	75. ○ A ○ B ○ C ○ D	105. ○ A ○ B ○ C ○ D	135. ○ A ○ B ○ C ○ D
16. ○ A ○ B ○ C ○ D	46. ○ A ○ B ○ C ○ D	76. ○ A ○ B ○ C ○ D	106. ○ A ○ B ○ C ○ D	136. ○ A ○ B ○ C ○ D
17. ○ A ○ B ○ C ○ D	47. ○ A ○ B ○ C ○ D	77. ○ A ○ B ○ C ○ D	107. ○ A ○ B ○ C ○ D	137. ○ A ○ B ○ C ○ D
18. ○ A ○ B ○ C ○ D	48. ○ A ○ B ○ C ○ D	78. ○ A ○ B ○ C ○ D	108. ○ A ○ B ○ C ○ D	138. ○ A ○ B ○ C ○ D
19. ○ A ○ B ○ C ○ D	49. ○ A ○ B ○ C ○ D	79. ○ A ○ B ○ C ○ D	109. ○ A ○ B ○ C ○ D	139. ○ A ○ B ○ C ○ D
20. ○ A ○ B ○ C ○ D	50. ○ A ○ B ○ C ○ D	80. ○ A ○ B ○ C ○ D	110. ○ A ○ B ○ C ○ D	140. ○ A ○ B ○ C ○ D
21. ○ A ○ B ○ C ○ D	51. ○ A ○ B ○ C ○ D	81. ○ A ○ B ○ C ○ D	111. ○ A ○ B ○ C ○ D	141. ○ A ○ B ○ C ○ D
22. ○ A ○ B ○ C ○ D	52. ○ A ○ B ○ C ○ D	82. ○ A ○ B ○ C ○ D	112. ○ A ○ B ○ C ○ D	142. ○ A ○ B ○ C ○ D
23. ○ A ○ B ○ C ○ D	53. ○ A ○ B ○ C ○ D	83. ○ A ○ B ○ C ○ D	113. ○ A ○ B ○ C ○ D	143. ○ A ○ B ○ C ○ D
24. ○ A ○ B ○ C ○ D	54. ○ A ○ B ○ C ○ D	84. ○ A ○ B ○ C ○ D	114. ○ A ○ B ○ C ○ D	144. ○ A ○ B ○ C ○ D
25. ○ A ○ B ○ C ○ D	55. ○ A ○ B ○ C ○ D	85. ○ A ○ B ○ C ○ D	115. ○ A ○ B ○ C ○ D	145. ○ A ○ B ○ C ○ D
26. ○ A ○ B ○ C ○ D	56. ○ A ○ B ○ C ○ D	86. ○ A ○ B ○ C ○ D	116. ○ A ○ B ○ C ○ D	146. ○ A ○ B ○ C ○ D
27. ○ A ○ B ○ C ○ D	57. ○ A ○ B ○ C ○ D	87. ○ A ○ B ○ C ○ D	117. ○ A ○ B ○ C ○ D	147. ○ A ○ B ○ C ○ D
28. ○ A ○ B ○ C ○ D	58. ○ A ○ B ○ C ○ D	88. ○ A ○ B ○ C ○ D	118. ○ A ○ B ○ C ○ D	148. ○ A ○ B ○ C ○ D
29. ○ A ○ B ○ C ○ D	59. ○ A ○ B ○ C ○ D	89. ○ A ○ B ○ C ○ D	119. ○ A ○ B ○ C ○ D	149. ○ A ○ B ○ C ○ D
30. ○ A ○ B ○ C ○ D	60. ○ A ○ B ○ C ○ D	90. ○ A ○ B ○ C ○ D	120. ○ A ○ B ○ C ○ D	150. ○ A ○ B ○ C ○ D

Self-Diagnostic Profile

How to Use the Self-Assessment Worksheet

1. Indicate on your answer sheet whether your answers are correct or incorrect.
2. Note the items you answered incorrectly.
3. Count the total number of items you answered incorrectly in each category.
4. Compare the total number of items you answered incorrectly in each category with the total number of items per category. This information will give you an idea of where you will need to focus your continued study.

Content Category	Questions Answered Incorrectly	Total Number of Questions Answered Incorrectly in Each Category	Total Number of Questions in Each CEN Content Category
Cardiovascular Emergencies			20
Respiratory Emergencies			16
Neurological Emergencies			16
Gastrointestinal, Genitourinary, Gynecology, and Obstetrical Emergencies			21
Psychosocial and Medical Emergencies			25
Maxillofacial, Ocular, Orthopedic, and Wound Emergencies			21
Environment and Toxicology Emergencies, and Communicable Diseases			15
Professional Issues			16

Practice Examination Answer Sheet

1. ○ A ○ B ○ C ○ D	31. ○ A ○ B ○ C ○ D	61. ○ A ○ B ○ C ○ D	91. ○ A ○ B ○ C ○ D	121. ○ A ○ B ○ C ○ D
2. ○ A ○ B ○ C ○ D	32. ○ A ○ B ○ C ○ D	62. ○ A ○ B ○ C ○ D	92. ○ A ○ B ○ C ○ D	122. ○ A ○ B ○ C ○ D
3. ○ A ○ B ○ C ○ D	33. ○ A ○ B ○ C ○ D	63. ○ A ○ B ○ C ○ D	93. ○ A ○ B ○ C ○ D	123. ○ A ○ B ○ C ○ D
4. ○ A ○ B ○ C ○ D	34. ○ A ○ B ○ C ○ D	64. ○ A ○ B ○ C ○ D	94. ○ A ○ B ○ C ○ D	124. ○ A ○ B ○ C ○ D
5. ○ A ○ B ○ C ○ D	35. ○ A ○ B ○ C ○ D	65. ○ A ○ B ○ C ○ D	95. ○ A ○ B ○ C ○ D	125. ○ A ○ B ○ C ○ D
6. ○ A ○ B ○ C ○ D	36. ○ A ○ B ○ C ○ D	66. ○ A ○ B ○ C ○ D	96. ○ A ○ B ○ C ○ D	126. ○ A ○ B ○ C ○ D
7. ○ A ○ B ○ C ○ D	37. ○ A ○ B ○ C ○ D	67. ○ A ○ B ○ C ○ D	97. ○ A ○ B ○ C ○ D	127. ○ A ○ B ○ C ○ D
8. ○ A ○ B ○ C ○ D	38. ○ A ○ B ○ C ○ D	68. ○ A ○ B ○ C ○ D	98. ○ A ○ B ○ C ○ D	128. ○ A ○ B ○ C ○ D
9. ○ A ○ B ○ C ○ D	39. ○ A ○ B ○ C ○ D	69. ○ A ○ B ○ C ○ D	99. ○ A ○ B ○ C ○ D	129. ○ A ○ B ○ C ○ D
10. ○ A ○ B ○ C ○ D	40. ○ A ○ B ○ C ○ D	70. ○ A ○ B ○ C ○ D	100. ○ A ○ B ○ C ○ D	130. ○ A ○ B ○ C ○ D
11. ○ A ○ B ○ C ○ D	41. ○ A ○ B ○ C ○ D	71. ○ A ○ B ○ C ○ D	101. ○ A ○ B ○ C ○ D	131. ○ A ○ B ○ C ○ D
12. ○ A ○ B ○ C ○ D	42. ○ A ○ B ○ C ○ D	72. ○ A ○ B ○ C ○ D	102. ○ A ○ B ○ C ○ D	132. ○ A ○ B ○ C ○ D
13. ○ A ○ B ○ C ○ D	43. ○ A ○ B ○ C ○ D	73. ○ A ○ B ○ C ○ D	103. ○ A ○ B ○ C ○ D	133. ○ A ○ B ○ C ○ D
14. ○ A ○ B ○ C ○ D	44. ○ A ○ B ○ C ○ D	74. ○ A ○ B ○ C ○ D	104. ○ A ○ B ○ C ○ D	134. ○ A ○ B ○ C ○ D
15. ○ A ○ B ○ C ○ D	45. ○ A ○ B ○ C ○ D	75. ○ A ○ B ○ C ○ D	105. ○ A ○ B ○ C ○ D	135. ○ A ○ B ○ C ○ D
16. ○ A ○ B ○ C ○ D	46. ○ A ○ B ○ C ○ D	76. ○ A ○ B ○ C ○ D	106. ○ A ○ B ○ C ○ D	136. ○ A ○ B ○ C ○ D
17. ○ A ○ B ○ C ○ D	47. ○ A ○ B ○ C ○ D	77. ○ A ○ B ○ C ○ D	107. ○ A ○ B ○ C ○ D	137. ○ A ○ B ○ C ○ D
18. ○ A ○ B ○ C ○ D	48. ○ A ○ B ○ C ○ D	78. ○ A ○ B ○ C ○ D	108. ○ A ○ B ○ C ○ D	138. ○ A ○ B ○ C ○ D
19. ○ A ○ B ○ C ○ D	49. ○ A ○ B ○ C ○ D	79. ○ A ○ B ○ C ○ D	109. ○ A ○ B ○ C ○ D	139. ○ A ○ B ○ C ○ D
20. ○ A ○ B ○ C ○ D	50. ○ A ○ B ○ C ○ D	80. ○ A ○ B ○ C ○ D	110. ○ A ○ B ○ C ○ D	140. ○ A ○ B ○ C ○ D
21. ○ A ○ B ○ C ○ D	51. ○ A ○ B ○ C ○ D	81. ○ A ○ B ○ C ○ D	111. ○ A ○ B ○ C ○ D	141. ○ A ○ B ○ C ○ D
22. ○ A ○ B ○ C ○ D	52. ○ A ○ B ○ C ○ D	82. ○ A ○ B ○ C ○ D	112. ○ A ○ B ○ C ○ D	142. ○ A ○ B ○ C ○ D
23. ○ A ○ B ○ C ○ D	53. ○ A ○ B ○ C ○ D	83. ○ A ○ B ○ C ○ D	113. ○ A ○ B ○ C ○ D	143. ○ A ○ B ○ C ○ D
24. ○ A ○ B ○ C ○ D	54. ○ A ○ B ○ C ○ D	84. ○ A ○ B ○ C ○ D	114. ○ A ○ B ○ C ○ D	144. ○ A ○ B ○ C ○ D
25. ○ A ○ B ○ C ○ D	55. ○ A ○ B ○ C ○ D	85. ○ A ○ B ○ C ○ D	115. ○ A ○ B ○ C ○ D	145. ○ A ○ B ○ C ○ D
26. ○ A ○ B ○ C ○ D	56. ○ A ○ B ○ C ○ D	86. ○ A ○ B ○ C ○ D	116. ○ A ○ B ○ C ○ D	146. ○ A ○ B ○ C ○ D
27. ○ A ○ B ○ C ○ D	57. ○ A ○ B ○ C ○ D	87. ○ A ○ B ○ C ○ D	117. ○ A ○ B ○ C ○ D	147. ○ A ○ B ○ C ○ D
28. ○ A ○ B ○ C ○ D	58. ○ A ○ B ○ C ○ D	88. ○ A ○ B ○ C ○ D	118. ○ A ○ B ○ C ○ D	148. ○ A ○ B ○ C ○ D
29. ○ A ○ B ○ C ○ D	59. ○ A ○ B ○ C ○ D	89. ○ A ○ B ○ C ○ D	119. ○ A ○ B ○ C ○ D	149. ○ A ○ B ○ C ○ D
30. ○ A ○ B ○ C ○ D	60. ○ A ○ B ○ C ○ D	90. ○ A ○ B ○ C ○ D	120. ○ A ○ B ○ C ○ D	150. ○ A ○ B ○ C ○ D

Self-Diagnostic Profile

How to Use the Self-Assessment Worksheet

1. Indicate on your answer sheet whether your answers are correct or incorrect.
2. Note the items you answered incorrectly.
3. Count the total number of items you answered incorrectly in each category.
4. Compare the total number of items you answered incorrectly in each category with the total number of items per category. This information will give you an idea of where you will need to focus your continued study.

Content Category	Questions Answered Incorrectly	Total Number of Questions Answered Incorrectly in Each Category	Total Number of Questions in Each CEN Content Category
Cardiovascular Emergencies			20
Respiratory Emergencies			16
Neurological Emergencies			16
Gastrointestinal, Genitourinary, Gynecology, and Obstetrical Emergencies			21
Psychosocial and Medical Emergencies			25
Maxillofacial, Ocular, Orthopedic, and Wound Emergencies			21
Environment and Toxicology Emergencies, and Communicable Diseases			15
Professional Issues			16

Practice Examination Answer Sheet

1. ○ A ○ B ○ C ○ D	31. ○ A ○ B ○ C ○ D	61. ○ A ○ B ○ C ○ D	91. ○ A ○ B ○ C ○ D	121. ○ A ○ B ○ C ○ D
2. ○ A ○ B ○ C ○ D	32. ○ A ○ B ○ C ○ D	62. ○ A ○ B ○ C ○ D	92. ○ A ○ B ○ C ○ D	122. ○ A ○ B ○ C ○ D
3. ○ A ○ B ○ C ○ D	33. ○ A ○ B ○ C ○ D	63. ○ A ○ B ○ C ○ D	93. ○ A ○ B ○ C ○ D	123. ○ A ○ B ○ C ○ D
4. ○ A ○ B ○ C ○ D	34. ○ A ○ B ○ C ○ D	64. ○ A ○ B ○ C ○ D	94. ○ A ○ B ○ C ○ D	124. ○ A ○ B ○ C ○ D
5. ○ A ○ B ○ C ○ D	35. ○ A ○ B ○ C ○ D	65. ○ A ○ B ○ C ○ D	95. ○ A ○ B ○ C ○ D	125. ○ A ○ B ○ C ○ D
6. ○ A ○ B ○ C ○ D	36. ○ A ○ B ○ C ○ D	66. ○ A ○ B ○ C ○ D	96. ○ A ○ B ○ C ○ D	126. ○ A ○ B ○ C ○ D
7. ○ A ○ B ○ C ○ D	37. ○ A ○ B ○ C ○ D	67. ○ A ○ B ○ C ○ D	97. ○ A ○ B ○ C ○ D	127. ○ A ○ B ○ C ○ D
8. ○ A ○ B ○ C ○ D	38. ○ A ○ B ○ C ○ D	68. ○ A ○ B ○ C ○ D	98. ○ A ○ B ○ C ○ D	128. ○ A ○ B ○ C ○ D
9. ○ A ○ B ○ C ○ D	39. ○ A ○ B ○ C ○ D	69. ○ A ○ B ○ C ○ D	99. ○ A ○ B ○ C ○ D	129. ○ A ○ B ○ C ○ D
10. ○ A ○ B ○ C ○ D	40. ○ A ○ B ○ C ○ D	70. ○ A ○ B ○ C ○ D	100. ○ A ○ B ○ C ○ D	130. ○ A ○ B ○ C ○ D
11. ○ A ○ B ○ C ○ D	41. ○ A ○ B ○ C ○ D	71. ○ A ○ B ○ C ○ D	101. ○ A ○ B ○ C ○ D	131. ○ A ○ B ○ C ○ D
12. ○ A ○ B ○ C ○ D	42. ○ A ○ B ○ C ○ D	72. ○ A ○ B ○ C ○ D	102. ○ A ○ B ○ C ○ D	132. ○ A ○ B ○ C ○ D
13. ○ A ○ B ○ C ○ D	43. ○ A ○ B ○ C ○ D	73. ○ A ○ B ○ C ○ D	103. ○ A ○ B ○ C ○ D	133. ○ A ○ B ○ C ○ D
14. ○ A ○ B ○ C ○ D	44. ○ A ○ B ○ C ○ D	74. ○ A ○ B ○ C ○ D	104. ○ A ○ B ○ C ○ D	134. ○ A ○ B ○ C ○ D
15. ○ A ○ B ○ C ○ D	45. ○ A ○ B ○ C ○ D	75. ○ A ○ B ○ C ○ D	105. ○ A ○ B ○ C ○ D	135. ○ A ○ B ○ C ○ D
16. ○ A ○ B ○ C ○ D	46. ○ A ○ B ○ C ○ D	76. ○ A ○ B ○ C ○ D	106. ○ A ○ B ○ C ○ D	136. ○ A ○ B ○ C ○ D
17. ○ A ○ B ○ C ○ D	47. ○ A ○ B ○ C ○ D	77. ○ A ○ B ○ C ○ D	107. ○ A ○ B ○ C ○ D	137. ○ A ○ B ○ C ○ D
18. ○ A ○ B ○ C ○ D	48. ○ A ○ B ○ C ○ D	78. ○ A ○ B ○ C ○ D	108. ○ A ○ B ○ C ○ D	138. ○ A ○ B ○ C ○ D
19. ○ A ○ B ○ C ○ D	49. ○ A ○ B ○ C ○ D	79. ○ A ○ B ○ C ○ D	109. ○ A ○ B ○ C ○ D	139. ○ A ○ B ○ C ○ D
20. ○ A ○ B ○ C ○ D	50. ○ A ○ B ○ C ○ D	80. ○ A ○ B ○ C ○ D	110. ○ A ○ B ○ C ○ D	140. ○ A ○ B ○ C ○ D
21. ○ A ○ B ○ C ○ D	51. ○ A ○ B ○ C ○ D	81. ○ A ○ B ○ C ○ D	111. ○ A ○ B ○ C ○ D	141. ○ A ○ B ○ C ○ D
22. ○ A ○ B ○ C ○ D	52. ○ A ○ B ○ C ○ D	82. ○ A ○ B ○ C ○ D	112. ○ A ○ B ○ C ○ D	142. ○ A ○ B ○ C ○ D
23. ○ A ○ B ○ C ○ D	53. ○ A ○ B ○ C ○ D	83. ○ A ○ B ○ C ○ D	113. ○ A ○ B ○ C ○ D	143. ○ A ○ B ○ C ○ D
24. ○ A ○ B ○ C ○ D	54. ○ A ○ B ○ C ○ D	84. ○ A ○ B ○ C ○ D	114. ○ A ○ B ○ C ○ D	144. ○ A ○ B ○ C ○ D
25. ○ A ○ B ○ C ○ D	55. ○ A ○ B ○ C ○ D	85. ○ A ○ B ○ C ○ D	115. ○ A ○ B ○ C ○ D	145. ○ A ○ B ○ C ○ D
26. ○ A ○ B ○ C ○ D	56. ○ A ○ B ○ C ○ D	86. ○ A ○ B ○ C ○ D	116. ○ A ○ B ○ C ○ D	146. ○ A ○ B ○ C ○ D
27. ○ A ○ B ○ C ○ D	57. ○ A ○ B ○ C ○ D	87. ○ A ○ B ○ C ○ D	117. ○ A ○ B ○ C ○ D	147. ○ A ○ B ○ C ○ D
28. ○ A ○ B ○ C ○ D	58. ○ A ○ B ○ C ○ D	88. ○ A ○ B ○ C ○ D	118. ○ A ○ B ○ C ○ D	148. ○ A ○ B ○ C ○ D
29. ○ A ○ B ○ C ○ D	59. ○ A ○ B ○ C ○ D	89. ○ A ○ B ○ C ○ D	119. ○ A ○ B ○ C ○ D	149. ○ A ○ B ○ C ○ D
30. ○ A ○ B ○ C ○ D	60. ○ A ○ B ○ C ○ D	90. ○ A ○ B ○ C ○ D	120. ○ A ○ B ○ C ○ D	150. ○ A ○ B ○ C ○ D

Self-Diagnostic Profile

How to Use the Self-Assessment Worksheet

1. Indicate on your answer sheet whether your answers are correct or incorrect.
2. Note the items you answered incorrectly.
3. Count the total number of items you answered incorrectly in each category.
4. Compare the total number of items you answered incorrectly in each category with the total number of items per category. This information will give you an idea of where you will need to focus your continued study.

Content Category	Questions Answered Incorrectly	Total Number of Questions Answered Incorrectly in Each Category	Total Number of Questions in Each CEN Content Category
Cardiovascular Emergencies			20
Respiratory Emergencies			16
Neurological Emergencies			16
Gastrointestinal, Genitourinary, Gynecology, and Obstetrical Emergencies			21
Psychosocial and Medical Emergencies			25
Maxillofacial, Ocular, Orthopedic, and Wound Emergencies			21
Environment and Toxicology Emergencies, and Communicable Diseases			15
Professional Issues			16

Practice Examination Answer Sheet

1. ○ A ○ B ○ C ○ D	31. ○ A ○ B ○ C ○ D	61. ○ A ○ B ○ C ○ D	91. ○ A ○ B ○ C ○ D	121. ○ A ○ B ○ C ○ D
2. ○ A ○ B ○ C ○ D	32. ○ A ○ B ○ C ○ D	62. ○ A ○ B ○ C ○ D	92. ○ A ○ B ○ C ○ D	122. ○ A ○ B ○ C ○ D
3. ○ A ○ B ○ C ○ D	33. ○ A ○ B ○ C ○ D	63. ○ A ○ B ○ C ○ D	93. ○ A ○ B ○ C ○ D	123. ○ A ○ B ○ C ○ D
4. ○ A ○ B ○ C ○ D	34. ○ A ○ B ○ C ○ D	64. ○ A ○ B ○ C ○ D	94. ○ A ○ B ○ C ○ D	124. ○ A ○ B ○ C ○ D
5. ○ A ○ B ○ C ○ D	35. ○ A ○ B ○ C ○ D	65. ○ A ○ B ○ C ○ D	95. ○ A ○ B ○ C ○ D	125. ○ A ○ B ○ C ○ D
6. ○ A ○ B ○ C ○ D	36. ○ A ○ B ○ C ○ D	66. ○ A ○ B ○ C ○ D	96. ○ A ○ B ○ C ○ D	126. ○ A ○ B ○ C ○ D
7. ○ A ○ B ○ C ○ D	37. ○ A ○ B ○ C ○ D	67. ○ A ○ B ○ C ○ D	97. ○ A ○ B ○ C ○ D	127. ○ A ○ B ○ C ○ D
8. ○ A ○ B ○ C ○ D	38. ○ A ○ B ○ C ○ D	68. ○ A ○ B ○ C ○ D	98. ○ A ○ B ○ C ○ D	128. ○ A ○ B ○ C ○ D
9. ○ A ○ B ○ C ○ D	39. ○ A ○ B ○ C ○ D	69. ○ A ○ B ○ C ○ D	99. ○ A ○ B ○ C ○ D	129. ○ A ○ B ○ C ○ D
10. ○ A ○ B ○ C ○ D	40. ○ A ○ B ○ C ○ D	70. ○ A ○ B ○ C ○ D	100. ○ A ○ B ○ C ○ D	130. ○ A ○ B ○ C ○ D
11. ○ A ○ B ○ C ○ D	41. ○ A ○ B ○ C ○ D	71. ○ A ○ B ○ C ○ D	101. ○ A ○ B ○ C ○ D	131. ○ A ○ B ○ C ○ D
12. ○ A ○ B ○ C ○ D	42. ○ A ○ B ○ C ○ D	72. ○ A ○ B ○ C ○ D	102. ○ A ○ B ○ C ○ D	132. ○ A ○ B ○ C ○ D
13. ○ A ○ B ○ C ○ D	43. ○ A ○ B ○ C ○ D	73. ○ A ○ B ○ C ○ D	103. ○ A ○ B ○ C ○ D	133. ○ A ○ B ○ C ○ D
14. ○ A ○ B ○ C ○ D	44. ○ A ○ B ○ C ○ D	74. ○ A ○ B ○ C ○ D	104. ○ A ○ B ○ C ○ D	134. ○ A ○ B ○ C ○ D
15. ○ A ○ B ○ C ○ D	45. ○ A ○ B ○ C ○ D	75. ○ A ○ B ○ C ○ D	105. ○ A ○ B ○ C ○ D	135. ○ A ○ B ○ C ○ D
16. ○ A ○ B ○ C ○ D	46. ○ A ○ B ○ C ○ D	76. ○ A ○ B ○ C ○ D	106. ○ A ○ B ○ C ○ D	136. ○ A ○ B ○ C ○ D
17. ○ A ○ B ○ C ○ D	47. ○ A ○ B ○ C ○ D	77. ○ A ○ B ○ C ○ D	107. ○ A ○ B ○ C ○ D	137. ○ A ○ B ○ C ○ D
18. ○ A ○ B ○ C ○ D	48. ○ A ○ B ○ C ○ D	78. ○ A ○ B ○ C ○ D	108. ○ A ○ B ○ C ○ D	138. ○ A ○ B ○ C ○ D
19. ○ A ○ B ○ C ○ D	49. ○ A ○ B ○ C ○ D	79. ○ A ○ B ○ C ○ D	109. ○ A ○ B ○ C ○ D	139. ○ A ○ B ○ C ○ D
20. ○ A ○ B ○ C ○ D	50. ○ A ○ B ○ C ○ D	80. ○ A ○ B ○ C ○ D	110. ○ A ○ B ○ C ○ D	140. ○ A ○ B ○ C ○ D
21. ○ A ○ B ○ C ○ D	51. ○ A ○ B ○ C ○ D	81. ○ A ○ B ○ C ○ D	111. ○ A ○ B ○ C ○ D	141. ○ A ○ B ○ C ○ D
22. ○ A ○ B ○ C ○ D	52. ○ A ○ B ○ C ○ D	82. ○ A ○ B ○ C ○ D	112. ○ A ○ B ○ C ○ D	142. ○ A ○ B ○ C ○ D
23. ○ A ○ B ○ C ○ D	53. ○ A ○ B ○ C ○ D	83. ○ A ○ B ○ C ○ D	113. ○ A ○ B ○ C ○ D	143. ○ A ○ B ○ C ○ D
24. ○ A ○ B ○ C ○ D	54. ○ A ○ B ○ C ○ D	84. ○ A ○ B ○ C ○ D	114. ○ A ○ B ○ C ○ D	144. ○ A ○ B ○ C ○ D
25. ○ A ○ B ○ C ○ D	55. ○ A ○ B ○ C ○ D	85. ○ A ○ B ○ C ○ D	115. ○ A ○ B ○ C ○ D	145. ○ A ○ B ○ C ○ D
26. ○ A ○ B ○ C ○ D	56. ○ A ○ B ○ C ○ D	86. ○ A ○ B ○ C ○ D	116. ○ A ○ B ○ C ○ D	146. ○ A ○ B ○ C ○ D
27. ○ A ○ B ○ C ○ D	57. ○ A ○ B ○ C ○ D	87. ○ A ○ B ○ C ○ D	117. ○ A ○ B ○ C ○ D	147. ○ A ○ B ○ C ○ D
28. ○ A ○ B ○ C ○ D	58. ○ A ○ B ○ C ○ D	88. ○ A ○ B ○ C ○ D	118. ○ A ○ B ○ C ○ D	148. ○ A ○ B ○ C ○ D
29. ○ A ○ B ○ C ○ D	59. ○ A ○ B ○ C ○ D	89. ○ A ○ B ○ C ○ D	119. ○ A ○ B ○ C ○ D	149. ○ A ○ B ○ C ○ D
30. ○ A ○ B ○ C ○ D	60. ○ A ○ B ○ C ○ D	90. ○ A ○ B ○ C ○ D	120. ○ A ○ B ○ C ○ D	150. ○ A ○ B ○ C ○ D

Self-Diagnostic Profile

How to Use the Self-Assessment Worksheet

1. Indicate on your answer sheet whether your answers are correct or incorrect.
2. Note the items you answered incorrectly.
3. Count the total number of items you answered incorrectly in each category.
4. Compare the total number of items you answered incorrectly in each category with the total number of items per category. This information will give you an idea of where you will need to focus your continued study.

Content Category	Questions Answered Incorrectly	Total Number of Questions Answered Incorrectly in Each Category	Total Number of Questions in Each CEN Content Category
Cardiovascular Emergencies			20
Respiratory Emergencies			16
Neurological Emergencies			16
Gastrointestinal, Genitourinary, Gynecology, and Obstetrical Emergencies			21
Psychosocial and Medical Emergencies			25
Maxillofacial, Ocular, Orthopedic, and Wound Emergencies			21
Environment and Toxicology Emergencies, and Communicable Diseases			15
Professional Issues			16

Practice Examination Answer Sheet

1. ○ A ○ B ○ C ○ D	31. ○ A ○ B ○ C ○ D	61. ○ A ○ B ○ C ○ D	91. ○ A ○ B ○ C ○ D	121. ○ A ○ B ○ C ○ D
2. ○ A ○ B ○ C ○ D	32. ○ A ○ B ○ C ○ D	62. ○ A ○ B ○ C ○ D	92. ○ A ○ B ○ C ○ D	122. ○ A ○ B ○ C ○ D
3. ○ A ○ B ○ C ○ D	33. ○ A ○ B ○ C ○ D	63. ○ A ○ B ○ C ○ D	93. ○ A ○ B ○ C ○ D	123. ○ A ○ B ○ C ○ D
4. ○ A ○ B ○ C ○ D	34. ○ A ○ B ○ C ○ D	64. ○ A ○ B ○ C ○ D	94. ○ A ○ B ○ C ○ D	124. ○ A ○ B ○ C ○ D
5. ○ A ○ B ○ C ○ D	35. ○ A ○ B ○ C ○ D	65. ○ A ○ B ○ C ○ D	95. ○ A ○ B ○ C ○ D	125. ○ A ○ B ○ C ○ D
6. ○ A ○ B ○ C ○ D	36. ○ A ○ B ○ C ○ D	66. ○ A ○ B ○ C ○ D	96. ○ A ○ B ○ C ○ D	126. ○ A ○ B ○ C ○ D
7. ○ A ○ B ○ C ○ D	37. ○ A ○ B ○ C ○ D	67. ○ A ○ B ○ C ○ D	97. ○ A ○ B ○ C ○ D	127. ○ A ○ B ○ C ○ D
8. ○ A ○ B ○ C ○ D	38. ○ A ○ B ○ C ○ D	68. ○ A ○ B ○ C ○ D	98. ○ A ○ B ○ C ○ D	128. ○ A ○ B ○ C ○ D
9. ○ A ○ B ○ C ○ D	39. ○ A ○ B ○ C ○ D	69. ○ A ○ B ○ C ○ D	99. ○ A ○ B ○ C ○ D	129. ○ A ○ B ○ C ○ D
10. ○ A ○ B ○ C ○ D	40. ○ A ○ B ○ C ○ D	70. ○ A ○ B ○ C ○ D	100. ○ A ○ B ○ C ○ D	130. ○ A ○ B ○ C ○ D
11. ○ A ○ B ○ C ○ D	41. ○ A ○ B ○ C ○ D	71. ○ A ○ B ○ C ○ D	101. ○ A ○ B ○ C ○ D	131. ○ A ○ B ○ C ○ D
12. ○ A ○ B ○ C ○ D	42. ○ A ○ B ○ C ○ D	72. ○ A ○ B ○ C ○ D	102. ○ A ○ B ○ C ○ D	132. ○ A ○ B ○ C ○ D
13. ○ A ○ B ○ C ○ D	43. ○ A ○ B ○ C ○ D	73. ○ A ○ B ○ C ○ D	103. ○ A ○ B ○ C ○ D	133. ○ A ○ B ○ C ○ D
14. ○ A ○ B ○ C ○ D	44. ○ A ○ B ○ C ○ D	74. ○ A ○ B ○ C ○ D	104. ○ A ○ B ○ C ○ D	134. ○ A ○ B ○ C ○ D
15. ○ A ○ B ○ C ○ D	45. ○ A ○ B ○ C ○ D	75. ○ A ○ B ○ C ○ D	105. ○ A ○ B ○ C ○ D	135. ○ A ○ B ○ C ○ D
16. ○ A ○ B ○ C ○ D	46. ○ A ○ B ○ C ○ D	76. ○ A ○ B ○ C ○ D	106. ○ A ○ B ○ C ○ D	136. ○ A ○ B ○ C ○ D
17. ○ A ○ B ○ C ○ D	47. ○ A ○ B ○ C ○ D	77. ○ A ○ B ○ C ○ D	107. ○ A ○ B ○ C ○ D	137. ○ A ○ B ○ C ○ D
18. ○ A ○ B ○ C ○ D	48. ○ A ○ B ○ C ○ D	78. ○ A ○ B ○ C ○ D	108. ○ A ○ B ○ C ○ D	138. ○ A ○ B ○ C ○ D
19. ○ A ○ B ○ C ○ D	49. ○ A ○ B ○ C ○ D	79. ○ A ○ B ○ C ○ D	109. ○ A ○ B ○ C ○ D	139. ○ A ○ B ○ C ○ D
20. ○ A ○ B ○ C ○ D	50. ○ A ○ B ○ C ○ D	80. ○ A ○ B ○ C ○ D	110. ○ A ○ B ○ C ○ D	140. ○ A ○ B ○ C ○ D
21. ○ A ○ B ○ C ○ D	51. ○ A ○ B ○ C ○ D	81. ○ A ○ B ○ C ○ D	111. ○ A ○ B ○ C ○ D	141. ○ A ○ B ○ C ○ D
22. ○ A ○ B ○ C ○ D	52. ○ A ○ B ○ C ○ D	82. ○ A ○ B ○ C ○ D	112. ○ A ○ B ○ C ○ D	142. ○ A ○ B ○ C ○ D
23. ○ A ○ B ○ C ○ D	53. ○ A ○ B ○ C ○ D	83. ○ A ○ B ○ C ○ D	113. ○ A ○ B ○ C ○ D	143. ○ A ○ B ○ C ○ D
24. ○ A ○ B ○ C ○ D	54. ○ A ○ B ○ C ○ D	84. ○ A ○ B ○ C ○ D	114. ○ A ○ B ○ C ○ D	144. ○ A ○ B ○ C ○ D
25. ○ A ○ B ○ C ○ D	55. ○ A ○ B ○ C ○ D	85. ○ A ○ B ○ C ○ D	115. ○ A ○ B ○ C ○ D	145. ○ A ○ B ○ C ○ D
26. ○ A ○ B ○ C ○ D	56. ○ A ○ B ○ C ○ D	86. ○ A ○ B ○ C ○ D	116. ○ A ○ B ○ C ○ D	146. ○ A ○ B ○ C ○ D
27. ○ A ○ B ○ C ○ D	57. ○ A ○ B ○ C ○ D	87. ○ A ○ B ○ C ○ D	117. ○ A ○ B ○ C ○ D	147. ○ A ○ B ○ C ○ D
28. ○ A ○ B ○ C ○ D	58. ○ A ○ B ○ C ○ D	88. ○ A ○ B ○ C ○ D	118. ○ A ○ B ○ C ○ D	148. ○ A ○ B ○ C ○ D
29. ○ A ○ B ○ C ○ D	59. ○ A ○ B ○ C ○ D	89. ○ A ○ B ○ C ○ D	119. ○ A ○ B ○ C ○ D	149. ○ A ○ B ○ C ○ D
30. ○ A ○ B ○ C ○ D	60. ○ A ○ B ○ C ○ D	90. ○ A ○ B ○ C ○ D	120. ○ A ○ B ○ C ○ D	150. ○ A ○ B ○ C ○ D

Self-Diagnostic Profile

How to Use the Self-Assessment Worksheet

1. Indicate on your answer sheet whether your answers are correct or incorrect.
2. Note the items you answered incorrectly.
3. Count the total number of items you answered incorrectly in each category.
4. Compare the total number of items you answered incorrectly in each category with the total number of items per category. This information will give you an idea of where you will need to focus your continued study.

Content Category	Questions Answered Incorrectly	Total Number of Questions Answered Incorrectly in Each Category	Total Number of Questions in Each CEN Content Category
Cardiovascular Emergencies			20
Respiratory Emergencies			16
Neurological Emergencies			16
Gastrointestinal, Genitourinary, Gynecology, and Obstetrical Emergencies			21
Psychosocial and Medical Emergencies			25
Maxillofacial, Ocular, Orthopedic, and Wound Emergencies			21
Environment and Toxicology Emergencies, and Communicable Diseases			15
Professional Issues			16

Practice Examination Answer Sheet

1. ○ A ○ B ○ C ○ D	31. ○ A ○ B ○ C ○ D	61. ○ A ○ B ○ C ○ D	91. ○ A ○ B ○ C ○ D	121. ○ A ○ B ○ C ○ D
2. ○ A ○ B ○ C ○ D	32. ○ A ○ B ○ C ○ D	62. ○ A ○ B ○ C ○ D	92. ○ A ○ B ○ C ○ D	122. ○ A ○ B ○ C ○ D
3. ○ A ○ B ○ C ○ D	33. ○ A ○ B ○ C ○ D	63. ○ A ○ B ○ C ○ D	93. ○ A ○ B ○ C ○ D	123. ○ A ○ B ○ C ○ D
4. ○ A ○ B ○ C ○ D	34. ○ A ○ B ○ C ○ D	64. ○ A ○ B ○ C ○ D	94. ○ A ○ B ○ C ○ D	124. ○ A ○ B ○ C ○ D
5. ○ A ○ B ○ C ○ D	35. ○ A ○ B ○ C ○ D	65. ○ A ○ B ○ C ○ D	95. ○ A ○ B ○ C ○ D	125. ○ A ○ B ○ C ○ D
6. ○ A ○ B ○ C ○ D	36. ○ A ○ B ○ C ○ D	66. ○ A ○ B ○ C ○ D	96. ○ A ○ B ○ C ○ D	126. ○ A ○ B ○ C ○ D
7. ○ A ○ B ○ C ○ D	37. ○ A ○ B ○ C ○ D	67. ○ A ○ B ○ C ○ D	97. ○ A ○ B ○ C ○ D	127. ○ A ○ B ○ C ○ D
8. ○ A ○ B ○ C ○ D	38. ○ A ○ B ○ C ○ D	68. ○ A ○ B ○ C ○ D	98. ○ A ○ B ○ C ○ D	128. ○ A ○ B ○ C ○ D
9. ○ A ○ B ○ C ○ D	39. ○ A ○ B ○ C ○ D	69. ○ A ○ B ○ C ○ D	99. ○ A ○ B ○ C ○ D	129. ○ A ○ B ○ C ○ D
10. ○ A ○ B ○ C ○ D	40. ○ A ○ B ○ C ○ D	70. ○ A ○ B ○ C ○ D	100. ○ A ○ B ○ C ○ D	130. ○ A ○ B ○ C ○ D
11. ○ A ○ B ○ C ○ D	41. ○ A ○ B ○ C ○ D	71. ○ A ○ B ○ C ○ D	101. ○ A ○ B ○ C ○ D	131. ○ A ○ B ○ C ○ D
12. ○ A ○ B ○ C ○ D	42. ○ A ○ B ○ C ○ D	72. ○ A ○ B ○ C ○ D	102. ○ A ○ B ○ C ○ D	132. ○ A ○ B ○ C ○ D
13. ○ A ○ B ○ C ○ D	43. ○ A ○ B ○ C ○ D	73. ○ A ○ B ○ C ○ D	103. ○ A ○ B ○ C ○ D	133. ○ A ○ B ○ C ○ D
14. ○ A ○ B ○ C ○ D	44. ○ A ○ B ○ C ○ D	74. ○ A ○ B ○ C ○ D	104. ○ A ○ B ○ C ○ D	134. ○ A ○ B ○ C ○ D
15. ○ A ○ B ○ C ○ D	45. ○ A ○ B ○ C ○ D	75. ○ A ○ B ○ C ○ D	105. ○ A ○ B ○ C ○ D	135. ○ A ○ B ○ C ○ D
16. ○ A ○ B ○ C ○ D	46. ○ A ○ B ○ C ○ D	76. ○ A ○ B ○ C ○ D	106. ○ A ○ B ○ C ○ D	136. ○ A ○ B ○ C ○ D
17. ○ A ○ B ○ C ○ D	47. ○ A ○ B ○ C ○ D	77. ○ A ○ B ○ C ○ D	107. ○ A ○ B ○ C ○ D	137. ○ A ○ B ○ C ○ D
18. ○ A ○ B ○ C ○ D	48. ○ A ○ B ○ C ○ D	78. ○ A ○ B ○ C ○ D	108. ○ A ○ B ○ C ○ D	138. ○ A ○ B ○ C ○ D
19. ○ A ○ B ○ C ○ D	49. ○ A ○ B ○ C ○ D	79. ○ A ○ B ○ C ○ D	109. ○ A ○ B ○ C ○ D	139. ○ A ○ B ○ C ○ D
20. ○ A ○ B ○ C ○ D	50. ○ A ○ B ○ C ○ D	80. ○ A ○ B ○ C ○ D	110. ○ A ○ B ○ C ○ D	140. ○ A ○ B ○ C ○ D
21. ○ A ○ B ○ C ○ D	51. ○ A ○ B ○ C ○ D	81. ○ A ○ B ○ C ○ D	111. ○ A ○ B ○ C ○ D	141. ○ A ○ B ○ C ○ D
22. ○ A ○ B ○ C ○ D	52. ○ A ○ B ○ C ○ D	82. ○ A ○ B ○ C ○ D	112. ○ A ○ B ○ C ○ D	142. ○ A ○ B ○ C ○ D
23. ○ A ○ B ○ C ○ D	53. ○ A ○ B ○ C ○ D	83. ○ A ○ B ○ C ○ D	113. ○ A ○ B ○ C ○ D	143. ○ A ○ B ○ C ○ D
24. ○ A ○ B ○ C ○ D	54. ○ A ○ B ○ C ○ D	84. ○ A ○ B ○ C ○ D	114. ○ A ○ B ○ C ○ D	144. ○ A ○ B ○ C ○ D
25. ○ A ○ B ○ C ○ D	55. ○ A ○ B ○ C ○ D	85. ○ A ○ B ○ C ○ D	115. ○ A ○ B ○ C ○ D	145. ○ A ○ B ○ C ○ D
26. ○ A ○ B ○ C ○ D	56. ○ A ○ B ○ C ○ D	86. ○ A ○ B ○ C ○ D	116. ○ A ○ B ○ C ○ D	146. ○ A ○ B ○ C ○ D
27. ○ A ○ B ○ C ○ D	57. ○ A ○ B ○ C ○ D	87. ○ A ○ B ○ C ○ D	117. ○ A ○ B ○ C ○ D	147. ○ A ○ B ○ C ○ D
28. ○ A ○ B ○ C ○ D	58. ○ A ○ B ○ C ○ D	88. ○ A ○ B ○ C ○ D	118. ○ A ○ B ○ C ○ D	148. ○ A ○ B ○ C ○ D
29. ○ A ○ B ○ C ○ D	59. ○ A ○ B ○ C ○ D	89. ○ A ○ B ○ C ○ D	119. ○ A ○ B ○ C ○ D	149. ○ A ○ B ○ C ○ D
30. ○ A ○ B ○ C ○ D	60. ○ A ○ B ○ C ○ D	90. ○ A ○ B ○ C ○ D	120. ○ A ○ B ○ C ○ D	150. ○ A ○ B ○ C ○ D

Self-Diagnostic Profile

How to Use the Self-Assessment Worksheet

1. Indicate on your answer sheet whether your answers are correct or incorrect.
2. Note the items you answered incorrectly.
3. Count the total number of items you answered incorrectly in each category.
4. Compare the total number of items you answered incorrectly in each category with the total number of items per category. This information will give you an idea of where you will need to focus your continued study.

Content Category	Questions Answered Incorrectly	Total Number of Questions Answered Incorrectly in Each Category	Total Number of Questions in Each CEN Content Category
Cardiovascular Emergencies			20
Respiratory Emergencies			16
Neurological Emergencies			16
Gastrointestinal, Genitourinary, Gynecology, and Obstetrical Emergencies			21
Psychosocial and Medical Emergencies			25
Maxillofacial, Ocular, Orthopedic, and Wound Emergencies			21
Environment and Toxicology Emergencies, and Communicable Diseases			15
Professional Issues			16

Practice Examination Answer Sheet

1. ○ A ○ B ○ C ○ D	31. ○ A ○ B ○ C ○ D	61. ○ A ○ B ○ C ○ D	91. ○ A ○ B ○ C ○ D	121. ○ A ○ B ○ C ○ D
2. ○ A ○ B ○ C ○ D	32. ○ A ○ B ○ C ○ D	62. ○ A ○ B ○ C ○ D	92. ○ A ○ B ○ C ○ D	122. ○ A ○ B ○ C ○ D
3. ○ A ○ B ○ C ○ D	33. ○ A ○ B ○ C ○ D	63. ○ A ○ B ○ C ○ D	93. ○ A ○ B ○ C ○ D	123. ○ A ○ B ○ C ○ D
4. ○ A ○ B ○ C ○ D	34. ○ A ○ B ○ C ○ D	64. ○ A ○ B ○ C ○ D	94. ○ A ○ B ○ C ○ D	124. ○ A ○ B ○ C ○ D
5. ○ A ○ B ○ C ○ D	35. ○ A ○ B ○ C ○ D	65. ○ A ○ B ○ C ○ D	95. ○ A ○ B ○ C ○ D	125. ○ A ○ B ○ C ○ D
6. ○ A ○ B ○ C ○ D	36. ○ A ○ B ○ C ○ D	66. ○ A ○ B ○ C ○ D	96. ○ A ○ B ○ C ○ D	126. ○ A ○ B ○ C ○ D
7. ○ A ○ B ○ C ○ D	37. ○ A ○ B ○ C ○ D	67. ○ A ○ B ○ C ○ D	97. ○ A ○ B ○ C ○ D	127. ○ A ○ B ○ C ○ D
8. ○ A ○ B ○ C ○ D	38. ○ A ○ B ○ C ○ D	68. ○ A ○ B ○ C ○ D	98. ○ A ○ B ○ C ○ D	128. ○ A ○ B ○ C ○ D
9. ○ A ○ B ○ C ○ D	39. ○ A ○ B ○ C ○ D	69. ○ A ○ B ○ C ○ D	99. ○ A ○ B ○ C ○ D	129. ○ A ○ B ○ C ○ D
10. ○ A ○ B ○ C ○ D	40. ○ A ○ B ○ C ○ D	70. ○ A ○ B ○ C ○ D	100. ○ A ○ B ○ C ○ D	130. ○ A ○ B ○ C ○ D
11. ○ A ○ B ○ C ○ D	41. ○ A ○ B ○ C ○ D	71. ○ A ○ B ○ C ○ D	101. ○ A ○ B ○ C ○ D	131. ○ A ○ B ○ C ○ D
12. ○ A ○ B ○ C ○ D	42. ○ A ○ B ○ C ○ D	72. ○ A ○ B ○ C ○ D	102. ○ A ○ B ○ C ○ D	132. ○ A ○ B ○ C ○ D
13. ○ A ○ B ○ C ○ D	43. ○ A ○ B ○ C ○ D	73. ○ A ○ B ○ C ○ D	103. ○ A ○ B ○ C ○ D	133. ○ A ○ B ○ C ○ D
14. ○ A ○ B ○ C ○ D	44. ○ A ○ B ○ C ○ D	74. ○ A ○ B ○ C ○ D	104. ○ A ○ B ○ C ○ D	134. ○ A ○ B ○ C ○ D
15. ○ A ○ B ○ C ○ D	45. ○ A ○ B ○ C ○ D	75. ○ A ○ B ○ C ○ D	105. ○ A ○ B ○ C ○ D	135. ○ A ○ B ○ C ○ D
16. ○ A ○ B ○ C ○ D	46. ○ A ○ B ○ C ○ D	76. ○ A ○ B ○ C ○ D	106. ○ A ○ B ○ C ○ D	136. ○ A ○ B ○ C ○ D
17. ○ A ○ B ○ C ○ D	47. ○ A ○ B ○ C ○ D	77. ○ A ○ B ○ C ○ D	107. ○ A ○ B ○ C ○ D	137. ○ A ○ B ○ C ○ D
18. ○ A ○ B ○ C ○ D	48. ○ A ○ B ○ C ○ D	78. ○ A ○ B ○ C ○ D	108. ○ A ○ B ○ C ○ D	138. ○ A ○ B ○ C ○ D
19. ○ A ○ B ○ C ○ D	49. ○ A ○ B ○ C ○ D	79. ○ A ○ B ○ C ○ D	109. ○ A ○ B ○ C ○ D	139. ○ A ○ B ○ C ○ D
20. ○ A ○ B ○ C ○ D	50. ○ A ○ B ○ C ○ D	80. ○ A ○ B ○ C ○ D	110. ○ A ○ B ○ C ○ D	140. ○ A ○ B ○ C ○ D
21. ○ A ○ B ○ C ○ D	51. ○ A ○ B ○ C ○ D	81. ○ A ○ B ○ C ○ D	111. ○ A ○ B ○ C ○ D	141. ○ A ○ B ○ C ○ D
22. ○ A ○ B ○ C ○ D	52. ○ A ○ B ○ C ○ D	82. ○ A ○ B ○ C ○ D	112. ○ A ○ B ○ C ○ D	142. ○ A ○ B ○ C ○ D
23. ○ A ○ B ○ C ○ D	53. ○ A ○ B ○ C ○ D	83. ○ A ○ B ○ C ○ D	113. ○ A ○ B ○ C ○ D	143. ○ A ○ B ○ C ○ D
24. ○ A ○ B ○ C ○ D	54. ○ A ○ B ○ C ○ D	84. ○ A ○ B ○ C ○ D	114. ○ A ○ B ○ C ○ D	144. ○ A ○ B ○ C ○ D
25. ○ A ○ B ○ C ○ D	55. ○ A ○ B ○ C ○ D	85. ○ A ○ B ○ C ○ D	115. ○ A ○ B ○ C ○ D	145. ○ A ○ B ○ C ○ D
26. ○ A ○ B ○ C ○ D	56. ○ A ○ B ○ C ○ D	86. ○ A ○ B ○ C ○ D	116. ○ A ○ B ○ C ○ D	146. ○ A ○ B ○ C ○ D
27. ○ A ○ B ○ C ○ D	57. ○ A ○ B ○ C ○ D	87. ○ A ○ B ○ C ○ D	117. ○ A ○ B ○ C ○ D	147. ○ A ○ B ○ C ○ D
28. ○ A ○ B ○ C ○ D	58. ○ A ○ B ○ C ○ D	88. ○ A ○ B ○ C ○ D	118. ○ A ○ B ○ C ○ D	148. ○ A ○ B ○ C ○ D
29. ○ A ○ B ○ C ○ D	59. ○ A ○ B ○ C ○ D	89. ○ A ○ B ○ C ○ D	119. ○ A ○ B ○ C ○ D	149. ○ A ○ B ○ C ○ D
30. ○ A ○ B ○ C ○ D	60. ○ A ○ B ○ C ○ D	90. ○ A ○ B ○ C ○ D	120. ○ A ○ B ○ C ○ D	150. ○ A ○ B ○ C ○ D

Self-Diagnostic Profile

How to Use the Self-Assessment Worksheet

1. Indicate on your answer sheet whether your answers are correct or incorrect.
2. Note the items you answered incorrectly.
3. Count the total number of items you answered incorrectly in each category.
4. Compare the total number of items you answered incorrectly in each category with the total number of items per category. This information will give you an idea of where you will need to focus your continued study.

Content Category	Questions Answered Incorrectly	Total Number of Questions Answered Incorrectly in Each Category	Total Number of Questions in Each CEN Content Category
Cardiovascular Emergencies			20
Respiratory Emergencies			16
Neurological Emergencies			16
Gastrointestinal, Genitourinary, Gynecology, and Obstetrical Emergencies			21
Psychosocial and Medical Emergencies			25
Maxillofacial, Ocular, Orthopedic, and Wound Emergencies			21
Environment and Toxicology Emergencies, and Communicable Diseases			15
Professional Issues			16